Disease and Fertility

This is a volume in

STUDIES IN POPULATION

A complete list of titles in this series appears at the end of this volume.

Disease and Fertility

Joseph A. McFalls, Jr.

Department of Sociology
Temple University
Philadelphia, Pennsylvania

Marguerite Harvey McFalls

Gladwyne, Pennsylvania

1984

ACADEMIC PRESS, INC.

(Harcourt Brace Jovanovich, Publishers)

Orlando   San Diego   San Francisco   New York   London
Toronto   Montreal   Sydney   Tokyo   São Paulo

ACADEMIC PRESS, INC.
Orlando, Florida 32887

United Kingdom Edition published by
ACADEMIC PRESS, INC. (LONDON) LTD.
24/28 Oval Road, London NW1 7DX

Library of Congress Cataloging in Publication Data

McFalls, Joseph A., Jr.
   Disease and fertility.

   (Studies in population)
   Includes bibliographical references and index.
   1. Fertility, Human. 2. Diseases--Complications
and sequelae. I. McFalls, Marguerite Harvey. II. Title.
III. Series. [DNLM: 1. Infertility--Etiology.
2. Communicable diseases--Complications. 3. Birth
rate. WP 570 M478d]
QP273.M38 1984   616.6'9   83-11835
ISBN 0-12-483380-2 (alk. paper)

For the late John Durand
J. A. M.

For my parents
M. H. M.

Contents

I
Introduction

II
Nonsexually Transmitted Diseases

7 African Sleeping Sickness

8 Chagas' Disease

III
Sexually Transmitted Diseases

9 Overview

10 Gonococcal and Nongonococcal Infections
and Their Complications

11 Syphilis

12 Genital Herpes

13 Genital Mycoplasmas

14 Genital Chlamydia

IV
Events Predisposing to Pelvic Inflammatory Disease and Other Reproductive Problems

V
Overview

VI
Appendixes

Preface

It has become increasingly apparent that subfecundity is a major determinant of individual and population fertility. However, the identity and/or fertility-inhibiting strength of the most important causes of population subfecundity have remained largely unknown. To improve this situation, a research project was undertaken which, during its earliest stages, identified and categorized those factors that could alter human reproductive potential at the population level. Five major categories emerged: genetic factors, disease, psychopathology, nutritional deficiencies, and other environmental factors. Upon completion of this preliminary task, the psychopathological factors that cause substantial population subfecundity—psychic stress, psychoses, sexual deviations, alcoholism, cigarette smoking, and illicit drug abuse—were studied comprehensively, and a monograph (McFalls 1979a) presenting the results of that work was written. The present volume deals with the principal diseases that cause population subfecundity.

Disease is a multipotent cause of individual subfecundity, capable of causing coital inability, conceptive failure, and pregnancy loss. It is highly prevalent in all societies and is thus an extremely important cause of population subfecundity. Of the five categories, disease has by far the most devastating impact on population fecundity. It has the potential literally to wipe out populations through subfecundity as well as through mortality. Indeed, in those societies where subfecundity has led or contributed to depopulation or to extraordinary levels of childlessness and low fertility, disease is invariably the paramount cause.

This book's first major objective is to identify diseases that can cause population subfecundity. The second major objective is to provide detailed information on each of these diseases that will help researchers and policymakers judge the quantitative impact of selected diseases on fecundity and fertility. Such information provides a ready resource with which to test hypotheses concerning the impact of a particular disease on the fertility of a specific population quickly and accurately. Moreover, such information, together with prevalence data, provides policymakers with an expedient means to help formulate and evaluate development policies in areas where subfecundity-producing diseases are prevalent. Without such information, control of disease might lead to unanticipated increases in fertility, with adverse effects on socioeconomic development. In sum, this monograph is a reference book designed to familiarize researchers and policymakers with those diseases that can cause substantial subfecundity and to help them estimate the quantitative impact of these diseases on population fertility.

This book concentrates only on the most important diseases that cause population subfecundity and divides them into three groups. The first group includes the nonsexually transmitted diseases: tuberculosis, malaria, filariasis, schistosomiasis, African sleeping sickness, and Chagas' disease. The second group is composed of the sexually transmitted diseases: gonorrhea, nongonococcal cervicitis and urethritis and their complications, syphilis, and genital herpes, mycoplasma, and chlamydia. The third group is composed not of actual diseases but of phenomena that can cause pelvic inflammatory disease and other adverse reproductive sequelae. These include induced abortion, childbirth, the intrauterine device, and female circumcision. Three other diseases, diabetes, sickle-cell hemoglobin, and smallpox, are discussed in appendixes. Other features of the book include a state-of-the-art review of the demography of subfecundity (Chapter 1) and a methodological discussion of pitfalls in population research (Chapter 20) that alerts researchers to problems encountered in trying to link a particular disease to the fertility of a specific population.

This book was written principally for three audiences. The first is population students, including those demographers, historical demographers, sociologists, economists, anthropologists, and historians concerned with population fertility. The second intended audience is the medical community, particularly workers in reproductive biology, obstetrics and gynecology, sexology, infertility, and medical history, as well as those specializing in any of the diseases mentioned earlier. The third target audience is professionals in disciplines that involve the study of both health and population; for example, public health workers, epidemiologists, and medical geographers.

Because this book is intended for nonmedical as well as medical professionals, the original intention was to write it without using medical terminology. However, once the actual writing began it soon became apparent that this goal was impractical and, in fact, undesirable. It was impractical because it would have made the text extremely wordy and unwieldy; a medical term frequently involves a concept that cannot be expressed by a single lay term but requires instead a phrase or even a sentence or two. A text dotted with such phrases and sentences becomes tedious reading, especially for persons familiar with the terminology. In addition, medical jargon is desirable here because it is our conviction that nonmedical professionals cannot do adequate research concerning disease and fertility at arm's length, but must familiarize themselves with all aspects of a disease by reading widely in the medical literature, where the same terminology will be encountered. Fortunately, the medical jargon in this book is not as imposing as it might seem at first glance. The nonmedical reader can navigate this book easily with a medical dictionary at hand. An excellent one available in virtually any library is *Dorland's Medical Dictionary*.

Some readers may be disappointed that this book does not include extended examples of the impact of each disease on specific populations. These were not included for two reasons, the most obvious one being space. This book is already lengthy, and such examples would push it well beyond the manageable stage. More important, there were few populations for which we were adequately familiar with all the biological and social variables that determine the impact a particular disease will ultimately have on fertility. However, a previous article (McFalls 1973) illustrates the relationship between particular diseases (gonorrhea and syphilis) and the fertility of a population familiar to us, namely, the U.S. black population. An elaboration of this example is presented in Chapter 19, along with an analysis of the impact of genital tuberculosis on the fertility of this population. This chapter not only provides a good example of the utility of the type of information developed in this book, but also contributes new and important substantive information concerning the 1880–1960 U.S. black fertility swing, a trend that to date has resisted adequate explanation. The reader will notice that just this single example requires a lengthy chapter and can therefore well understand why it was impractical to have such an extended discussion for each disease.

Acknowledgments

We express our gratitude to those institutions and individuals who have advised and assisted us in this research. We are especially indebted to the Ford and Rockefeller Foundations, which supported this research with a grant under their Research Program on Population and Development Policy. We would also like to thank the Ford Foundation for an additional grant to finish this book, and Timothy P. Rice, who helped make that grant possible. Other support for this project came from the Population Studies Center of the University of Pennsylvania under funds granted by the Rockefeller Foundation. Etienne van de Walle was responsible for this support and has our gratitude for it as well as for his advice on drafts of two chapters and for several recommendations. We are also grateful to George Masnick, Richard Easterlin, and the late John Durand for reading drafts of two chapters and for their advice and recommendations. Dr. Durand always took a personal interest in the first author and his work (including this project), and of all the author's professors had the greatest influence in shaping his professional life. Dr. Durand knew well before he died that this book would be dedicated to him, and it seemed to give him great pleasure. We also express our gratitude to those who read and advised us on other chapters, including Achilea Bittencourt, Herman Buyst, Willard Cates, Allen Cheever, John Eaton, Marsh Edwards, Stanley Engerman, Thomas Klein, Richard Lewis, William Mosher, George Nelson, R. B. Patel, and Jean van der Tak. We thank Gloria Basmajian and her staff at Temple University's Word Processing Center for typing the manuscript, Jean McFalls for her help with the proofreading, and many people at Academic Press for their support and patience in producing this book.

Finally, special thanks are due to Hal Winsborough, who was gracious enough to include this book in his fine Studies in Population series.

Note on Terminology

Fecundity is used here to mean reproductive ability as opposed to *fertility*, which denotes actual childbearing. *Subfecundity* refers to the diminished capacity to reproduce. The most severe form of subfecundity is *infecundity*, the total inability to reproduce both currently and in the future. Infecundity may develop in an individual who in the past was fecund and perhaps even had children. A *subfecundity factor* refers to a cause of subfecundity, such as disease or psychic stress.

Subfecundity results from impairment of any of the biological aspects of reproduction—coitus, conception, and the carrying of a conceptus to a live birth. *Coital inability* is defined as the inability to perform normal heterosexual intercourse. It afflicts both men and women, especially the former, and can be chronic or temporary. *Infertility* is defined as the diminished ability to conceive or to bring about conception. Thus, infertility refers here only to conceptive difficulties, although the term has been used elsewhere to cover pregnancy loss and even coital problems. Another term for infertility is *conceptive failure*. *Sterility* is the complete inability to conceive or bring about conception; it is simply the lowest point on the infertility continuum. Infertility is an important cause of subfecundity in both men and women and, like coital inability, can be chronic or temporary. Finally, *pregnancy loss* refers to the involuntary termination of a pregnancy before a live birth. In includes spontaneous abortion (miscarriage), late fetal death, and stillbirth, but not induced abortion or neonatal mortality (death in the first 4 weeks of life). Although primarily a form of female subfecundity, some pregnancy loss may be due to defective sperm and thus may also be a form of male subfecundity. *Perinatal mortality*, a joint term for late fetal mortality and neonatal mortality, is also discussed with respect to the findings of studies that do not differentiate between these two components.

I

Introduction

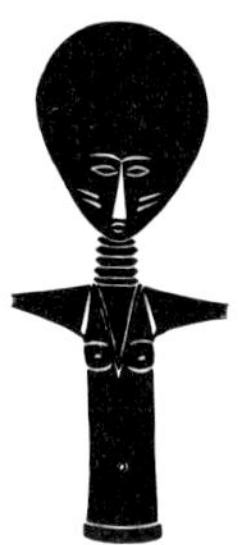

CHAPTER 1

The Demography of Subfecundity

General Introduction

A population's fecundity is the average fecundity of its individual members. Individual fecundity varies widely. Some women are unable to have children throughout their reproductive lives. Others are superfecund, giving birth to more than 30 children. Pearl (1939:36), for instance, mentioned one woman who had 32 children by age 40, thus, individual fecundity varies from zero to more than 30 children. Maximum population fecundity falls somewhere between these extremes. It is impossible to calculate actual population fecundity, but by splicing together the highest age-specific fertility rates on record and considering other hypothetical models, most authorities (see Hansluwka 1975:203; Petersen 1975:199) estimate maximum population fecundity to be about 15 children per woman. In other words, a population of women who engage in regular sexual intercourse from menarche to menopause without using any form of birth control would, under the most favorable reproductive circumstances, average about 15 children per woman. A population is subfecund to the extent that it is biologically incapable of achieving this roughly estimated average. No population enjoys completely favorable reproductive circumstances. Some causes of subfecundity—genetic, disease, nutritional, environmental, or psychopathological—are present in all real populations, and hence all are subfecund according to this definition (see McFalls 1979a). It is their relative ability to achieve this standard of maximum fecundity, however, that is pertinent and of demographic significance.

If population fecundity is seen as a continuum, the Hutterites, a small religious sect scattered in the United States and the prairie provinces of Canada, would establish the upper extreme, and the population of the Bas-Uele district of Zaire would perhaps represent the lower extreme. Among the latter, subfecundity is rampant, as evidenced by the nearly 50% rate of childlessness for women aged 30–34 during the 1960s (Romaniuk 1968:328). By contrast, only 2% of one cohort of ever-married Hutterite women were childless (Eaton and Mayer 1954:20). The Hutterites have extraordinarily high fecundity because they are subject to few of the causes of subfecundity. They are probably genetically superfecund, virtually all individuals being the offspring of parents with eight or more children. They are prosperous enough to provide each individual with a nutritionally adequate diet and have a social system that ensures that each person receives it. They avail themselves of two of the world's most advanced health care systems (those of the United States and Canada), which minimizes disease and its consequences. They have extraordinarily low rates of psychopathology. And, as inhabitants of simple farm communities, they avoid most of the environmental factors that depress fecundity (Eaton and Mayer 1954; Eaton and Weil 1955). By contrast, poverty deprives inhabitants of Bas-Uele of proper nutrition and health care; malaria and other subfecundity-producing diseases are endemic and epidemic, and the devastating social forces at work in this rapidly changing society probably ensure substantial rates of psychic stress and other forms of psychopathology. Virtually all other populations experience a degree of fecundity somewhere along the continuum bounded by the high-fecundity Hutterites and the low-fecundity inhabitants of Bas-Uele.

Population subfecundity thus varies widely among populations because populations experience diverse sets of subfecundity factors whose number, mix, and prevalence within a set are variable. This results in substantial population differences in rates of coital inability, conceptive failure, and pregnancy loss, and in the length of time between puberty and the climacteric in men and between menarche and menopause in women. The average length of the reproductive period, for instance, is greater in developed than in developing societies. Subfecundity also varies over time for a given population. German women at the turn of the century, for example, had a reproductive span 10 years shorter than they have presently. On the average, they now reach childbearing age at 12 and cease at age 52; 75 years ago, their reproductive lifetime stretched only from ages 15 to 45.

The relative contribution of male disorders and female disorders to subfecundity is difficult to pinpoint because of male reluctance to admit responsibility for a couple's subfecundity, particularly in developing societies (Ladipo 1980).[1] Less is therefore known about the prevalence of male subfecundity, but experts estimate that male subfecundity accounts in whole or in part for 20 to 60% of the subfecundity in various populations (Amelar *et al.* 1977). In the United States, the consensus is that men contribute to subfecundity in 30 to 40% of cases, and women in 60 to 70%. Similar proportions have been estimated for Cameroon, a country in central Africa (Guest 1978:25).

Effect of Subfecundity on Fertility

Even though maximum population fecundity is about 15 children per woman, the actual fertility of almost all populations ranges from only 1 to 8 children per woman (Bongaarts 1976:227), with about 4 being the worldwide average in 1982. Of course, subfecundity accounts for only some of the difference between this performance and the 15-child estimate of maximum fecundity. As demographers Davis and Blake (1956) pointed out in a classic article, in addition to subfecundity a society's fertility level is determined by various forms of birth control and by the fact that much of an individual's reproductive period is spent without regular coital activity (see Table 1.8). One of the basic tasks of fertility studies is to determine the relative impact of these subfecundity, birth control, and mate exposure factors that Davis and Blake characterized as intermediate variables.

Though subfecundity is just one of several factors that hold fertility to only a fraction of its theoretical maximum, it is a major determinant of fertility in most, if not all, populations (Bongaarts 1976:227). This is true even in the group reproducing closest to the maximum rate—the Hutterites. But the power of subfecundity to affect fertility is most vividly seen in essentially noncontracepting societies with unexpectedly low fertility. These populations frequently reveal extraordinarily high rates of subfecundity. Africa presents a poignant example of this. In parts of Gabon, Cameroon, Zaire, the Central African Empire (now the Central African Republic), the Sudan, and elsewhere across central Africa,

---

[1]Although both men and women can be subfecund, most fertility specialists prefer to focus on the couple because the couple's subfecundity is frequently the result of several defects, often minor, in both partners. Also, two otherwise fecund individuals may form a subfecund couple due to various biological incompatibilities. A woman, for instance, may produce antibodies against her partner's sperm. The emperor and empress of France, Napoleon and Josephine, may have been a classic case of such situational subfecundity; both were fertile with another mate but were unable to have children together.

20–50% of women aged 50 and older have never borne children, and subfecundity is recognized as an acute problem (Guest 1978:23).

As the following discussion will show, subfecundity was an important determinant of fertility in historical societies both before and during modernization and is important today in developed and developing societies, both those that are demographically and economically stagnant and those undergoing modernization. And subfecundity will doubtless remain an important determinant of fertility in the developed and developing societies of the future.

Historical Societies

Subfecundity has undoubtedly depressed fertility since the human race began. During most of this time the rate of population growth was scarcely above zero. For such a low growth rate to be sustained, fertility and mortality had to be roughly the same. Experts conclude that for much of world history the average life expectancy was about 20 years. To offset this mortality, women would have had to average six to seven children, that is, substantially fewer than the biological maximum. Birth control and mate exposure variables probably accounted for much of this fertility deficit, but subfecundity undoubtedly also played an important role in curtailing fertility and holding down population growth. Indeed, Frisch (1975:21) suggested that subfecundity may be even more important in premodern societies than is usually assumed: It could be responsible for some of the shortfall usually credited to the other factors, especially traditional forms of birth control such as abstinence and prolonged breast-feeding.

Population history prior to the eighteenth century can be divided into two periods, one extending back to about 8000 B.C. when agriculture was introduced and the other from 8000 B.C. to the beginning of humanity. Subfecundity influenced fertility in both periods although the leading causes were probably different. Subfecundity in historical preagricultural societies may have been similar to that observed among some contemporary hunting and gathering societies. The !Kung tribe of Africa's Kalahari Desert, for instance, has moderate fertility with relatively long intervals between births. This may be partly due to poor nutrition and low body weight, conditions that reduce fecundity and may have also been common in historical preagricultural societies. The village life of the agriculturalists, on the other hand, brought comparatively many individuals close together, facilitating the spread of many diseases that cause subfecundity. Also, by relying more on crops for survival, agriculturalists became more vulnerable to crop failure, which led to unpredictable and catastrophic famines and the gross malnutrition that is a potent cause of subfecundity. Thus, chronic undernutrition may have been a relatively more important cause of subfecundity in the preagricultural period, and disease and starvation may have been relatively more potent in the agricultural period.[2] (This capsule description of population history glosses over the short-term variations in growth, death, and birth rates that occurred in many societies in response to changes in the food supply and disease rates; subfecundity also fluctuated with the ups and downs of the food supply and disease rates.)

Research in historical demography has found a surprisingly wide variation in the level of fertility in various historical societies. Indeed, as van de Walle and Knodel (1980:12) noted, the remarkable variation in natural fertility levels is one of the most important findings of this body of literature. Subfecundity undoubtedly is one of the important factors that account for these differences, as many studies of specific historical societies attest. Flandrin (1979, cited in Marcy 1981:320), for instance, concluded that subfecundity was an important reason for unexpectedly low fertility in a number of eighteenth-century French towns and villages in the Parisian basin. Knodel and Wilson (1981:54) provided another European example in their study of the reproductive histories of couples married between 1750 and 1899 in 14 German villages. They found more subfecundity among couples living toward the beginning of this period than among those living near the end and attributed this temporal increase in fecundity to increased conceptive ability. A third example was furnished by Coale (1978:411), who reported that subfecundity helped depress the fertility of married women in the central Asian republics of the Soviet Union prior to 1926.

Fertility studies of historical U.S. populations have also found that subfecundity was an influential fertility depressant among both the white (Ridley 1981:101) and black (McFalls and Tolnay, forthcoming) populations. Ridley, for instance, using a conservative measure of subfecundity, classified as subfecund about 20% of women aged 30 in a sample of white women born between 1900 and 1910—the lowest-fertility white cohorts in U.S. history. By age 45 less than half of this cohort were classified as fecund (Ridley 1981:101).

---

[2]For a fuller discussion of the historical information in this and the preceding paragraph, see Coale (1974:40–51).

Developing Societies

Subfecundity is also an important determinant of fertility in contemporary developing societies. It is the cause of profound personal tragedy for couples who are rendered childless or subfertile, especially in the many developing societies that highly value childbearing (Belsey 1978:1).

Prevalence of Subfecundity

Because specific information on the level of subfecundity in developing societies is rarely available, most estimates use the childlessness rates of women who have completed their reproductive periods as an expedient though imperfect proxy. The childlessness rate is a fairly good proxy for a measure of primary infecundity in the largely pronatalist developing countries because voluntary childlessness is not very common. But it is not as good a proxy for the rest of subfecundity—that part which affects the fertility of the nonchildless population (McFalls 1979b:227).

High rates of childlessness have been reported in many developing societies in recent decades. Childlessness has been prevalent in Jamaica, for instance, where about 13% of married women aged 30–34 years in the 1960s had never had a live birth (Tekse 1968). And in Zanzibar, an island off the east coast of Africa and now part of Tanzania, 25% of women over 46 years of age in one region and 38% in another were reported childless in 1960 (Blacker 1962).

Subfecundity has been especially prevalent during the present century over great areas of West, Central, and East Africa, notably in northern Zaire, the eastern Central African Republic, southwest Sudan, Gabon, mainland Equatorial Guinea or Rio Muni (now Mbini), southeast Cameroon, and parts of Chad (Caldwell 1981:109; Frank 1983:137; Gwatkin 1977:7). In these areas, a large proportion of women complete their reproductive years without giving birth to a live child (see Figure 1.1), and many others finish with fewer children than they desire (Haupt 1980:13; *Population Reports* 1979a:135). This situation is mostly due to subfecundity, as shown by the intense concern felt in these areas over childlessness and low fertility and by the large number of indigenous specialists who treat subfecundity complaints (Caldwell 1981:109, 1974:7; Frank 1983:140). It is noteworthy and paradoxical that such areas of high subfecundity exist on the continent with the world's highest birth rate.[3]

---

[3]Africa's total fertility rate in 1982 was 6.5 compared to 4.2 for Asia, 1.9 for North America, 4.4 for Latin America, 1.9 for Europe, and 2.7 for Oceania (Population Reference Bureau 1982).

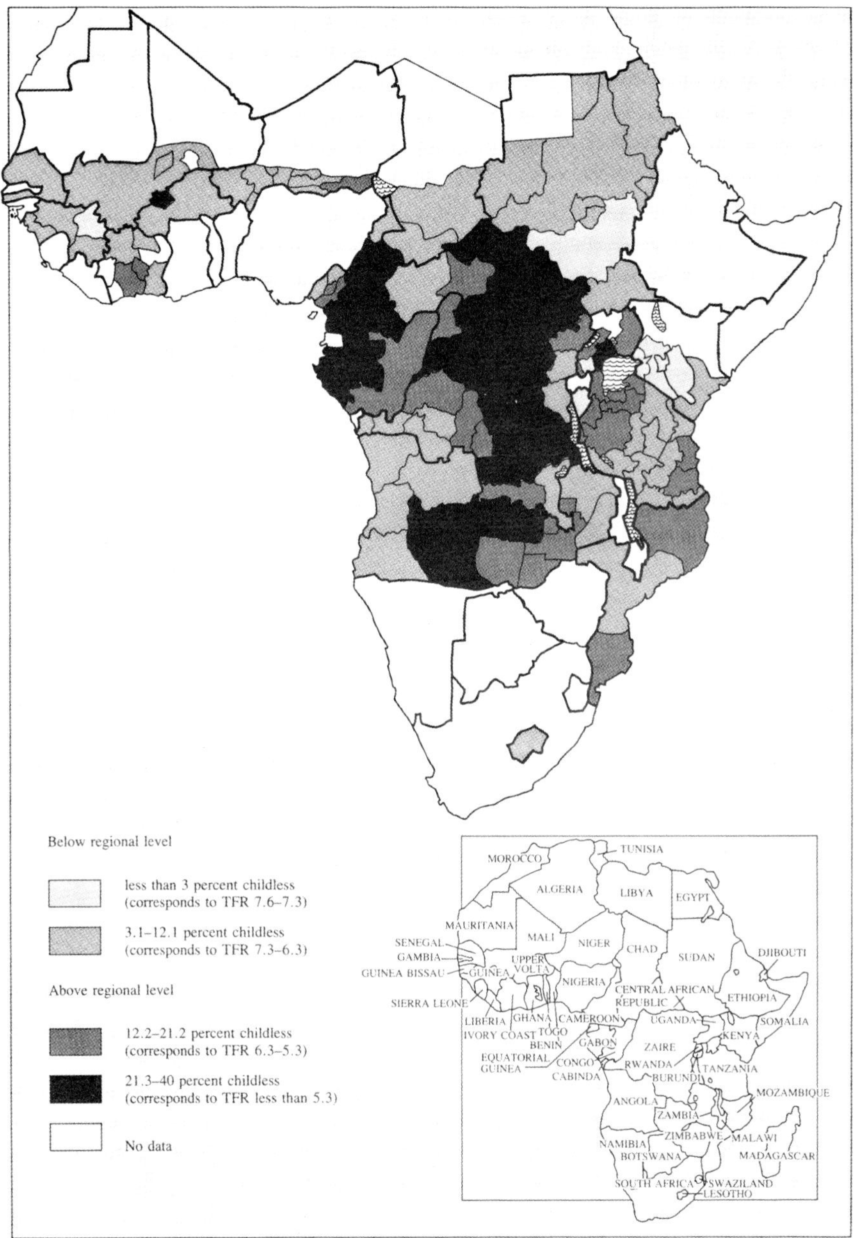

Figure 1.1 Levels of childlessness among women aged 45–49 (or closest age group) in 21 countries of sub-Saharan Africa, various years. TFR denotes total fertility rate. Source: Frank (1983:139).

This indicates that high fertility and considerable subfecundity can exist side by side—a topic that will be discussed later in this chapter.

Another imperfect but useful proxy for subfecundity is the percentage of noncontracepting, continuously married women who do not have a child for a certain number of years. This proxy variable for subfecundity is inversely related to the number of years chosen, longer intervals resulting in fewer women being classified as subfecund. Vaessen used a very conservative 5-year interval in an analysis of World Fertility Survey data from 27 developing countries and still found that subfecundity was extremely common in many of them. For example, the proportion of noncontracepting, continuously married women aged 35–39 who did not have a child for the previous 5 years was 31% in Lesotho, 26% in Senegal, 20% in the Sudan, 19% in Kenya, 25% in Guyana, 15% in Paraguay, 28% in Indonesia, 24% in Bangladesh, 23% in Nepal, 21% in Pakistan, 19% in Sri Lanka, 18% in Malaysia, and 17% in Jamaica (*Population Reports* 1983). These percentages would be very much higher if the 1-year interval used in many other studies had been employed.

The impact of subfecundity on fertility often varies by region within countries (Frank 1983; Hull and Tukiran 1976; Lantum 1979; Leke and Nash 1981; Retel-Laurentin 1974). Although this is true of all countries, it is particularly true of developing countries, especially those in Africa. This observation is supported by Table 1.1, which presents data on childlessness, population size, and fertility for many countries and regions of central and western Africa, compiled by Belsey (to whom we are indebted for much of the information in this section). Table 1.1 shows that the proportion of women childless at age 50 or over varies from 7 to 23% in Cameroon, from 10 to 19% in the Central African Republic, from 8 to 46% in Gabon, from 2 to 21% in the Sudan, and from 3 to 40% in Zaire.

The effect of subfecundity on fertility also varies substantially by district and tribe within the regions of many developing societies (Frank 1983:140). In three southern regions of the Sudan (see Figure 1.2), for instance, the percentage childless among women completing reproductive age varies by district from 1 to 42% (Belsey 1976:323). Similarly, in Zaire's Equateur province, childlessness in women 45–49 years of age varies from a low of 6% among the Batwa-Batshwa and Ngbaka peoples to a high of 65% among the Mbelo (Sala-Diakanda 1981). The !Kung of the Kalahari Desert region of Botswana provide an example of a tribe with a high level of subfecundity in a country with a total fertility rate of 6.5 (see Howell 1979).

Although subfecundity varies by tribal and ethnic group in developing societies, these associations are probably not genetic but rather

Table 1.1

Indices of Infertility and General Fertility in Central and West Africa[a]

Country and/or region	Population (in 1,000)	General fertility rate (No. births per 1,000 women aged 15–44 years)	Crude live birth rate per 1,000 population	Percentage of childless women aged 25–29 years	Percentage of childless women aged 50+ years
Cameroon					
West region	1,025	196	49.8	7.0	6.7
Southeast region	1,185		36.4	28	23
North region	1,395		41.0	21	15
Central African					
Republic	1,021	157	48	25.2	13.6
Banda	318	122	40.6		
Nzakara	30	48	20.0		
Baya	294	194	54.6		
Center region	240	125	41.0	34.7	15.0
West region	643	187	53	19.4	10.4
River region	134	101	36	36.3	19.0
Gabon	440	116	35	34	31.9
Wolen N'tem	78	122	37		31.2
Ogoone Lolo	37	80	25		46.2
Nyanga	37	170	52		17.8
Upper Volta	4,440	194	49.6	7.2	6
Niger	2,600	232	50.55	12.8	5.2
Mali (Tuareg)	76	209	52	26	15
Senegal	3,049	178	43.3	12	5.6
Sudan	10,262		51.7		9.6
Bahr el Ghazal	991		84.6		4.2
Blue Nile	2,070		45.7		8.4
Darfur	1,329		41.8		7.3
Equatoria	904		54.1		21.2
Kassala	941		42.6		13.5
Khartoum	505		40.7		9.7
Kordofan	1,762		50.0		9.9
Northern region	873		43.0		7.8
Upper Nile	889		69.3		2.3
Zaire	21,800	171	42.7	22.1	17.6
Kwango	466	203	48.1	6.8	3.4
South Kivu	831	211	52.3	7.1	4.6
Equateur	302	133	33.7	39.1	40.0
Tshuapa	395	113	30.5	44.1	33.0
Kisangani (formerly Stanleyville)	635	123	34.0	34.4	23.3
Bas-Uele	468	64	19.1	50.7	37.3
Haut-Uele	589	83	23.2	46.2	36.9
Nanie-Ma	447	129	34.3	27.9	23.5
Congo[b]		145	41.1	17	15

[a]Source: Belsey (1976:321).
[b]Excludes Brazzaville and Pointe Noire.

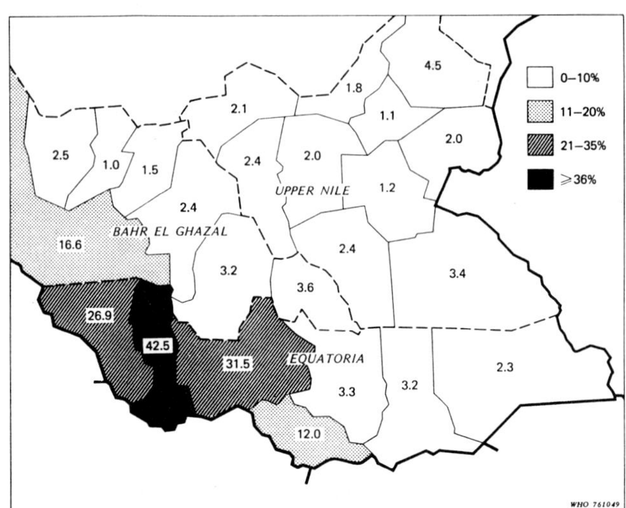

Figure 1.2 Percentage childlessness among women completing reproductive age in the districts of three southern Sudan provinces. Source: Belsey (1976:323).

are primarily a function of differing locales, social factors, and other health- associated conditions (Belsey 1976:323). Henin's (1969) study of childlessness among the settled and nomadic members of two tribes in the Sudan illustrates this point. He found that the prevalence of childlessness among ever-married women 20–49 years of age was 5% or less in the settled communities but 13–18% in the nomadic groups. The level of subfecundity among women with children also seemed to differ in the nomadic and settled groups. The age-adjusted mean number of births of the two nomad groups were 3.13 and 3.37 respectively, whereas they were 5.19 and 4.45 respectively for the two settled groups for the same tribes. The nomad women had higher rates of infertility and pregnancy loss and a longer interval between marriage and first pregnancy than did settled women.

Finally, there are substantial urban–rural differences in subfecundity in some developing societies (Blacker 1962; Dankoussou *et al.* 1975; Mosley *et al.* 1982; Romaniuk 1980b; Tabutin 1982). Belsey (1978:4) noted that the higher levels of either childlessness or nulliparity in the urban areas of some developing countries such as Colombia suggest that some of the causes of subfecundity, such as pelvic inflammatory disease, may be more common in these areas than in rural areas. In particular, sexually transmitted diseases may be more prevalent in the cities of some developing nations (Arya and Lawson 1977), and may spread quickly through the ranks of unmarried rural to urban migrants or those migrants temporarily separated from their spouses (Bennett 1962; Verhagen 1974; World Health Organization 1975). (Voluntary childlessness and low fertility undoubtedly are also involved in these differentials.) In other developing countries there is more subfecundity in rural than in urban areas. In a study of the sterility among the Nzakara tribe of the Central African Republic, Correa (1969) found that those who had moved to an urban area were generally more fertile than their rural counterparts. Isely (1980:11) suggested that urbanization in this case may have resulted in less subfecundity because of greater access to medical services.

In sum, subfecundity is an important fertility depressant in developing societies, and its power to affect fertility is often far stronger at the regional, district, or tribal level than it is at the national level. In the past, national data have often masked the severity of the problem at the local level, leading to a lack of public health action. More recently, however, there has been considerable effort to alleviate subfecundity and childlessness. As a result the proportion of individuals currently in their reproductive years who are affected by subfecundity is declining (see Belsey 1976:322–324).

Subfecundity affects fertility more in developing than in developed societies (Caldwell 1974:12). This is primarily due to two situations. First, in developing societies there are fewer social checks on fertility such as effective contraception and thus more fertility potential for subfecundity to negate. Second, these societies are far more exposed to powerful causes of subfecundity, particularly disease and malnutrition. This situation is compounded (and perpetuated) by the relative absence of high-quality health care and facilities.

Impact of Health Care on Subfecundity

Health conditions are extremely poor in most developing nations, particularly for the most impoverished groups and especially for children (Bell 1980:63). Almost 1 billion of the inhabitants of these societies still have no access to any health care at all, and more than 80% have no access to any permanent form of health care (Mahler 1979:25). The great shortage of trained medical personnel in developing societies can be seen in Table 1.2 and Figure 1.3. Not only are there few physicians, but those present are concentrated in the cities, especially the capital cities (Potts and Selman 1979:326). Nevertheless, medical care even in the cities is grossly inadequate by western standards. In Cali, Colombia, for instance, the patient-to-doctor ratio is 900:1; 17% of children never see a physician during their fatal illness and an additional 19% do not see one during the 48 hours preceding death (C. Smith 1972:4). African nations have by far the poorest ratios of health personnel and facilities

Table 1.2

Health Manpower by Occupation and Rate per 100,000 Population,
Availability of Data, and Population Covered by the Data: Circa 1975[a]

| | World[b] | | | | | Developed | |
| | | | *Availability of data* | | | | |
Health occupation	*Number*	*Rate per 100,000 population*	*Number of countries or areas*	*Population covered (in 1,000s)*	*% of world population*	*Number*	*Rate per 100,000 population*
Physicians	3,037,674	76.86	193	3,952,295	99	2,089,319	190.65
Medical assistants	676,016	82.00	56	824,436	21	624,609	168.96
Multipurpose health auxiliaries	1,820,134	160.24	20	1,135,911	29	—	—
Midwives and assistant midwives	790,145	29.31	161	2,695,448	68	484,579	59.87
Nurses and assistant nurses	6,904,613	174.75	193	3,951,132	99	5,035,582	459.52
Traditional medical practitioners	596,967	33.61	14	1,776,308	45	3,715	6.01
Dentists	551,211	18.64	188	2,957,702	75	437,372	42.09
Dental operating auxiliaries and dental hygienists	55,398	5.30	61	1,045,448	26	51,363	11.64
Dental laboratory technicians	95,886	9.04	79	1,060,908	27	91,553	13.92
Pharmacists	691,873	23.39	178	2,958,038	75	518,439	47.97
Pharmaceutical assistants	297,045	20.42	114	1,454,452	37	240,364	40.36
Laboratory technicians and assistant technicians	476,622	16.81	176	2,835,121	71	418,385	47.31
X-ray technicians and assistant technicians	211,226	7.95	162	2,658,210	67	174,968	19.88
Sanitarians and assistant sanitarians	153,527	6.80	156	2,256,924	57	73,474	12.41

[a]Source: World Health Organization (1980:268).

[b]Excluding Bhutan and Democratic People's Republic of Korea (North Korea). Data for China were provided by the State Statistical Bureau and the Ministry of Public Health, Beijing, and relate to 1978.

Table 1.2 (*Continued*)

| | countries | | | | | Developing countries | | |
| | Availability of data | | | | | | Availability of data | |
Number of countries or areas	Population covered (in 1,000s)	% of world population	Number	Rate per 100,000 population	Number of countries or areas	Population covered (in 1,000s)	% of world population
39	1,095,899	100	948,355	33.18	154	2,858,307	99
8	369,687	34	51,407	11.31	48	454,699	16
—	—	—	1,820,134	160.24	20	1,135,911	40
33	809,400	74	305,566	16.87	128	1,811,667	63
39	1,095,841	100	1,869,031	65.46	154	2,855,291	99
1	61,832	6	593,252	34.60	13	1,714,476	60
38	1,039,153	95	113,839	5.93	150	1,918,349	67
15	441,145	40	4,036	0.67	46	604,310	21
16	657,838	60	3,284	0.81	63	403,070	14
37	1,080,708	99	173,434	9.24	141	1,877,330	65
25	595,564	55	56,681	6.60	89	858,888	30
31	884,307	81	58,237	2.99	145	1,950,814	68
28	879,902	81	36,258	2.04	134	1,778,308	62
25	591,906	54	80,053	4.81	131	1,665,018	58

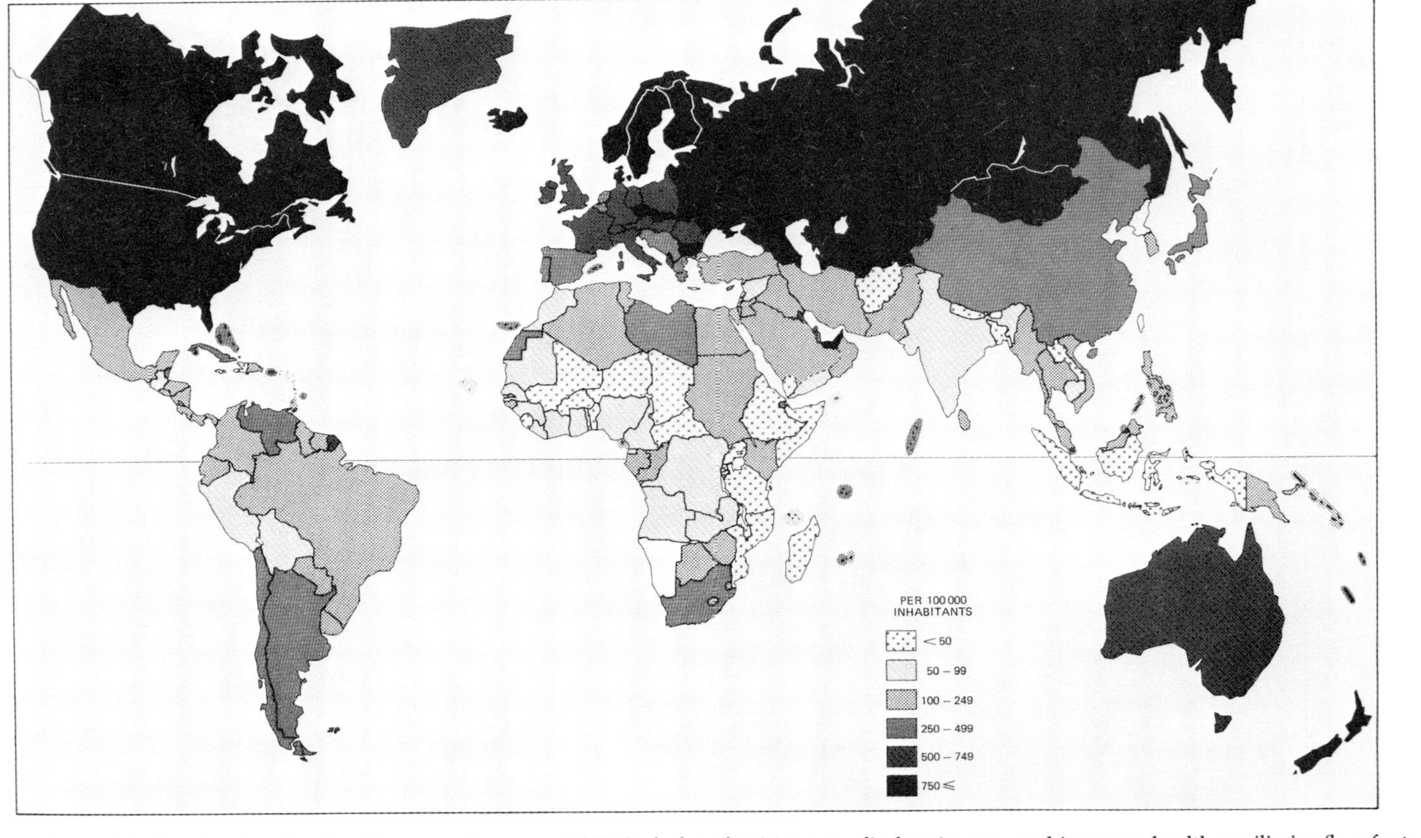

Figure 1.3 Density of certain health occupations circa 1975. Includes physicians, medical assistants, multipurpose health auxiliaries (barefoot doctors, village health auxiliaries, etc.), professional midwives, assistant midwives, traditional birth attendants, professional nurses, assistant nurses, and traditional medical practitioners. Source: World Health Organization (1980:276).

to population of any continent (Cassen 1978:338). This is particularly true of the 49 sub-Saharan countries, which contain about four-fifths of Africa's 500 million people. These nations have only 2–7 physicians per 100,000 people. But because physicians are concentrated in the urban areas, even these extremely low ratios greatly exaggerate actual availability. In the rural areas, where about 80% of African populations reside, the ratios are more like one or fewer physicians per 100,000 people (Mosley 1983:49).

Whereas the level of general health care and patient–doctor ratios are very unfavorable in the developing world, deficiencies are even more marked in the case of subfecundity-related specialties such as obstetrics and gynecology. Trained midwives also are often in short supply. In Iran, for instance, there are only 700 fully trained midwives (Potts and Selman 1979:326). As a result of this scarcity of physicians and trained midwives at least 50%, and in some instances as many as 85%, of births in many developing societies are assisted by untrained traditional birth attendants or relatives. In a rural area in Nigeria, 2% of deliveries were attended by a physician (or at least took place in a hospital), 52% by an untrained midwife, 40% by a family member, and 6% by only the woman herself (World Health Organization 1980:138).

Also relevant to subfecundity is the availability of antenatal care, which varies greatly both among and within developing countries. In the Americas, for instance, the proportion of women receiving such care ranges from 14% in Uruguay to 98% in Trinidad. In some developing countries antenatal care is available but underutilized. Studies in India found that in urban Delhi and in a rural area with a clinic, 64% and 69% of pregnant women, respectively, eschewed available antenatal care (World Health Organization 1980:138).

Antenatal and delivery care, like general health care, are much more available in the cities of the developing world than in the rural areas. For example, 49% of the births in urban Korea are attended by a physician or midwife compared to only 6% in rural Korea. There are also vast differences by district in many countries. The percentage of institutional deliveries in the districts of Uganda varies from 5% to 66% (World Health Organization 1980:138). But even in those places where services are available, the demand is often so great that the care is necessarily brief, unsophisticated, and frequently inadequate. Potts and Selman (1979:27) described the delivery situation in hospitals of the developing world as follows.

> Sometimes the hospitals are so busy that women are only in them for the hours of labour and for a few hours afterwards, as in the great obstetric hospitals of Caracas, Tehran, or Kinshasa. Often the women lie two in a bed, head to toe with their

babies between them before being discharged to make room for the next woman. In Saigon, women used to sit in the street during the first stage of labour and were only admitted into the hospital after an examination to prove that the cervix had begun to dilate.

In sum, there is a tremendous lack of high-quality health care, both general and obstetrical, in the developing world. And although there are significant regional differentials in the level of health care available, almost nowhere does it match the customary standards of developed societies. The result is that many causes of subfecundity in the developing world are not effectively challenged, moderated, or eliminated.

The impact on population fecundity of obstetrical difficulties, for example, is greater where health services are less accessible. Workers therefore believe that in many developing societies where antenatal and delivery care are scarce or nonexistent, the role of obstetric difficulties in causing subfecundity is undoubtedly considerable (World Health Organization 1975:17). In addition, the inadequate care that does exist in many areas may itself actually produce subfecundity. For instance, traditional midwives often fail to use aseptic procedures and follow a variety of other practices, including the use of herbs with oxytocic properties to speed labor, that increase pregnancy loss and subsequent infertility (see *Population Reports* 1980b:450).

However, it is clear that health services in the developing world are expanding and improving. The proportion of women receiving antenatal care and the proportion of deliveries attended by trained personnel is rising steadily in many developing countries. As one case in point, the proportion of women in Botswana given antenatal care increased from 40% in 1973 to 70% in 1977 (World Health Organization 1980:138). Demographers (e.g., Hull and Tukiran 1976:21; Romaniuk 1981:164) have been quick to notice the positive impact of such improvements on the fertility of specific populations. However, improved health can bring with it, ironically, its own subfecundity problems. For instance, mothers who were chronically malnourished in childhood but who now get good nutrition during pregnancy have a high risk of obstructed labor because of cephalo–pelvic disproportion (Mosley 1979:1). Thus the positive impact of health improvements on fertility is dampened in some areas by countervailing effects.

Transitional or Modernizing Societies

In the previous two sections, it has been shown that health conditions prejudicial to fecundity were common in some developed societies prior to modernization[4] and are common in some developing societies today. Therefore, the possibility exists that improvement in health during modernization might lead to a reduction of subfecundity and to a subsequent rise in fertility. This possibility has been raised often in the population literature (e.g., Birdsall 1980:32; Cassen 1978:339; Frank 1983:143; Freedman 1963:54; Henin 1969; *Intercom* 1978c:13; Kirk 1971; Langford 1981:292; Preston 1978; Ridley *et al.* 1967; Romaniuk 1981; Taylor *et al.* 1958:115) and is the subject of this section.

Modernization affects the level of fertility by working through the Davis–Blake intermediate variables, which, as noted earlier, can be divided into three groups: subfecundity, mate exposure, and birth control variables (see Table 1.8). When modernization begins public health improves, and if reproductive problems are prevalent subfecundity declines. If this were all that occurred, fertility would certainly rise. But modernization also leads to a variety of other social, economic, and health changes that tend both to increase and to decrease fertility. For instance, improved health increases the duration of marital unions, a pronatalist force, but it also increases the survival of children, an antinatalist force. It is the net effect of all these countervailing effects and their timing that determines whether fertility rises or falls at any given time in the modernization process.[5] If fertility does rise due to a reduction in subfecundity, this usually occurs in the early stages of modernization before birth control becomes widely and effectively practiced.

There is evidence that a number of developed societies experienced fertility increases during modernization (Petersen 1975:450–463; Tabah 1977:7). Many studies in historical demography have found that although natural fertility varied widely before modernization, it typically rose substantially once that process began (Mosk 1981:28). This occurred in Japan and in a variety of other Asian countries (Mosk 1981:28). Similarly, Knodel and Wilson (1981:54) reported that there was probably a substantial rise in fecundity in a sample of German villages at the onset of their modernization. England's birthrate apparently increased in the second half of the eighteenth century as modernization got under way (Glass 1965:241; Habakkuk 1965:280; Krause 1963:589; McKeown, 1978:538). Eversley (1963:576) and Krause (1963:589) argued that the sub-

---

[4]The process of modernization is defined loosely by Nag (1980:571) as including some of the following: industrialization, urbanization, spread of education, improvement of health and nutrition, control of epidemic diseases, increase in communication, erosion of traditional values, and secularization. This definition is adopted here.

[5]Cassen (1978:338) concluded that in high-mortality countries in the near future, the impact of reduced subfecundity on fertility will more than offset the impact of improved prospects for child survival.

stantial increase in England's population during this period was primarily due to rising fertility rather than falling mortality (Nag 1980:572). Fertility also rose in some areas of France between 1856 and 1876 and subsequently declined (van de Walle 1974:176–179). Finally, the fertility of married women in the central Asian republics of the Soviet Union increased by nearly 50% between 1926 and 1970, partly because of improvements in health and nutrition (Coale 1978:411).

However, it should be noted that not all studies of historical societies found increases in fertility during modernization. No such increases were found in studies based on eighteenth- and nineteenth-century natality data for Sweden (Hofsten and Lundstrom 1976), Italy (Livi-Bacci 1977), Portugal (Livi-Bacci 1971), Belgium (Lesthaeghe 1977), France (Bourgeois-Pichat 1965), and Germany (Knodel 1974) (see Nag 1980:571–572).

There is mounting evidence that substantial increases in fertility have taken and are now taking place in various parts of the developing world (Caldwell 1981:109; Knodel and Wilson 1981:53). This includes countries in Africa, Asia, and Latin America. In Africa, increases in fertility have been reported in northern and central regions. Modernization in Algeria (see Table 1.3) and Kuwait was accompanied by increases in fertility over the past few decades (Allman 1980:8). Total fertility in Kenya also rose steadily over the same period (Mosley 1979:1; Mott and Mott 1980:28). Kenyan women reportedly averaged 6.8 births in 1962, 7.6 in 1969, and 8.1 in 1978 (*Intercom* 1979:3). The percentage of childlessness has dropped by over 50% and there has been a rise in the percentage of women with parity 8 or above (Mosley 1979:1). There was a similar rise in fertility in Zaire, where the crude birthrate rose from about 41 per 1000 in the early 1930s to about 48 per 1000 in the 1960s (Romaniuk 1980b:306). In addition, there is evidence that Egypt, Mauritius, and Réunion experienced the same phenomenon (see Table 1.3).

In several Latin American countries undergoing modernization fertility rose before it began a steady decline (Nag 1980:572). Table 1.4 documents this trend for 11 countries between 1950 and 1973. The data in Table 1.4 underestimate the rise in fertility for some of these countries because much of it occurred prior to 1950. For example, the crude birthrate in Guyana rose 43% between 1909–1913 and 1957; in Jamaica, it increased 22% between 1941–1944 and 1964; and in Trinidad and Tobago, it rose 37% between 1929–1933 and 1955 (Nag 1980:572).

There are also reports that substantial increases in fertility have occurred in the developing countries of Asia including Korea, Taiwan (Knodel and Wilson 1981:53), Malaysia, Singapore (see Table 1.4), and in some countries in the Middle East (Allman 1980:1). In rural India, the

Table 1.3
Variation of Crude Birth Rates in Selected African and Asian Countries, 1919–1973[a]

	1919–1955	Peak	1968–1973
Algeria	45.0 (1950)	52.1 (1963)	45.8 (1970)
Egypt	43.8 (1955)	46.7 (1961)	40.6 (1968)
Malaysia	35.4 (1930–1934)	44.0 (1955)	34.0 (1970)
Mauritius	30.9 (1930–1934)	49.7 (1950)	22.7 (1973)
Réunion	42.4 (1946–1949)	51.3 (1952)	28.1 (1973)
Singapore	27.9 (1919–1923)	43.4 (1950)	22.1 (1970)

[a]Source: United Nations data, cited in Nag (1980:572). From *Current Anthropology*, published by The University of Chicago.

fertility of couples married after 1930 was higher than that of those married before 1930. And a comprehensive review of two surveys conducted in Karnataka (formerly Mysore) in 1951 and 1975 showed that fertility increased among women in most age groups in both rural and urban areas (Nag 1980:573). As these last two surveys indicate, the rise in fertility accompanying modernization is not just a rural phenomenon. There have long been indications that some urban areas in developing countries have higher fertility than the rural areas in their vicinity and that this is due in part to better health conditions (Cassen 1978:338).

These data on fertility increases accompanying modernization in historical and developing societies must be viewed cautiously (see Romaniuk 1980a:584; van de Walle 1980:584). A portion of the increase in fertility may be more apparent than real, and most of the cited studies

Table 1.4
Variation of Crude Birth Rates in Selected Latin American Countries, 1950–1973[a]

	1950	Peak	1970–1973
Chile	35.2	38.3 (1960)	27.4
Costa Rica	42.9	48.2 (1959)	31.3
Cuba	29.6	36.3 (1964)	25.3
El Salvador	48.7	50.9 (1957)	40.7
Guyana	40.4	44.3 (1952)	34.3
Jamaica	33.1	42.0 (1960)	31.3
Panama	31.3	40.0 (1962)	33.2
Surinam	39.0	49.0 (1959)	36.5
Trinidad and Tobago	37.5	41.9 (1954, 1955)	25.1
Uruguay	18.6	25.3 (1962)	22.6
Venezuela	42.6	46.0 (1960)	36.8

[a]Source: United Nations data, cited in Nag (1980:572). From *Current Anthropology*, published by The University of Chicago.

carefully point out potential problem areas. One such problem is that the reporting of fertility may improve over the period, which can create an apparent natality increase when none exists or exaggerate the magnitude of one that does exist.

Nevertheless, despite such problems most authors (e.g., Romaniuk 1980a:584) conclude that genuine increases do occur and, in fact, are probably more prevalent than is generally assumed. And, according to Romaniuk (1980b:307), "there can be little doubt that the potential for natural fertility to increase as a result of modernization is significant." Sometimes such a rise is not due to improved health and lower subfecundity but to changes in other fertility-inhibiting customs. For instance, fertility increased among a group of Canadian Indians during the early stage of modernization, but the main factor underlying this trend was a massive shift from breast-feeding[6] to bottle-feeding, which occurred prior to widespread use of birth control (Romaniuk 1981:168). But in many other situations the increases in fertility undoubtedly reflect changes in fecundity (see Allman 1980:8; *Intercom* 1979:3; Knodel and Wilson 1981:53; Mosley 1979:1). This is particularly true in Africa where increases in fertility are primarily caused by improvements in health and, more specifically, by reductions in sterility (Romaniuk 1981:158).

In sum, if subfecundity is prevalent prior to modernization, its reduction during the process leads to either a rise in fertility or at least to a slower decline than otherwise would have occurred. Indeed, many developing countries that now seem poised on the verge of sustained fertility declines may hover there for longer than expected due to the impact of reduced subfecundity on fertility (Cassen 1978:338).

Developed Societies

Although their virulence and prevalence seldom reach the levels seen in developing societies, subfecundity factors in developed societies are still demographically important (see Leridon 1982). This situation has been increasingly recognized. For instance, referring to the United States, Mosher (1982a:318) noted:

> A number of social and demographic trends have made fecundity impairments important issues in recent years. These include the postponement of marriage and childbearing by many women; increasing uncertainty and controversy over the plausibility of birth expectations and fertility projections; the possibility that in-

---

[6]Breast-feeding lowers fertility but does not lower fecundity (i.e., the innate ability to have children). It does not cause subfecundity although it does, like contraception, lower the probability of conception.

creasing proportions of women will remain permanently childless; a shortage of adoptable babies associated with the availability of legal abortion and with more effective contraception; the potential reproductive effects of occupational and environmental hazards on the growing number of working women; and the tripling in the annual number of reported cases of gonorrhea, from 325,000 in 1965 to one million in 1975. All these developments make it increasingly important to document the levels, trends and differentials in fecundity impairments in the United States. [Reprinted with permission from *Family Planning Perspectives*, Volume 14, Number 6, 1983.]

Prevalence of Subfecundity

Subfecundity is surprisingly common in developed countries such as the United States. Indeed, even though the major U.S. fertility surveys of the past several decades have tended to omit subfecund women (McFalls 1979a:29), they still found extraordinarily high rates of subfecundity among their respondents. About one-third of the married white couples of reproductive age surveyed in the 1941 Indianapolis Study (Whelpton and Kiser 1946–1958) and in the 1955 and 1960 Growth of American Families Studies (Freedman *et al.* 1959; Whelpton *et al.* 1966) were considered subfecund. Harter (1970) also classified 33% of a New Orleans sample as subfecund.

The best study of the current level of subfecundity in the United States is that of William Mosher and William Pratt (1982). The estimates of subfecundity used in this study were based on findings obtained from the 1976 National Survey of Family Growth (NSFG) (see Grady 1981). Mosher and Pratt (1982:20) found that about 7 million couples—some 25.3% of all U.S. couples with wives aged 15–44 in 1976—were classifiable as subfecund (if women who were sterilized for noncontraceptive reasons are included)[7] (see Table 1.5). This 25.3% figure actually substantially underestimates subfecundity in the entire U.S. population because it does not include the subfecund hidden among either

[7]The rationale for including under the definition of subfecundity women who are sterilized for noncontraceptive reasons is that such women do have a diminished capacity to reproduce. Indeed, the vast majority are infecund, being totally unable to reproduce both presently and in the future. The fact that this condition was caused by medical surgery rather than by some natural process seems of little import. The key factor is that these sterilizations are almost always due to involuntary pathological factors such as disease. Thus, the real cause of the sterility is the pathological factor, not the medical solution. Moreover, many of these individuals were already subfecund prior to the sterilizing operation. Chronic pelvic inflammatory disease, for example, is a powerful cause of subfecundity. It is also a serious health problem in other ways, and its resolution may require surgical procedures that would result in sterility. But this sterility is often redundant because it is placed on top of pre-existing subfecundity.

Table 1.5

Number of Currently Married Women Aged 15–44 Years and Percentage Distribution by Fecundity Status, by Age: United States, 1976[a]

| | | | | | Subfecund | | | | |
Age	Number of women (in 1,000s)	Total	Fecund	Contraceptively sterile	Noncontraceptively sterile	Nonsurgically sterile	Other problems[b]	Long birth intervals[c]	Total
All women	27,488	100.0	56.1	18.5	9.6	1.3	10.4	3.9	25.3
15–24	6,030	100.0	85.3	3.5	0.4	0.2	9.8	0.8	11.2
15–19	1,043	100.0	90.1	0.8	0.2	—	8.8	0.1	9.1
20–24	4,977	100.0	84.3	4.0	0.5	0.3	10.0	1.0	11.7
25–34	12,179	100.0	58.7	19.1	6.8	1.3	11.5	2.6	22.3
25–29	6,443	100.0	68.7	12.5	4.0	1.3	11.1	2.3	18.7
30–34	5,736	100.0	47.5	26.4	9.8	1.3	12.0	2.9	26.0
35–44	9,288	100.0	33.9	27.6	19.4	2.1	9.3	7.7	38.5
35–39	4,814	100.0	36.3	28.8	16.4	2.3	9.9	6.2	34.8
40–44	4,474	100.0	31.2	26.4	22.6	1.8	8.7	9.3	42.4

[a]Source: Constructed from Mosher and Pratt (1982:20).

[b]The "Other problems" category consists of women for whom it is difficult but perhaps not impossible to conceive and/or carry a pregnancy to term.

[c]The "Long interval" category consists of women who were not surgically sterile and who, during the 3 years of continuous marriage before the interview, did not use contraception and did not become pregnant. They are presumably sterile, although some might conceive in the future.

contraceptive users or those sterile for contraceptive reasons.[8] It also understates subfecundity because the NSFG entirely excluded the unmarried and those not married for the entire 12 months preceding the interview, groups that are probably disproportionately subfecund.

It is also informative to look at the number of couples classified as fecund in this study. As Table 1.5 shows, the proportion of all couples aged 15–44 who were fecund in 1976 was only 56%. By age 40–44, only 31% of these women were still fecund.

It is also possible to appreciate the prevalence of subfecundity in the United States by looking at the prevalence of its three components—coital inability, infertility, and pregnancy loss. Coital inability is particularly rife in the United States. Sex researchers Masters and John-

[8]Contraceptive surgical sterilization masks subfecundity in two instances. First, some individuals who are already subfecund but not necessarily infecund choose sterilization as a certain form of birth control. Second, some individuals who are fecund at the time of sterilization would have eventually become subfecund later in life anyway. These two categories of subfecundity are not counted as such in the Mosher and Pratt study and in many similar ones.

son (1970:369) estimated—conservatively, they said—that half of U.S. couples experience sexual dysfunction sometime during their lives. This seems confirmed by the work of many other sex researchers. Frank *et al.* (1978), for example, found that among white, well-educated, and happily married U.S. couples, a startling 40% of men and 63% of women reported coital difficulties or sexual dysfunction.

Infertility (i.e., conceptive difficulty) is also prevalent in the United States, and again, the 1976 NSFG is the best source for data on infertility. Mosher (1982b) analyzed these data and in the process classified couples as infertile if they were not surgically sterile and if, during the 12 months preceding the interview, they had been continuously married, had not used contraception, and had not conceived. This measure underestimates infertility in the U.S. population because, as noted earlier, surgical sterilization and contraception mask subfecundity in some couples, and the NSFG study did not include the unmarried and other relatively infertile groups in its sample. Nevertheless, as indicated in Table 1.6, about 2.8 million couples—10% of all married couples with wives aged 15–44—were classified as infertile in 1976. Based on data from the National Fertility Study (see Ryder and Westoff 1971), the comparable figure for 1965 was 11%. For women aged 40–44, the figures were 16% in 1976 and 20% in 1965.

Pregnancy loss is also common in the United States. Each year at least 800,000 pregnancies, approximately 15–20% of all conceptions, end as spontaneous abortions and another 33,000 result in stillbirths (Hacker 1981:D1). The NSFG found that in 1976 about one-third of currently married women had at least one spontaneous loss by ages 35–44 (Mosher 1982a:318).

Thus it is clear from all the major U.S. fertility surveys and from a variety of other studies that subfecundity is prevalent in the U.S. population. Indeed, it is likely that nearly all U.S. couples experience some form of subfecundity at one time or another during their reproductive careers. The situation in other developed societies is probably similar.

Impact on Fertility

Because the majority of couples in developed countries choose low fertility and are able to obtain it through birth control, the impact of subfecundity on fertility is not as substantial as it is in developing societies. However, it is still very important. If subfecundity were eliminated in developed societies, fertility would certainly rise. Involuntarily childless couples or those who have fewer children than desired due to subfecundity would increase their fertility. Mosher and Pratt (1982:2)

Table 1.6

Percentage of Infertile Currently Married Couples by
Age and Race of Wives: United States, 1965 and 1976[a]

	% infertile	
Race and age of wife	*1965*	*1976*
Total 15–44[b]	11.2	10.3
15–19	0.6[c]	2.1[c]
20–24	3.5[c]	6.4
25–29	6.5	9.0
30–34	11.6	10.3
35–39	14.2	12.5
40–44	20.2	15.9
White 15–44	10.5	9.4
15–19	0.6[c]	2.0[c]
20–24	3.4	5.6
25–29	6.1	8.4
30–34	10.8	9.5
35–39	13.4	11.4
40–44	18.5	14.6
Black 15–44	16.3	18.1
15–19	0.0[d]	3.7[c]
20–24	3.4	15.4
25–29	7.1	11.2
30–34	15.7	18.1
36–39	24.4	23.3
40–44	39.0	28.8

[a]Source: Mosher (1982b:24). Reprinted with permission from *Family Planning Perspectives*, Volume 14, Number 1, 1982.

[b]Includes races other than white and black.

[c]Percentage has a standard error that is greater than or equal to 25% of the estimate itself.

[d]Percentage based on fewer than 100 cases.

provided an indication of just how many births would result. Without considering the desires of the 2.7 million U.S. couples who are surgically sterilized for noncontraceptive reasons, they found that 47% of the remaining 4.3 million subfecund couples (or about 2 million couples) wanted to have a baby or another baby. This included about 840,000 couples who had no children, about 641,000 who had one child, and about 556,000 who had two or more. The fertility desires of those surgically sterilized for noncontraceptive reasons would add substantially to these already sizable figures. Thus, the elimination of subfecundity would have a significant impact on U.S. fertility—without even considering increases in fertility among those other subfecund couples who do not want more children and for whom subfecundity is a blessing. Undoubtedly, there would be large increases in unwanted as well as wanted births.

Moreover, within contracepting developed societies there are often significant subgroups not practicing effective birth control whose fertility would rise appreciably if subfecundity were not present. Indeed, it could be that many subfecundity factors are disproportionately prevalent among such groups. As Freedman noted (1963:51), "Health conditions and poor nutrition may affect the fecundity of the whole society or may affect the lowest stratum with special force as a result of the operation of the economic distribution."

In the United States such subgroups include immigrant groups (e.g., Haitians), lower-income whites and blacks, and teenagers. The black population in particular has had higher levels of subfecundity than the general population, at least since Emancipation (see McFalls 1973; McFalls and Tolnay, forthcoming). And even today their level of subfecundity is much higher than that of the white population. Again, the best study on current racial differentials in subfecundity is that of Mosher and Pratt (1982:22–23). Using the definition of subfecundity adopted earlier, 31.5% of black couples and 24.6% of white couples in the NSFG can be classified as subfecund (compared to 25.3% for all couples).

Another subgroup in the United States with relatively poor health and undoubtedly higher subfecundity is the American Indian. The age-adjusted death rate for Indians in 1975 was 30% higher than that for the entire U.S. population, and infant mortality was 10% higher. The prevalence of subfecundity factors such as tuberculosis, influenza, alcoholism, and malnutrition, to mention just a few, is also unusually high among the Indians. Those still living on reservations where health conditions are especially bad also suffer from higher rates of venereal disease (Klimas 1982:2, 10, 15).

The elimination of subfecundity in developed societies would also increase, at least temporarily, the fertility of those subgroups that have not yet undergone modernization and that remain largely outside the central culture. This is the same phenomenon discussed in the previous section on transitional and modernizing societies. There already are a number of examples of this in the literature. Romaniuk (1974:344) found that the fertility of the Indians of Canada's James Bay area rose with the onset of modernization and concluded that a reduction in subfecundity was a key factor. Another example is the increase in Alaska Native fertility during the 1950s and early 1960s, which resulted from substantial improvement in the level of health care (Blackwood 1981:177). Similar increases in fertility have been shown for groups in the central Asian republics of the Soviet Union between 1926 and 1970 (Knodel and Wilson 1981:53).

As in developing societies, lack of medical care is an important cause of subfecundity among the underprivileged in developed societies (Poston and Kramer 1980:17). Even in the United States, with its relative abundance of medical professionals, medical care is spotty; it is unavailable on a regular basis, for instance, to 10 million underprivileged children. Only about 60% of American children have been fully immunized against childhood diseases, some of which, such as mumps and rubella (German measles), can cause subfecundity. In many inner-city neighborhoods, less than half the children have been immunized (Maize 1978:22).

Other developed countries besides the United States continue to have substantial health and medical care problems related to subfecundity both at the national and subgroup levels. The Soviet Union, for instance, experienced a phenomenal rise in infant mortality in the 1970s (Davis and Feshbach 1980:12–14), which means that subfecundity has undoubtedly also risen because many of the same factors (e.g., diet, smoking, alcoholism, induced abortion,) lead to both infant mortality and pregnancy loss.

In sum, subfecundity is a very important determinant of fertility in developed societies, even those with the highest standards of living. As in developing societies, subfecundity's power to affect fertility varies by region and subgroup and is particularly evident among the underprivileged. Differing health conditions and medical care contribute to this variation.

High-Fertility Societies and Subgroups

It is generally thought that subfecundity is only an important determinant of natality in noncontracepting, low-fertility societies and subgroups. This is not the case in either the developing or the developed world. Subfecundity can have a sizable impact on the natality of high-fertility societies and subgroups as well, and because of the prevailing misconception it is worth making a special point of this. Indeed, as noted previously, subfecundity exerts a sizable impact even on the fertility of the Hutterites, the group reproducing closest to the maximum fertility rate. Their increasing fertility from generation to generation during the first half of this century was partly due to improvements in health conditions that affect fecundity[9] (see Eaton and Mayer 1954:20). Subfe-

---

[9]Hutterite fertility has apparently been declining over the past several decades due to postponement of marriage (Peter 1981:9).

cundity had its greatest impact on the Hutterites during the second half of their reproductive careers. Of Hutterite women aged 35–39, 22% were permanently sterile during the first half of the twentieth century (Tietze 1957, cited in Bongaarts 1982:76). If this subfecundity had not been present, their record high fertility would have been significantly even higher.

The same is true of another high-natality subgroup in the developed world, the Older Order Amish of the United States. Recent cohorts have completed childbearing with a mean family size of 7 children compared to 2.7 for comparable national cohorts. The fertility of the Amish has been increasing over the past 100 years and childlessness has been declining. Ericksen and associates (1979) argued that this is chiefly due to reductions in subfecundity, noting the group's willingness to take advantage of modern medical technology as soon as it appears. They also observe that whereas the Amish have an average of 7 children, the number varies greatly among families, probably due mostly to subfecundity. Even in one sample of particularly high-fertility Amish women, which happened to include no childless women, 10% of the women could be classified as significantly subfecund on the basis of conception problems alone. (An even higher figure might have been obtained if pregnancy loss had also been considered.) These subfecund women finished childbearing with only 4.6 children on average compared to 9.4 for the sample as a whole. In short, the authors concluded that the extraordinarily high fertility of the Amish would have been still higher had subfecundity not existed.

Other subgroups with both high fertility and high subfecundity exist currently and have existed historically in developed countries, and several have already been used as examples earlier in this chapter (e.g., Alaskan Natives; American blacks after Emancipation). Note has also been made of the fact that the fertility of some of these subgroups increases temporarily as they undergo modernization and subfecundity declines.

Similarly, subfecundity can have a significant effect on the fertility of high-natality developing societies (Mosley *et al.* 1982). For instance, the married Yoruba women in Ibadan, Nigeria, average about 6 children per woman. Yet by age 45 8% are involuntarily childless and another 25% have had fewer than 4 live births in a society where 4 or more living children is considered the ideal. The low fertility of these women has been attributed to subfecundity (Arowolo 1978:13). If this apparent subfecundity were not present, the already high fertility of the whole population would rise materially. Another example is the western tribe of the Republic of Upper Volta. Though they have a high crude birth rate (45.4), 12% of the women are childless due undoubtedly to subfecundity (Brass 1968:365–367). Finally, Frank (1983:142) estimated that high subfecundity lowers the total fertility rate (TFR) of 17 high-fertility sub-Saharan African nations by an average of 1 birth per woman—a reduction in the average rate from 7.6 to 6.6. Frank also concludes that Gabon, with a 1982 TFR of 4.7, might have more than 3 more births per woman if its extremely high subfecundity were eliminated.

Future Societies

It was noted previously that in developing societies as a whole subfecundity has been declining recently due to the improvement and expansion of health services. In the future many developing countries will continue their struggle against the causes of subfecundity, particularly infectious diseases. Further improvements seem inevitable in the long run, but progress may be slow in the short run and there may even be some backsliding (see Frank 1983:143). Indeed, there are indications that the trend toward reduced subfecundity in many developing countries has recently abated.

One way to determine if the health of a population is improving is to check trends in life expectancy. Despite its limitations, life expectancy at birth has proven to be the most important single measure of a population's health[10] (World Health Organization 1980:237). It is noteworthy then that after decades of large increases in life expectancy in the Third World, the increases have declined and even vanished in some countries (Arriaga 1982:1; Bell 1980:63; Gwatkin 1980:615, 637, 1981:8; Tabah 1980:372). In Gwatkin's (1980:615) words, ''the suggestion emerging from recent findings is that the remarkably rapid rates of mortality decline that have prevailed since World War II have begun to falter, to give way to a confused, diverse, ambiguous situation marked by unexpected slowdowns in the pace of health improvements observed in many large areas of the developing world.'' In most Third World countries there continues to be some improvement in life expectancy, although the rate of progress is slowing and is substantially below earlier predictions. But in some countries, including Sri Lanka and Bangladesh, the death rate has actually increased. Because subfecundity and mortality are caused by many of the same factors (e.g., malaria, tuberculosis

---

[10]The relationship between mortality and morbidity is not the same everywhere. In developed countries both have declined fairly proportionately, but in poor developing countries much of the medicine practiced is therapeutic rather than preventive. This means that the death rate may be reduced with little change in morbidity, resulting in a large burden of chronic ill health allied with nutritional deficiencies (Keyfitz 1981:15). Thus, change in life expectancy is in some respects a conservative proxy for change in the subfecundity level.

[TB]), these mortality trends undoubtedly took place in tandem with a slowdown in the reduction of subfecundity in some areas, and even with an increase in subfecundity in others.

Recent experience has demonstrated that the difficulties involved in eliminating subfecundity factors in the developing world should not be underestimated. The conquest of subfecundity factors such as malaria and schistosomiasis will be a long and arduous task challenging both public health ingenuity and political determination. The extent to which countries succeed will depend heavily on changes in the political situation and the socioeconomic setting. Many developing countries undoubtedly will not reduce subfecundity to levels experienced in developed societies without the removal of the main causes of poverty and underdevelopment (World Health Organization 1980:241). It is probably fair to say that many developing countries will continue to experience high levels of subfecundity far into the future.

There is reason to believe that in recent years subfecundity has been rising, or at least not declining much, in developed countries. There is no good time series study to confirm this, but there is information for the U.S. population on the trend in infertility, one of subfecundity's key components. These infertility data come from the 1976 National Survey of Family Growth and the 1965 National Fertility Study. Using the same definition of infertility as in the Mosher and Pratt (1982) study discussed earlier, Mosher (1982b:24) conservatively classified 11% of U.S. married couples as infertile in 1965 and 10% in 1976 (see Table 1.6). Although there was no statistically significant change in the proportion of white or black couples classified as infertile between 1965 and 1976, this apparent overall stability was produced by increases in infertility among younger couples—especially those with wives aged 20–24—and decreases among older couples.[11] Because there is a growing tendency for older couples in the United States to mask their infertility by entering the ranks of the surgically sterile, Mosher's figures suggest that infertility for the entire U.S. population is actually on the rise.

The increase in infertility among the younger couples was quite substantial. Whereas 482,000 couples with the wife younger than age 30 were classified as infertile in 1965, this number grew to approximately 920,000 by 1976. The most striking component of this trend is the sharp increase in the proportion of black couples aged 20–24 who were infertile

---

[11]Older couples in 1965 may also have been more subfecund than those in 1976 because the former passed through some of their early reproductive period when subfecundity-producing infectious diseases were common and when their treatment was less effective.

(see Table 1.6). This proportion swelled from 3% in 1965 to 15% in 1976 (Mosher 1982b:24).

Subfecundity is probably also moving upward in the Soviet Union where there has been recent deterioration in both the infant mortality rate and life expectancy,[12] two phenomena closely linked to subfecundity. These are both remarkable and disturbing reversals that mark a sharp departure from the prevailing trend of steady improvement during the twentieth century (Cusick 1981:11).

The fact that subfecundity is holding steady or even rising in the developed world is attributed to a variety of causes. One factor is the dramatic increase in venereal disease, which can seriously damage reproductive potential. Another is the widespread use of the intrauterine contraceptive device (IUD), which can cause problems for women who later hope to bear children. Increasing levels of stress, environmental pollutants, alcohol and drug abuse, and a variety of other factors have also been cited (see McFalls 1979a).

It is remarkable that subfecundity has remained fairly stable in developed countries, even though medical advances in the treatment of subfecundity have been proceeding at a prodigious rate. Only 10% of the subfecund couples seeking treatment 40 years ago could be helped to achieve pregnancy. Today 40–70% of subfecund couples can be helped (Gorman 1982:63; Mazor 1979:104). There have been tremendous treatment advances in all three components of subfecundity—coital inability, conceptive failure, and pregnancy loss.

Much coital inability, particularly impotence and dyspareunia (painful coitus), stems from psychosexual disorders. The pioneering work in sex therapy of Masters and Johnson (1966, 1970), together with more conventional types of psychiatric treatment, have brought tremendous improvements in this area of reproduction. And for those men whose impotence results from a physical problem and for those whose problem is psychological but not helped by psychotherapy there are now several implantable mechanical devices that can mimic a natural erection.

A variety of new techniques are available to reduce conceptive failure including (1) hormone and other drug therapies to deal with such problems as spermatogenic and ovulatory failure,[13] secretion of anti-

---

[12]Interestingly, life expectancy at birth in the United States also was down slightly in 1980 to 73.6 years from a record 73.8 in 1979. This was probably due to a 14% increase in deaths from influenza and pneumonia, two diseases that also affect fecundity adversely (National Center for Health Statistics, cited in *Philadelphia Bulletin* 1981a:A4).

[13]The more powerful of the so-called fertility drugs have the ability to increase individual fecundity greatly by increasing the number of multiple births. Some women have

spermal antibodies, and endometriosis, (2) microsurgery to correct obstructed sperm ducts, blocked fallopian tubes, and varicocele, and to reverse sterilization, and (3) innovative psychotherapy to remedy psychosexual disorders such as ejaculatory incompetence, premature ejaculation, and anovulatory amenorrhea. There is also in vitro fertilization, a process in which a mature egg is removed from a woman's ovary, fertilized in a glass dish, and transferred to the woman's uterus about 36 hours later. If the embryo successfully implants itself, the pregnancy may proceed normally. The process has begun to be used for women whose fallopian tubes, the egg's normal conduit from ovary to uterus, are missing or irreparably blocked.

New medical technology and practices can also minimize the probability of pregnancy loss (and neonatal mortality [Henig 1981]) due to spontaneous abortion and stillbirth. The increased use of cesarean sections, for example, has dramatically improved the outcome of high-risk deliveries, such as those involving premature babies. The cesarean rate in the United States rose from 5% in 1965 to about 18% in 1980. During that period infant mortality dropped from about 25 per 1000 births to about 12. In California in 1977, cesarean section was used in 25% of births, an increase of 6% a year over the previous 2 decades. Perinatal mortality fell 48% over the same period due in part to the increased use of this technique. Pregnancy loss can also be averted by new forms of drug therapies. For instance, by giving heart medicine (digoxin) to an expectant mother it is now possible to treat congestive heart failure in the fetus successfully. And a new drug, ritodrine, has been successfully used to ward off premature labor, the single biggest problem in obstetrics in the 1980s and a prime cause of or contributor to late fetal death and stillbirth.

New forms of intrauterine diagnostic and surgical techniques have also been developed that help decrease pregnancy loss. Amniocentesis, the laboratory analysis of a small sample of the amniotic fluid drawn from the sac surrounding the baby in the womb, can alert physicians to serious and potentially life-threatening disorders. An even more recent diagnostic aid is fetoscopy, a technique that permits physicians actually to see the fetus in the uterus and spot certain physical defects as well as to take blood and tissue from the fetus to aid in the search for other

---

produced up to 15 nonviable fetuses at a time. Although not enough women are currently using these drugs to alter population fertility rates, the ratio of multiple births to all births has apparently been affected. For example, in Western nations 1 in every 8 million confinements currently results in quintuplets; in the 1930s it was 1 in every 20 million (Shearer 1980a:13).

problems.[14] Surgery is now being performed on the fetus still in the womb, and even more remarkably outside the womb. In the latter situation, the fetus is then returned to its mother's uterus where it continues to term.

Another new practice that helps avert pregnancy loss, especially among habitual aborters and women with histories of problem pregnancies, is the use of high-risk pregnancy monitoring systems. These programs give specialized care throughout those pregnancies that pose danger to either the child or the mother. Such pregnancies are disturbingly common in the United States where there are as many as 50,000 perinatal deaths per year. Women who benefit most from these programs have problems such as hypertension, diabetes, alcohol and drug abuse, and kidney disease. The tremendous improvement in fetal survival among diabetic women whose pregnancies are closely supervised is an excellent example of the effectiveness of these monitoring systems.

Medical advances in the treatment of subfecundity will continue to proceed rapidly well into the future. Several promising devices are on the horizon to help solve male coital inability. One is an electronic genital stimulator, which will be placed inside the body to remedy impotence through the use of electrical impulses. There are also drugs such as yohimbine being tested that may be used in the future to improve coital ability.

Conceptive failure will be combated by a tiny electronic microchip called the sexometer, which will indicate when the optimum phase for conception has been reached. This device will not only help couples having difficulty conceiving but will also double as an effective contraceptive aid. Another promising advance is the low tubal ovum transfer, which will aid women with blocked fallopian tubes (*Intercom* 1980:2). In this process, an egg is extracted from a ripening follicle with a hollow needle and immediately reinserted into the fallopian tube below the blockage point. This permits normal in vivo fertilization to take place. As noted earlier, fallopian tube blockage—the most common cause of infertility in women—can now be repaired by surgery, but conception occurs in only about 25% of cases. Currently, the only possible recourse

---

[14]Amniocentesis and fetoscopy have an effect on another intermediate variable besides subfecundity, induced abortion. If Down's syndrome, Gaucher's disease, or some other disorder is diagnosed, prospective parents sometimes opt for induced abortion. On the other hand, the absence of such a diagnosis sometimes saves fetuses that would otherwise be aborted due to a suspected though actually nonexistent problem.

in women with irreparable tubal blockage is in vitro fertilization, but conception rates are very low with this method also. The success rate for low tubal ovum transfer should be much higher than either of these methods, judging from experiments on monkeys.

Physicians are already freezing human embryos to be thawed and implanted later in infertile women. By 1983, in Australia an embryo had been successfully implanted in its mother's womb, and there was an unconfirmed report from India of the birth of a child who was frozen prior to implantation. In the future, couples and even individuals may routinely freeze away fertilized eggs early in their reproductive careers for later implantation. This practice would have many implications for fecundity. It would permit childbearing among those who become infertile in the freezing–implantation interval; it may even have the minor effect of decreasing pregnancy loss because the egg providing the basis for the embryo would not age as much biologically due to its frozen state and because it would be subject to fewer harmful influences than if it had not been frozen during the interval.

The more distant future will include such techniques as genetic engineering and possibly even genuine conception-to-term test tube babies. It is probably fair to say that techniques will be developed in the future that will permit physicians to eliminate or sidestep most forms of subfecundity.

Much of this new technology has been in service for several decades, so why has it not substantially reduced subfecundity in the United States? There are several reasons. First, as noted earlier, many of the causes of subfecundity in the United States are increasing. Second, some of the new technology can actually cause subfecundity, although this is a minor point. For instance, fetoscopy causes spontaneous abortion in about 5% of cases and amniocentesis does so in about 1% of cases. Third, for a variety of reasons ranging from embarrassment to ignorance, not all subfecund couples seek treatment. Others, especially those who already have the number of children they desire, actually view their subfecundity as a blessing in disguise freeing them from the practice and problems of birth control. Fourth, much of the present technology—and the same will be true, for a long time, of the future technology—is not available to large segments of the U.S. population. For instance, fetoscopy is still experimental and as of 1982 had only been used on a few hundred women. Similarly, the high-risk pregnancy monitoring systems are not widely available. There are too few doctors and nurses with the skills needed to staff these programs, and consequently they are often situated at scattered medical centers not easily accessible to the women who most need them.[15] Likewise, in vitro fertilization—the test tube method for circumventing damaged or missing fallopian tubes—is offered in only a handful of clinics in the United States, and its widespread use is still a long way off. Thus for almost all of the 600,000 U.S. couples who could benefit from it, in vitro fertilization remains a tantalizing, unavailable remedy.

Even when some of this technology is available, it is very expensive and many couples cannot afford it (Poston and Kramer 1980:17). Psychotherapy for psychosexual disorders is costly and often not included in health insurance and medical plans. In 1980, rod implant surgery to counter impotence cost about $3500, including hospitalization, and the cost could go as high as $9000 for the inflatable prosthesis. These expenditures again are frequently not covered by medical insurance. In 1982, the sexometer cost $240; cesarean delivery cost $4200; test tube babies cost at least $3500 (and in some clinics $10,000 or more). And high-risk pregnancy monitoring systems could run into tens of thousands of dollars including the fragile newborn's stay in an intensive care unit. It is ironic that although the United States pioneered much of this new technology to thwart subfecundity, it lags behind many other developed countries in making it available to its citizens. This explains in part why, for instance, the United States has a higher perinatal (and neonatal) mortality rate than a dozen other countries (Population Reference Bureau, 1982).

In sum, although tremendous progress has been made in recent decades in reducing subfecundity in the developing and developed worlds, the pace of that progress has slowed recently almost everywhere. It is also clear that both areas of the world will continue to experience high levels of subfecundity; this is particularly true of the developing world, which still lags substantially behind the developed world in fecundity. The modern advances in the treatment of subfecundity discussed here are virtually nonexistent in most countries in the developing world where even rudimentary obstetrical care is often absent. And these advances are also unavailable or unaffordable to large

---

[15]A well-publicized case (see *Philadelphia Bulletin* 1982:A3) of a premature baby unable to find care in Florida dramatized the fact that neonatal as well as prenatal care of children in the United States is frequently unavailable to low-income groups. In this instance, a premature baby whose parents were unemployed and without insurance was denied desperately needed care at 26 Florida hospitals and probably would have died without the intercession of the president of the United States. That child's struggle, which left the parents with $100,000 in medical bills, focused attention on the state's deficient neonatal care system. An organization that places critically ill babies in Florida reported that between February 1979 and November 1981 it was unable to find room for 410 of 1607 premature babies in Florida. Of the 410 who were not placed, 212 died.

segments of the populations of the developed world. So subfecundity will continue to exert an influence on fertility far into the future. Indeed, one expert (Mosley 1979:2) suggested that, at least in the developed world, given current trends in controlled fertility wanted pregnancies will be a future health problem of greater magnitude than unwanted pregnancies.

Subfecundity and the Timing of Fertility in Developed Societies

Some might argue that most subfecund women in developed societies still have the number of children they want; it just takes them longer. In other words, subfecundity would not affect completed fertility. This position denies the reality documented earlier that substantial fractions of ever-married women in developed societies are involuntarily and permanently childless and that large numbers with children can have no more. It also ignores the effect of the timing of fertility on completed family size. For example, many women in the United States are now postponing childbearing until their late 20s and early 30s. This gives them fewer years to achieve their desired fertility and also requires that they do so in the face of the lower fecundity characteristic of these years that is due to aging and accumulated subfecundity from causes such as disease.[16] About the much-speculated-upon possibility that many U.S. women will try to have their quota of two children late in their reproductive careers, demographer Taeuber (cited in Blackman 1975:WA2) has commented: ''It's a pretty cloudy crystal ball. If women have these two children, we're bound to see the number of births go up. . . . But there is some reason to believe that some women will be disappointed and find that they can't have these children.''

Much attention has been given to an article by Schwartz and Mayaux (1982) suggesting that the risk of permanent sterility (infertility)[17]

[16]Postponements of childbearing can eventually lead to voluntary childlessness and low fertility as well as to involuntary restriction on childbearing due to subfecundity. See Poston and Kramer (1980:25, 26, 60) for a review of the literature.

[17]Schwartz and Mayaux did not really measure the risk of permanent sterility, but rather that of infertility. This is because they limited the study period to a single year of attempted pregnancy. Some women who fail to conceive during a 12-month period are not permanently sterile, however; they become pregnant in subsequent years. Thus, although all these women are infertile (i.e., they have a difficult time becoming pregnant), not all are sterile. Hendershot *et al.* (1982), although mindful of this distinction, used this same 12-month measure of infertility to compare women in the NSFG directly to those in the Schwartz and Mayaux study.

increases sharply not only after age 40, as previously thought, but starting as early as age 30 (see Table 1.7). If this were true it would have
profound implications for the temporal pattern of childbearing, and possibly also for individual and societal goals concerning the education,
training, and labor force participation of women. However, the Schwartz
and Mayaux findings have been challenged by a number of critics (see
Bongaarts 1982; Webster 1982), and it is generally agreed that the study
does contain some methodological flaws that could lead to an overstate-
ment of the risk of infertility. Nevertheless, despite these flaws Hendershot and associates (1982) argued persuasively that the actual pattern
of infertility by age in women in the developed world may not be too
different from the Schwartz and Mayaux pattern. Using 1976 NSFG data,
Hendershot *et al.* derived infertility rates for U.S. married women that
are very close to those given in the Schwartz and Mayaux study, except
for ages 20–24 (see Table 1.7).[18] The data from this hypothetical exercise
also follow the same pattern as the Schwartz and Mayaux data, with
infertility rising sharply through the 30s.

Two additional observations on the Hendershot *et al.* data are worth
making. First, the NSFG data used by Hendershot *et al.* actually underestimate infertility (and subfecundity) for the reasons already discussed earlier in this chapter. Correcting for this understatement would
boost the rates. Second, if Hendershot *et al.* had presented the NSFG
data for high-subfecundity subgroups such as U.S. blacks, the infertility
rates probably would have exceeded those in the Schwartz and Mayaux
study across the board.

Thus, subfecundity increases with age in developed societies, and
the present phenomenon of postponing childbearing for a variety of personal, social, and economic reasons contributes to the number of individuals who have problems having children. The longer the decision to
have children is delayed, the greater the risk of subfecundity and even
infecundity. Although the risks of subfecundity and infecundity may
not increase as sharply as the Schwartz and Mayaux study suggested,
they do rise substantially between the early 20s and late 30s, especially
among high-subfecundity subgroups.

Incidentally, subfecundity also increases with age in developing societies, and in some at a far faster rate than in developed ones. Here too
subfecundity's rise with age affects the timing and level of fertility. In
high-subfecundity societies with strong pronatalist values, the threat of
future subfecundity can increase the pressure to marry and begin child-

[18]The Hendershot *et al.* (1982) rates are based on the assumption that the proportion
of contraception users who would discover they were infertile if they tried to become
pregnant is half that of nonusers.

Table 1.7

Percentage of Infertile Nonsterile Currently Married Women Aged
15–44 by Woman's Age Group in Two Studies[a]

	% infertile	
Age group	*Schwartz and Mayaux*[b]	*Hendershot et al.*[c]
20–24	27	14
25–29	26	22
30–34	39	37
35–39	44	48

[a]*Infertile* are those who did not conceive in 12 months of unprotected intercourse.

[b]Source: Schwartz and Mayaux (1982:404). Reprinted, by permission of the *New England Journal of Medicine* (Volume 307).

[c]Source: Hendershot *et al.*(1982:288). Reprinted with permission from *Family Planning Perspectives*, Volume 14, Number 5, 1982. Rates are based on the assumption that the proportion of contraception users who would discover they were infertile if they tried to become pregnant is half that of nonusers.

bearing near the age of menarche (Cassen 1978:338; *Population Reports* 1979a:134).[19] Families concerned about low fertility and childlessness want to maximize the fertility of their children, and the children themselves are reluctant to postpone childbearing for fear of becoming barren in the meantime. This is particularly true of societies where descent is patrilineal (Mosk 1981:31). Thus, the prospect of subfecundity lowers the age at marriage and the age at first birth. Whether this early start at childbearing leads to higher completed fertility depends on many factors, including the nature and prevalence of the prevailing causes of subfecundity, the presence of and allegiance to such norms as fidelity, and adjustments in other intermediate variables. This last factor is of key importance. Early marriage does not commit a couple irretrievably to a large family, because many other ways of reducing fertility (e.g., abstinence, contraception, and abortion) are used after this point (Davis and Blake 1956:215). Also important is that early age at marriage in some areas of developing countries often leads to early pregnancy loss and subsequent infertility (Adadevoh 1974). This will be discussed in more detail later. In any event, subfecundity and the threat of subfecundity may be partly responsible for the lack of an association between age at

[19]Early marriage is not just a hedge against subfecundity, it is a hedge against mortality as well (Davis and Blake 1956:215). In fact, mortality is probably a stronger threat than subfecundity; it is a threat both to the parents themselves and to the potential offspring. An early marriage makes it more likely that the young adults will have some children before they die and enough children to help guarantee that some will survive to adulthood.

marriage and total fertility in the developing world (*Population Reports* 1979a:134).

Subfecundity can also indirectly affect fertility in developed societies by influencing the timing of early fertility. Delays in early childbearing due to subfecundity can provide women with the opportunity to develop a life-style other than that of becoming the mother of a large family (Presser 1971:336). Also, the presence of subfecundity during the early reproductive years can allow progress to be made toward learning effective birth control, which would reduce unwanted fertility or give a woman time to consider what her reproductive goals really are and then attempt to stick by them (see Masnick and McFalls 1976, 1978). The subfecundity produced by syphilis, for instance, can provide such a delay. Usually contracted early in reproductive life, syphilis causes high rates of pregnancy loss during the 2 years following infection. However, even untreated syphilis has little effect on pregnancy outcome after this period, so a direct effect on completed fertility would be unlikely for couples with low or moderate family size desires. But the 2-year respite during the peak reproductive years provided by the subfecundity gives a woman the opportunity to revise her reproductive goals.

Although not so important demographically, it is worth noting that subfecundity can also affect fertility indirectly by influencing the timing of late fertility. Delays in second or later children can result in lower lifetime fertility. Subfecundity used to be responsible for a considerable proportion of two-family women—those who had children early, stopped childbearing for many years for a variety of reasons including subfecundity, and then had other children who were far younger than the first group. With increased availability of induced abortion and better contraceptives, women now more often forego the second family in favor of other life-styles. If it were not for subfecundity in the middle years, many of these women, especially those who had not yet achieved their desired family size, might well have had additional children spaced close to the first set. Thus subfecundity, by altering when women are able to have their higher order children, may alter completed family size as well.

Impact of Subfecundity on Birth Control and Mate Exposure

Subfecundity affects fertility directly through its components—coital inability, conceptive failure, and pregnancy loss. But it can also have important indirect effects on population fertility. One group of such indirect effects, the influence of subfecundity on the timing of fertility, was discussed in the previous section. This section focuses on another group, the ability of subfecundity to influence fertility behaviorally through the other Davis–Blake intermediate variables (see Table 1.8). The following discussion provides examples of how subfecundity can affect each of these variables. The emphasis here is on that portion of subfecundity pertaining to the reduced ability to have children, not to the complete inability (infecundity), because the latter can have no further effect on fertility.

The first intermediate variable is age of entry into sexual unions (see Table 1.8). It has been noted above that subfecundity and the threat of subfecundity frequently lower the age of marriage. Subfecundity can also lead to permanent celibacy, the second variable. Temporary or intermittent causes of subfecundity such as relative impotence, premature ejaculation, and other psychosexual disorders are so disturbing to some

Table 1.8

The Davis–Blake Intermediate Variables through Which Social Factors Influence Fertility by Phase of Fertility and by Subfecundity–Birth Control–Mate Exposure Categories[a]

Phase of fertility

I. Factors affecting exposure to intercourse (intercourse variables)
  A. Those governing the formation and dissolution of unions in the reproductive period
   1. Age of entry into sexual unions
   2. Permanent celibacy: proportion never entering sexual unions
   3. Amount of reproductive period spent after or between unions
    a. When unions are broken by divorce, separation, or desertion
    b. When unions are broken by death of spouse
  B. Those governing the exposure to intercourse within unions
   4. Voluntary abstinence
   5. Involuntary abstinence (from impotence, illness, unavoidable but temporary separations)
   6. Coital frequency (excluding periods of abstinence)

II. Factors affecting exposure to conception (conception variables)
   7. Conceptive failure (infertility, sterility)
   8. Use or nonuse of contraception
    a. By mechanical and chemical means
    b. By other means (rhythm, withdrawal)
   9. Fecundity or infecundity as affected by voluntary causes (sterilization, subincision, medical treatment, etc.)

III. Factors affecting gestation and successful parturition (gestation variables)
   10. Fetal mortality from involuntary causes
   11. Fetal mortality from voluntary causes

(Continued)

Table 1.8 (Continued)

Subfecundity–Mate Exposure–Birth Control

I. Subfecundity
    1. Involuntary abstinence due to coital inability
    2. Conceptive failure (infertility, sterility)
    3. Fetal mortality from involuntary causes (pregnancy loss)

II. Mate exposure
    A. Those governing the formation and dissolution of unions in the reproductive period
        4. Age of entry into sexual unions
        5. Permanent celibacy: proportion never entering sexual unions
        6. Amount of reproductive period spent after or between unions
            a. When unions are broken by divorce, separation, or desertion
            b. When unions are broken by death of spouse
    B. Those governing the exposure to intercourse within unions
        7. Voluntary abstinence
        8. Involuntary abstinence due to reasons other than coital inability (unavoidable temporary separations)
        9. Coital frequency (excluding periods of abstinence)

III. Birth control
    10. Use or nonuse of contraception
    11. Fecundity or infecundity, as affected by voluntary causes (sterilization, subincision, medical treatment, etc.)
    12. Fetal mortality from voluntary causes (induced abortion)

---

[a]Source: Modified from Davis and Blake (1956:212). From *Economic Development and Cultural Change*, published by The University of Chicago. © 1956 by The University of Chicago.

sufferers that they choose to withdraw from all sexual contacts and live celibate lives (see McFalls 1979b).

Subfecundity's most important indirect effect on fertility is its ability to affect the amount of the reproductive period spent after or between unions. This works in several ways. First, subfecundity can lead to any of the forms of marital disruption—separation, divorce, or desertion (Isely 1980:B8, B9; Rozat 1980:418). In societies that value women in direct proportion to their fertility, subfecundity and especially childlessness represent a social stigma, usually borne by the woman alone. In such cultures the failure to bear children is an accepted basis for marital disruption (Belsey 1978:1), and this disruption can occur early in a marriage. Isely (1980:4) reported that childlessness for just 2 years can lead to marital instability, infidelity, and sexual promiscuity, and childlessness for longer than 5 years, to separation and divorce. The subfecund wife cast out by a disappointed husband has been a familiar tragedy throughout history and still is in many developing societies. The population literature is replete with studies reporting a negative impact of subfecundity on marital stability. In a study based on interviews with 17 sterile women in Buganda, Bennett (1965) found much evidence of marital instability. The 17 women had 43 sexual partners, and their current husbands had 37 sexual partners. Ampofo (1977) found a high degree of marital instability among 202 subfecund women in Ghana, about half of whom were completely sterile. Only 16% of them had been married for more than 10 years, and only 40% for 1 to 5 years. Henin (1969) reported that barrenness was cited by Sudanese nomads as a cause of divorce in 25% of cases, and Roberts and Tanner (1959) found that low fertility correlated with short duration of marriage and conjugal mobility in several communities of present-day Tanzania. The latter authors also observed that subfecund marriages terminated in divorce more often than did fertile marriages of the same duration. Armagnac and Retel-Laurentin (1981) found that a history of subfecundity increased marital instability among the members of an Upper Volta tribe. They noted that every reproductive-aged male and female in the tribe is on the lookout for a fecund partner. Correa (1969) also concluded that subfecundity destabilized marriages among the Nzakara of the Central African Republic. He reported that married women had less subfecundity than unmarried women. Finally, Retel-Laurentin (1972), in another study of the Nzakara, found that subfecundity was related to multiple marriages and nonmarital sexual unions and to unions of short duration. Women with more than two unions, especially if marital mobility had been rapid before age 20, had particularly high rates of infertility and pregnancy loss as well as high rates of such subfecundity factors as venereal disease and pelvic infections.

Besides causing marital disruption, subfecundity can also diminish the possibility of remarriage for subfecund individuals or those who were previously married to a subfecund person. Meuwissen (1966:156, 1967b:1205) found this to be true in Ghana, where those subfecund individuals who succeed in remarrying often do so with others of proven or suspected subfecundity. This is important because this nonrandom mating pattern minimizes the impact of subfecundity on a population's fertility wherever it occurs.

The final way subfecundity can increase the time spent after or between unions is by causing the death of a spouse. For instance, women with scarred fallopian tubes often experience pregnancy loss due to ectopic pregnancies. This form of subfecundity is a life-threatening condition in both the developed and developing worlds, but particularly in the latter with its relative lack of health care.

Subfecundity can also lead to several other intermediate variables: voluntary abstinence, contraception, and sterilization. For example, some habitual aborters—women who have more than two consecutive spontaneous abortions—choose voluntary abstinence, contraception, or sterilization rather than taking the chance of suffering another traumatic miscarriage. Voluntary abstinence is more often the choice in societies or subgroups opposed to contraception and sterilization. And sometimes just the prospect of subfecundity can result in voluntary abstinence or contraception. For instance, a person may choose abstinence or a prophylactic contraceptive rather than contract or spread a subfecundity-producing disease. This behavior may have averted a substantial number of births in historical societies and in present-day developing ones where treatment is not immediately available. Spreading the disease, however, would also have averted births.

In the developing world subfecundity affects the use of birth control in yet another way. In a sense, birth control is an opportunity cost of subfecundity because the latter consumes a large proportion of the reproductive health service resources that could otherwise be used to increase the use and effectiveness of the former. A number of African studies specify that up to one-third of family planning or gynecological consultations deal with subfecundity complaints (Belsey 1978:4). Subfecundity retards the expansion of birth control in the developing world in still another way. Reproductive dysfunction is attributed in some places to the use of contraception and this interferes with family planning programs (Hopcraft *et al.* 1973:581). Hence, there are countervailing effects, with subfecundity having both a positive and a negative effect on fertility via the birth control intermediate variable.

Subfecundity may also increase or decrease coital frequency.[20] Couples who have problems conceiving but who are not sterile often increase coital frequency to the level that maximizes fecundity. On the other hand, individuals who suffer from such subfecundity problems as habitual abortion, intermittent or marginal potency, and premature ejaculation may sharply reduce coital frequency in order to lessen anxiety, embarrassment, or the chances of a miscarriage.

The last nonsubfecundity intermediate variable is induced abortion or voluntary fetal mortality. Many of the causes of subfecundity, particularly of pregnancy loss, also compel women to have induced abortions. Examples such as toxic chemicals (e.g., PVC [polyvinyl chloride], DBCP [dibromochloropropane]), infectious diseases (e.g., rubella), and

---

[20]It is worth stressing that coital frequency is not a determinant of subfecundity, though it is a factor in natural fertility. A person may be highly fecund, for example, but have low fertility due to infrequent coitus. But, although low and even too-high coital frequency may depress fertility (see Amelar *et al.* 1977:206), it is a behavioral phenomenon independent of an individual's innate capacity to reproduce.

psychopathological factors (e.g., psychic stress, illicit drug abuse) come readily to mind (see McFalls 1979a, 1979b). But it is difficult to offer a common example of subfecundity itself leading to induced abortion. One possibility is the situation in which a woman has an induced abortion upon learning through fetoscopy or amniocentesis that her unborn child will likely be stillborn (pregnancy loss).

Therefore, it is clear that subfecundity can influence fertility indirectly through each of the other intermediate variables. Some of these relationships are far more important than others. In general, subfecundity affects fertility to a greater extent through the mate exposure variables than through the birth control ones (see Table 1.8).

Impact of Mate Exposure and Birth Control on Subfecundity

It is important to recognize that the mate exposure and birth control variables may themselves cause subfecundity and thus affect fertility in this way also. The following discussion provides examples of these relationships.

An early age of entry into sexual unions can cause subfecundity (Adadevoh 1974:10, 16; Ibeziako 1974:92). Physical maturity, especially of the pelvis, occurs later than the ability to conceive. This means the pelvis and its outlet may not be ready for pregnancy and delivery in women who marry early. If a pregnancy occurs, spontaneous abortion, obstetrical complications, stillbirth, puerperal infection, fistulas, subsequent infertility, and maternal death often follow, especially in the developing world and particularly in Africa. These conditions are common, for instance, among the Isoko tribe of Nigeria. Although these problems are substantially less important where adequate medical care is available, even in the United States rates of stillbirth, prematurity, neonatal mortality, and serious physical or mental handicaps are much higher for the very young mother than for women in their 20s (Menken 1972:45).

Also, a young age of entry into sexual unions can lead to subfecundity in societies where venereal disease is prevalent: Women who enter a series of early fleeting relationships before marriage have a greater chance of contracting these infections and impairing their fecundity (Isely 1980:21). There is some evidence that this is happening in the United States, where adolescent sexual activity is on the increase, aided by access to oral contraceptives. Many infertility specialists conclude that this increased adolescent sexual activity has resulted in a marked rise in gonorrheal salpingitis and tubal adhesions. This example also illustrates the impact on fecundity of another intermediate variable, contraception. Indeed, one of the inventors of the pill, Min-Cheuh Chang, has lamented the fact that his invention has led to increased promiscuity and subfecundity.

But the association between age at first coitus and subfecundity may not always be a negative one. Age at first coitus was positively associated with the incidence and degree of infertility in at least one study. Cutler *et al.* (1979a) found that infertility patients reported later first coital ages than routine gynecological patients in a sample of 792 women.

Voluntary abstinence can lead to subfecundity in societies that enforce long periods of sexual abstinence during pregnancy and lactation. Husbands who seek sexual relations outside marriage not infrequently contract subfecundity-producing diseases, which they may later pass on to their wives (Frank 1983:140; Isely 1980:21). Likewise, too-high or too-low coital frequency can cause subfecundity under certain circumstances. Too-frequent intercourse during the final 6 months of pregnancy may lead to pregnancy loss by producing one of three disorders that cause nearly half of all fetal and neonatal deaths: infection of the amniotic fluid, separation of the placenta from the uterine wall, and premature rupture of the fetal membranes. On the other hand, too-infrequent or sporadic intercourse is associated with an increased likelihood of long menstrual cycles, and these cycles tend to be anovulatory. Thus infrequent coital activity probably leads to infertility (Cutler *et al.* 1979b:214, 1979c:307). Too-infrequent coital activity may also cause prostatitis in men (Nass *et al.* 1981:494), but probably not prostate cancer as had been previously thought.

The birth control intermediate variables have many ways of increasing or decreasing subfecundity. A minority of women develop anovulatory amenorrhea after discontinuing use of oral contraceptives; in some of these women the amenorrhea may persist for years. But the condition nearly always cures itself or is responsive to drug treatment (*British Medical Journal* 1972b:59). In predisposed women, use of the pill may also lead to overt diabetes with all the subsequent risks to fecundity (Tyson and Felig 1971:956). The termination of use of another chemical contraceptive, Depo-Provera, can result in anovulatory amenorrhea for up to 2 years (*Intercom* 1978d:9, 1982:14; Woodall 1982:K1). And male pills, which are still experimental, can cause impotence and sterility (World Health Organization Task Force on Psychosexual Research in Family Planning, 1982).

The IUD has been linked to an increase in ectopic pregnancies, spontaneous abortions, and sterility-threatening pelvic infections. Such infections are three to nine times as likely to develop in women using an IUD as in sexually active women using another contraceptive method. One of these devices, the Dalkon Shield, is particularly hazardous. Under certain conditions, including pregnancy, its complex multifilamented tail contributes to the transmission of bacteria from the vagina into the uterus. This device was withdrawn from the market, but not before a score of deaths and hundreds of septic abortions had been attributed to its use (Tatum 1977:194).

Induced abortion can also have a negative effect on fecundity. Illegal or "back-street" induced abortion can lead to all the forms of subfecundity: coital inability (dyspareunia), sterility, and pregnancy loss. These consequences have been recognized as long as this ancient method of birth control has been practiced. With the ever-increasing number of abortions in countries where restrictive laws have been eased, it appears that even legal abortions carry some risk. Although pelvic infection and its sequelae—coital inability (dyspareunia) and sterility—are rare following legal induced abortion, a number of studies have suggested some increased risk of pregnancy loss. Cervical damage is believed to be one important cause of this pregnancy loss. Indeed, researchers now believe that the cervical dilatation method is more important than the uterine evacuation method in determining future fecundity following legal induced abortion.

In sum, subfecundity can affect fertility indirectly by acting through one of the other Davis–Blake intermediate variables. Conversely, these other intermediate variables may themselves cause subfecundity and thus also affect fertility. Not infrequently a reciprocal or circular relationship exists (Rozat 1980:418). For instance, subfecundity may lead to divorce and the inability to marry. This in turn drives some women to prostitution, which increases their own subfecundity and contributes to the dissemination of venereal disease and subsequent subfecundity in the population as a whole (Belsey 1978:1). Another example of circularity can be found in those societies in which a subfecund woman is forced to leave her husband and return to her village of origin. The style of life thrust upon a single, unmarriageable woman often involves poverty, malnutrition, unhygienic surroundings, and other negative health circumstances, increasing the likelihood that the subfecundity will continue and grow worse (Isely 1980:18). Population fertility and the role subfecundity plays in it cannot be fully understood unless the complex interrelationships among subfecundity, mate exposure, and birth control are sorted out and taken into consideration. However, this is rarely attempted and as a result the impact of subfecundity on population fertility is generally underestimated in the population literature.

Current Research Project

It has become increasingly apparent that subfecundity is a major determinant of fertility in developed, developing, and historical societies, and that it is important to understand its determinants (see Allman 1980:4, 8; Bongaarts 1976:227; Hesser *et al.* 1976:73; Menken 1979:10; Mosher 1982a:318). Population students, however, know very little about the fundamental causes of subfecundity (Easterlin *et al.* 1976:46; Hansluwka 1975:203; Menken 1979:9; Mosley 1979:1; World Health Organization 1975:6). Most research to date has focused more on the measurement of subfecundity than on its causes. For instance, advances have been made in understanding how subfecundity manifests itself in the elongation of birth intervals and their components (see Leridon 1977), but not much research has gone beyond this to identify the fundamental causes of subfecundity and to quantify their impact on fertility (Mosher 1982a:318). Thus one authority (Hansluwka 1975:205) concluded, ''the gaps in our knowledge are too large to permit the construction of a reasonably plausible model of the effects of health on fertility via fecundity.''

To improve this situation, a research project was undertaken to identify those factors capable of causing population subfecundity and to provide information with which population students can judge the quantitative impact of these subfecundity factors on individual fecundity and, ultimately, on population fecundity as well. These factors were divided into five categories: (1) psychopathology, (2) disease, (3) nutritional deficiencies, (4) environmental factors, and (5) genetic factors. The importance of these factors varies tremendously among populations and within populations by subgroup and by time, and this variation can cause substantial fertility differentials.

An overview of this research project and each of the five categories of subfecundity factors is available elsewhere (McFalls 1979a). More detailed findings on the factors in each of the five categories will be presented separately. A monograph (McFalls 1979b) on the importance of psychopathological factors—psychic stress, psychoses, sexual deviations, alcoholism, cigarette smoking, and illicit drug abuse—has already been completed. This volume deals with the principal diseases that cause population subfecundity.

CHAPTER 2

Disease and Subfecundity: An Introduction

"We are often inclined to view the salutary effects of health measures upon mortality to the exclusion of effects upon fertility," recently stated Lessa and Myers; "our evidence suggests the fallibility of such conclusions." Furthermore, while certain diseases tend to affect fertility and mortality comparably, it seems clear that certain diseases . . . principally affect fertility . . . and that others principally affect mortality. Unfortunately, however, systematic research in this field which would throw light on the quantitative or statistical relationships between different diseases and fecundity is still quite inadequate. . . . The findings of such research may be quite relevant for the undertaking of reliable demographic projections and the formulation of effective population policies.

[*Tabbarah (1971:268)*. From *Economic Development and Cultural Change*, published by *The University of Chicago.* © 1971 by The University of Chicago.]

Introduction

Disease is a ubiquitous variable in demography. It is closely related to each of the discipline's three core variables: migration, mortality, and fertility. Disease is often both a cause and a consequence of migration (Basch 1978:321–327; Roundy 1976: 103). Large numbers of people have been known to flee from disease-ridden areas, and others with diseases such as leprosy and filariasis have been forced to migrate because of their disease. For instance, the islanders of Addu Atoll believe filariasis to be contagious, and anyone showing permanent swellings is transferred to an island used especially for this purpose, where all the adults have elephantiasis. On the other hand, migrants spread diseases prevalent in their place of origin to populations in their place of destination

(Howe 1977:10). Indeed, refugee populations present important disease problems in many parts of the world. This is particularly true in the developing world, where refugees are numerous and diseases rampant. During the 1960s, for instance, about 1 million Africans were forced to take refuge in other countries (C. Smith 1972:3). And during the 1970s and early 1980s sizable numbers of persons from Southeast Asia and the Caribbean immigrated to the United States, bringing with them significant health problems that have the potential to spread throughout the U.S. population. Southeast Asians have brought with them high rates of hepatitis B and Haitians have been scrutinized as the possible source of the new and terrifying acquired immune deficiency syndrome (AIDS), which leaves its victims extremely susceptible to many diseases including cancer.[1]

Nevertheless, when population students think of disease, it is invariably in relation to mortality—largely because disease has always been and probably always will be its principal architect. Indeed, the history of mortality in advanced nations can be divided into three stages—the ages of pestilence and famine, of receding pandemics, and of degenerative and man-made diseases—based on the changing patterns of disease (Omran 1971). The developing world is currently undergoing the same epidemiological transition.

Disease is also an important determinant of fertility in many, if not all, societies; however, this relationship, like that involving migration, receives only a small share of the attention population students devote to disease. Nevertheless, disease can affect fertility in many ways—including mortality, which can remove individuals from the population before they have completed or even begun their reproductive careers (Bongaarts 1978:120; Gwatkin 1977:11). Widows in many populations

[1]The Haitians have been suspect because Kaposi's sarcoma, a rare skin cancer that is seen in some AIDS victims, is known to occur among Haitians. It is theorized that AIDS was introduced by Haitians into the homosexual community of Miami and subsequently spread to the homosexual communities of Los Angeles and New York. However, a 1983 study (Pape et al. 1983:943) conducted in Haiti states that AIDS probably did not exist there until 1978, the same year the first U.S. case was reported, suggesting that the disease could not have originated in that Caribbean country. It is now recognized that AIDS, like hepatitis B, is transmitted primarily via blood or its products, and the list of victims now includes drug addicts (from contaminated syringes) and hemophiliacs (from frequent blood transfusions). Indeed, the American Red Cross, alarmed by the news that AIDS is being transmitted by blood transfusions, has drawn up strict guidelines regarding transfusions. (Why homosexuals experience significantly higher rates of both AIDS and hepatitis B, both of which are believed to be transmitted by blood or blood products, is not known. It is theorized that anal intercourse is more traumatic than vaginal intercourse and that resulting tiny breaks in the mucous membrane might predispose to transmission.)

(Nag 1980:579; Tolnay 1980:257), for example, have fewer births than women living with a spouse. Disease can also influence fertility through migration. For example, persons moving to escape subfecundity-producing diseases often carry the disease with them, thereby lowering the fertility of the population at their point of destination.

In addition, disease can affect fertility through any of the Davis–Blake intermediate variables (see Table 1.8). Many of these relationships are obvious. Disease can delay or permanently deny entry into marriage and can bring about marital disruption through divorce, separation, desertion (Crain *et al.* 1971:247), or death of a spouse (Bongaarts 1978:120). Likewise, it can lead to voluntary abstinence to avoid transmitting an infection and to involuntary abstinence for reasons such as hospitalization. Disease may also increase the use of contraception to avoid infecting a spouse and/or fetus or to avoid childbearing while burdened by a debilitating illness. Sterilization may also be employed for this last reason. Furthermore, any chronic debilitating disease is likely to lessen or abolish sexual desire, resulting in lower coital frequency (Hansluwka 1975:206; Money 1967:270; Nag 1962:85; Procci *et al.* 1978:402).

Disease can affect fertility via another intermediate variable—induced abortion. This effect is becoming increasingly important as the number of countries that permit abortion grows. The identification of diseases harmful to the fetus and better detection of these diseases (Chedd 1981) together with readily available abortions have undoubtedly raised rates of fetal wastage. For example, pregnant women who contract German measles (rubella) face an increased risk of spontaneous abortion (Barrett-Connor 1969:277), but the induced abortions obtained by infected women who fear their offspring might be malformed by this virus account for far greater amounts of pregnancy wastage. Even inadvertent vaccination of pregnant women with the attenuated virus of German measles, though not conclusively known to cause malformations in the fetus, is a frequent cause of induced abortion. In one series 50% of vaccinated women sought abortions, yet not one of the continued pregnancies ended in congenital rubella (Kuhr 1973:1357). Similarly, pregnant women who have had cancer often unnecessarily choose induced abortion for fear of the effect of the disease or its treatment on the health of any future children (Blatt *et al.* 1980:828). But a study of 103 women 40 years of age or less who were treated for Hodgkin's disease with radiation, chemotherapy, or both found that of the 26 who tried to become pregnant, 20 were successful and all 20 delivered children without defects (*Philadelphia Inquirer* 1981:3D).

Finally, disease can affect the fertility of a population through the three subfecundity intermediate variables—coital inability, conceptive

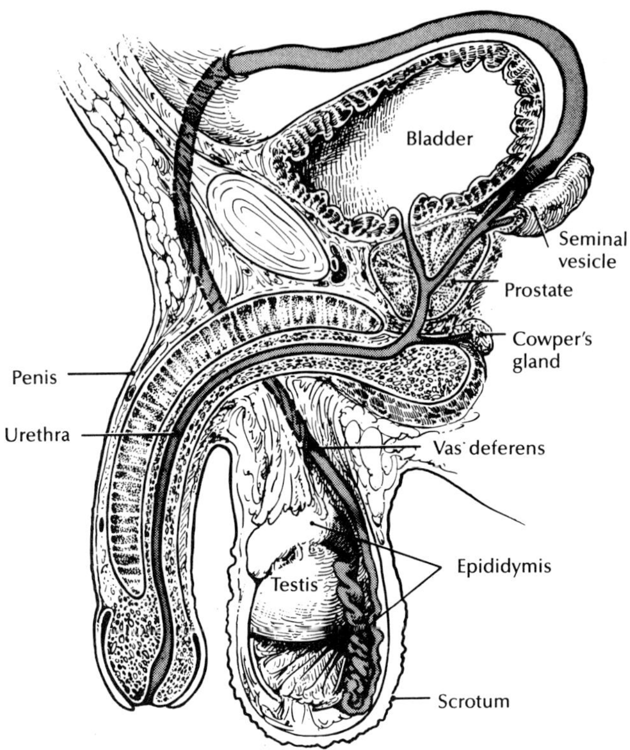

Figure 2.1 The male reproductive tract. From *Population Reports*, Series L, Number 4, Population Information Program, the Johns Hopkins University, Baltimore, Maryland 21205.

failure, and pregnancy loss. This relationship—the effect of disease on population fecundity—is the principal subject of this book. The male and female reproductive systems are shown in Figures 2.1 and 2.2, respectively, to help the reader visualize the structures that are discussed in this and subsequent chapters.

Effect on Individual Fecundity

The identification of diseases that adversely affect fecundity is an ongoing task of biomedical science. It has been generally known for centuries that such diseases exist. As early as 1702 Duttle realized that maternal smallpox could be transmitted to the fetus, resulting in pregnancy loss. However, it was discovered in only comparatively recent times that rubella causes pregnancy loss (Penrose 1971:112). Even today knowl-

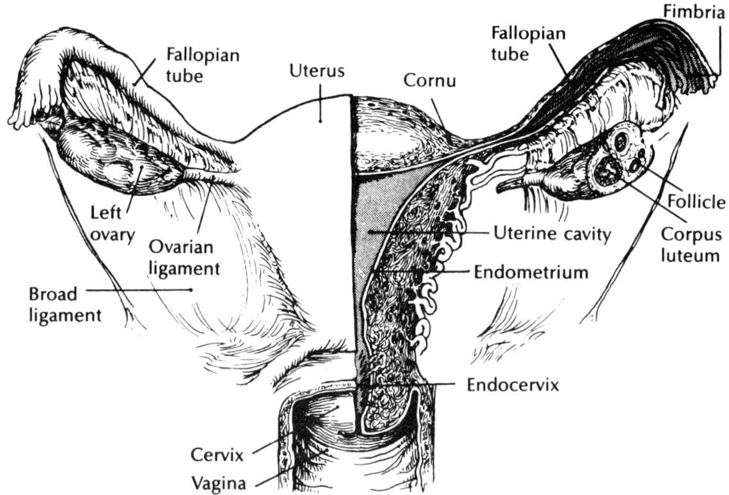

Figure 2.2 The female reproductive tract. From *Population Reports*, Series L, Number 4, Population Information Program, the Johns Hopkins University, Baltimore, Maryland 21205.

edge about the effect on fecundity of many diseases is incomplete (Bongaarts 1976:229; World Health Organization 1975:15). Nevertheless, it is clear that disease can have a pronounced effect on individual fecundity.

Coital Inability

The role of disease in coital inability is not disputed, although few data concerning specific diseases are available (Gebhard 1965:484). A review of the literature published before 1940 revealed an almost complete lack of professionally meaningful discussions of sexuality in relation to any illness (Sha'ked 1978:x), and although the pace of research has quickened since then there is still much to be learned. Disease causes coital inability in men through impotence (the inability to achieve and/ or maintain an erection sufficient to accomplish successful intercourse), dyspareunia (difficult or painful coitus), and genital deformities such as penile elephantiasis, and in women through dyspareunia and genital deformities such as vulval elephantiasis or a large schistosomal pseudotumor of the vulva.

In general, health is of primary importance in sexuality, and almost any disease can diminish sexual responsiveness and capacity (Gebhard 1965:484; Sha'ked 1978:x). Impotence may develop with any debilitating disease, metabolic disorder, central nervous system disease, or cardiovascular disorder (Cross 1973:1), and with certain forms of cancer such as prostate cancer (Katchadourian and Lunde 1980:192). Acute and chronic infections of any kind, even infected tonsils, can have an adverse effect on sexual functioning (Stone 1954:737). The prostatitis frequently seen in acute male genital tract infections such as gonorrhea is often accompanied by pain upon ejaculation, and chronic infections involving the upper genital tract of the female are extremely important causes of dyspareunia (Masters and Johnson 1970:284–285).

Specific diseases that impair coital ability include, for example, African sleeping sickness (African trypanosomiasis) and leprosy, which often lead to impotence in men. And male and female coital ability may be reduced by the painful blisters in the genital area that accompany recurrent attacks of genital herpes. Dyspareunia may also be an outcome of septic abortion and of female circumcision.

Conceptive Failure

Whereas chronic illness may lead to a variety of conceptive disorders such as anovulatory amenorrhea, the principal way disease causes conceptive failure is by interfering with the production of viable sperm by the male or eggs by the female, or with their proper transport. Any infection accompanied by high fever may temporarily halt spermatogenesis, and sperm production can be reduced or stopped completely by direct infection of the testes, as happens in a certain type of leprosy (Belsey 1976:331). A number of diseases such as gonorrhea can hinder the proper transport of sperm through the epididymis (sperm duct) of a male and of the egg through the fallopian tube of a female, because the resulting scarring can partially or completely block these tubes.

It is also worth noting that some diseases may affect the growth processes such that menarche is markedly delayed (Johnston 1974:165; Petersen 1975:193), and others can bring on early menopause.

Pregnancy Loss

Some of the same diseases that can damage the fallopian tubes and a woman's ability to conceive may also cause pregnancy loss. For example, if the fallopian tube remains open but the lining is distorted or the transport mechanism impaired, the egg may be fertilized but instead of being carried through the fallopian tube into the uterus it is trapped in the tube and implants there. Such pregnancies almost always end as spontaneous abortions or must be removed surgically. Thus gonorrheal inflammation, if treated before the fallopian tubes are completely blocked, can lead to a tubal pregnancy.

Pregnancy loss due to disease may also occur if the disease results in anemia, because severe anemia can result in spontaneous abortion and stillbirth (Lawson 1967d:66). Anemia is very common in persons infected by *Plasmodium falciparum* malaria, for instance. In addition, some diseases can precipitate pregnancy loss by affecting the unborn fetus. German measles (rubella) caught early in pregnancy can be transmitted to the fetus with disastrous results, including miscarriage. Toxoplasmosis, a parasitic disease acquired by close contact with infected cats or the consumption of undercooked meat containing toxoplasma cysts, is also generally thought to result in fetal infection and subsequent pregnancy loss only during a woman's initial infection. But some researchers feel that in some chronic infections the parasites form cysts in the uterus and thus many fetuses are infected and pregnancy loss occurs repeatedly (Belsey 1976:332). And in malaria, an intense infection of the placenta with the *P. falciparum* parasite can interfere with the flow of oxygen and nutrients to the fetus and pregnancy loss occurs.

Many diseases such as malaria, filariasis, and African sleeping sickness are associated with high fevers and this can be yet another cause of pregnancy loss. Also, obstetric complications occur in nearly every woman who has been circumcised and this, too, can cause pregnancy loss. Scar tissue resulting from the circumcision can leave the vagina so inelastic that passage of the baby is impossible. And frequently the tissue is so devitalized by the long and difficult labor that vulnerability to postpartum infection is increased.

Thus, individual fecundity is seriously affected by many diseases. This is a powerful threat for five reasons. First, many diseases such as pelvic inflammatory disease (PID) do not just reduce fecundity, they frequently obliterate it. Second, disease can exert a potent negative influence on reproduction anywhere from coitus to childbirth. It is a major cause of each of the principal components of subfecundity (coital inability, conceptive failure, and pregnancy loss). Some diseases like diabetes affect all three. Third, disease can reduce or destroy the reproductive ability of both men and women. Fourth, many diseases such as malaria occur early in life and persist for much, and sometimes all, of the reproductive period. Thus, subsequent subfecundity may also be prolonged. Fifth, many diseases such as genital herpes are incurable, which means their impact on fecundity cannot be eliminated. And with other diseases such as genital tuberculosis, although the pathogen can be eliminated and the patient cured tubal damage cannot be reversed and permanent sterility is usual. Still others, like hypertension or kidney disease, can be kept in check, but the treatment itself causes subfecundity (Levy 1978:591). For these reasons, disease is clearly an important cause of individual subfecundity.

Prevalence

Historical Societies

Subfecundity-producing diseases were prevalent in many past societies, at least as far back as the beginning of recorded history and undoubtedly beyond (Brothwell and Sandison 1967). A partial list of these diseases includes present-day ones like African sleeping sickness, malaria, schistosomiasis, tuberculosis, and leprosy, as well as endocrine diseases and some now-extinct diseases like smallpox.

Developing Societies

Disease is highly prevalent throughout the world. Diseases that cause subfecundity affect millions and probably even billions of people. Many of the diseases considered to pose the greatest threat to public health and survival, such as tuberculosis, malaria, and syphilis, are also causes of subfecundity. Their prevalence is high and remains so because of inadequate health care and a variety of behavioral phenomena (e.g., reluctance to seek treatment).

Subfecundity-producing diseases are especially prevalent in the developing world where they are also frequently a country's number-one health problem (Baird 1979:193; C. Smith 1972:3). They are particularly widespread in Africa south of the Sahara and in other developing areas where there is, not surprisingly, a high prevalence of subfecundity and childlessness. Diseases common in Nigeria, for instance, include malaria, dysentery, measles, gonorrhea, pneumonia, chicken-pox, whooping cough, schistosomiasis, filariasis, tuberculosis, and syphilis (Ajaegbu and Mann 1972:125), almost all of which can cause subfecundity. Subfecundity-producing diseases can be prevalent in both rural and urban areas. The staggering lack of medical care in both areas guarantees that there are tremendous numbers of individuals with largely curable or preventable subfecundity-producing diseases (C. Smith 1972:4).

Developed Societies

Subfecundity-producing diseases are not nearly as prevalent in developed societies as they are in developing ones. But some, like the sexually transmitted diseases, are still very prevalent. Indeed, 10–15 million people in the United States contract some form of sexually transmitted disease every year. Over 75% of these cases occur in 15- to 30-year-olds, with 15- to 24-year-olds accounting for the majority (Nass *et al.* 1981:474). Thus, subfecundity-producing diseases are commonplace in the prime reproductive age groups. These diseases are also disproportionately prevalent in some population subgroups, particularly the poor.

Other subfecundity-producing diseases such as malaria, tuberculosis, and filariasis may be prevalent in local populations, especially those with many immigrants and refugees (Barrett-Connor 1978:1901). These diseases have been increasing recently due to changes in the traditional pattern of immigration. The 1965 federal immigration law allowed people from developing countries where these diseases are rampant to enter the United States in increased numbers. Refugees from Southeast Asia and Cuba also helped create sizable pockets of these diseases. There are now, for instance, 4200 reported cases of leprosy in the United States, most of which are concentrated in pockets in California, Hawaii, Texas, and New York. There was a 500% increase in new cases from 1960 to 1980.

Future Societies

The future prevalence of subfecundity-producing diseases is uncertain. Through vaccination and other public health measures smallpox and some other diseases were successfully eliminated, and public health officials have now begun programs to eliminate such diseases as measles and tuberculosis through the immunization of every child. Some advanced nations are well on their way to achieving these goals. The United States, for instance, may have eradicated measles as a native disease by the mid-1980s. Moreover, research continues on vaccines for stubborn tropical diseases. Such vaccines could profoundly affect the lives of millions of people. In the coming decades many developing countries will undoubtedly continue their struggle against infectious diseases, often giving them first priority.

In 1977 the United Nations, the World Bank, and the World Health Organization (WHO) set up a joint program for research and training in tropical diseases. They focused on seven diseases: malaria, schistosomiasis, filariasis, African sleeping sickness, Chagas' disease, leprosy, and leishmaniasis. A report (World Health Organization, World Bank, and United Nations 1982:8) on the program's first 5 years noted there are good grounds for optimism that research can develop new tools to improve disease control. It pointed to the remarkable advances in fundamental biomedical sciences in areas such as genetic engineering, hybridoma technology, and technical methodology; of course, these advances had yet to be exploited in the field of tropical disease control.

In any event, there is reason to hope that the prevalence of subfecundity-producing diseases will decline in the future; but such optimism must be closely guarded. The joint program report (World Health Organization, World Bank, and United Nations 1982:5) noted that the degree of damage to health caused by the major tropical diseases had actually changed little since 1977 and that the situation remained a major challenge to health authorities in many tropical countries. Indeed, some experts believe that mankind may now be actually losing the battle against many of these diseases (Agarwal 1980:5; Schmeck 1978:18E). Malaria, for example, seemed almost vanquished during the 1950s, but since then mosquitoes have become resistant to pesticides, the malarial parasite has learned to cope with some of the widely used drugs, and the prevalence of malaria has rebounded. The experience of India is a grim example. Prevalence went from 75 million cases in 1947 to only about 60,000 in 1962 when a nationwide control program was at peak effectiveness. However, by the mid-1970s the prevalence had climbed to more than 4 million cases as the dollar cost of eradication soared and the disease became more resistant to public health measures. The experience of India is not exceptional; in many other countries there was a 30- to 40-fold increase in malaria cases in the 1970s (Agarwal 1980:5). Schistosomiasis is another subfecundity producer that is increasing in prevalence in many areas (Schmeck 1978:18E). It increased in the Sudan and Egypt after the Aswan High Dam was built, and in Ghana, Nigeria, and the Gezira region of the Sudan after other water and irrigation projects were constructed. Filariasis, yet another parasitic disease, may also increase in the future because there are signs that the insect that carries this dreaded disease is becoming resistant to insecticides (Agarwal 1980:5).

The prevalence of bacterial diseases may also increase in the future because available antibiotics are becoming less and less successful in treating them. And as new antibiotics come into use (and abuse), nature simply responds once again by producing more resistant bacteria. For instance, both tetracycline and penicillin, once completely effective against gonorrhea, now have more than a 20% failure rate against certain strains. It is conceivable that in the future 80–90% of infections will be resistant to all known antibiotics.

Another alarming trend is the resurgence of sexually transmitted diseases in the developed world, a trend that is almost certain to continue (Holmes and Puziss 1980:640), and the expansion of these diseases into populations where they were almost unknown before (Jacobs 1978:10).

In broader terms, the future prevalence of subfecundity-producing diseases is dependent to a large degree on trends in such areas as population, economic development, energy use and development, and agricultural productivity. If the worst scenarios of *The Global 2000 Report* (Council on Environmental Quality and the United States Department of State 1981) and similar forecasts come true, then these diseases and a host of other subfecundity factors will be more prevalent in the future than they are now. These scenarios envision great masses of people living at subsistence levels in sprawling urban ghettos with few public services or resources—in short, natural breeding grounds for disease with little or no health care available.

One other factor is worth considering. Though entirely new diseases are rare (C. Smith 1972:6), they do occur. Legionnaires' disease serves as a reminder of this. It is also possible that some new subfecundity-producing infectious disease may evolve (or be created through genetic engineering) just as venereal syphilis did—appearing very suddenly in the late 1400s in Europe. The acquired immune deficiency syndrome (AIDS), which has baffled physicians and experts at the U.S. Centers for Disease Control, is a frightening example of what can happen in the future. This new disease makes the individual much more susceptible to other diseases like genital herpes or cytomegalovirus and makes these secondary problems very difficult to cure. As of 1983, AIDS had a survival rate after 2 years of less than 20%, far exceeding the rate smallpox had before a vaccine was discovered.

In sum, diseases that cause subfecundity were prevalent in many historical societies and are widespread in present-day developing and developed societies. They will undoubtedly also continue to plague future societies.

Importance of Disease as a Cause of Population Subfecundity

Disease is a multipotent cause of individual subfecundity, and is highly prevalent in many societies. It is therefore an extremely important cause of population subfecundity. Indeed, of the subfecundity project's five categories—psychopathology, disease, nutritional deficiencies, environmental factors, and genetic factors—it has by far the most devastating impact on population fecundity. Disease has the potential literally to wipe out populations through subfecundity as well as through mortality. Indeed, in those societies where subfecundity has led or contributed to depopulation or to extraordinary levels of childlessness and low fertility, disease is invariably the paramount cause.

Despite the fact that it is the pre-eminent cause of subfecundity, disease has received relatively little attention in the population literature. Population students have spent far more time studying the effects of nutritional deficiencies on fecundity than those of disease. Malnutrition has been the primary interest because it is exceedingly prevalent and can have a negative effect on individual fecundity. However, the balance of research indicates that the impact of malnutrition on individual fecundity is not nearly so great as previously suspected (Bongaarts 1980; Marcy 1981; McFalls 1979a; Menken *et al.* 1981; Mosley 1978; Nag 1980). Thus, its stature as a major cause of population subfecundity has appreciably eroded, leaving disease more clearly than ever the most important subfecundity cause. Indeed, malnutrition's greatest impact on fecundity is probably its tendency to increase susceptibility to subfecundity-causing diseases and to increase the seriousness of these diseases (Ajaegbu and Mann 1972: 127; P. Lee 1977: 295; McKeown 1976: 134; Pollard 1979:65; World Health Organization 1966). However, researchers (Eaton *et al.* 1976:758) have noted at least one fascinating exception to this rule. It is now believed that a deficiency of vitamin E can actually protect against *P. falciparum* malaria by increasing cell membrane fragility and thereby increasing the likelihood that a malaria-infected red blood cell will burst prematurely, causing the release of immature parasites incapable of propagating the infection. It has been observed in some areas of endemic malaria that malnourished herding people whose diet is normally low in vitamin E are relatively resistant to severe malaria. Feeding these people with cereal grains, a rich source of vitamin E, causes a recrudescence of previously undetected malaria infections.

Because subfecundity-producing diseases have been prevalent for thousands of years, they undoubtedly have had a significant impact on the fecundity of numerous historical societies. However, it is difficult to gauge the importance of this relationship because few studies have addressed it. One disease that may have had an important impact is tuberculosis. Smallpox may have also considerably reduced the fecundity and fertility of historical populations, as Razzell (1977:vi) felt it did in Britain before 1850. One study (Hotelling and Hotelling 1931) of English birthrate fluctuations from 1838 to 1914 concluded that much of the variance can be explained by epidemics of smallpox, influenza, cholera, and dysentery, which increased pregnancy loss and thereby reduced births

7–9 months later. Leridon (1973) also found that influenza had a strong negative impact on fertility 9 months later, adding support to the hypothesis that this disease may have been an important natality force in past societies.

Diseases that cause subfecundity are important fecundity depressants in developing countries where they are widespread and, in some areas, actually increasing. Rampant untreated disease is the most important reason for the subfecundity that afflicts such developing societies as the band of central African countries with unexpectedly low fertility and high childlessness (Caldwell 1981:109; *Population Reports* 1979a:135). Disease is also an important cause of subfecundity in some South Pacific and Caribbean societies (Gwatkin 1977:7). In parts of the developing world sudden declines in the prevalence of subfecundity-producing diseases have been accompanied by a rise in fertility. This also happened in Europe during the nineteenth century (Tabah 1977:7; Taylor *et al.* 1958:115).

Disease is also an important cause of subfecundity in developed societies such as the United States. Although there are few major subfecundity producers prevalent there, the ones that do exist are among the most powerful. These, of course, are the sexually transmitted diseases (STDs), many of which are epidemic in the United States. One investigator (Curran 1980:848) estimated that if trends in STDs and PID persist in the United States, by the year 2000 11% of women in the 1955 birth cohort will be involuntarily sterile and 3% will have experienced an ectopic pregnancy as a result of these diseases alone.

Thus, population fecundity is seriously threatened by many diseases in both the developing and developed worlds. This was also true in the past and will continue to be true in the future. The extent of such diseases varies greatly among populations so the amount of subfecundity attributable to them is also a population variable.

In evaluating the impact of subfecundity-producing diseases on fertility, it is important to recognize that some of these diseases are among those that can depress fertility in the other ways outlined in the beginning of this chapter. For instance, many can also affect fertility through mortality. Some, like varicella (chicken pox) and influenza, can cause not only fetal but also maternal mortality. One reason for this is that these diseases are more severe in pregnant women than in the remainder of the population. Influenzal pneumonia was significantly associated with pregnancy in the 1918 pandemic and again in the 1957 Asian A epidemic. In the latter outbreak, pregnant women made up almost 50% of childbearing-age women who died from influenza in New York City and Minnesota (Barrett-Connor 1969:275). Other subfecundity-producing diseases like gonorrhea can cause maternal mortality via ectopic pregnancy.

In addition, some subfecundity-producing diseases are among those that affect fertility through the other intermediate variables. Diabetes is a prime example. Besides causing coital inability, conceptive failure, and pregnancy loss (and incidentally mortality), diabetes traditionally led to voluntary childlessness or low fertility in pre-insulin days (before 1921) because of the risk pregnancy posed to the mother's life—maternal mortality approached 50%. In the past physicians strongly advised diabetic women not to get pregnant, and as a result sterilization, contraception, voluntary abstinence, and induced abortion were used to a greater extent than in the population at large (McKay 1981:B4). With the introduction of insulin maternal mortality abruptly fell to 2%. Nevertheless, many diabetic women still avoided pregnancy because of persisting high perinatal mortality rates. As late as the 1950s 25% of children of diabetic women died in the perinatal period. Not until the 1960s could diabetic women be encouraged about their prospects of having a live healthy infant. At this time full medical supervision of the diabetic pregnancy using the high-risk monitoring system discussed in Chapter 1 became available, and perinatal mortality dropped precipitiously to 5%. However, in many parts of the world insulin and these monitoring systems are unavailable, and diabetes continues to exert its effects on fecundity and fertility (see Appendix A).

In sum, disease is the most important cause of population subfecundity and therefore is an important determinant of fertility. Moreover, many of those diseases that cause subfecundity are also among those that depress fertility through mortality and nonsubfecundity intermediate variables, thus giving them a multiple negative impact on fertility. This impact was undoubtedly felt in many historical societies and continues to be experienced today in developing and developed nations. The same will be true in the foreseeable future.

Handling of Disease
in the Population Literature

Research specifying the relationship between disease and population fecundity and the fertility of current and historical societies is scarce and often defective (Hansluwka 1975:203; Knodel and Wilson 1981:53; Tabbarah 1971:268; Weisbrod *et al.* 1973:17). Much of the available materials are articles simply listing diseases thought to have the potential to depress population fecundity (e.g., Hansluwka 1975; Taylor *et al.* 1976) and sources devoting several paragraphs to a very generalized discussion of the impact of such diseases on fecundity (e.g., World Health Organization 1975, 1976). Few studies discuss the impact of a particular disease on the fecundity and fertility of a specific population, and many of the discussions that do exist can be characterized in one of three ways.

First, the possibility is raised that a disease is the cause of a population's low fertility, but is quickly dismissed without evidence being brought to bear. Blake (1961:13), for instance, in trying to answer the question of why the Jamaican birthrate was so modest for such a poor agrarian country, noted that "the answer is sometimes sought in sterility and spontaneous abortion on the grounds that Jamaican women are especially subject to fibroid tumors and that venereal disease is prevalent on the island." However, she quickly discounted venereal disease (VD) by stating that "proof is hard to find" and cited Roberts (1957:207–215) as the source for this appraisal. However, Roberts primarily discussed the relationship between the control of syphilis and mortality; his research was not designed to address the issue of whether VD was an important determinant of the fertility level. It is also noteworthy that Roberts was discussing only syphilis, not all venereal diseases. Gonorrhea may have been important even if syphilis was not.

The second way the relationship between subfecundity and disease is treated is speculative in nature. Hypotheses are advanced that are incidental, casual, and conjectural and these are followed by little, if any, discussion (Nag 1980:573). It is clear in such instances that the authors are interested only in covering all possibilities and have no intention of rigorously exploring the hypothesis. This is the most common form the discussion of disease takes in the literature. An example of this treatment is a study by Allman and May (1979:510), which simply mentions filariasis and gonorrhea and other venereal diseases as possible contributors to the surprisingly moderate birthrate in Haiti.

The final form taken by discussions concerning disease and subfecundity is that of the residual hypothesis. These hypotheses are interjected into the discussion when other research hypotheses are tested and found wanting. An example of such treatment is the VD hypothesis (see subsequent discussion) used by many authors to explain the trend in U.S. black fertility from 1880 to 1960.

There are a few medically oriented studies that go beyond these approaches in attempts to specify the relationship between diseases and the fertility of particular populations. Most of these studies concern populations in Africa (e.g., Ampofo 1977; Arya and Taber 1974; Correa 1969; Griffith 1963; Lwanga 1977; Meuwissen 1966; Retel-Laurentin 1972, 1978) and the South Pacific (e.g., Scragg 1957; Lessa 1955; Lambert 1934). Though these studies provide valuable evidence and insight into the relationship between diseases and fertility, they often contain a variety of methodological problems: considerable selectional bias in their study groups, absence of controls, and small samples (Isely 1980:17). The medical techniques used and their interpretation have also been frequently criticized (Adadevoh 1974:15).

Another problem with this body of literature is its overemphasis on VD at the expense of other diseases and of psychopathological, nutritional, genetic, and environmental factors as well (Adadevoh 1974:16; Belsey 1978:9; Caldwell 1981:109). This is a problem that runs through all of the population literature. When widespread subfecundity is evident in a society population students think first, and usually only, of VD. Thus, it is not coincidental that most of the studies used as examples in this chapter, with the notable exception of that by Weisbrod *et al.* (1973), all deal with VD as a possible fertility depressant. What is happening is that much subfecundity caused by other diseases is ascribed to VD. For instance, in those areas where both tuberculous and gonococcal infections are common the difficulty in resolving the precise origin of tubal disease serves to underestimate the importance of genital tuberculosis (TB), because the tendency is to assign the tubal pathology in such areas to the more familiar gonococcal salpingitis (Charlewood 1956:37; Middlemiss 1972:255).

There is no doubt that the venereal diseases are the most important subfecundity-producing diseases. In fact, gonorrhea may be the single most powerful cause of population subfecundity. But there are other important causes. Belsey (1978:9) underscored this fact in the following passage:

> The high levels of infertility in certain areas of Africa remain an enigma to research. . . . Two well recognized processes may well contribute in some areas to part of the problem: the consequences of postpartum and postabortal sepsis affecting the woman, and the consequences of sexually transmitted diseases affecting either the man or the woman. But neither of these two phenomena appear capable of completely explaining the problem as seen in many African countries. There are many countries and regions both within and outside Africa where high levels of sexually transmitted diseases are found or where inadequate obstetric care is common. Yet infertility is not of a magnitude to affect 20%, 30%, or even 40% of couples in these areas.

Just how important VD is relative to other subfecundity causes is uncertain. It is worth noting that some estimates attribute about one-third of the total subfecundity in central African countries to VD (Gwatkin 1977:7), although these estimates could be wide of the mark.

The use of involuntary childlessness as a proxy measure for subfecundity is another common problem besetting the population literature on disease and fertility. Involuntary childlessness is a poor proxy for subfecundity: The effect of subfecundity on population fertility is not limited to producing childlessness, because it can cause other individuals to have fewer children than they would have had otherwise. Some diseases like gonorrhea are major causes of both childlessness and low fertility. A study that uses childlessness as a proxy for subfecundity would therefore underestimate the true impact of gonorrhea on the population's fertility. Other problems like postpartum infections produce infecundity after childbearing has occurred. The effect of these infections on a population's fertility are missed altogether when childlessness is used as an indicator of subfecundity. Finally, there are some diseases like syphilis that depress fecundity without completely eliminating the ability to bear children. The effect of these diseases is also omitted when childlessness is the proxy.

Consequences of Deficient Research

The past lack of rigorous research into disease as a cause of subfecundity has led to two important research problems. First, it is not known what diseases are actually capable of materially affecting population fecundity. Researchers are often unable to specify causality even when they are sure a disease is an important fertility determinant. For example, in trying to establish the causes for the unusually low fertility of the Afro–Arab population of the city of Zanzibar, Blacker (1962:265) was almost certain that subfecundity played a major role but was unable to specify the cause of the subfecundity. Venereal disease and malaria, two of only a handful of diseases capable of impairing fecundity commonly known to population students, were not sufficiently prevalent to be major determinants. Blacker was apparently at a loss to suggest and investigate any other disease or cause of subfecundity, his analysis was truncated, and the causes of the subfecundity in Zanzibar remain obscure. Similarly, in an interesting study of Alaska Native fertility trends between 1950 and 1978 Blackwood (1981:177) concluded that a reduction of subfecundity accounted in part for the increase in fertility during the 1950s and early 1960s. But Blackwood failed even to speculate about what subfecundity-producing diseases or other subfecundity causes were involved, perhaps because it is not generally known in population studies what the potential factors might be. Thus, there is a clear need to identify the important diseases that cause population subfecundity to aid hypothesis formation. As Hawthorn (1970:11) aptly stated, "Until we know the biological factors contributing to [subfecundity] we shall not be able to interpret properly the checked performance that we in fact observe almost everywhere, and in particular, we shall not be able to disentangle these [subfecundity] factors from social ones." Identification of diseases that cause subfecundity will also eliminate the previously discussed preoccupation of most population students with venereal diseases.

The second research problem stemming from the past lack of research is that little or nothing is known concerning even the approximate quantitative relationship between disease and subfecundity (Hansluwka 1975:206). Thus, even in studies where a disease has been identified and is known to be important, it is usually impossible for researchers to estimate its absolute importance or its significance relative to other factors (Isely 1980:17). Lessa and Myers (1962:250), for example, in a study of the 1904–1949 fertility decline in Ulithi (Micronesia), reached the conclusion that it was due to widespread gonorrhea. However, their conclusion would have been more satisfying if they had estimated the impact of the disease on individual fertility and, together with prevalence data and other information, related these findings to the fertility trend. Without such quantitative estimates, it is easy to misinterpret the causal strength of such factors. Perhaps gonorrhea was only half as powerful as Lessa and Myers believed, and other factors escaped unnoticed because the effect of gonorrhea was overstated. Without quantification there is no certain way to check the validity of conclusions.

A good illustration of why it is necessary to estimate the quantitative impact of disease on fertility is the VD hypothesis that has been used to explain the U.S. black fertility trend from 1880 to 1960. Essentially this hypothesis stipulates that the prevalence of VD increased among blacks from 1880 to 1936, thereby severely reducing their fecundity and subsequent fertility. In addition, the hypothesis attributes the subsequent black natality rise to a fall in VD prevalence, which resulted from the discovery of superior treatment methods and their simultaneous application to large numbers of people through the creation of government VD control programs. This hypothesis was first introduced in a speculative fashion with no accompanying attempts at validation (Grabill *et al.* 1958:217; Thompson and Whelpton 1933:284). Then Farley (1970), having investigated other explanations and found them wanting, advanced it as a residual hypothesis.

Both in its speculative and residual forms, the VD hypothesis suggests that venereal disease was the principal architect of the black fertility trend. However, no adequate attempt was made to measure the quantitative impact of these diseases on fecundity and to relate such information to the fertility trend. Once this effort was made (McFalls 1973), it became clear that VD was actually a minor though probably still-significant determinant of the fertility trend. This quantification process not only placed the role of VD in its proper perspective, but also drew attention to the fact that a new explanation for the black fertility trend was required (see also Chapter 19).

If researchers are to be able to identify diseases and to quantify their impact on population fecundity and fertility, they must study potentially important diseases in depth, determining whether and to what extent they can cause coital inability, conceptive failure, and/or pregnancy loss.[2] Such determinations, which should be made for men as well as for women, require an understanding of diseases that can only be gained from intensive research into the medical literature or consultation with appropriate health specialists. Failure to proceed in this manner often leads to disappointing results.

One study that did not proceed in this manner was that of Weisbrod and associates (1973), which investigated the relationship between schistosomiasis and fertility, as well as other variables, on the island of Saint Lucia where *Schistosoma mansoni* is prevalent. This study was prompted by the widely accepted notion that schistosomiasis causes mass chronic invalidism. The research hypothesis was that the purported physical and mental defects associated with the disease would have a quantifiable negative effect on natality as well as on mortality, academic performance, and numerous economic variables. Before conducting the study the authors checked the literature to verify the a priori sensibility of their research hypothesis—that schistosomiasis affects demographic and social variables through chronic ill health. But they

---

[2]Though neonatal mortality is not a component of subfecundity, it should also be investigated in studies of subfecundity-producing diseases for several reasons. First, because some research focuses on perinatal mortality it may be impossible to separate neonatal from late fetal mortality. Second, information about neonatal mortality is often better than that on late fetal mortality. Because deaths that occur before and those that occur after delivery can often be ascribed to the same etiology (Babson and Benson 1971:10), knowledge that a disease causes neonatal mortality is sometimes also useful in inferring a probable impact on pregnancy loss. Finally, population students investigating the causes of the unexpectedly low fertility observed in some societies may jump to the conclusion that the fertility deficit is entirely due to subfecundity if a disease known to cause subfecundity is prevalent. Any neonatal mortality caused by such a disease might be overlooked because underreporting of deaths among very young children is common. Thus some information on neonatal mortality would help population students avoid this error of possibly overestimating the subfecundity effects of disease (Shapiro *et al.* 1968:42).

found little supporting evidence, and argued that there had been "extremely little careful research on these matters" (Weisbrod *et al.* 1973:11). Thus, they had to underpin their research hypothesis with remarks made almost 25 years earlier about schistosomiasis causing mental retardation and being the possible cause of the physical defects observed in Egyptian army recruits.

In their initial discussion of the effects of schistosomiasis on natality, the authors gave three reasons for expecting a negative impact: They felt that a deteriorating general health in severe cases would increase conceptive failure and pregnancy loss, that parasites would irritate the biological system and divert essential nutrients away from childbearing, and that in persons of ill health the probability of marrying and the frequency of intercourse would be reduced. But their data did not show the anticipated negative relationship between schistosomiasis and fertility and, in fact, showed a slightly positive one. In order to square this unexpected finding with the study hypothesis they then contended that chronic invalidism could indeed lead to higher natality rates. They reasoned that schistosomiasis might actually increase coital frequency rather than lowering it as they previously thought, because coitus might become one of the few sources of gratification in the otherwise limited existence of persons weakened by these parasites (Weisbrod *et al.* 1973:65). But all this is just speculation and not grounded in a scientific understanding of the disease and its consequences.

Further research failed to show any negative effect of schistosomiasis on mortality, academic performance, or economic variables (Weisbrod *et al.* 1973:81). The question was then raised whether schistosomiasis was severe enough in Saint Lucia, but the researchers were advised that the island was a representative area of modern severity (Weisbrod *et al.* 1973:84). They finally concluded that schistosomiasis, even when moderately severe, has only a modest effect on physical and mental health (Weisbrod *et al.* 1973:89). In sum, the data did not support their original hypothesis—that schistosomiasis would, because of assumed deleterious effects on health, adversely affect demographic and social variables. Thus, the researchers in the Saint Lucia study were incorrect when they initially identified schistosomiasis, specifically *S. mansoni,* as a cause of physical and mental illness grave enough to be reflected in demographic and social variables (see Chapter 6).

On the other hand, Farley (1970: 222–226) did not accurately quantify the impact of a correctly identified subfecundity factor, VD, which he advanced as the major factor in the 1880–1936 U.S. black fertility decline. Unlike other proponents of the VD hypothesis, Farley, at least with respect to syphilis, did attempt to go beyond the fact that syphilis causes subfecundity via pregnancy loss to an understanding of just how much subfecundity it could produce. Unfortunately, his conclusions were based on data from early sources, which estimated that "a syphilitic woman, untreated, has only one chance in six of bearing a live healthy infant" (Moore 1941:474, as cited in Farley 1970:222). However, more recent sources whose data are based on a more scientific understanding of the pathological changes associated with each stage of syphilitic disease limit fetal infection, even in untreated women, to the 2 years following initial infection (early syphilis) (Kissane and Smith 1967:58).[3] Such findings substantially reduce the estimate of impact of syphilis on population fecundity and seriously challenge the VD hypothesis.

In sum, there is a clear need for research to identify those diseases capable of causing population subfecundity and help determine the quantitative impact of such diseases on population fecundity. Such research requires an in-depth study of each disease.

Objectives and Methodology

This book is an in-depth study of the effects of disease on population fecundity and fertility. Its first major objective is to identify diseases that can cause population subfecundity. Such diseases must not only be capable of depressing individual fecundity but also must be sufficiently prevalent to merit consideration on the population level. This identification process is not as elementary as it may appear. Indeed, there is disagreement whether even major public health threats such as malaria have this potential.

The book's second major objective is to provide information with which population students can judge the quantitative impact of selected diseases on fecundity and fertility. Such information would aid researchers to test quickly and accurately their hypotheses concerning the importance of a particular disease as a determinant of a specific population's fertility. If, for example, proponents of the VD hypothesis had had access to this kind of population-related discussion of syphilis and gonorrhea, their research time would have been shortened and faulty conclusions based on misinformation may have been avoided. Or if Weisbrod and associates (1973) had had access to this kind of discus-

---

[3]Some more recent material may also be misleading. For instance, Brown *et al.* (1970:26, 27) noted that syphilis causes abortions and stillbirths but failed to mention that such outcomes are limited to early syphilis.

sion of schistosomiasis, they would have known before conducting their study that the disease was not a grave cause of physical and mental illness and they might well have changed the focus of their study. Moreover, such information, together with prevalence data or estimates, would provide policymakers with a ready resource to help formulate and evaluate development policies in areas where subfecundity-producing diseases are prevalent. Without such information control of disease might lead to unanticipated increases in fertility, with adverse effects on socioeconomic development. In sum, this monograph is designed to help population students identify diseases that cause subfecundity and estimate their quantitative impact on population fecundity.

It is not possible to cover in depth all diseases that cause population subfecundity. This book concentrates only on the most important ones; these are divided into three groups. The first group includes the nonsexually transmitted diseases: tuberculosis, malaria, filariasis, schistosomiasis, African sleeping sickness, and Chagas' disease. The second group is composed of the sexually transmitted diseases: syphilis, gonorrhea, nongonococcal cervicitis and urethritis, genital herpes, mycoplasma, and chlamydia. The third group comprises, rather than actual diseases, phenomena that can result in PID and other adverse reproductive sequelae. These include childbirth, induced abortion, the intrauterine device, and female circumcision. Three other diseases—diabetes, sickle-cell hemoglobin, and smallpox—could not be covered in the body of the text, but because they are demographically interesting they are discussed briefly in Appendixes A, B, and C, respectively.

Although some of the diseases covered in this book were prevalent in historical societies and are common in current developed countries, they have had their greatest impact on the fecundity and fertility of developing societies, particularly those in Africa. Thus this book can contribute to an understanding of fertility levels and trends in developed, developing, and historical populations, but it is most pertinent to developing nations where these diseases are most influential and very often the direct or indirect target of population and development policies.

The reader should not infer that these are the only diseases that can significantly affect the fecundity and fertility of populations. There are others that can be very important at the regional level, though they do not usually have global or even national significance. Still others that are not normally major causes of subfecundity can periodically strike with ferocity. For instance, epidemics of influenza and measles in the Cocos Islands had a sizable though temporary effect on the birthrate there (Smith 1960:116). The influenza epidemic struck in August 1929. In the months of March, April, and May 1930—9 months after the epidemic—only 4 births out of a normal yearly total of 62 births occurred. Similarly, a measles epidemic began in March 1945 and in October, November, and December 1945 and January and February 1946—again about 9 months after the epidemic—only 7 births occurred, one-fifth the expected number. These were just two of many epidemics that struck the Cocos Islanders, a population particularly susceptible to contagious diseases brought by ships (Smith 1960:99).

To accomplish this study's objectives, potentially important diseases were studied in depth. Determinations were made as to whether and to what extent they can cause coital inability, conceptive failure, and/or pregnancy loss. Attention was devoted to the mechanisms through which such effects occur. In addition, other aspects of the disease were investigated that have a great bearing on its impact on fecundity and fertility. Questions that were asked include, for instance, (1) does the disease have different stages, (2) how does the effect on fecundity differ among stages, (3) does it affect the fecundity of both men and women, (4) does the effect on fecundity invariably occur or is it a feature of a particular complication, (5) do reinfections occur, (6) can immunity develop, (7) is there the possibility of spontaneous cure, (8) what is the nature and effectiveness of treatment, (9) does a treatment or diagnostic method associated with the disease itself cause subfecundity,[4] and (10) does the disease substantially influence fertility through intermediate variables other than subfecundity? Prevalence data were also investigated to find out if the disease is prevalent enough to be of interest on the demographic level.

Ironically, many of the very diseases that have the most significant impact on population fecundity are the ones about which least is known (Hansluwka 1975:193; World Health Organization 1980:210). It must be recognized that most research on disease is carried out in developed nations and it centers on diseases that affect them. Diseases such as schistosomiasis that are rare in developed nations receive very little attention, and research on diseases such as TB that have been almost eradicated in developed nations but are still widespread in developing

---

[4]The treatment of many diseases is associated with side effects that can cause subfecundity. Drugs such as quinine (malaria), diethylcarbamazine (filariasis), and pentamidine (African sleeping sickness) can cause pregnancy loss, and others such as niridazole (schistosomiasis) can depress sperm counts. And surgical repair of a hydrocele (filariasis) may be followed by testicular atrophy. On the other hand, some treatments may actually increase fecundity in unexpected ways. A report in the *British Medical Journal* (see Shearer 1980b:14) suggested that the antibiotic tetracycline, commonly used to treat gonorrhea and other bacterial infections, may neutralize the contraceptive effects of the low-dose estrogen pills, permitting conception to occur.

nations has come to a virtual halt. Little research was carried out on filariasis until U.S. soldiers were exposed to it during World War II. In all, only about 1% of the money spent on biomedical research throughout the world is devoted to malaria, schistosomiasis, and other major disease problems of poor nations.[5]

The lack of research makes the objectives of this book difficult to attain. Nevertheless, enough information to evaluate roughly the impact of these diseases on population fecundity and fertility is available, though not in a readily usable form. It is scattered throughout various publications, mostly medical journals, or embedded in data sets awaiting discovery, retrieval, and analysis. A World Health Organization group (1975:230) concerned with advancing knowledge on population subfecundity recommended that this information be further studied and analyzed. This book followed that recommendation and its data were obtained through careful study, analysis, and evaluation of such sources as journals in medicine and the biological sciences as well as epidemiological reports, demographic data, vital statistics, and many other research materials.

---

[5]Few drugs have been developed by pharmaceutical companies to deal with these so-called orphan diseases. The reason for this neglect is probably largely economic. Pharmaceutical houses have not found it profitable to develop medicines for diseases that strike the impoverished.

II

Nonsexually Transmitted Diseases

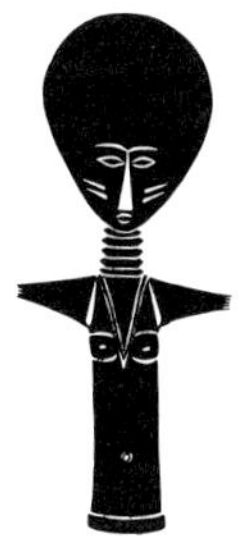

CHAPTER 3

Tuberculosis

Introduction

Population students have always recognized tuberculosis (TB) as an important cause of mortality trends and differentials. McKeown (1976:92), for instance, referring to the mortality trend in England and Wales since 1838, noted: "This is the disease [TB] which, if any, was critical for the fall of the death rate. It was much the largest single cause of death in the mid-nineteenth century, and it was associated with nearly a fifth of the total reduction of mortality since then." Although TB is rarely seen today in western Europe, the United States, and Australia (see Figure 3.1), it remains an important cause of morbidity and mortality in much of the world. Approximately 3.5 million persons develop tuberculosis each year, and more than 500,000 die of the disease (World Health Organization 1980:89). But, as with most diseases, population students have largely ignored any impact of TB on fecundity and fertility (Hansluwka 1975:203; Tabbarah 1971:268). Most available references in the literature either simply list TB as a disease thought to have the potential to depress population fecundity (e.g., Hansluwka 1975:206; Hesser *et al.* 1976:73; Isely 1980:16; Petersen 1975:192; Potts and Selman 1979:25; Stone 1954:737; Taylor *et al.* 1976:95) or devote only one or several paragraphs to a very generalized discussion of the relationship between TB and fecundity (e.g., Belsey 1976:330–331; Gray 1977:29, 1979:242; World Health Organization 1975:14). In-depth research specifying the nature of the relationship between TB and population fecundity is scarce, which prohibits the quantification of this relationship

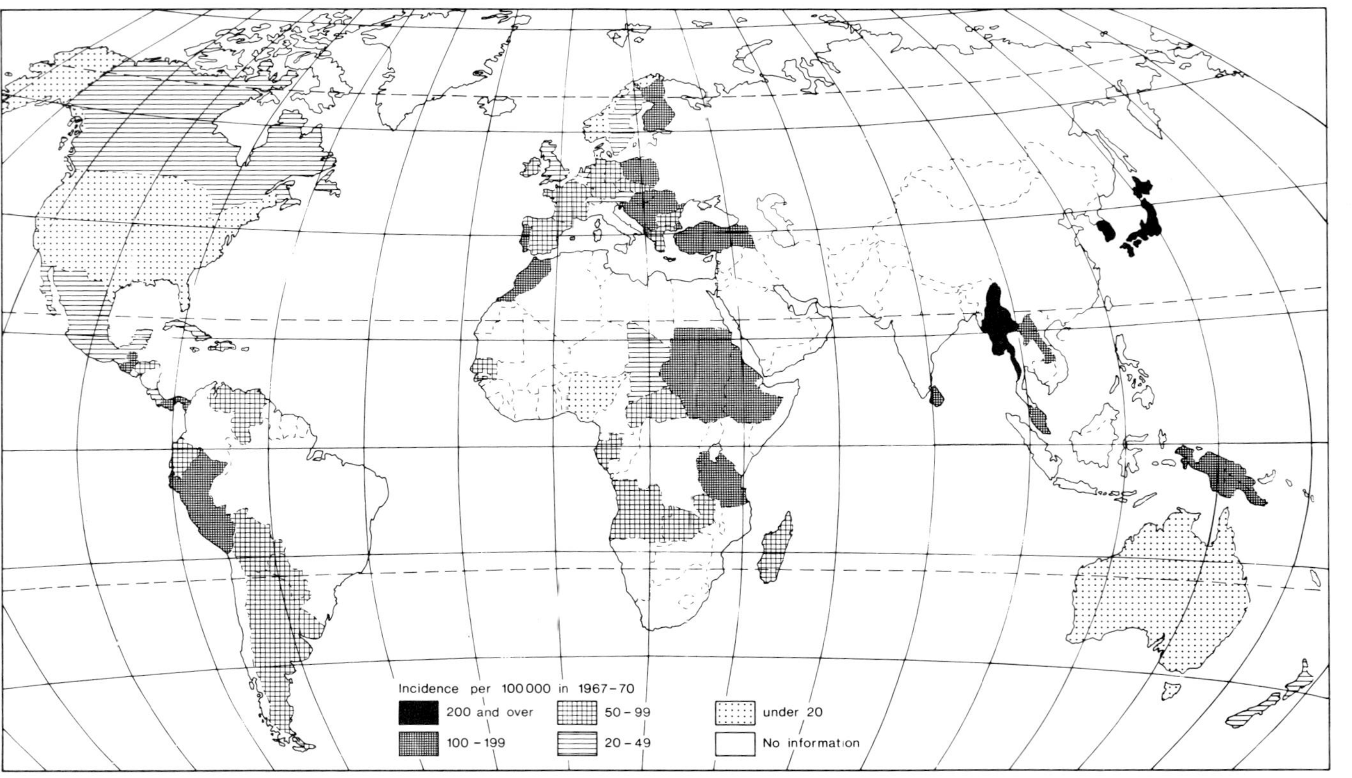

Figure 3.1 Tuberculosis incidence: newly reported cases in 1 year (between 1967 and 1970; based on WHO data). Source: Sutherland 1977:182. Reprinted with permission from ''Tuberculosis and leprosy.'' In G. Howe (ed.), *A world geography of human diseases*. Copyright: Academic Press Inc. (London) Ltd.

(Hansluwka 1975:206). This chapter is an effort to fill a portion of this research gap.

Pathophysiology

TB is a chronic infectious disease caused by a rod-shaped bacterium, either *Mycobacterium tuberculosis* or, less frequently, *Mycobacterium bovis*. The body responds to invasion by the bacillus by initiating a fibrous tissue reaction at the infection site, which results in the formation of nodular lesions called tubercles. The sites of initial (primary) infection are commonly the lung and less frequently the gastrointestinal tract when the infection is of the bovine type caused by *M. bovis*. The bacilli multiply and enter the lymph and vascular systems and thereby seed distant organs including the reproductive organs. As the individual's immunological defenses rise, most bacilli are eventually killed and the majority of persons never develop tuberculous disease.[1] Even the lesions in the lung (primary complex) may be so insignificant as to not be visible on X rays. A positive reaction to extracts of killed bacilli, the tuberculin test, is often the only clinical indication that infection has occurred. However, in the presence of certain conditions that suppress the immune system—these include malnutrition (Bhuyan 1976:275; Malaviya 1976:203), leprosy (Revillard 1971:167), early syphilis (Revillard 1971:167), malaria (*Lancet* 1978a:975; Voller 1974:181; Williamson and Greenwood 1978:1328), and African sleeping sickness (Goodwin 1974:109)—a few of the bacilli that have not been destroyed may be reactivated. Progressive disease then develops, usually in the lungs. But disease can arise in any of the seeded organs as well, independent of any lung involvement.

Effect on Fecundity

Genital TB, one of the many extrapulmonary forms of TB, may cause subfecundity by increasing rates of coital inability, conceptive failure, and pregnancy loss. Painful coitus (dyspareunia) may occur in both men and women with genital TB. Genital tubercles may interfere with the passage of gametes through the male and female genital tracts, resulting

---

[1]Progressive primary disease occurs mostly in children who have little or no acquired resistance to the disease.

in lower conception rates (Amelar 1966:17; Snaith and Barns 1962:715). Or they may interfere with the proper passage of the fertilized ovum through the fallopian tubes and/or the implantation of this ovum in a suitably prepared uterus (Snaith and Barns 1962:715–716), thereby increasing rates of pregnancy loss.

Coital Inability

In men, genital TB may be a cause of seminal vesiculitis, orchitis, or chronic prostatitis, and hence of dyspareunia and impotence (Masters and Johnson 1970:184). Similarly, women with genital TB may experience pelvic pain, which may be aggravated by coitus (Feldman 1977:30). Genital TB is therefore a cause of coital inability in both men and women.

Even if the genital organs are not directly involved in the tuberculous process, coital ability may be diminished. Advanced cases of pulmonary TB may be associated with such shortness of breath on exertion that coitus becomes impossible. Also, decreased libido and decreased sexual potency have been reported in men with pulmonary TB and a decreased interest in sex in similarly affected women. Fear and anxiety about sexual functioning causes further impairment. Eventually a cyclical relationship is established and serves to perpetuate the sexual dysfunction (Feldman 1977:29).

Fortunately, none of the drugs used in the treatment of TB has any specific deleterious effects on sexual functioning (Feldman 1977:30).

Conceptive Failure

Male

It has been suggested (Gow 1971:615; Stewart 1967c:451) that genital TB in the male is usually associated with infection of the kidneys. One autopsy series (Medlar *et al.* 1949:1080) noted that the kidneys were involved first in almost all cases of male genital TB, the infection reaching the reproductive organs by contiguous spread. Similarly, Feldman (1977:30) stated that the sequence of involvement is lungs to kidney to prostate to seminal vesicles to epididymis. On the other hand, others (e.g., Amelar and Dubin 1977:84; Israel 1967:546) have held that the prostate and seminal vesicles are the first pelvic organs involved. And Monif (1974:225) stated that if there is pelvic dissemination of bacilli, the epididymis will be the initial site of infection. Indeed, clinical studies support the notion that infection of the kidneys is neither a necessary nor a usual precursor of genital infection. An African study (Pieterse

1973:2418), for example, showed renal involvement in less than 10% of cases of tuberculous epididymitis. Hence, the results of Medlar *et al.*'s autopsy series may not be applicable to clinical cases of genital TB (see also Kondo 1971:139).

Characteristically, the infection spreads to involve the entire genital tract. Involvement of either the genital ducts or the accessory glands may lower conceptive ability. Because bilateral involvement is the rule in male genital TB (Medlar *et al.* 1949:1088; Pieterse 1973:2418), complete tubal occlusion means sterility. Sterility may also follow extensive destruction of the functional cells of the prostate because of resulting low semen volume (Feldman 1977:30). More subtle changes in the prostate or seminal vesicles may lead to a dimunition of fertilizing capacity because of chemical alterations in the seminal fluid (Eliasson 1975:113ff; Greenberg 1979:318). Thus, genital TB has been observed to depress sperm motility as well as sperm count (Ross *et al.* 1961:664–665). Although chemotherapy is usually sufficient to arrest the disease, conceptive ability is seldom regained, even with surgery (Amelar 1966:17).

It is unfortunate that so little has been reported concerning genital TB in the male. As a result this study focuses primarily on female genital TB and is able to draw only the broadest hypothetical conclusions about the impact of male disease. Nevertheless, we and others (e.g., Paulsen 1977:464) believe that male genital TB is responsible for a sizable portion of male infertility where TB is a prevalent disease. Indeed, genital TB and subsequent sterility may occasionally be important even in areas where TB is not a major problem. For example, Pomerol and Marina (1974:498–501), investigating 79 male patients in Barcelona—the vast majority of whom were complaining of infertility—found 13 with acquired obstruction of the spermatic ducts. In 9 of the 13 the obstruction was at the epididymal level, and among these men a previous history of TB was the most important finding in the clinical history.

Female

In women, primary tuberculous infection of the genitalia may occur if bacilli are present in the semen of a male with genital TB (Amelar 1966:17; Amelar and Dubin 1977:84). This is, however, a very unusual route of infection. Usually the infection is a secondary one, the result of the spread of bacilli through the lymph and vascular systems to the pelvic area following a primary pulmonary infection[2] (Monif 1974:223; National Tuberculosis and Respiratory Disease Association 1969:11). Infection starts at the end of the fallopian tube nearest the ovary and

[2]Genital TB secondary to active pulmonary disease is discussed in Chapter 19.

spreads slowly but continuously toward, and, in some cases, into, the uterus; tubercles are formed along the way (Israel 1967:463).

A minority of experts believe that endometrial TB can exist without tubal involvement. Snaith and Barns (1962:715) cited three reports which found isolated endometrial lesions in 20 to 25% of cases of genital TB. Nevertheless, tubal involvement in genital TB cases is generally felt to be almost universal (Monif 1974:225; Snaith and Barns 1962:715). However, the incidence of endometrial involvement is still a matter of lively debate. A review by Snaith and Barns (1962:715) quoted figures of 100%, 83%, and their own figure of 43% involvement. Similar figures of 80% (Botella-Llusia 1967:519) and 50% (Klein *et al.* 1976:102) have also been reported. A figure of 50% is the most widely encountered (e.g., Belsey 1976:331; Klein *et al.* 1976:102).

As with men, tubal involvement is usually bilateral, being so in 90% (Browne 1943:128) to 93% (Wood 1953, cited in Snaith and Barns 1962:715) of cases. The fibrosis may be so intense as to result in tubal closure (Rozin 1968:214). Or the tubes may remain patent, as they do in 15 to 50% of cases (Rozin 1968:213; Snaith and Barns 1962:715) and may appear normal, but the lining of the fallopian tube may be so involuted that spermatozoa are delayed or trapped and degenerate before reaching the ovum (Snaith and Barns 1962:715).[3] Or, more subtly, tubal motility may be impaired because of damage to the ciliated cells that line the fallopian tube. In any case, sterility is the most probable result once the tubes are involved in the fibrotic process (de Carle 1955:535; Falk *et al.* 1980:977; Hallo 1971:138; Rozin 1968:214; Snaith and Barns 1962:715).

Pregnancy Loss

Conceptions have been recorded in women with treated genital TB, although conception rates are less than 10% (Monif 1974:229; Snaith and Barns 1962:716). Fertility depends on the extent of damage prior to treatment, for although the chemotherapeutic agents introduced in the late 1940s can effectively eradicate the infectious agent they cannot reverse the damage resulting from fibrosis. And if conception should occur, the pregnancy will probably terminate unsuccessfully—50% (Monif 1974:229) to 66% (Snaith and Barns 1962:716) will end as ectopic pregnancies or spontaneous abortions. Ectopic pregnancies are common because residual fibrosis impairs tubal patency and motility, favoring a

---

[3]This proliferation of mucosal folds is similar to that seen in patients with tubal adenocarcinoma (Mardh 1980:944).

tubal implantation. And even if the conceptus should reach the uterus, endometrial lesions may prevent the hormonal stimuli necessary for implantation, and abortion will result (Snaith and Barns 1962:714–716). In one series of over 7000 women with treated genital TB, there was a successful pregnancy in only 2% of cases (King and Burkman 1977:427).

Although untreated genital TB is usually viewed as conferring a state of sterility, conceptions have been recorded in such women. A full-term pregnancy in an untreated woman is rare (Gupta 1957:191), however, because the pregnancy is almost always extrauterine (Browne 1943:129; de Carle 1955:535; Gupta 1957:191; Hallo 1971:138; Snaith and Barns 1962:714–715).

Genital TB has been cited as an important cause of tubal pregnancy in areas where there is a high incidence of pulmonary TB (Hallo 1971:138; Schut 1971:140). But the fact that conceptions are so infrequent in both treated and untreated cases of genital TB makes any substantial role for TB in the etiology of ectopic pregnancy unlikely. Other inflammatory diseases of the tubes (i.e., gonorrheal salpingitis and postabortal and postpartum sepsis) are probably of much greater importance. Interestingly, in some tropical countries where a ruptured tubal pregnancy is the commonest surgical emergency among women, only half the extirpated tubes show histological evidence of any inflammatory process (Stewart 1967b:371), indicating that much remains to be learned about the etiology of ectopic pregnancy.

It is also worth noting that some drugs used to treat TB can adversely affect the fetus (Zellweger 1974:338).

Thus, TB is capable of producing genital lesions that usually render affected individuals permanently infecund even in the face of modern chemotherapy. Yet a comprehensive study of genital TB and its impact on population fecundity is lacking. This is particularly surprising because TB is both historically and currently a very prevalent disease.

The Development
of Genital Tuberculosis

That genital TB should be fairly widespread in areas where TB is prevalent is supported by the natural history of tuberculous infection. Importantly, the bacillus is able to disseminate lymphohematogenously (through the lymph and blood systems), especially during a primary infection when resistance levels are lowest (National Tuberculosis and Respiratory Disease Association 1969:11). The frequency with which a primary infection results in lesions in distant organs is a pivotal issue in determining the frequency of genital TB. Unfortunately, it is an issue that has not been resolved. An extensive autopsy study showed post-primary seeding of distant organs in only 4% of cases of TB infection in which there was no progressive tuberculous disease (Medlar 1955:32). In cases where minimal disease (usually pulmonary) was present, this figure rose to 12% (Medlar 1955:39). Yet Rich (1951:797) stated that bacilli "commonly" find their way to the circulation and are deposited in distant organs during a primary infection. This view is the more frequently encountered one (see Malaviya 1976:198; Sartwell 1965:212).

This seeding of distant organs including the genitals may occur regardless of the seriousness of the primary infection. In fact, in most cases of female genital TB the primary infection has been so mild as to go unnoticed (Klein *et al.* 1976:99; Novak and Woodruff 1967:267). The lesions resulting from postprimary seeding are few in number and most of the bacilli in these lesions are eventually killed as the individual's defenses rise. But in a significant proportion of infected persons, resistance does not rid the body of the invading organisms (Comstock 1975:368), and some lesions, though quiescent, harbor viable bacilli. These may be reactivated[4] anytime by a collapse of the individual's immunological defenses to form progressive disease independent of any disease at the primary infection site (National Tuberculosis and Respiratory Disease Association 1969:11; Rich 1951:797, 827). Once involved, the genital tissues are frequently the sites of progressive destructive lesions because they are excellent sustainers of bacillus multiplication (Rich 1951:321).

In the developed world, the eradication of TB from dairy herds and the widespread pasteurization of milk has meant that today few cases of tuberculosis in these areas are the result of *M. bovis* infection. However, this organism is not an uncommon etiological agent of TB and genital TB in less-developed countries lacking facilities for the pasteurization of milk (Monif 1974:223). This disease, which is identical to that caused by the human bacillus, is contracted by drinking milk from an infected cow (Myers and Steele 1969:65). The primary infection site is the gastrointestinal tract. The establishment of infection is more difficult by this gastrointestinal route, and therefore most bovine infections are

---

[4]Medlar (1955:48–49) stated that his autopsy series found no evidence for reactivation disease and that any tuberculous disease that did not progress from a primary infection (childhood-type tuberculosis) was the result of a reinfection. However, the National Tuberculosis and Respiratory Disease Association (1969:11) and others (e.g., Malaviya 1976:199; Sartwell 1965:212) have maintained that most tuberculous disease arises from reactivation of latent lesions, not from reinfection.

seen in children because of their lower resistance and their ingestion of greater quantities of milk (Rich 1951:60).

Is bovine TB, because of the proximity of the primary infection site to the genitals, more likely than human-type TB to result in genital TB? No hard evidence exists to support this notion. One early (prior to 1927) literature survey found that infection with the human bacillus resulted in urogenital TB approximately four times more often than infection with the bovine bacillus (see Rich 1951:58). However, some later studies in England and Scotland suggest that the proportion of cases of urogenital TB caused by the bovine bacillus was a fair reflection of the proportion of all cases of TB caused by this organism (Myers and Steele 1969:187–188; O'Rear 1947:381).

Problems in Estimating the Prevalence of Genital Tuberculosis

Why, considering the high prevalence of TB historically and currently and the potential for genital TB to occur and lead to permanent infecundity, has the role of this disease in population fecundity been overlooked?[5] The answer likely arises from the problems associated with obtaining any reliable prevalence data for genital TB. Several factors account for this. First, genital TB is usually a silent disease, producing minor symptoms if any. Second, confirmation of a diagnosis of genital TB is difficult. Last, although the prevalence of genital TB in a population is directly related to the prevalence of extragenital TB, the proportion of infected individuals who develop genital TB is not constant but depends on such variables as age at primary infection and perhaps race.

Lack of Symptoms

Female

The most important reason the prevalence of genital TB is so difficult to gauge is that latent cases far exceed those showing definite clinical signs (Rozin 1968:209). Latent cases outnumber clinical ones by estimates of 5:1 (Medlar *et al.* 1949:1088) to 30:1 (Bonafos *et al.* 1967:308).

---

[5]For a more general discussion of the reasons population students have conducted little research into the causes of population subfecundity like TB, see McFalls (1979b:9–17).

In addition, there usually are no palpable or visible abnormalities of the female reproductive organs; amenorrhea and subfecundity are often the only indications that pathology exists (Israel 1967:421).

Menstrual disorders, particularly amenorrhea,[6] are seen in a substantial percentage of cases of genital TB (Durgamba *et al.* 1972:37). This amenorrhea is not caused by ovulatory failure, as is so often the case, but is the result of damage to or actual destruction of the endometrium by the tuberculous process (Rozin 1968:215). Amenorrhea is estimated to occur in 5 to 50% of cases (Rozin 1968:214). It has been suggested that the proportion of cases that exhibit amenorrhea varies by race (Francis 1964:420). For example, in India 50% of cases reported are so affected, whereas in Germany only 4% are (Ojo *et al.* 1971:285). (Variations in nutritional status may be an important contributing factor in such differentials.) But despite an association between menstrual disorders and genital TB, at least half the women with genital TB give no clues as to the cause of their infertility because they have no menstrual problems and appear to be in excellent health (Stallworthy 1963:291).

Infertility is probably the most common reason women with genital TB seek medical attention. Cases of primary sterility are far more numerous than those of secondary sterility (World Health Organization 1975:14), for reasons that are discussed later. In many reported series (e.g., Bonafos *et al.* 1967:308; Rozin 1968:214) cases of primary sterility outnumber those of secondary sterility by 4 or 5:1. Some series (e.g., Rajan *et al.* 1974:11) have reported lower ratios, and a minority of researchers (e.g., Durgamba *et al.* 1972:34) have even reported that secondary sterility is more frequently encountered.

The total incidence of sterility among women with proved cases of genital TB has been recorded as 55% (Gupta 1957:186), 57% (Stallworthy 1952, cited in Ojo *et al.* 1971:285), 62% (Russell *et al.* 1951, cited in Ojo *et al.* 1971:285), 70% (Ojo *et al.* 1971:282), and 80–85% (Gupta 1957:186). The fact that not all women with genital TB are recorded as being sterile is contrary to earlier statements that a diagnosis of genital TB almost totally excludes the possibility of conception (or a successful pregnancy). Are these earlier statements invalid? Stallworthy (1963:291, 293) felt that they may be. He noted that those women who are investigated have a complaint (infertility, amenorrhea, etc.), and that just because pregnancy cannot occur in this group does not mean that it cannot occur in women with genital TB who have no symptoms. Nevertheless, the con-

[6]Some researchers (e.g., Klein *et al.* 1976:100; Rajan *et al.* 1974:11; Stewart 1967c:453) have reported that abnormal bleeding is more often associated with genital TB than is amenorrhea. Still others (e.g., Schaefer and Birnbaum 1956:182) have said that amenorrhea is not a prominent symptom at all.

sensus is that genital TB, unless detected and treated in the very earliest stages when tubal involvement is minimal, confers a state of complete sterility in the vast majority of cases and that when conception does occur, the pregnancy usually terminates unsuccessfully with an abortion or ectopic nidation (Falk *et al.* 1980; Schaefer 1964). Indeed, Schaefer (1964:87ff) noted that many reports of successful pregnancy following treatment of genital TB are in error because a diagnosis of genital TB was frequently made without sufficient confirmatory evidence.

Male

In men the symptoms of genital TB are also elusive; painful urination is sometimes the only indication of disease (Christensen 1974:379). In one autopsy study (Medlar *et al.* 1949:1088) clinical recognition of male genital TB was accomplished in only 18% of cases despite advanced disease.

It should also be noted that a history (patient recall, radiographic evidence, etc.) of extragenital TB is usually unobtainable in male or female patients with genital TB, and is therefore not very helpful in identifying persons at risk. In an Indian study (Krishna 1979b:506) X-ray evidence of old pulmonary TB was apparent in only one-third of cases of genital TB. In an African study (Ojo *et al.* 1971:284) only 22% of women with genital TB gave a previous history of extragenital TB. And a U.S. study (Klein *et al.* 1976:99) obtained a history of TB in only 25% of female genital TB cases.

Problems of Diagnosis

As noted earlier, many women with genital TB have no pelvic abnormality palpable on physical exam. And even if laparoscopy is performed and tubal thickening, peritubal adhesions, and so on are observed, a conclusive diagnosis still cannot be made because chronic gonococcal salpingitis presents the same picture (Mardh 1980:944). Hence, it is necessary to use laboratory methods, primarily bacteriology (identification of the organism in cultures of menstrual blood, endometrium, prostatic and seminal secretions, etc.) and histology (microscopic identification of tuberculous lesions in tissue sections of fallopian tube, endometrium, epididymis, etc.) to confirm the diagnosis. Even these methods are riddled with problems. Because the lesions of TB may resemble those produced by other diseases such as sarcoidosis, only bacteriologic methods offer absolute proof of tuberculous infection (T. Klein, personal communication, 1981). But identification of the mycobacterium is laborious and time consuming (Mardh 1980:947). And although one worker (Francis 1964:427) feels that bacteriology is the superior method—that employment of histological methods will miss 50% of cases of genital TB—most authorities disagree and feel that many more cases of genital TB can be confirmed by histological methods. In a Nigerian study (Ojo *et al.* 1971:284) bacteriologic confirmation was possible in only 13% of histologically confirmed cases of genital TB. In a long-term (1968–1977) Swedish study, bacteriologic confirmation was possible in only 29% of confirmed cases of genital TB (Falk *et al.* 1980:975). And in a U.S. study (Klein *et al.* 1976:99) histological methods gave positive results in twice as many cases of genital TB as did bacteriological methods. It seems, then, that histological methods are superior, though the best results are obtained when both methods are employed. And some workers such as Morris and associates (1970:89) have stated that inoculation of guinea pigs with biopsy material should also be done. In their series 16 to 31 women with endometrial TB would have been missed if culture and/or histology had been relied upon and guinea pig inoculation not done.

Although examination of the fallopian tubes is necessary for a diagnosis of tuberculous salpingitis, the premier cause of TB-associated subfecundity, such specimens are usually obtainable only at the cost of mutilation (Bonafos *et al.* 1967:308). Thus, endometrial specimens are most often studied. But this severely restricts the number of confirmable cases, as surgical and autopsy material has shown that the endometrium is not involved in approximately one-half of cases of genital TB (Klein *et al.* 1976:102). And technical difficulties ensure that the actual incidence of positive endometrial samples is even lower than 50%.[7] Bacteriological confirmation may fail because often few bacilli reach the uterus from the fallopian tubes and these may grow slowly (Klein *et al.* 1976:102). Likewise, endometrial lesions may be scanty[8] and the chances of obtaining negative histological results are substantial for any one sample[9] (Klein *et al.* 1976:102; Rajan *et al.* 1974:13; Sutherland 1960:491).

[7]How the sample is procured is very important. In one study (Padubidri *et al.* 1980:323–324) biopsy missed 25% of cases of endometrial TB diagnosed from material aspirated from the uterus. This was probably because aspirated tissue represents a wider endometrial surface than that obtained by the limited curetting employed in biopsy procedures.

[8]Even when tubal material is available for histological analysis, tubercles may be scanty (Novak and Woodruff 1967:269) and have a limited distribution (Mardh 1980:944). Hence, the pathologist must carefully examine several sections of the tube or the diagnosis can be missed (Krishna 1979b:509).

[9]One researcher (Botella-Llusia 1967:515, 520) has maintained that in some countries the growing incidence of endometrial tuberculosis is more apparent than real, reflecting a greater precision in identifying characteristic tubercles in endometrial tissue.

Table 3.1

Investigation of a Woman with Genital TB: Common Clinical and Laboratory Findings

Investigative procedure	*Findings*
Recording of symptoms	None except infertility
Recording of patient history	Negative for TB
Pelvic examination	Normal
Chest X ray	Negative
Laparoscopy	Gross lesions (thickening of tubes, peritubal adhesions) may resemble chronic gonococcal salpingitis
Laboratory tests on endometrial tissue[a]	
Culture	Negative
Histology[b]	Positive if several sections carefully examined
Guinea pig inoculation	Positive

[a]More positive results can be expected with tissue samples acquired by endometrial aspiration than with smaller samples acquired by simple biopsy because aspirated tissue represents a wider endometrial surface (Padubidri *et al.* 1980:324).

[b]Must exclude other diseases that produce similar granulomatous lesions such as sarcoidosis (Klein, personal communication, 1981).

(See Table 3.1 for a summary of typical clinical and laboratory results in an investigation of a woman with genital TB.)

In men, diagnostic confirmation of genital TB is even more difficult. It is impossible to examine the epididymis histologically for indications of tuberculosis without compromising fecundity. And bacteriological confirmation is difficult because the bacillus can rarely be demonstrated in prostatic and seminal fluids (Pieterse 1973:2418).

In those areas of the world where both tuberculosis and gonorrhea are common, much difficulty may be encountered in making a differential diagnosis of tubal disease because the clinical (Rozin 1968:209) and pathological (Novak and Woodruff 1967:269) pictures in tuberculous and gonorrheal salpingitis may be quite similar.

Population Variability in the Ratio of Extragenital to Genital Tuberculosis

The third reason for deficient data on the prevalence of genital TB is that, given the prevalence of TB in a population, there is no pat equation for estimating the prevalence of genital TB in that population accurately. Although one researcher (Cameron, cited in Gupta 1957:182) estimated that in men 5% of all tuberculous lesions are of the genitals and that in women the incidence is higher yet, it is generally recognized that the incidence of genital TB in a tuberculous population varies with certain demographic characteristics of the population, particularly age at first infection.[10] Race and sex may also be important in determining whether or not genital TB will develop.

Age

Age at primary infection (when seeding of distant organs occurs) seems to be the most important determinant for the development of genital TB. It is generally agreed that the closer to menarche the primary infection occurs, the more likely it is that genital TB will follow[11] (Monif 1974:220; Rozin 1968:210–211). It has been suggested that the greater vascularity of the genital tract at this time is responsible (Jedberg 1950), greater numbers of lymphohematogenously borne bacilli gaining access to the reproductive organs.[12] This is consistent with the observation that disseminated bacilli settle in tissues with a high oxygen content, that is, well-vascularized tissue. Because the genital tissues are otherwise relatively deficient in the ability to remove bacilli from the circulation (Rich 1951:321), seeding of the genitals may be effectively limited to this period of life.

Although progressive disease may develop at this time (Snaith and Barns 1962:715), more commonly it will occur later as reactivation disease (National Tuberculosis and Respiratory Disease Association 1969:11). The age at actual onset of tuberculous disease of the genitals, though estimated by some to be the early 20s (Rajan *et al.* 1974:12), is difficult to determine as pathology and subfecundity are often present years before the disease is recognized. But data for extragenital TB show that tuberculous disease is most likely to develop between the ages of 12 and 24 (Comstock 1975:374). And Jedberg (1950) noted that genital

[10]In Sweden 5–10% of all cases of TB in the 1970s were urogenital TB, according to a study conducted from 1950 to 1979 (Mardh 1980:944). However, it would be incorrect to assume from this that in the past 5–10% of TB in Sweden was urogenital because, unlike other forms of TB such as pulmonary and bone TB, urogenital TB is often silent and may remain undetected for many years. Indeed, 20% of the cases of urogenital TB were caused by the bovine bacillus. Because TB in cows had been eradicated many years earlier it was apparent that these infections had been acquired long ago. And a similar study (Falk *et al.* 1980:976) noted that although most cases of genital TB in the past were diagnosed during childbearing age, most cases are now diagnosed after menopause, again indicating long-standing infections.

[11]Primary infection during pregnancy has also been suggested as predisposing to genital TB (Snaith and Barns 1962:715).

[12]In two other diseases, schistosomiasis and filariasis, the same phenomenon occurs; significant involvement of the internal reproductive organs does not occur until after the onset of puberty.

TB was diagnosed during childbearing age in 98% of all women with this disease.

Race

Race may also be important in determining whether or not genital TB will develop. Blacks are believed more likely to develop extrapulmonary forms of the disease (Long 1971:300). However, this may not necessarily be due to a racial factor, but may be the result of introducing the disease into a previously unexposed population. In this regard, McNeill (1976:61) noted that extrapulmonary TB was extremely common in a tribe of Canadian Indians exposed to the bacillus for the first time, but that the disease accommodated itself after several generations to the more familiar target organ, the lung (see also footnote 14).

One autopsy series (Medlar *et al.* 1949:1081) showed genital TB to be 50% more common in blacks than whites. But, as mentioned earlier, caution must be used when generalizing from such an autopsy series because the pathological picture may be quite different between cases of genital TB detected in clinical practice where dysuria or infertility may be the only complaint, and cases investigated in autopsy series biased toward persons who had advanced tuberculous disease (Kondo 1971:139). Nevertheless, an inspection of TB infection rates for the United States during the first half of this century points to one reason why genital TB could indeed have been more common in U.S. blacks. These data show that many more blacks than whites were infected before age 20 (Payne 1949:333). Thus a larger proportion of blacks were experiencing their primary infection at a time in their lives when post-primary dissemination of bacilli was most likely to set the stage for genital tuberculosis.

Data from Africa (e.g., Charlewood 1956:32) also indicate a greater prevalence of genital TB in African natives than in Europeans. Although most workers agree that this manifestation of the disease is seen with greater frequency in blacks, one research team in Africa (Gelfand *et al.* 1973:74) did report higher genital TB rates in Europeans than in African natives.

Sex

Sex differences in the prevalence of genital TB have been recorded. Some researchers (e.g., Gow 1970:648) say that men are predominantly affected. Others (e.g., Bruce 1970:638) believe that men and women are affected in approximately equal numbers. But the most frequently encountered opinion (e.g., Fritjofsson and Kollberg 1973:292; Gupta 1957:182) is that genital TB strikes women more often than men.

Genital Tuberculosis
in Selected Populations

From the preceding discussion a profile can be drawn of an individual likely to develop genital TB. This individual lives in an area where TB infection is common and nutritional and health levels are so low that immunological defenses may be suppressed to the point where active disease can develop. If this individual was first infected with the bacillus in early adolescence and, perhaps, if they are black or female the chances are increased that the tuberculous disease that develops will be of the genitals.

Developing Societies

Such persons are likely to be encountered in developing societies where open pulmonary TB is a serious problem. McNeill (1976:283–284) underscored the importance of TB in developing societies:

> In much of Oceania, Asia, and Africa, tuberculosis remains a major source of human debility and death. The development of antibiotic drugs, during and after World War II, that were capable of attacking the bacillus without doing damage to the human body, meant that in places where modern medical services were available the disease lost its former importance. But since the dramatic retreat of malaria in the post-World War II years, tuberculosis has remained probably the most widespread and persistent human infection in the world at large. [Excerpt from *Plagues and People* by William H. McNeill. Copyright © 1976 by William H. McNeill. Reprinted by permission of Doubleday & Company, Inc.]

Tuberculosis is one of the few communicable diseases that is a major public health problem in all World Health Organization (WHO) regions, and the TB situation in the developing world is not improving very rapidly. This is due to the specific epidemiological dynamics of the disease as well as to the difficulties many developing nations face in applying the available control techniques. Morbidity from TB is particularly high in such developing countries as Burma, East Timor, Macao, the Philippines, and the Republic of Korea (South Korea) (World Health Organization 1980:89–90).

The ubiquitousness of TB infection in developing societies and the low nutritional and health levels of these areas make development of tuberculous disease in many individuals highly probable. That most persons in developing societies are infected early in life (70% are infected before the age of 14 [Gallagher 1969:174]) leaves the door open for a substantial number of cases of genital TB. Indeed, Hajj (1978:289) stated that genital TB is ''common'' in developing countries. In Africa, rates of genital TB could be especially high because blacks may be predisposed to this form of the disease. In what is probably the most extensive study of disease frequency in Africa, TB was found in over 20% of all persons dying traumatically in Kinshasa, Zaire (Smith *et al.* 1976:641). Thus it is likely that at least a portion of the large amount of tubal disease in women in the Kinshasa study—20% of all women over age 10 had active or healed pelvic inflammatory disease (Smith *et al.* 1976:642)—is attributable to genital TB.

Given these circumstances, genital TB is likely to have a strong impact on the fecundity and fertility of some developing societies.[13] Indeed, it has been cited as one significant cause of subfecundity in tuberculous areas (Muir and Belsey 1980:918; Paulsen 1977:464), and even as the most important cause of subfecundity in the low-fertility, tuberculosis-ridden areas of Africa, specifically Cameroon and the adjacent areas of low fertility (Nasah *et al.* 1974:75). Genital TB has also been mentioned as a possible cause of the involuntary childlessness common in Indonesia (Hull and Tukiran 1976:21). A report from Algeria (Bonafos *et al.* 1967:308) stated that 25% of the sterility in that country was the result of genital TB. And Ledward (1980:118) reported that TB remains a high possibility as an etiological factor in infertility in Saudi Arabia. Table 3.2 presents some reported data on the incidence of genital TB in other developing countries.

In Table 3.2 there is great variation in the genital TB rates reported by different authors working in the same countries at about the same time. This is somewhat disturbing. But because each study population is unique and methods of diagnosing genital TB vary, such fluctuations should be expected. However, every study should be the object of much critical evaluation. Factors to be considered include the prevalence of TB infection in the study area; the race, age at initial infection, and nutritional and health status of the study population; whether the study population consists of unselected women or those with fertility problems; what methods of diagnostic confirmation are being relied upon; and what other infections are common in the study population that could make a differential diagnosis difficult. This last factor is a very important one because in many populations both tuberculous and gonococcal infections of the genitals, which present a very similar clinical picture (Rozin 1968:209), are common. In such populations it is difficult to resolve the precise origin of tubal disease (Middlemiss 1972:255). Even when direct visualization of the tubes is possible, the appearance may be similar in both diseases. In some cases of genital TB the tubes, aside from

---

[13]The contribution of genital TB to the pelvic inflammatory disease (PID) problem in any given country depends on the prevalence of TB in that country versus the prevalence of other PID factors such as gonorrhea and postpartum and postabortal infection (see Muir and Belsey 1980).

Table 3.2
Incidence of Genital TB in Sterility Cases in Developing Countries

Country	Author	Year	Endometrial TB (%)	Minimum estimate of genital TB (%)[a]
India	Gupta	1957	17.4	34.8
	Malkani and Rajani[b]	1959	8.5	17.0
	Isaac	1971	1.6	3.2
	Ganguly[c]	1972	2.1	4.2
	Panda and Dey[c]	1972	2.2	4.4
	Saxena and Pathak[c]	1972	5.1	10.2
	Krishna *et al.*	1979a	—	10.3
Kenya	Chatfield *et al.*	1970	2.0	4.0

[a]These studies (except for Krishna *et al.*) report the incidence of endometrial TB in sterile women. Because endometrial TB is present in only half the cases of genital TB and technical difficulties may preclude its detection even when present, doubling the rate of endometrial TB gives a minimum estimate of the rate of genital TB in these women. In the Krishna *et al.* study, a diagnosis of genital TB was made on the basis of laparoscopy, clinical findings, and patient history.

[b]Cited in Rozin (1968).

[c]Cited in Padubidri *et al.* (1980).

an occasional tubercle in the mucous membrane, present an appearance not different from chronic gonorrheal salpingitis (Novak and Woodruff 1967:269). These similarities serve to underestimate the importance of genital TB because the tendency among medical workers is to assign the tubal pathology to the more familiar gonorrheal salpingitis (Charlewood 1956:37). Perhaps this explains why demographers have focused on venereal disease (VD) as a cause of population subfecundity to the virtual exclusion of other diseases like genital TB.

Tuberculosis has undoubtedly played an important role in the depopulation of some primitive societies where the disease is reported to be widespread (Howe 1974:29; Nag 1962:41; Petersen 1975:382; Scragg 1957:70). However, most workers conceive of TB's role in depopulation as solely one of increasing mortality rates, though it is clear from this discussion that it also can exert a strong influence on fertility via subfecundity. Two workers who did recognize the potential role of TB in decreasing fertility in depopulating societies are Fujii (cited in Nag 1962:41) and Scragg (1957:93). The latter concluded, however, that TB did not contribute materially through subfecundity to the depopulation of highly tuberculous New Ireland. This conclusion was based on curettings on less than one-third of selected sterile women (Scragg 1957:87). Perhaps closer inspection of many tissue sections would have yielded positive results, but this is only conjecture.

Developed Societies

The prevalence of TB, both extragenital and genital, is today far lower in developed than in developing societies. Yet TB was widespread in the developed world in the first half of this century, and, according to Falk *et al.* (1980:974), "A few decades ago, genital tuberculosis in women [in developed countries] was very common and was considered a possible diagnosis in every gynecologic investigation." Even today TB is still fairly prevalent in particular population groups such as the Celtic people in France, Wales, Ireland, and Scotland, whom some observers regard as being inherently more susceptible to the disease, and in American Indians in the United States (Klimas 1982:10). But even in these and other hard-hit groups improvements in living conditions and efforts in fighting the disease have led to substantial prevalence declines in recent years (Pettigrew 1964:84). Active TB is currently a problem in the United States among illegal immigrants from Mexico and other Central American countries (*Intercom* 1978a:15). Pockets of TB have emerged in southern California where the number of pulmonary TB cases rose 36% between 1970 and 1974 (Klein *et al.* 1976:99). Health workers in this area have been advised to consider genital TB as a possible cause of any infertility in their foreign-born patients (Klein *et al.* 1976:99). In 1980, 2% of Southeast Asian refugees to the United States had TB and another 50% had a positive skin test to tuberculin (*Philadelphia* Bulletin 1980b:A6). Indeed, TB is by far the most common infection imported by these refugees into the United States (Barrett-Connor 1978:1901). As a result of these legal and illegal migration streams, the incidence of TB in the U.S. population began to grow in 1980 after years of steady decline, and the incidence may continue an upward swing for years to come. This problem is not confined to the United States, however. Immigrants to other developed nations such as Britain have a considerably higher prevalence of TB than the indigenous populations (C. Smith 1972:5).

Table 3.3 presents reported data on the incidence of genital TB in sterility cases in selected developed countries. The rates for countries such as Spain and Sweden are surprisingly high, especially when compared to those presented in Table 3.2 for developing nations such as Kenya where open pulmonary TB and tubal occlusion are major health problems (Chatfield *et al.* 1970:213–215). The authors of the Kenya study (Chatfield *et al.* 1970) were themselves puzzled by the low incidence of genital TB in this country as compared with some developed nations. No completely satisfactory explanation is available for this observation. However, it is noteworthy that in one of the Spanish studies reporting a high incidence of genital TB (Botella-Llusia 1967), repeated examina-

Table 3.3

Incidence of Genital TB in Sterility Cases in Developed Countries

Country	Author[a]	Year	Endometrial TB (%)	Minimum estimate of genital TB (%)[b]
Argentina	Murray	1950	1.6	3.2
Australia	Townsend	1955	.7	1.4
Belgium	Schockaert and Ferin	1947	6.0	12.0
England	Haines	1958	4.0	8.0
France	Palmer	1950	3.0–5.0	6.0–10.0
Hungary	Selmeci *et al.*	1960	7.6	15.2
	Szereday and Matz	1961	4.2	8.4
Israel	Rabau	1950	3.5	7.0
	Halbrecht	1951	4.5	9.0
Japan	Shinagawa and Ono	1960	5.5	11.0
Scotland	Sharman	1962	5.7	11.4
Spain	Lopez de la Osa	1953	14.8	29.6
	Botella-Llusia	1967	10.6	21.2
Sweden	Liljendahl and Hyden	1951	10.1	20.2
	Rubin	1954	19.0	38.0
United States	Foss *et al.*	1958	.6	1.2
	Israel *et al.*	1963	.3	.6

[a]All cited in Rozin (1968) except Haines, Sharman (cited in Chatfield *et al.*, 1970), Botella-Llusia, and Rubin (cited in Gupta, 1957).

[b]Cases of endometrial TB represent fewer than half the cases of genital TB.

tion of several sections of tissue for evidence of TB yielded substantially more (30%) cases of genital TB than would ordinarily have been found. Perhaps, then, a greater proportion of genital TB cases in the developed countries are being unearthed because more effort and money are invested in their detection.

Historical Societies

TB is of such great age that it was afflicting the human race before written history. Indeed, skeletons of prehistoric humans have included some with TB-twisted spines (Gallagher 1969:167). It is probable that after 500 A.D., TB may have exerted demographic effects in Eurasia comparable to or exceeding those of smallpox and plague (McNeill 1976:145). These would likely include effects on both mortality and fertility. Tuberculosis was very prevalent in Europe prior to the twentieth century (McNeill 1976:283), and Gray (1977:29) has suggested that genital TB may have been a significant cause of subfecundity during this period.

E. van de Walle (personal communication, 1978) commented on this possibility:

> A surprising and unexplained set of differential marital fertility rates have been recorded in Western Europe before the demographic transition. A great deal of work has gone into trying to explain why natural fertility is so diverse. Among the explanations, we have looked at factors such as different length or intensity of lactation and nutrition. A large part of the variance remains to be explained, for example among countries of Europe, for provinces in the same country, urban vs rural, etc. The relation of fertility to disease is practically unexplored, although allusions have occasionally been made to VD. As far as I know, TB is not mentioned in the historical literature on fertility. This, however, is a researchable topic, since there are nineteenth century cause of death statistics relating to a time prior to the secular decline of mortality.

In sum, it is possible and, we believe, likely that TB exerted a significant impact on the fecundity and fertility of numerous historical populations.

It is also possible that TB had a substantial impact on the natality history of the U.S. black population over the past 100 years. Although many antebellum physicians felt that TB was almost unknown among slaves—a judgment shared by most modern authorities—several medical historians, notably Savitt (1978) and Kiple and King (1981), have argued that TB afflicted slaves at a rate equal to or greater than it did southern whites. However, because southern TB rates were only a small fraction of northern rates (Kiple and King 1981:140), a reflection of the largely rural nature of the South, the black race as a whole suffered less than the white race prior to 1865. However, following Emancipation TB grew at an alarming rate among blacks. Census reports in 1870 and 1880 indicated a dramatic upsurge in Negro mortality from the disease, and predictions of the Negroes' extinction began to circulate (Torchia 1977:261). A number of factors may have facilitated rising TB morbidity (and mortality) among freed blacks. One was increased infection rates due to increased exposure to tuberculous whites. This was particularly true for blacks who moved into urban areas where TB rates were higher. Another factor was the crowded, unsanitary conditions that were the norm for urban blacks and that facilitated the spread of the tubercle bacillus. And development of tuberculous disease, which is more serious in blacks[14] than whites, was facilitated by poor nutrition, high rates of

---

[14]TB occurs with greater frequency and severity in blacks (Long 1971:300; Medlar *et al.* 1949:1080). It is believed that resistance has not yet developed in blacks as it has in whites, in whom natural selection against the disease has been operating for centuries (McKusick 1964:120–121). Other researchers (e.g., Payne 1949:335, 338) believe that the disease is more serious in blacks because they are the more intensely exposed group. That is, because of their living and working conditions blacks are less likely to encounter the small doses of bacilli that lead to development of acquired immunity. Rather, they are

diseases such as syphilis,[15] and the stress associated with social disorganization (Lowell *et al.* 1969:84)—all of which blacks endured throughout this period in varying degrees.

It was not until the late 1930s that health conditions for blacks greatly improved and a precipitous fall in the number of cases of TB was recorded. Intriguing then is the possibility that changes in the prevalence of TB, and consequently genital TB, were *partly* responsible for the dramatic changes in the fertility rates (see Figure 19.1) and childlessness rates of the U.S. black population between 1880 and 1960, patterns that are still largely unexplained. That is, perhaps the steep decline in black fertility and the concomitant rise in childlessness between 1880 and 1936 are attributable partly to the tremendous increase in TB among blacks during this period. And similarly perhaps the 1936–1960 increase in fertility and decrease in childlessness were due partly to the declining prevalence of TB. These possibilities are explored further in Chapter 19.

Effect on Other Davis–Blake Intermediate Variables

Before closing it is worth noting briefly that TB can depress fertility not only through subfecundity, but through many other Davis–Blake (Davis and Blake, 1956) intermediate variables as well.

TB can certainly affect fertility by reducing mate exposure. For instance, TB may increase both voluntary and involuntary celibacy. In the early twentieth century, some U.S. physicians were advising TB sufferers not to marry, largely for eugenic reasons (*Eugenical News* 1936). Moreover, as with many other maladies TB makes an individual less attractive as a potential mate. TB also leads to increased separation. The systematic effort in Western nations after 1880 to isolate TB patients in sanatoriums (McNeill 1976:283) resulted in separation from mates or

---

more likely to receive a massive dose, which in the nonimmune leads rapidly to serious disease. It is likely both these factors are important in explaining the greater virulence of TB in blacks.

[15]Syphilis was a frequent and serious complication of TB in blacks (Torchia 1977:266). Syphilis was prevalent among blacks throughout the 1880–1950 period. There is good evidence that prior to 1940 as many as 27% of blacks aged 21–35 were infected. No firm figures exist for the late nineteenth century, but they are probably somewhat lower (McFalls 1973:5,16).

from the usual opportunities of finding a sexual partner (McKeown 1976:118; Money 1967:268). This separation, together with the TB itself, can also lead to higher rates of divorce. At least one researcher (Jansen 1952) noted hospitalized TB patients in the United States had unusually high rates of separation and divorce. Finally, TB can result in substantial time outside of a union for the nontuberculous spouse when the union is broken by the death of the tuberculous spouse.

Tuberculosis can also lower coital frequency. The notion that TB is conducive to eroticism and increased coital frequency, an idea reinforced by Thomas Mann's novel *The Magic Mountain,* is fallacious (see Haggan 1944). This misconception probably stems from observation of well-fed and rested patients in a state of symptom remission relaxing in a resort hotel environment (Gebhard 1965:484). But in fact pulmonary TB, which comprises about 93% of all clinically recognized TB (Long 1971:299), would be expected to diminish coital frequency due to associated symptoms such as fatigue, decreased libido, and decreased sexual potency—concomitants of many chronic debilitating diseases (Feldman 1977:29; Gallagher 1969:176). Interestingly, Henin (1969:196) noted that TB was partly responsible for the apparent low coital frequency among nomadic groups in the Sudan and may have contributed to their unexpectedly low fertility.

TB can also lower fertility through birth control, including contraception, sterilization, and induced abortion. In some women, pregnancy can reactivate dormant TB and can cause an already active case to worsen. Just how frequently these phenomena occur is still a matter of disagreement, although the consensus seems to be that they are not as common as was previously thought. Because of the earlier thinking, however, physicians advised tuberculous women to prevent pregnancy through contraception (Knopf 1915, 1932). In one study (Haggan 1944:55) 33 of 50 women with TB reported use of contraception. Other physicians recommended sterilization for the woman's protection and for eugenic reasons (*Eugenical News* 1936; Robitscher 1973). Still others advised pregnant tuberculous women to undergo therapeutic induced abortion (*Newsweek* 1947:53; Rosenback and Gangemi 1956).

In evaluating the impact of TB on fertility, especially in historical societies, it is important to understand how TB was viewed and how these conceptions influenced the intermediate variables. In the late nineteenth century in the United States, for instance, TB patients, and sometimes their families, were shunned in much the same way as lepers were shunned (Mooney 1979). This treatment no doubt had a depressing effect on the TB sufferer's fertility.

Conclusions

Genital TB is a disease that almost always causes primary sterility in affected men and women. Its prevalence varies with the prevalence of extragenital TB, and it has been considered an important cause of subfecundity where TB is a common disease. It has thus been implicated as a cause of the low fertility in certain tuberculous areas of present-day Africa and in numerous historical populations that had high TB rates.

Proving these contentions conclusively is problematic because of the silent nature of the disease and the difficulties encountered in making a definitive diagnosis. But the pathophysiology of the disease suggests that the seeding of distant organs, including the genitals, with bacilli occurs not infrequently during primary infection. Some of the lesions formed at this time harbor live bacilli and, though quiescent, these lesions may be reactivated by such factors as undernutrition and immunosuppressive diseases such as (early) syphilis, causing active disease to develop. If the affected individual experienced the primary infection during puberty, is black, or is female, chances are increased that any tuberculous disease that develops will be of the genital type. Thus it is likely that genital TB is a demographically significant cause of subfecundity in the tuberculous areas of Africa and was important in some historical populations. It is proposed here that genital TB played a significant role in the decline in fertility and the rise in childlessness among U.S. blacks between 1880 and 1936 and in the subsequent reversal of these trends (see Chapter 19).

CHAPTER 4

Malaria

Introduction

Of all the infectious diseases, malaria is today the greatest killer, claiming the lives of 1 million children in Africa alone each year (*Intercom* 1977a:11). Indeed, malaria is possibly the single greatest infectious killer of all time (Garnham 1966, cited in Livingstone 1971:33). This disease has been known for at least 2500 years. References in hieroglyphics indicate that malaria was present in ancient Egypt, and references to the disease may also be found in pre-Christian writings in China and India. The great ancient civilizations of Greece and Rome were affected by malaria and the disease may have played a major role in their declines (Livingstone 1971:33).

Malaria was a global disease until the eradication programs of the twentieth century dramatically reduced its range. Before that time malaria was found as far north as the northern part of Russia and, on the other side of the world, as far south as southern Argentina (*Journal of Tropical Medicine and Hygiene* 1977:229). In 1940 the incidence of malaria perhaps reached its peak. It was then common in all the temperate as well as tropical and subtropical regions of the world and claimed about 3 million lives each year (Jones 1967:25). But because of the post-World War II global eradication program of the World Health Organization (WHO), malaria is today primarily a disease only of the tropical and subtropical zones. Hopes that the disease would also become extinct in these areas were dashed in the 1970s because the malaria parasite and its mosquito vectors have evolved resistant strains capable of evading the arsenal of antimalarial drugs and insecticides that humans had, at first with so much success, aimed at them.

Species and Life Cycle

Human malaria is caused by four major species of Protozoa that belong to the genus *Plasmodium,* namely *P. falciparum, P. vivax, P. malariae,* and *P. ovale.* The latter three parasites are similar in morphology and life cycle; only the *P. falciparum* parasite is nonconforming and, as a result, has sometimes been classified in a different genus (Livingstone 1971:39). *Plasmodium vivax* was the first major human malaria parasite and the primary one in ancient civilizations (Livingstone 1971:41). *Plasmodium vivax* has become the most widespread of the malaria parasites, and is found in most of the malarious areas of the world with the important exception of Africa (Gear 1974:1082). *Plasmodium ovale,* on the other hand, is the rarest of all the malaria parasites and is confined to West Africa (Livingstone 1971:41). *Plasmodium malariae* is seen most often in areas surrounding the Mediterranean Sea, and *P. falciparum,* which requires higher temperatures for optimum development, is effectively limited to the tropical areas of the world (Young and Taliaferro 1971:670). Because of the overlapping geographical distributions of the malaria parasites, mixed infections are common. *Plasmodium vivax* and *P. falciparum* have the widest distributions and account for most of the cases of human disease (Hall 1976:323).

The life cycle of the malaria parasite is important to review because vital clues as to pathology and immunity are found in the different stages of development. The cycle usually begins when an *Anopheles* mosquito takes a blood meal from an infected human. In this meal are asexual parasite forms called merozoites and sexual forms called gametes. The gametes unite in the gut of the mosquito and form a zygote. This zygote undergoes many divisions to form several thousand sporozoites, which pass into the insect's blood stream and eventually accumulate in the salivary gland. When the mosquito bites a person, these sporozoites enter the human bloodstream and circulate for a few minutes before becoming localized in the liver where the pre-erythrocytic (pre-red blood cell) stage of development occurs. In the liver the sporozoites develop into merozoites that, when released into the peripheral circulation, infect red blood cells, thus beginning the erythrocytic stage of development. Within the red blood cell the merozoite undergoes a process of multiple fission called schizogony. During schizogony a merozoite is first cleaved into small ring forms that eventually develop into larger, mature schizonts. The red cell, swollen by the presence of these intracellular parasites, bursts open (lyses), releasing 12–18 new merozoites or, occasionally, some gametes. The gametes serve to complete the parasite's life cycle when ingested by an *Anopheles* mosquito, whereas the merozoites invade fresh red cells and schizogony is repeated and repeated. As schizogony becomes synchronized and a sufficient concentration of parasites is attained in the blood, the human host begins to suffer the paroxysms of malaria—alternating chills, fever, and sweating (Jones 1967:14–15; Spingarn and Edelman 1965:693). The periodicity and length of these febrile attacks is different for each of the species of malaria, although cases conforming to textbook descriptions are seldom seen clinically (Gear 1974:1081).

The number of parasites in the blood never reaches its theoretical maximum because parasites and parasitized cells are constantly being removed from the circulation. A few are destroyed when they are phagocytosed (engulfed) by cells in the spleen, a normal function of the spleen that occurs even in the absence of an infection. Many more are destroyed by any one of a number of host defense mechanisms that eventually gain control and lead to an abrupt drop in the number of parasites (Voller 1974:177). The erythrocytic phase of the disease is now complete. For *P. falciparum* malaria, all the parasites have disappeared and the infection has run its course. But in the other three types of malaria the merozoites can continue to reinfect the liver cells (exoerythrocytic stage) and the infection becomes chronic with the potential for future relapses (Livingstone 1971:57). There is one other important difference between the life cycle of *P. falciparum* and the other parasites. For *P. vivax, P. malariae,* and *P. ovale,* the entire process of schizogony takes place in the well-oxygenated peripheral blood. However, *P. falciparum*-infected red cells lodge in the deep vessels of the internal organs once parasite development has gone beyond the small ring forms. Here in the relatively poorly oxygenated vessels of the spleen, bone marrow, liver, and brain the later stages of parasite development take place (Pasvol *et al.* 1978:702).

Prevalence

Approximately one quarter of the world's population live in areas where malaria is transmitted; these areas include many parts of Africa, Central America, South America, Asia, and Oceania (Schultz 1977:1259) (see Figure 4.1 and Table 4.1). Although there are malaria eradication programs in most of these areas, 350 million people live in malarious

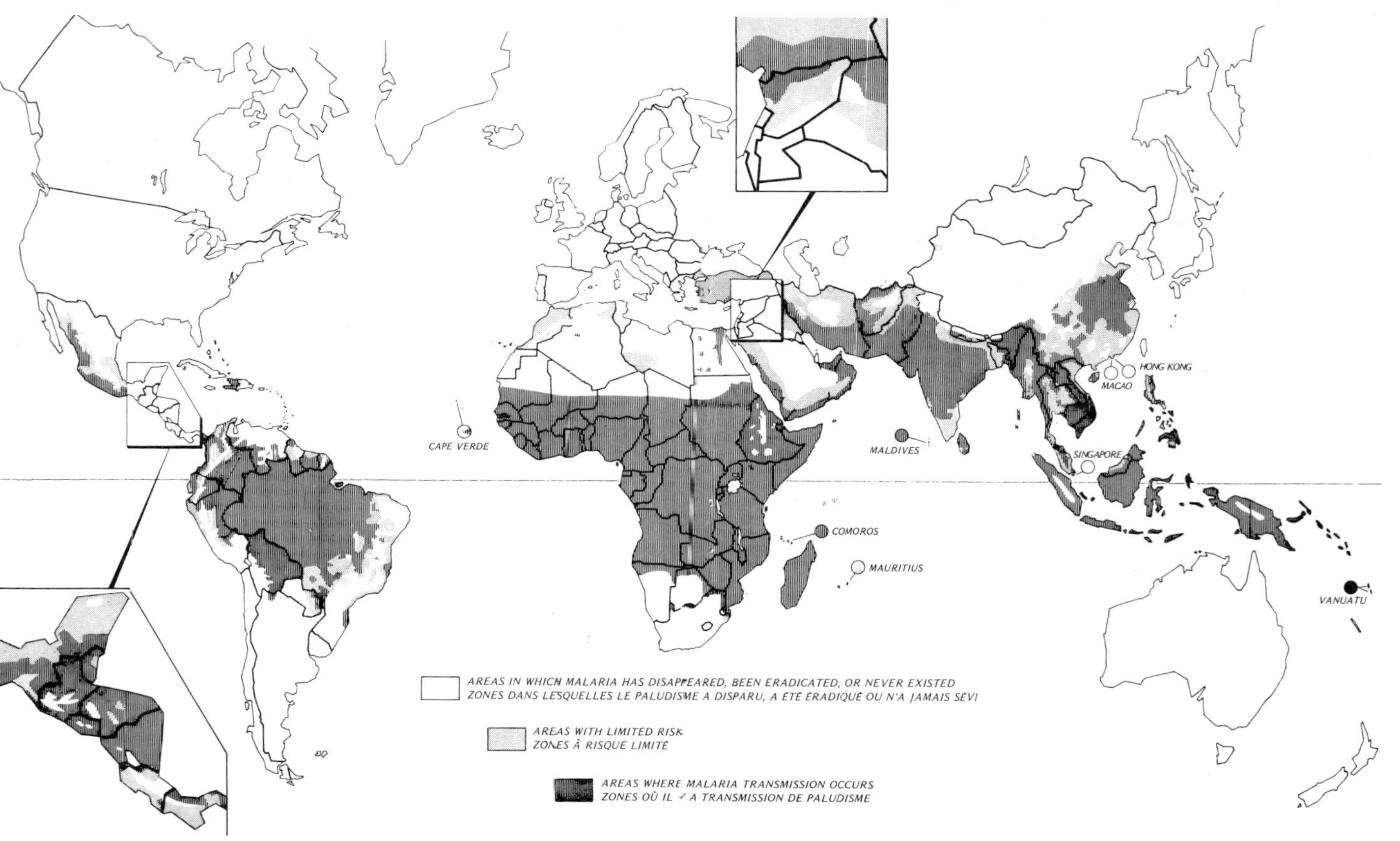

Figure 4.1 Epidemiological assessment of the status of malaria, 1981. Source: *Weekly Epidemiological Record* (1983:12–13).

Table 4.1

Summary of Malaria Situation According to Level of Malaria Risk (Midyear 1978) by Region[a]

| | | | | | Countries or areas where malaria was endemic[b] | | | | | |
| | | | | | Risk nil | | Risk minimum | | Risk moderate to high | |
Region	Total number of countries or areas	Estimated population[c]	Total number of countries or areas	Population originally at risk	Countries or areas	Population	Countries or areas	Population	Countries or areas	Population
Africa	47	336.18	43	292.65	2	1.37	3	9.73	38	281.55
Americas	49	586.50	34	220.17	12	73.21	4	15.44	18	131.52
Southeast Asia	10	992.02	8	918.72	0	—	0	—	8	918.72
Europe	38	822.57	17	376.22	14	309.67	2	23.34	1	43.21
Eastern Mediter- ranean	24	249.20	23	224.14	4	5.72	4	48.95	15	169.47
Western Pacific[d]	38	303.57	18	98.03	5	10.79	2	13.33	11	73.91
Total	206	3290.04	143	2129.93	37	400.76	15	110.79	91	1618.38

[a]Population given in millions. Source: Lepes 1981:10.
[b]Taking 1947 as reference year.
[c]Based on *United Nations Monthly Bulletin of Statistics* (1979).
[d]Excluding China.

regions unprotected by specific antimalarial measures (*Intercom* 1977a:11; World Health Organization 1978d:9). A record 400 million persons suffered from malaria in 1982 (*Time* 1982:67), and that number is likely to increase because malaria is resurging in many countries.

After World War II the World Health Organization initiated a global attack on malaria. Residual spraying of mosquito breeding areas with DDT and the discovery and use of synthetic antimalarial drugs led a combined assault on the disease. Although the disease remained deeply entrenched in sub-Saharan Africa and some parts of Asia, malaria was eradicated in Australia, the United States, the major Caribbean Islands, and all but one European country, and substantial reductions in morbidity and mortality were achieved in North Africa and Central and South America (World Health Organization 1974a:479). However, since 1970 the situation has deteriorated badly and malaria began raging in countries where a few years earlier eradication seemed about to be attained. In India, for example, there were only 125,000 cases in 1965, down from a high of 75 million cases in 1947. But by the mid-1970s 4 million cases per year were being reported. Malaria has re-established itself with particular vengeance in Turkey, India, Pakistan, and countries in Southeast Asia and Latin America (*British Medical Journal* 1976b:1029; World Health Organization 1978c:226).

There are several reasons for this resurgence. In India the rise in the number of cases of malaria is blamed in part on the complacency that followed early success. In the late 1960s DDT-spraying programs were phased out after malaria almost completely disappeared from formerly uninhabitable areas. But because the *Anopheles* mosquito had not been eradicated the spraying slowdown only allowed the insect to thrive and multiply in great numbers once again. Because of success with the synthetic drug chloroquine, the cultivation of the *Cinchona* tree (from whose bark quinine is made) was not encouraged. The disease began to show a resistance to chloroquine and there was not enough quinine available. The worldwide economic situation contributed further to the problem; the insecticide DDT skyrocketed in price, as did all petrochemicals, after the mid-1970s. In the other hard-hit countries the story was much the same—the cost of spraying programs, the resistance of mosquitoes to DDT, and the resistance of the malaria parasite to many of the antimalarial drugs combined to make malaria once again a menace. The most that many of these countries can hope for is to contain the disease reasonably; none expects to eradicate malaria as it is too well entrenched to be defeated by present control methods. That new methods will be found to fight malaria seems remote because so little money is spent on research. In 1976 $40 million was spent worldwide for research on all the parasitic diseases, whereas in the United States alone $800 million was spent that year on cancer research (Schultz 1977:1259). Hope for a breakthrough in malaria control now rests heavily on the development of an effective vaccine. Yet scientists have serious reservations about both the effectiveness and the safety of a malaria vaccine. The changing antigenic nature of the parasite (so-called antigen drift) may make development of an effective vaccine very difficult, and there are fears of the possibility of the development of immune nephritis in well-immunized individuals who subsequently develop malaria; the latter has actually been observed in an animal model (Eaton, personal communication, 1981).

Sequelae of Infection

Mortality

Of the 200 million people who suffer malaria attacks each year about 2 million will die (Lantum 1971:285), and most of these will be children. Malaria takes a particularly heavy toll in tropical Africa; about 15% of all clinical illness there is malaria and each year 1 million persons, again mostly children, die of the disease (Cohen 1978:476). Malaria is very serious in tropical Africa because *P. falciparum* infections are so frequently seen there. Infections with *P. falciparum* malaria offer a poor prognosis because death from malaria is directly related to the concentration of parasites in the blood (Firschein 1961:249) and the highest parasite densities are reached in *P. falciparum* infections (Spingarn and Edelman 1965:693). Although the other three malaria infections are generally not life threatening except in the very young or in patients with a concurrent disease, the case fatality rate among untreated children and nonimmune adults exceeds 10% for *P. falciparum* malaria (Benenson 1975:189). Thus, although all four human malarias are accompanied by considerable morbidity and some mortality, it is *P. falciparum* infections that are especially life threatening.

Mortality rates from malaria are probably higher than many statistics indicate. In some areas malaria mortality rates recorded prior to eradication do not agree with the reduction in the crude mortality rates that followed malaria control, the latter indicating a much larger role for malaria (Livingstone 1971:38). This gap has been partially explained by the fact that malaria contributes to death from other causes such as kidney failure (Livingstone 1971:39), and this is especially true in areas where *P. malariae* is common (Giglioli 1972:201). Death due to anemia and pneumonia may also accompany malaria infections (Lantum 1971:287).

Morbidity

Although a fair proportion of infected persons do die as a result of malaria, particularly *P. falciparum* malaria, the vast majority survive but are intermittently disabled by fevers, chills, and headaches. These symptoms, together with the anemia that may accompany malaria because of massive red cell destruction, are responsible for the observation that malaria drains the strength and ambitions of entire populations (Gallagher 1969:3). When considering the effects of malaria on fecundity, fever and anemia are extremely important. Thus, the pathophysiology of these concomitants of malaria infection will be briefly discussed, as will placental parasitization. Although the latter does not cause any disability in the host, it may have a substantial negative impact on the offspring.

Fever

As indicated earlier, the fevers associated with malaria are initiated when the concentration of parasites in the blood reaches a critical level. The severity of these fevers is directly related to the level of parasitemia (Eaton and Mucha 1971:456). Because the highest levels of parasitemia are reached in *P. falciparum* infections the fevers are highest in those cases, which accounts for the high mortality rates associated with this form of malaria (Hall 1976:323; Livingstone 1971:39). High fevers may also have serious implications for fecundity; this will be discussed later.

Anemia

The anemia associated with malaria is part and parcel of the infection and the host's attempts to control it. The replication of malaria parasites within the red blood cell eventually destroys it, releasing infective merozoites. Parasitized red cells may also be destroyed by the host's defense system before they unload their deadly cargo. Parasitized red cells possess parasite-specific proteins (antigens) on their surface, which elicit antibody production in the host; host antibody attaches to the antigen and the red cell subsequently is either lysed while circulating in the peripheral blood (Lewis *et al.* 1973:698; McGregor 1974:262) or is engulfed in the host's spleen by cells called macrophages, which are members of the body's immune system (McGregor 1974:262; Woodruff *et al.* 1979:1057). But these known mechanisms for red cell destruction are not sufficient to account for the degree of anemia that may develop in malaria infections, especially *P. falciparum* infections (Lawson 1967d:61). And, in fact, considerable red cell destruction has been noted even after all parasites have been eradicated from the blood (Woodruff *et al.* 1979:1057). Thus, it has been theorized (Greenwood *et al.* 1978:384; *Lancet* 1978a:974; Lawson 1967d:61) that the destruction of nonparasitized red cells must occur. It has been suggested (Woodruff *et al.* 1979:1057) that proteins from dead parasites can absorb onto the surface of normal red cells. The host now sees this cell as being infected and deals with it accordingly. However, Houba (1981:3) felt there is only indirect evidence for such an event and suggested two other possibilities: (1) adsorption of immune complexes onto the surface of red cells with subsequent immune-mediated hemolysis and (2) depression of erythropoiesis.

Some degree of anemia will develop even in the mild types of malaria such as *P. vivax* and *P. ovale*. But because total red cell destruction is related to the severity of infection (i.e., the level of parasitemia), severe anemia occurs most frequently in *P. falciparum* infections (Hall 1976:325; Spingarn and Edelman 1965:693; Woodruff *et al.* 1979:1057). The severe hemolytic anemia that accompanies *P. falciparum* infections causes stress on the heart, lungs, bone marrow, spleen, and, perhaps most important, the kidneys; death may be caused by kidney failure (Reese *et al.* 1978:5665). In malarious areas the anemia associated with *P. falciparum* is a major hazard for pregnant women (Voller 1974:182). The possible effects on pregnancy will be discussed later.

Placental Parasitization

The placenta is an additional site where malaria parasites may be found. This organ consists of maternal and fetal components. The fetal blood vessels from the umbilical cord form branching processes or villi in the placenta, and the maternal blood circulates through the intervillous spaces. In the placenta important exchanges take place between the maternal and fetal compartments, the maternal blood giving up oxygen and nutrients to the fetal blood while removing the waste products of fetal metabolism. In women infected with *P. falciparum*, however, these normal exchange functions may be impaired as the intervillous spaces become the site of parasite replication and destruction.

Placental parasitization is particularly characteristic of *P. falciparum* (Lawson 1967d:63; Lewis *et al.* 1973:698) and not the other human malarias because, as mentioned earlier, only in *P. falciparum* malaria does parasite multiplication and growth take place in the deep vessels of the internal organs rather than in the peripheral circulation. Thus, the intervillous spaces of the placenta offer an additional site for *P. falciparum* replication. But parasites and parasitized red cells are also engulfed and destroyed in the placenta. Yet despite intense phagocytic activity by placental macrophages, *P. falciparum* can reach very high densities, and the placenta must therefore be considered an "immunologically protected site" in regard to falciparum malaria (Voller 1974:182). In many cases the intervillous spaces of the placenta may be so packed with parasites and macrophages that it is difficult to understand how the fetus can be nourished (Lawson 1967d:63; Macgregor and Avery 1974:436). Under such conditions pregnancy loss would be anticipated and, indeed, increased rates of abortion, stillbirth, and perinatal mortality have been suggested by some early studies of placental parasitization (Livingstone 1957:762). Most of the more recent studies (Jelliffe 1975:821; Lawson 1967d:65; Lewis *et al.* 1973:698; Llewellyn-Jones 1974:484; Monif 1974:195), however, have concluded that placental parasitization is primarily responsible for low-birth-weight infants. All the possible pregnancy outcomes in cases of placental parasitization will be discussed in detail later.

Immunity

Although the fevers and anemia associated with *P. falciparum* malaria may be life threatening and, together with placental parasitization, are potentially hazardous to reproductive ability, their impact on affected populations is not nearly so devastating as might be anticipated. This is because most persons living in areas where malaria is common possess a degree of immunity to the disease. Much of this immunity is acquired, either passively by transplacental transmission of maternal antibodies during fetal life and/or actively by individuals producing their own antibodies in response to repeated infection. Some of the immunity is, however, innate—that is, inherited. An individual's immunity is the sum total of his or her acquired and inherited immunity, and determines how well that person will be able to survive in malarious areas.[1]

Acquired Immunity

Passive

Most infants born to mothers with high levels of immunity to malaria are themselves immune to malaria at birth because of the transplacental transmission of maternal antibodies.[2] But these antibodies are degraded during the early weeks of life and antibody negative sera become more and more common as time passes (McGregor 1974:263). The length of time that the infant is protected by passively acquired immunity is usually placed at 3 to 6 months (Lantum 1971:288; Ringelhann *et al.* 1976:277; Spingarn and Edelman 1965:694). However, during these months an infant, though bitten by infected mosquitoes, is protected against dangerously high levels of parasitemia and is gradually able to develop a degree of active immunity. Whether or not a child in a highly malarious area will succumb to malaria depends in large part on how rapidly he or she is able to acquire a protective level of active immunity. The high malaria mortality rates for children less than 5 years old is grim evidence that the race between malaria and immunity is often won by the disease.

Active

Active immunity to malaria is slowly acquired in response to the parasitemia that accompanies infection. In highly malarious areas where the native population is continuously being infected, antibody produc-

---

[1]Factors such as nutritional status and health status do, however, impinge on the body's ability to produce antibody. For example, an individual who normally enjoys a high degree of immunity to malaria but is suffering from African sleeping sickness would, because of the exhaustion of the immune system associated with sleeping sickness, be unable to mount a substantial defense against malaria. Iron-deficiency anemia, such as that resulting from heavy infestation with intestinal parasites, has been noted to increase susceptibility to malaria, particularly during iron-replacement therapy (Masawe *et al.* 1974:314). Also, a decrease in normal levels of immunity is often seen during pregnancy; hence the frequent observation that pregnancy exacerbates malaria. And malnutrition, particularly lack of protein, is known to diminish immune responsiveness. On the other hand, there are some indications that deficiencies of certain important nutrients may actually protect the individual against severe malaria (see footnotes 3 and 4).

[2]In one study of the Ivory Coast 75–80% of newborns had malaria antibodies (Reinhardt *et al.* 1978:81).

tion is ongoing and therefore antibody levels are always quite high. Exposure to infection is so pervasive that 90–100% of children at age 3 possess some level of active immunity and this prevalence is maintained throughout life. Antibody titers (concentrations) rise more slowly, however, and peak titers are not attained until adult life (McGregor 1974:263).

This scenario describes only areas where there is intense transmission of malaria, so-called holo- and hyperendemic areas. In areas of the most intense transmission, for example, every person is bitten by an infected mosquito every 10 days or less (Livingstone 1971:34). In many malarious areas, such as the mesoendemic and hypoendemic areas, transmission is not nearly so intense. Antibody prevalence and titers vary greatly between areas of different endemicity, and the subsequent effects of malaria on morbidity and mortality vary accordingly.

Endemicity levels have been defined in many different ways. Parasitemia rates and densities were classically used to define endemicity levels. In hyperendemic areas, for example, parasitemia should be prevalent and dense in young children and often associated with clinical illness, and in older children prevalence should remain high while density declines. Parasitemia in adults in such areas should be infrequent and scanty and clinical illness rare (McGregor 1974:263). This way of defining endemicity has been abandoned by malariologists for two reasons: The widespread and sometimes irregular use of antimalarial drugs have made the method inaccurate for many populations (McGregor 1974:263), and parasite rates and densities may vary seasonally depending on local transmission patterns (Lantum 1971:286).

The spleen usually increases in size in malarial infections, partially due to an increase in the number of splenic macrophages (Voller 1974:180), and thus the number of children aged 2–9 with enlarged spleens has been a popular way of defining malaria endemicity. In holoendemic areas, for example, more than 75% of children constantly have enlarged spleens, and in hyperendemic areas 50–75% do. In meso- and hypoendemic areas the rates are 10–50% and up to 10% respectively (Lantum 1971:286). But using spleen rates to define endemicity has some of the same pitfalls as using parasite rates and densities. Antibody profiles—prevalence and titers—are considered the most accurate way to assess endemicity because these are the least affected by seasonal fluctuations in malaria transmission and the use of antimalarials shows readily (McGregor 1974:263).

Once the endemicity level of a population has been determined using one of these methods, what degree of morbidity and mortality should be anticipated in that population? Unfortunately, this issue is still not settled (Livingstone 1971:35). Some researchers believe that in hyperendemic areas solid immunity is acquired in childhood with little effect on the health of the population, and that morbidity and mortality rates are lower than in areas of lesser endemicity. Other researchers believe that the more malaria there is in a population, the higher the morbidity and mortality rates from the disease will be. Generally it is believed that in hyperendemic areas morbidity and mortality rates are quite high among children, but that these rates greatly decrease with age such that by adult life, despite continuous reinfection, parasite densities are low and by extension so are morbidity and mortality rates (Lantum 1971:286; Livingstone 1971:34). Where malaria transmission is less intense (such as mesoendemic areas), morbidity and mortality rates, though lower among children, will be greater in adults because immunity falters when there is not continuous reinfection, allowing parasite rates and densities to increase with all the subsequent risks (Livingstone 1971:34). For example, morbidity and mortality rates for adolescents and adults are reported to be higher in areas of Asia with moderate endemicity than in the more malarious parts of Africa (World Health Organization 1974a:479).

All the areas described so far are areas of stable malaria; transmission rates may be high or low, but malaria is always present to some degree in the population. But when transmission is interrupted for a considerable length of time population immunity falls to almost nil, and an unstable condition exists where the introduction of malaria could lead to an epidemic in which all segments of the population would be about equally affected and overall morbidity and mortality rates would be high (Livingstone 1971:34).

In conclusion, it can be said that in areas of greatest endemicity malaria morbidity and mortality fall hardest upon the children; adults suffer only from periodic fevers of marginal clinical significance. With declining endemicity, however, a number of adults will experience such serious symptoms as high fevers and anemia and there will be some adult mortality. These different adult reactions to malaria are associated with vastly different effects on reproductive potential. Knowing the level of malaria endemicity in a population is therefore crucial to estimating the impact of malaria on that population's fecundity. Also important to know is whether or not, in addition to acquired immunity (which is dependent on the endemicity level), there is any inherited immunity in the population that could mitigate disease consequences and therefore the reproductive outlook.

As an aside, it should be noted that acquired immunity is strain-specific, that is, immunity exists only to the local strain of, say, *P. falciparum.* The high level of immunity in adults from hyperendemic areas will not serve to protect them if they should visit an area where a different strain of *P. falciparum* exists (Lantum 1971:286; Lawson 1967d:59). Thus, increasing mobility in developing nations means a greater risk of serious disease if populations are unprotected by antimalarial efforts.

Inherited Immunity

According to Charles Darwin, W. C. Wells was the first to espouse the principle of natural selection when he proposed that populations in Africa had been selected for resistance to local disease (see Miller *et al.* 1976:302). His proposal has been verified for at least one disease, malaria: According to Livingstone (1971:33), "As a leading cause of human morbidity and mortality, malaria has undoubtedly been a major agent of natural selection and consequently a determinant of man's genetic evolution."

Genetically determined resistance to malaria could operate at many levels: There could be variation in the amount of antibody produced; the ability of the spleen to remove parasitized red cells could vary, as could the ability of the spleen to provide a suitable environment for the pre- and exoerythrocytic stages of parasite development. Most studies to date have focused on genetically determined variations in the red blood cell that could alter its ability to be penetrated by and support the development of malaria parasites (Luzzatto 1974:196). This is the basis for the "malaria hypothesis," the idea that a genetically determined variation in the human red cell can affect susceptibility to malaria. The first advocate of the malaria hypothesis was Haldane, who in 1949 introduced the notion that a red cell defect known as thalassemia offered protection against the ravages of malaria. However, the argument was first convincingly presented in 1954 by Allison with respect to the red cell defect that produces sickling, hemoglobin S (HbS). Since that time other red cell variations—glucose-6-phosphate dehydrogenase (G6PD) deficiency, hemoglobin C (HbC), hemoglobin E (HbE), ABO blood type, elliptocytosis, and low intraerythrocytic adenosine triphosphatase (ATPase) levels—have come under scrutiny as possibly altering susceptibility to malaria (Luzzatto 1974:197); the basis for many of these theories will be discussed later. It is interesting to note that of the many infectious diseases that W. C. Wells thought capable of exerting selective pressure in Africa, malaria is to date the only disease that has been conclusively demonstrated to influence population genetics (Miller *et al.* 1976:302).

Hemoglobin S

The malaria hypothesis grew out of two observations: (1) Areas of the world with a high frequency of the *S* gene (the gene that codes for sickle hemoglobin) coincide with areas where *P. falciparum* malaria is endemic, and the greater the level of malaria endemicity, the higher the *S* gene frequency; and (2) the *S* gene persists at high frequencies despite loss of the gene because of high early mortality due to severe anemia among persons with only sickle hemoglobin, HbSS homozygotes. Allison's pioneering work explained these observations by showing that the HbAS heterozygote, who has both normal hemoglobin (HbA) and sickle hemoglobin (HbS), has a survival advantage over normal HbAA individuals in malarious areas—an advantage great enough to offset the loss of the *S* gene through early death of the HbSS homozygote. Allison's data showed that heterozygous children had a lower frequency of malaria parasitemia, and that in heterozygous adults infections with *P. falciparum* malaria were neither as frequent nor as severe as in normal adults. These two phenomena would result in lower morbidity and mortality rates for heterozygotes.

Allison's points have been tested by many malariologists, and although many agree with his observations others do not. Despite contradictory evidence (cf. Johnson 1977:1535; Livingstone 1971:45), most studies do show a differential mortality rate from *P. falciparum* for sicklers (HbAS) and nonsicklers (HbAA), especially among children (Livingstone 1971:45). More recent studies on the frequency of parasitemia in sicklers and nonsicklers are less conclusive than the mortality studies, but most do tend to show lower rates for sicklers (Livingstone 1971:45). And although there are also conflicting data on whether parasite densities are lower in HbAS individuals, it is generally agreed that those with severe infections (> 100,000 parasites/cc of blood) are less frequently heterozygotes (Jilly 1969, cited in Livingstone 1971:46; Ringelhann *et al.* 1976:277).

Further, it is believed that for the *S* gene to attain the high frequencies seen in many hyperendemic areas the heterozygote must enjoy not only a lower malaria mortality rate, but also a higher fertility rate. And it is likely there are other undefined factors at work (Livingstone 1957:762). For example, it has been noted that malaria infections are associated with a general immunosuppression, and epidemiological data suggest that development of Burkitt's lymphoma, a virus-induced tumor that claims many young lives in Africa, may be related to this immunosuppression (*Lancet* 1978a:975; Voller 1974:181; Williamson and Greenwood 1978:1328). Because a significant correlation exists between the level of parasitemia and the degree of immunosuppression (Voller 1974:181; Williamson and Greenwood 1978:1328), it has been hypothesized that fewer heterozygotes get this tumor, and this may be yet another factor contributing to a greater survival of the HbAS genotype. (Preliminary results of a study in Uganda indicate that the risk of Burkitt's lymphoma is twice as great in persons with normal hemoglobin as compared to the HbAS heterozygote [Learmonth 1972:150].) By the same line of reasoning, because malaria-induced immunosuppression may also contribute to the high incidence of bacterial infections observed among children in the tropics and may interfere with vaccination programs (Williamson and Greenwood 1978:1328), the HbAS genotype again would probably be less affected and thus more likely to survive to reproductive age.

Although numerous mechanisms have been advanced to describe how HbS protects against malaria (see, for example, Laser and Klein 1979:614; Roth *et al.* 1978:652), that proposed by Pasvol *et al.* (1978) is the most satisfying. Their experiments show that under conditions of low oxygen tension there is a striking retardation of parasite growth in both HbAS and HbSS red cells, whereas in HbAA red cells growth is unaffected. Thus, in *Plasmodium falciparum* malaria, in which the latter part of the erythrocytic stage of development takes place in the deep vessels of the internal organs where oxygen tensions are low, parasite growth is likely to be retarded if the red cell contains sickle hemoglobin. This theory is attractive for several reasons. First, it explains the observation that HbS protects only against *P. falciparum*, as this is the only malaria parasite in which part of the erythrocytic stage is confined to tissues where oxygen tensions are low. Second, it explains why the heterozygote remains susceptible to infection but experiences lower parasite densities and thereby lower mortality rates (Pasvol *et al.* 1978:702–703).

Thus, in areas where *P. falciparum* malaria is highly endemic and has been present for a long time, selective pressures have been acting favorably for the survival of the S genotype.[3] In some hyperendemic

---

[3]A fascinating link among sickle hemoglobin, resistance to malaria, and nutrition has been described by William Durham, an anthropologist. He observed that in some West African societies persons with sickle-cell anemia (HbSS) live longer than most victims of this extremely serious disorder. He theorized that persons in these societies eat more yams, which contain thiocyanate, and this prevents the red blood cells from assuming a sickle shape, thereby protecting persons with sickle-cell anemia from the worst effects of their disease. But this would increase their chances of dying of malaria because sickling of red cells causes their destruction, thereby truncating the parasite's life cycle. However, Durham observed that yams were not eaten during the malaria season because of religious proscriptions. Hence, the victims' red cells would sickle during the rainy season, helping to protect them from malaria (*Philadelphia Bulletin* 1981b:A15).

areas of Africa up to 40% of the population are heterozygotes (Lehmann and Raper 1956, cited in Firschein 1961:247), and the effects of malaria on population morbidity and mortality are mitigated by this fact. In some highly malarious areas, however, the disease has only recently been introduced, and there has not been time for any inherited red cell variation to reach frequencies at which a substantial proportion of the population could enjoy its protection. The effects of malaria on morbidity and mortality in such populations, despite endemicities similar to those in the former areas, would be more severe. And, as will be discussed later, so will be many adverse affects of the disease on reproductive ability.

Hemoglobin F

Thalassemia was the first red cell defect to be proposed as offering a relative resistance to malaria (Haldane 1949), but at that time no mechanism was offered to support the proposal. A peculiarity of thalassemia and related red blood cell disorders (i.e., the persistence of fetal hemoglobin, HbF, during early life) now appears to be the cause of the resistance according to experimental evidence. These experiments show (1) that because *P. falciparum* malaria parasites preferentially invade young erythrocytes, red cells containing HbF, being older, are somewhat spared (Wilson *et al.* 1977:183), and (2) that *P. falciparum* growth is retarded in HbF-containing cells (Pasvol *et al.* 1976:1269). Additional experiments (see Cao *et al.* 1977:202) suggest that red cells with HbF can resist *P. malariae* as well. In either case, persons with such red cell defects are offered some resistance to severe malaria infection during infancy, allowing them more time to acquire a protective level of active immunity.

Glucose-6-Phosphate Dehydrogenase Deficiency

Persons whose red cells lack the enzyme glucose-6-phosphate dehydrogenase (G6PD) are also believed to enjoy some protection against *P. falciparum* (Gear 1974:1083; Luzzatto 1974:198). A possible mechanism for such protection has been suggested by studies showing that the *P. falciparum* parasite itself lacks G6PD activity (World Health Organization 1978d:16) and thus requires a G6PD-positive red cell for development. Alternately, experiments have shown that G6PD deficiency predisposes erythrocytes to oxidant-induced hemolysis; because the malaria parasite exerts an oxidant stress on infected red cells, premature lysis of malaria-infected erythrocytes might occur in persons with G6PD deficiency, thus limiting the severity of the infection by causing the release of immature parasites incapable of propagating the infection (Eaton *et al.* 1976:758).[4] Observations in malaria-endemic areas suggest that only females heterozygous for the deficiency are protected (Luzatto 1974:200; Luzatto and Bienzle 1979:1184; Martin *et al.* 1979a:526; Ringelhann *et al.* 1976:277); no males are believed protected because the trait is found only on the X chromosome and male heterozygosity is therefore not possible (Martin *et al.* 1979a:525). However, the experimental evidence cited earlier regarding sensitivity to oxidant-induced stress in G6PD-deficient red cells suggests that hemizygous Gd($-$) males might also be protected. In either case, resistance is weaker than that associated with the abnormal hemoglobins (Ringelhann *et al.* 1976:277), which partly explains why there is generally a low correlation between the endemicity of malaria and the frequency of G6PD deficiency (Bottini *et al.* 1978:363).

Other Red Cell Polymorphisms

Other red cell polymorphisms that might possibly offer protection against *P. falciparum* malaria are hemoglobins C and E (Livingstone 1971:52; Ringelhann *et al.* 1976:276), low levels of the enzyme adenosine triphosphatase (ATPase) (Livingstone 1971:43), and elliptocytosis (oval cell) (Livingstone 1971:54). A study of the Temuan in West Malaysia, for example, showed that persons with G6PD deficiency and elliptocytosis had a selective advantage in that malarious jungle environment (Baer *et al.* 1976:187). Although there were preliminary indications that blood group B offered protection against malaria, data from more extensive studies failed to show any association between ABO blood type and malaria (cf. Livingstone 1971:44; Martin *et al.* 1979b:216; Mourant *et al.* 1978:19).

Duffy Blood Type and Plasmodium vivax

It has been known since the 1930s that a high percentage of African and U.S. blacks are completely resistant to infection with *P. vivax* (Gear 1974:1082; Martin *et al.* 1979b:218; Miller *et al.* 1976:302).[5] And since 1955 it has been known that the vast majority of African and U.S. blacks are Duffy blood group negative (Fy Fy), lacking the Duffy blood group de-

---

[4]Experiments have shown that vitamin E deficiency also predisposes red cells to oxidant-induced hemolysis. Evidence from some areas of endemic malaria suggests that malnourished African herding peoples, whose diet is low in vitamin E, are relatively resistant to severe malaria infections, a resistance that disappears when their diet is supplemented with foods rich in vitamin E (Eaton *et al.* 1976:758).

[5]Others (e.g., Livingstone 1971:43; Luzzatto 1974:199) have felt that this is not an absolute resistance.

terminants Fy^a or Fy^b (Martin *et al.* 1979b:218; Miller *et al.* 1976:302). These two observations were linked by the hypothesis of Miller and associates (1976:304) that the Duffy determinants Fy^a and Fy^b may be necessary for *P. vivax* infection, acting as receptors for the attachment of *P. vivax* merozoites onto the red blood cell. Still problematic is how so benign a disease as *P. vivax* malaria could exert such selective pressures. It has been suggested that perhaps this selection took place long ago, when *P. vivax* malaria might have been a more serious disease (Martin *et al.* 1979b:218), or that the disease, though infrequently a cause of death in otherwise healthy persons, could decrease survival in children with high rates of other endemic diseases (Miller *et al.* 1976:304).

Summary

The immunity level of a population is thus the sum total of acquired and inherited immunity. Most infants born to immune mothers are themselves immune at birth due to antibodies passively acquired in utero. But this immunity disappears rapidly and is gone by 6 months of age. Meanwhile active immunity is being acquired in response to repeated episodes of infection. The level of acquired immunity depends on the endemicity of malaria in that population. In areas where endemicity is high, the intense level of malaria transmission results in high childhood mortality. But those who survive childhood will have high levels of immunity and as adults will suffer few clinical symptoms of malaria. In less endemic areas the lower level of transmission means less childhood mortality. But because many persons will survive to adulthood without acquiring high levels of immunity, more adults in such populations will suffer malaria attacks of some severity and there will be some adult mortality. Thus, the higher the endemicity, the higher population immunity will be. Because acquired immunity is strain-specific—that is, it is usually effective only against local parasite strains to which a population has been exposed—movement into a region where there is a different strain of parasite or introduction of a new strain will leave that population unprotected.

Inherited immunity against the most serious of the human malarias, *P. falciparum* malaria, has been proven to a statistical level of significance only for the sickle hemoglobin gene.[6] The strongest evidence is for a differential mortality rate for the HbAS heterozygote. In malarious areas the heterozygote is not only less likely to die from the direct effects of

---

[6]Evidence is also quite strong for a very high level of protection against *P. vivax* by the Duffy blood group negative genotype.

malaria, but is also possibly less likely to die from indirect effects, such as Burkitt's lymphoma and bacterial infections. The case for a differential fertility rate and the HbAS genotype is less strong, but there is still compelling evidence that because parasitemia in the heterozygote is less dense, the concomitants of *P. falciparum* that negatively affect fertility (i.e., fever, anemia, and placental parasitization) are less severe. Most of the evidence that fertility is higher in heterozygotes comes from mesoendemic areas where adult immunity is lower and the benefits of inherited immunity are therefore more obvious. For example, among the Black Caribs of Belize (formerly British Honduras), an area of mesoendemic malaria, Firschein (1961:251) noted that women heterozygous for sickle hemoglobin had a fertility rate 1.45 times higher than women with normal hemoglobin.

Population immunity to malaria is not a constant. Although inherited immunity is unchangeable, acquired immunity (i.e., antibodies) may break down under certain conditions. If, for example, transmission should be interrupted for a period of time, acquired immunity will falter. Also, acquired immunity is so labile that certain conditions such as surgery (Spingarn and Edelman 1965:694) or concomitant infections such as measles and pneumonia or malnutrition (Lantum 1971:286) can cause a decline. Most important, pregnancy is often associated with a breakdown of acquired immunity to malaria (Lantum 1971:286; Lewis *et al.* 1973:698; Spingarn and Edelman 1965:694). The mechanism involved in the loss of immunity is not known (Voller 1974:182), but it has been observed that during pregnancy there is a dramatic increase in both parasite rates and densities (Lawson 1967d:60; Voller 1974:181–182). More pregnant women than nonpregnant women have attacks of malaria and these will be more severe (Lewis *et al.* 1973:698). Severe anemia can develop (Voller 1974:182) and the intermittent episodes of parasitemia that were hardly noticed before may be obvious febrile attacks similar to those experienced in childhood (Lawson 1967d:60). The breakdown of malaria immunity is most marked in first pregnancies (Hamilton *et al.* 1972:598; Lawson 1967d:60). Although the reason for this is not known, it is suspected that this is just a concomitant of age; younger women, who make up the majority of primigravidas, have lower immunity than do their older counterparts. It has also been observed that the pregnancy-associated breakdown in malaria immunity is more severe after the first trimester (Hamilton *et al.* 1972:598–599; Lawson 1967d:60); thus, accidents of pregnancy common to the last 6 months of gestation might be more frequently encountered.

The fact that acquired immunity breaks down during pregnancy makes any inherited immunity doubly important for the reproductive well-being of a population. Thus, if one area has holoendemic malaria and a high S gene frequency and a second area also has holoendemic malaria but a low S gene frequency, the effects of malaria on fecundity will probably be more severe in the latter. It is interesting to note that populations in West Africa, Cameroon, and the Congo (now Zaire) have holoendemic malaria and very low S gene frequencies (Livingstone 1971:37), and these are among the same areas noted by Belsey (1976:322) as being among the low-fertility regions of Africa.

But exactly what are the effects of malaria on reproductive potential and how are these effects altered by immunity, both acquired and inherited? The following section will explore the effects of malaria on coital ability, conceptive ability, and pregnancy loss and will attempt to show how immunity levels can alter these effects.

Effects on Fecundity

Coital Inability

Although one early researcher (Cilento 1928, cited in Scragg 1957:69) stated that malaria "has a markedly depressing effect on . . . potency," the pathophysiology of the disease does not suggest that coital ability should be affected. But surely the fevers and anemia associated with attacks of malaria drain the victim's strength and could result in a lower frequency of coitus. This would probably be true only for those persons with low levels of immunity, and would be especially important among nonimmunes during a malaria epidemic.

Conceptive Failure

Although some authors (e.g., Gallagher 1969:78; Siegler 1944:27) have reported that malaria causes infertility, the notion that conceptive ability in the male or female should be affected by malaria has generally been dismissed. Rather, any differentials in birthrates between areas of different malaria endemicity, or between immunes and nonimmunes in areas of similar endemicity, have almost always been ascribed to differences in rates of pregnancy loss, not conception rates. Some more recent studies have suggested, however, that malaria may impact substantially on conceptive ability.

Male

In 1941 MacLeod and Hotchkiss (1941, cited in Eaton and Mucha 1971:456) showed that if scrotal temperature exceeds 37°C (35°C is normal) for more than 45 minutes, azoospermia will result, followed by a recovery period of reduced sperm count (oligospermia) lasting for 2 months. Indeed, it is now recognized that a number of febrile illnesses—pneumonia, recurrent familial Mediterranean fever, mononucleosis, hepatitis, chicken pox—are associated with reduced sperm count (Amelar *et al.* 1977:71–72). Eaton and Mucha (1971:456) have shown that malaria can be included with these. They noted that even immune adults in hyperendemic areas suffer about two malaria attacks yearly, and because the fevers that accompany these attacks of malaria, though moderate, are still of sufficient height and duration to cause this effect (fevers often exceed 40°C and last 8 hours), the fertility of many men in these areas may be depressed for 2 to 4 months each year. The importance of this observation to population fertility is potentially great because oligospermia is, according to one author (Guest 1978:25), the most common cause of male infertility in Africa. In measuring sperm densities in an area of endemic malaria in Nigeria, Chukudebelu (1978:239) found that 55% of men tested had fewer than 20 million sperm/ml (i.e., oligospermic levels).

Not all adult men in hyperendemic areas are equally affected. The more immune, who are better able to limit parasitemia and therefore experience lower fevers, are less affected. For example, Eaton and Mucha suggested that men who are heterozygous for sickle-cell hemoglobin, because of their greater ability to limit parasitemia, are less likely to experience a fever-induced reduction in sperm count and hence are more fertile in malarious areas than men with normal hemoglobin. They proposed that this fertility differential between HbAS and HbAA men acts in tandem with the mortality differential in maintaining a high S gene frequency in malarious areas. Interestingly, Allard (1955, cited in Eaton and Mucha 1971:456) reported 15 years earlier that HbAS men in the Belgian Congo (now Zaire) had significantly higher fertility than their HbAA counterparts.

In areas of lower endemicity male fertility is probably also affected. Because transmission is less intense in a mesoendemic area, fewer adults are likely to suffer febrile episodes, but of those that do the lower immunity level of the average individual means that the fever will certainly be severe enough to lower sperm count. Even men heterozygous for sickle hemoglobin will probably not be able to hold fevers below that level capable of adversely affecting spermatogenesis.

The number of men in a given area whose fertility will be adversely affected depends, therefore, on two factors—the level of malaria endemicity in the area and the frequency of the *S* gene. Compare, for example, three areas: one holoendemic for malaria with a 40% *S* gene frequency, one holoendemic with a 15% *S* gene frequency, and one mesoendemic with a 15% *S* gene frequency. In the first holoendemic area, about 60% of the male population will experience fevers sufficiently high to alter spermatogenesis, and in the second holoendemic area about 85% will. In the mesoendemic area, despite higher fevers among infected persons and insufficient protection offered by sickle hemoglobin, certainly many fewer than 60% of males suffer malaria fevers each year and, therefore, the effect on male fertility is less than in either of the more endemic areas.

Female

Although it has been speculated that some women may be unable to conceive during an attack of malaria (Gray 1977:23), evidence for any direct role for malaria in female conceptive ability has not been forthcoming. However, two indirect roles for the disease have been proposed. First, malaria is an important cause of maternal anemia in the developing world, and puerperal sepsis with the possibility of subsequent sterility is much more frequent in anemic women (Lawson 1967a:86; Lewis *et al.* 1973:698). Second, in malarious areas a high fever in the postpartum period is too frequently ascribed to malaria when, in fact, it could be a symptom of puerperal sepsis. The use of antimalarials instead of antibiotics increases the chances that the infection will worsen and the new mother will be rendered sterile (Lawson 1967d:62).

Pregnancy Loss

The fever, anemia, and placental parasitization associated with malaria can all contribute to pregnancy loss. But, as previously emphasized, the immunity level of the population being studied must be known before the impact of these concomitants of infection can be assessed. And because *P. falciparum* malaria is associated with the highest fevers, the most severe anemia, and the highest rates of placental parasitization, populations affected by this species of malaria will be the most seriously affected by far.

Fever

It is known that in pregnant women high fevers, such as those associated with influenza, typhoid fever, pneumonia, and malaria, can cause spontaneous abortion, stillbirth, and premature birth. And maternal hyperpyrexia during the first trimester has been implicated in congenital anomalies, particularly facial and central nervous system abnormalities (Pleet *et al.* 1981:788, 786). Research has shown that *sustained* maternal temperature increases of 1.5 to 2.5°C can result in (1) spontaneous abortion due to increased uterine activity, fetal hypoxia, placental necrosis, or embryonic damage incompatible with life, or (2) birth of an infant with congenital abnormalities. The particular outcome depends on (1) the stage of gestation—early pregnancy is more sensitive to temperature variations, (2) the height of the fever—low fevers are more likely to result in deformed offspring and higher fevers in abortion, and (3) the duration of fever—prolonged temperature elevations of 1 or 2 days are generally believed to be necessary to cause adverse effects, although they have been noted following spikes of temperature caused by certain infections or by sauna bathing or hot tubs (Arora *et al.* 1979; Morishima *et al.* 1975; Pleet *et al.* 1981). One researcher (Edwards, personal communication, 1981) believes that embryonic or fetal death, followed by resorption or abortion, is probably more common than congenital malformation under natural (versus experimental) conditions, where temperature height and duration are not tightly controlled. This idea has been supported by a study by Clarren *et al.* (1979:81–82) in which only .3% of 55,000 women at midgestation reported a temperature ≥ 38.9°C. This is a very low incidence and the authors believe that many pregnant women with fevers never entered the study because their pregnancies were lost before midgestation. Because loss may occur very early in pregnancy with subsequent fetal resorption, some cases of pregnancy loss due to high fever undoubtedly go unnoticed.

Falciparum malaria, which is associated with the highest fevers of the four species of human malaria, is a widely cited cause of pregnancy loss (Lawson 1967d:63; Lewis *et al.* 1973:698; Monif 1974:194). (The fevers associated with *P. vivax* have also been noted to cause abortion and prematurity [A. Smith 1972:793].) Indeed, the low fertility observed in some areas has been attributed to interruption of pregnancy caused by malaria (Prothero 1972:106; Roberts 1965:4; Tabbarah 1971:267). And studies in the Sudan (Henin 1969, cited in Prothero 1972:106) and the Kalahari Desert region of Botswana (Dyson 1980:412) have suggested that the higher fertility of the settled versus the nomadic peoples of certain population groups is due to the fact that the nomads, exposed to many different strains of *P. falciparum*, are unable to produce protective levels of antibody to all these strains; therefore, they suffer higher levels of pregnancy loss than their settled counterparts who, exposed to only one or two strains of parasite, are able to produce protective antibody levels to the few local strains. And studies of fertility changes following eradication, though mixed (Gill 1940; Gray 1974), seem to indicate that malaria eradication does indeed lead to a rise in fertility (Langford 1981; Newman 1970).

Whether or not malaria is a cause of pregnancy loss in an area depends on the immunity level of the population. Fevers sufficiently high to precipitate an abortion or premature labor are uncommon in highly immune women, even during pregnancy (Lawson 1967d:63).[7] Thus, in holo- and hyperendemic areas malaria would not be an important cause of pregnancy loss, except in nomadic women who, as noted, rarely have protective levels of antibody to any of the many strains of parasite they encounter. However, in mesoendemic areas, where clinical illness is seen among adults, fevers sufficiently high to cause pregnancy loss would be more frequent. Firschein (1961:251) has further clarified the effect of malaria on pregnancy loss in his study of the Black Caribs of Belize. These people are biologically an African population with a high S gene frequency that has been transported to the New World. His data show that under the existing conditions of mesoendemic *P. falciparum* malaria in Belize, women heterozygous for sickle hemoglobin have a fertility rate 1.45 times that of normal homozygotes.

As would be expected, fertility differentials between heterozygous and homozygous women in highly endemic areas show only the smallest advantage, if any, for the heterozygote (Firschein 1961:250; Livingstone 1971:46). Thus, in areas of hyperendemic malaria population immunity is so high that even though immunity falters under the stress of pregnancy, it is still at a level that prevents the fevers of malaria from reaching a height sufficient to activate the uterus. In such areas, the extra protection against high parasitemia and high fevers offered by sickle hemoglobin is not necessary to prevent fetal loss. However, in mesoendemic areas, where average adult immunity is much lower, fevers capable of causing pregnancy loss do occur and under these conditions the extra protection offered by sickle hemoglobin is important in holding fevers below a critical level.

---

[7]It would be interesting to investigate whether the incidence of those congenital abnormalities associated with elevated maternal temperature is greater in these areas.

Anemia

Anemia is a common feature of *P. falciparum* malaria because red cell destruction is often so intense that although the body has the ability to replenish the red cell supply, it cannot do so quickly enough. In pregnant women this hemolytic anemia may be complicated by a second type of anemia, megaloblastic anemia, which is caused by a deficiency of folic acid (a nutrient essential to the manufacture of red blood cells). Pregnant women in malarious areas are particularly prone to this type of anemia because they must provide folic acid for the replenishment of destroyed adult red cells and for the development of fetal red cells (Lewis *et al.* 1973:698). In areas of West Africa the situation is particularly grave because the normal dietary sources of folic acid—fresh vegetables and meat—are subjected to prolonged cooking that destroys the folic acid (Lawson 1967c:77). But the problem of maternal anemia due to malaria is also common in central Africa (McFee 1973:167) and in many other malarious areas (Giglioli 1972:195; Harrison and Ibeziako 1973:799; Mati *et al.* 1971:3).

Fortunately, the use of antimalarial drugs is usually sufficient to resolve the anemia, although in some severe cases folic acid supplements must be given as well. But many women in developing countries do not receive prenatal care, and anemia, which usually appears after the 20th week of pregnancy (Lewis *et al.* 1973:698), may go untreated. Severe anemia, defined as a hemoglobin value of less than 45% or alternately of less than 6.5 gm of hemoglobin/100 cc of blood (Lawson 1967a:74), may develop in untreated cases and cause substantial fetal and maternal mortality (Lawson 1967d:61). Second trimester abortion, intrauterine death with a macerated stillbirth, and fresh stillbirth due to intrapartum asphyxia are all possible results of severe maternal anemia (Lawson 1967d:66; Lewis *et al.* 1973:698).

Immunity levels are important in determining whether or not severe anemia will develop, although the relationship between parasite density and level of anemia is not extremely strong (Lawson 1967d:61; Voller 1974:182), certainly not as strong as that between parasite density and level of fever. However, the fact that primigravidas in malarious areas are the most likely to develop anemia during pregnancy (Lawson 1967d:61; Reinhardt *et al.* 1978:83) indicates that immunity levels are important in limiting anemia. Also, Fleming *et al.* (1968, cited in Livingstone 1971:46) found that in malarious areas anemia in pregnancy was significantly less frequent in sicklers. Thus, women with high degrees of acquired and/or inherited immunity are less likely to suffer from severe anemia than are their less immune counterparts.

Placental Parasitization

Placental infection with malaria parasites is frequently seen in malarious areas and has been shown to be one of the main reasons for the low-birth-weight neonate so common in tropical areas. Some early researchers (e.g., Blacklock and Gordon 1925, cited in Macgregor and Avery 1974:436) felt that *P. falciparum* malaria infection of the placenta was a cause of abortion, stillbirth, and neonatal death. Clark (1915, cited in Macgregor and Avery 1974:436) noted, for example, that the rate of placental infection in normal deliveries was only 3%; in cases where the pregnancy ended as an abortion, stillbirth, or premature infant, this rate was 18%. Even some more recent reports (Lawson 1967d:65; Lewis *et al.* 1973:698; Spingarn and Edelman 1965:694) have noted that placental infection may cause intrauterine death with a macerated stillbirth or a fresh stillbirth due to intrapartum asphyxia. However, most researchers have generally discounted a significant role in pregnancy loss and have concentrated almost exclusively on the effects of placental parasitization on intrauterine growth retardation. Nevertheless, it does seem probable that in cases of heavy placental infection fetal loss could occur (Gray 1977:22).

Intrauterine Growth Retardation, Prematurity, and Perinatal Mortality

Placental Parasitization

Placental parasitization with *P. falciparum* has an extremely important influence on fetal well-being in tropical areas. First, it is a widespread problem; in Africa placental infection is present in an estimated 15 to 30% of all births (Llewellyn-Jones 1974:484). Second, it is well documented (Cannon 1958:877; Lawson 1967d:65; Lewis *et al.* 1973:698; Spitz 1959:242) that placental parasitization causes intrauterine growth retardation and thereby contributes to high perinatal mortality rates. Despite its overwhelming importance, there are still aspects of placental parasitization that are incompletely understood, such as who is most likely affected and why. These topics will be discussed and an attempt made to reconcile some conflicting points of view.

As mentioned earlier, *P. falciparum*, because of its unique life cycle, is the species of *Plasmodium* most often found in placental tissue, although the other three species are occasionally observed there also. Placental parasitization is usually seen in the second half of pregnancy (Lawson 1967d:63; Lewis *et al.* 1973:698; Macgregor and Avery 1974:434), so any adverse effects on pregnancy are effectively limited to this period. Microscopic observation reveals placental villi packed not only with parasites and parasitized red cells, but also with host defender cells (i.e., macrophages). The latter may form an almost solid mass of cells, prompting observers to question how the fetus can be nourished at all.

Unlike the fevers and anemia associated with malaria, placental parasitization is believed rare in susceptible nonimmunes although it is common in women with well-developed immunity (Lawson 1967d:63). But within the group of immune women, those with the lowest level of immunity (i.e., primigravidas) have the highest frequency of placental involvement (Cannon 1958:878; Lawson 1967d:63; Reinhardt *et al.* 1978:82). It is difficult to reconcile these two apparently contradictory observations. And, certainly, parasites are present in the placentas of a fair number of nonimmunes; the presence of congenital malaria in 1 to 4% of their offspring attests to that (Reinhardt *et al.* 1978:81). Perhaps if more nonimmune women were examined for placental parasitization—we have not seen a study on this yet, just the statement that it is rare in such women—this seemingly paradoxical situation could be resolved.

Nevertheless, for immune women in hyperendemic areas data supporting a negative correlation between the level of immunity and the rate of placental parasitization are very persuasive. Using parity as a proxy for age and therefore for immunity, these data show that as parity increases the frequency of placental parasitization decreases. Summary figures from three African studies show that whereas 37% of parity 1 women had infected placentas, only 23% of parity 2 and 15% of parity 3 were so affected (Morley *et al.* 1964:668). Thus, the older, higher parity woman who has acquired a greater degree of immunity is, according to these data, more able to prevent parasitemia in placental blood.[8]

At first glance, the presence of malaria parasites in the placenta would seem to pose a significant threat of transplacental passage and subsequent congenital infection. Transplacental passage, as determined at birth by parasites in umbilical cord blood, is a frequent occurrence in

[8]Some authors believe there is little (e.g., E. Jelliffe 1967:20) or no (e.g., Macgregor and Avery 1974:436) correlation between peripheral parasitemia and placental parasitemia and that examining the peripheral blood for parasites will offer few clues as to whether or not the placenta is infected. Other authors (e.g., Logie *et al.* 1973:549; Spitz 1959:242) suggest there is a correlation by showing that in a study population rates of peripheral and placental parasitemia are roughly the same. Unfortunately, they fail to say how many women actually had both peripheral and placental parasitization. However, the observations of Reinhardt *et al.* (1978:82) that rates of peripheral and placental infection fall in tandem with increasing parity imply that the two are inextricably related. Thus, it should be possible to identify most women who are at risk of having placental malaria by checking their peripheral blood for parasites.

placental malaria, according to Reinhardt *et al.* (1978:81). Their data show that in 20 to 60% of cases of placental parasitemia, the cord blood also contains parasites. It may be that this very high rate reflects damage to the placenta during delivery, or it could reflect actual penetration of the placental villi by the parasites. Generally, it is thought that the parasites do enter the fetal circulation during gestation but that no infection results because the fetus is protected by maternal antibodies (Logie *et al.* 1973:547, 553; Reinhardt *et al.* 1978:81). For this reason, congenital malaria is rare—about .03% of all births—in hyperendemic areas, despite a very high frequency of placental malaria (Cannon 1958:878; Logie *et al.* 1973:547; Reinhardt *et al.* 1978:81: Spingarn and Edelman 1965:694; Spitz 1959:244). The fetus of a nonimmune mother is left unprotected, however, and congenital malaria among these infants occurs in 1 to 4% of all such births (Reinhardt *et al.* 1978:81; Spingarn and Edelman 1965:694).

Although congenital malaria is not a threat to the offspring of highly immune women, intrauterine growth retardation due to the physical interference by parasites and macrophages with placental function poses grave danger to fetal well-being. The major observation has been that infants born to mothers with placental malaria have a lower average birth weight than infants born to mothers with uninfected placentas. In various studies in Africa the birth weights of infants born with infected placentas were anywhere from 114 to 312 gm lower than those of infants with uninfected placentas (Cannon 1958:877). Both mosquito eradication programs and the use of antimalarial drugs have proved useful in raising birth weights. A study by Macgregor and Avery (1974:435) showed that malaria eradication in the British Solomon Islands resulted in a 165 gm increase in the average infant birth weight. And in an area of southern Nigeria where there is holoendemic *P. falciparum* malaria, women who took malaria suppressive drugs during pregnancy gave birth to babies weighing 156 gm more than did women who were untreated (Morley *et al.* 1964:668).

Not infrequently the infant birth weight is 2500 gm or less and thus the infant is, according to WHO standards, classifiable as premature. Using this criterion 27% of newborns in eastern Nigeria with uninfected placentas were premature, whereas 41% of those with infected placentas could be so classified (Spitz 1959:242). In western Nigeria, Cannon (1958:877) reported that 12% in the uninfected group and 37% in the infected group were premature. However, both researchers argued that not all such babies are truly premature, that is, expelled from the uterus before the end of the normal gestation period. The WHO standard is an international one; although an infant weighing 2500 gm in England, where the average is about 3200 gm, would quite likely be gestationally premature, one in Nigeria, where the average is only 2800 gm, may very well be full term. And because most African women have no record of their last menstrual period there is no way for the physician to determine accurately the length of gestation. Thus, it is best not to use the term *premature* to describe the major effect of placental parasitization. Most discussions in the literature use the term *low birth weight,* but this term is too nonspecific; a premature infant, for example, can be described as being low birth weight. The best term to describe the effect of placental parasitization on the fetus is *intrauterine growth retardation.* It does not suggest that the baby was prematurely expelled from the uterus or suggest that the child is small (low birth weight) without telling why. It does indicate, however, that the infant is probably full term but is small because intrauterine growth was retarded.

The problem of intrauterine growth retardation should not be underestimated. In the studies cited earlier, as many as 30% of all births were affected by placental malaria. These births are characterized by intrauterine growth retardation, which in about 40% of cases is so severe that the newborn weighs less than 2500 gm. Intrauterine growth retardation poses particular hazards for the newborn, especially in tropical areas where there are so many endemic diseases. Cannon (1958:877) noted, for example, that the neonatal period is particularly hazardous for the Nigerian infant born with an infected placenta: Mortality in the first week of life is twice that for an infant born with an uninfected placenta. This relative disadvantage may persist for some time, making placental malaria a major contributor to the high infant mortality rates present in developing countries. However, in some cases the smallness of the baby may actually increase its chances for survival. This occurs when the mother's pelvis is so small because of prior nutritional deficiencies that serious mechanical difficulties during labor are anticipated. In fact, contracted pelvis is so common in tropical areas that there were some misgivings about whether or not the control of malaria would result in more or less perinatal mortality. But it was concluded that "despite the problem which cephalo-pelvic disproportion poses in many African communities most tropical obstetricians would appear to agree that anti-malarial drugs would prove beneficial" (E. Jelliffe 1967:34).

As discussed earlier, primigravidas, because of their lower immunity levels, are the most frequently affected by placental malaria. But do their lower immunity levels mean that parasite densities within the placenta are higher as well, indicating a more serious effect on fetal outcome? Probably not. Because parasite densities within the placenta are generally much higher than would be anticipated merely from retreat from the peripheral circulation, it seems that parasites within the placenta are so little affected by circulating antibodies[9] that the placenta has been called an "immunologically protected site" (Voller 1974:182). Thus, despite their lower antibody levels primigravidas should experience parasite densities within the placental villi that are no higher than those of more immune multigravidas. Intrauterine growth retardation secondary to placental parasitization should, therefore, occur more frequently in primigravidas but should be no more severe.

But what about women who are more immune to malaria because they are heterozygous for sickle hemoglobin? How will placental parasite rates and densities differ between these women and less immune homozygotes? This situation is quite different because the protection against malaria conferred by the HbAS genotype is not dependent on circulating antibodies but is a characteristic of the red blood cell. Although the HbAS red cell is about equally as well penetrated by the malaria parasite as is the HbAA red cell, *P. falciparum* growth and multiplication (schizogony) is much reduced in the former when the cell experiences lower oxygen tensions as it retreats from the peripheral circulation to the internal organs, including the placenta. Indeed, the entire malaria hypothesis rests not on lower frequencies of infection in the heterozygote but on lower parasite densities because *P. falciparum* schizogony is truncated. Thus, because frequency of infection does not differ significantly between the HbAS and HbAA genotypes, it would be expected that frequency of placental parasitization also does not differ. Indeed, two studies (Cannon 1958:877; E. Jelliffe 1967:37) showed that the frequency of placental parasitization differs little between sicklers and nonsicklers. However, the unique ability of the HbAS genotype to limit parasite growth and multiplication within the placenta means that parasite densities should be lower in the heterozygote and that subsequent intrauterine growth retardation should be less severe. Hamilton *et al.* (1972:600) disputed this hypothesis; they found no difference in the outcome of pregnancy, the baby's weight, or other important factors between sicklers and nonsicklers in a malarious area. But another study by Edington (1955, cited in Livingstone 1957:762) noted a more favorable pregnancy outcome and higher birth rates among sicklers. Whether heterozygotes are less severely affected by placental malaria will remain conjecture, however, until parasite densities are included with parasite rates as a routine part of investigations of placental parasitization.

[9]Significant amounts of antibody do reach and circulate within the placenta, however, as evidenced by maternal antibodies in fetal blood.

Anemia

Severe maternal anemia, already mentioned as a cause of pregnancy loss during the second half of gestation, has also been linked to an increase in premature babies and a rise in perinatal mortality. Lawson (1967a:86) noted that 20% of infants born to women with severe anemia were premature as opposed to only 7% born to control women, and perinatal mortality rates were doubled if the mother was severely anemic. Less severe anemia may, on the other hand, be an important cause of intrauterine growth retardation. Because maternal anemia and placental parasitization often coexist (E. Jelliffe 1967:30), Harrison (1974:229) speculated that many cases of intrauterine growth retardation may be blamed on placental parasitization when anemia may actually be at fault. In his study in Nigeria, Harrison noted that whereas 53% of anemic women gave birth to intrauterine-growth-retarded infants, only 35% of matched nonanemic women did so. Other studies (e.g., E. Jelliffe 1967:37) have also noted an association between maternal anemia and subsequent delivery of an intrauterine growth retarded infant. It is quite likely that intrauterine growth retardation is caused by maternal anemia as well as placental parasitization, and that those most severely affected with either or both of these concomitants of malaria infection will experience the most marked intrauterine growth retardation.

Fever

The ability of malarial fevers to cause fetal loss has already been extensively discussed in the section "Pregnancy Loss." If the malaria attack occurs late in pregnancy the child may be born alive. Thus, the fevers associated with malaria may be an important cause of prematurity, especially when immunity levels are low.

Summary

The preceding discussion makes clear that malaria, most especially *P. falciparum* malaria, has the potential to depress fecundity severely. The fevers, anemia, and placental parasitization that are concomitants of the disease may cause temporary azoospermia and oligospermia as well as abortion and stillbirth. Malaria may also affect fertility by lowering coital frequency. It also contributes to neonatal mortality through an increased number of premature births and intrauterine growth retarded infants. Considering the very high prevalence the disease can reach, even a modest effect on individual fertility translates into a significant demographic impact (Gray 1977:23).

Whether or not malaria will have a substantial impact on the fecundity or fertility of any given population depends on two factors: the species of malaria and the level of acquired and inherited immunity in the population. *Plasmodium falciparum* malaria is associated with the highest fevers, the most severe anemia, and the highest rates of placental parasitization, so unfavorable effects are most likely in areas where this species of malaria is present. Because acquired and inherited immunity can limit fevers, anemia, and placental parasitization, the immunity level of a population must also be known before the effects of the disease can be assessed.

The fevers associated with malaria have the most varied effect on human fecundity. Although they do not affect coital ability, the severe episodes of fever seen in poorly immune or nonimmune persons are debilitating and can certainly lower coital frequency. Spermatogenesis may be impaired by only moderate elevations in body temperature, so even the fertility of immune men in hyperendemic areas may be affected. But adult males in such areas who are sicklers experience somewhat lower fevers and are thus spared this assault on their fertility. In mesoendemic areas adult fevers are quite high, and male fertility is undoubtedly affected in those men who suffer malaria attacks whether or not they possess sickle hemoglobin.

A fever must be quite high to be capable of causing pregnancy loss. Such fever levels are common in women in mesoendemic areas but are not reached by women from highly endemic areas, even under the stress of pregnancy. Sicklers in mesoendemic areas, however, have lower fevers than nonsicklers and are therefore more able to complete their pregnancies successfully. Thus, among a people living in one mesoendemic area, the fertility of HbAS women was 1.45 times that of HbAA women (Firschein 1961:251).

Severe maternal anemia is associated with fetal loss in the second half of pregnancy and with increased rates of prematurity and perinatal mortality; less severe anemia may have a role in causing intrauterine growth retardation. Whether or not anemia will develop in a woman from a malarious area and the severity of the anemia depend, again, on immunity levels. Primigravidas, who have lower levels of acquired immunity than older multigravidas, are more likely to develop anemia. Sicklers, on the other hand, are less likely to be anemic.

Placental parasitization is the concomitant of malaria infection that has received the most attention. Heavy infections may result in fetal loss during the second half of pregnancy. Most emphasis has been, however, on its role in intrauterine growth retardation, with the threat this poses to infant survival. The relationship between immunity and placental parasitization remains somewhat confusing. In contrast to malarial fevers and anemia, which are most common in nonimmunes, placental parasitization is stated to be rare in nonimmunes. It is common, however, in immune women; the least immune among these, the primigravidas, are the most often affected whereas the more immune multigravidas are much less often affected. We have hypothesized that because the placenta is an immunologically privileged site the severity of infection is not altered by antibody levels and, therefore, placental densities should be comparable in primi- and multigravidas. However, we feel that sicklers, though as frequently infected as nonsicklers, are better able to limit placental parasite densities because their red cells are less able to support parasite growth in the placenta. As yet there is no hard evidence to support or refute this hypothesis.

Diagnosis, Treatment, and Control

Although malaria can often be diagnosed on the basis of the characteristic periodic attacks of fevers, chills, and sweating, blood films are used to confirm the diagnosis and identify the species of parasite. A thin film of peripheral blood is normally used to identify the species of parasite, and thick blood films will determine parasite densities (Hall 1976:323).

Once a positive diagnosis is made and the species of parasite is known, the physician can employ any one of a number of antimalarial drugs. Properly used, these drugs can eradicate the infection. The patient may then use these same drugs on a routine basis to prevent subsequent infection.

The first effective antimalarial drugs were obtained from the bark of the *Cinchona* tree. This class of drugs includes quinine and related substances, and since 1640 they have been used against the erythrocytic stage of the disease. In the 1920s and during World War II new synthetic drugs were introduced including chloroquine, amodiaquin, and primaquine (Jones 1967:19–20). Some of these drugs (e.g., primaquine) are effective against the exo-erythrocytic stage of malaria and are, therefore, particularly important in preventing relapses from *P. vivax*, *P. malariae*, and *P. ovale* infections (Monif 1974:195).

Unfortunately, many parasites have developed drug-resistant

strains and these may be expected to become more numerous. *Plasmodium falciparum* strains in Southeast Asia and Central and South America are already resistant to chloroquine and amodiaquin (Peters 1977:1261). Although Africa was reported to be untouched by this problem, several *P. falciparum* infections with a low level of resistance to chloroquine have been confirmed in east Africa, and in time widespread chloroquine resistance will become a major problem there also (*Lancet* 1979:1329).

Many antimalarials have the disadvantage of being toxic, and this is particularly true with regard to the fetus. Chloroquine, the most widely used and effective of all the antimalarials, may cause serious eye, ear, and central nervous system defects in the offspring of pregnant women (Lewis *et al.* 1973:699). Quinine, which has been increasingly relied upon in recent years because of the proliferation of chloroquine-resistant parasite strains, is extremely dangerous to the fetus. Fetal death following its use has been reported (Hall 1976:326; A. Smith 1972:793) and may be the basis of reports (see Hansluwka 1975:206) that extensive use has been shown to have a depressing effect on fecundity.

The world economic situation, the lack of funding for malaria research, the cost and problems associated with the application of DDT, mosquito resistance to insecticides, the irregular application of antimalarial drugs, and the development of drug-resistant parasites are all responsible for the resurgence of the disease. Some researchers believe that an immunological solution is necessary because neither insecticides nor antimalarial drugs will be sufficient to control, much less eradicate, the mosquitoes and parasites now present. A vaccine effective against malaria is the best hope for elimination of the disease and some developments have brought that hope ever closer to reality. The first step was taken when scientists at Rockefeller University grew *P. falciparum* in tissue culture, thus providing a large amount of material potentially suitable for vaccine production (Auerbach 1976:A9). Subsequent work by Reese *et al.* (1978:5668) has demonstrated that the parasite material obtained from this in vitro cultivation can induce protective immunity in monkeys. And workers at the University of Hawaii Medical School have a vaccine prepared against *P. falciparum* ready for trial on humans (Nelson 1978:1, 2). It is hoped that a safe and effective vaccine will emerge from this research that will place malaria alongside smallpox, a deadly disease made extinct.

CHAPTER 5

Filariasis

Introduction

Several parasitic worms of the superfamily Filarioidea may infect humans. The more medically important of these are *Loa loa*, also known as the West African eye worm, *Onchocerca volvulus*, which causes the dreaded "river blindness," and *Wuchereria bancrofti*, *Brugia malayi*, and *B. timor*, which cause systemic disease and have elephantiasis as their most remarkable symptom.

Wuchereria bancrofti and *B. malayi* have attracted the most attention largely because of the grotesque appearance of those sufferers who develop elephantiasis and whose limbs or genitals are therefore grossly enlarged and covered by a thick elephantlike skin. As early as 1500 B.C. elephantiasis was graphically depicted by the Egyptians, and in A.D. 1 Greco–Roman authors described elephantiasis and other sequelae of filarial infection (Schacher and Sahyoun 1967:234). Until the 1940s, consideration of filariasis in the temperate zone was confined to an occasional picture of elephantiasis in a textbook on tropical medicine. Filariasis was viewed as an exotic disease and was of only casual interest to those not living in endemic areas. This attitude changed abruptly in the 1940s when a large percentage of U.S. troops stationed in the Pacific became infected with *W. bancrofti* and feared they might develop elephantiasis.

The focus of this chapter is on *W. bancrofti* because many of the lesions associated with this type of filariasis affect the genitals. Although *B. malayi* causes a disease fundamentally similar to Bancroftian filariasis, the genitals are rarely involved. For example, whereas *W. bancrofti* causes elephantiasis of the genitals and limbs, *B. malayi* typically causes elephantiasis of the limbs only (Hunter *et al.* 1976:506). And hydrocele, a condition in which fluid collects in the membranous sac that envelops the testes, is common in Bancroftian filariasis but rare in Malayan (Edeson 1972:62; World Health Organization 1967:10). Other filarial parasites such as *L. loa* and *O. volvulus* may cause genital abnormalities (Gratama 1966:32, 34; 1969b:265; Hunter *et al.* 1976:512), but these occur in only a small minority of infected persons and are not interesting at the population level. In all, filariasis, especially Bancroftian filariasis, is one of the major diseases of the developing world (Nelson 1979:1136), and its ability to cause genital abnormalities has prompted the World Health Organization (WHO) (1974b:22) to urge research into the impact on fertility of this disease.

Life Cycle

The life cycle of filariasis has particular importance to tropical medicine because this branch of medicine emerged as a distinct discipline when Patrick Manson discovered in 1877 that the parasite that causes elephantiasis in humans is transmitted by mosquitoes (Nelson 1979:1136). The life cycle of the filarial parasite was understood by the first part of the twentieth century.

Development of the parasite in the vector begins when a suitable mosquito takes a blood meal from an infected individual whose blood contains prelarval parasite forms called microfilariae. These microfilariae penetrate the insect's stomach wall and lodge in the thoracic muscles where they undergo molting as they develop into first-stage, second-stage, and then third-stage larvae. The third-stage larvae migrate to the proboscis and penetrate the skin of the host when the mosquito takes another blood meal.

The first stages of development in the human host are not clearly defined, but studies suggest that the third-stage (infective) larvae enter the lymphatics at the site of inoculation and within 5 to 18 months develop into mature filiform worms 19–60 mm in length. If a male and female worm are present in the same place at the same time, mating may occur with the production of offspring (i.e., microfilariae). At the lymph nodes, where lymph and blood vessels converge, the microfilariae can move from the lymph into the blood and are thereafter detectable in the general circulation. Although their life span is only several months (Brown 1975:143), microfilariae may be found in the blood several years after the infective bite because the adult worms may live and reproduce for more than 20 years.

An interesting feature of microfilariae is their periodicity. During certain periods of the day large numbers of microfilariae appear in the circulation, but at other times their numbers there are low. Nocturnal periodicity is the most common case, and that of *W. bancrofti*. During the day when the host is active the parasites lodge in the lung, but during the evening, at times of rest, they can be found in the general circulation—sometimes in huge numbers. Thus, from 10 P.M. to 4 A.M. chances are greatest of finding microfilariae of *W. bancrofti* in the blood. This periodicity corresponds to the biting time of the mosquito vector, and this inborn rhythm is therefore an evolutionary adaptation that ensures parasite survival.

Prevalence

Although prevalence estimates vary considerably, it is likely that more than 300 million people are infected with filarial parasites and that two-thirds of these are infected with *W. bancrofti* or *B. malayi* (World Health Organization 1974b:6, 1981:87; Schultz 1977:1260). Some estimates (e.g., Grove *et al.* 1978:975) have placed the number infected with *W. bancrofti* at 250 million, making this disease one of the major diseases of the developing world. *Wuchereria bancrofti* is widespread throughout the tropical and subtropical world; it is found in tropical Africa, Southeast Asia, China, Korea, the southwestern Pacific Islands, eastern South America, Central America, the Caribbean area, and on the Indian subcontinent (see Figure 5.1).

The prevalence of the disease within these areas differs. In the Americas, for example, the prevalence of *W. bancrofti* is much lower than in many populous areas of Africa and Asia (Hawking 1975:16). But the situation is not a static one and filariasis appears to be on the increase in many endemic areas; the population at risk doubled in the period between 1960 and 1970 (World Health Organization 1974b:8). The increase is primarily the result of a population explosion in areas where the disease is endemic (Nelson 1979:1136), but several other factors play a role. Population mobility is important, and with the increased mobility of people throughout the world, infected individuals may now appear in any country (Iturregui-Pagan *et al.* 1976:207). Indeed, the disease was brought to the Americas by the slave trade from West Africa (Beaver 1970:181; Hawking 1975:16). This spread is further facilitated by the fact that those species of mosquito that carry the disease—*Anopheles*, *Aedes*, and *Culex*—are distributed throughout the world. And the numbers of

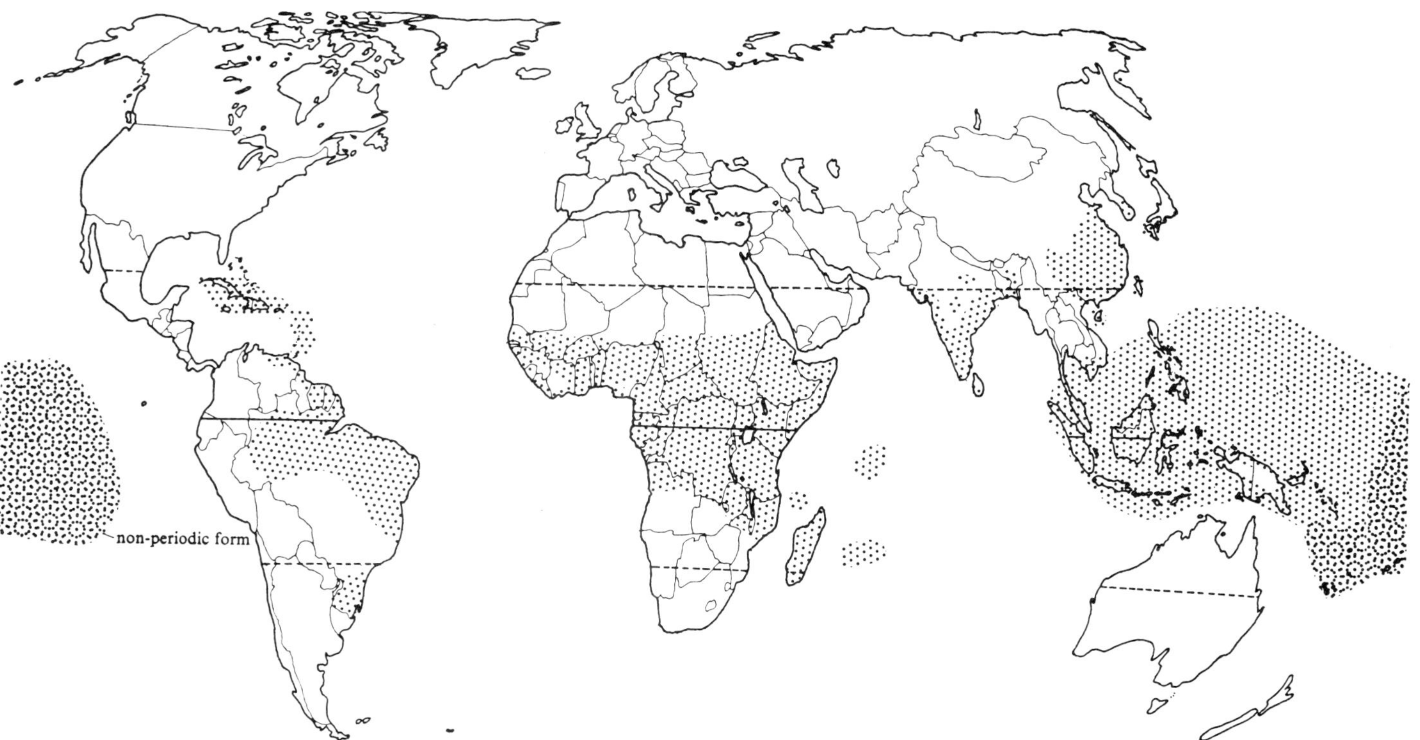

Figure 5.1 Global distribution of Bancroftian filariasis. Source: Muller 1975:95.

these vectors is increasing in the developing world. The *Anopheles* mosquito has found new breeding areas in waters dammed for irrigation or hydroelectric projects and also in the pools and streams of areas deforested for agricultural purposes. The *Culex* mosquito thrives in septic tanks and pit latrines that, ironically, were built at the urging of health officials to control intestinal parasites (World Health Organization 1974b:8–9). Filariasis may be a serious problem in any area that fulfills the two requirements for high prevalence: a large reservoir of infected persons and abundant vector breeding. These requirements are most often met in developing countries where there is a heavy population density and inadequate sanitation favoring mosquito breeding. This is particularly true in areas undergoing rapid urbanization (C. Smith 1972:4;World Health Organization 1974b:8).

Although filariasis is definitely on the upswing, some of the "new" foci of filariasis are not new at all but have been newly discovered because of improved diagnostic techniques and increased awareness of the clinical signs of the disease (World Health Organization 1974b:9). The membrane filtration technique that concentrates microfilariae in a blood sample is much more sensitive than the older blood smear method for detecting persons with patent infections, and is particularly useful when parasite densities are low (i.e., among children and treated adults) (World Health Organization 1974b:23). By using the filtration technique very high infection rates have been noted in communities where there were no previous records of filariasis (Nelson 1979:1137). In addition, local physicians are becoming increasingly aware that many of their patients are suffering from filariasis. Nevertheless, reports still appear indicating that many tropical physicians do not recognize that many of the disorders they are treating have a filarial origin (Nelson 1979:1136; Spencer 1974:26). One research team (Satti and Abdel Nur 1974:314–315) was told by local Sudanese physicians that filariasis was never found in the area, yet they found evidence of infection in about 25% of the population.

Proposed Effects of Filariasis
on Fecundity

Filariasis is suspected of being able to influence population fecundity for two reasons: (1) Hundreds of millions of persons are affected and (2) the genitals are often the site of filarial lesions. Remarkably, however, the impact of filariasis on population fecundity has been virtually ignored in the demographic literature. Two notable exceptions are Caldwell (1981:109), who believed it may be important in parts of Africa, and

Allman and May (1979), who contended it may help explain the unexpectedly moderate fertility in Haiti.

The details of filarial infection will be discussed later. But it is useful here to discuss briefly the nature of Bancroftian filariasis, specifically as it affects the genitals, to illustrate at the outset why it should be studied as a potential population subfecundity factor.

The lesions associated with filariasis arise in the lymph vessels (and perhaps nodes) where the adult worms spend their lives. The disease is potentially important to human reproductive ability because the worms are frequently found in the lymph vessels that drain the male and female genital tissues and, according to some reports (Reddy *et al.* 1974:494; Wartman 1947:374), in the lymph vessels lying within the genital tissues themselves. Specifically, the lymphatics of the scrotum, penis, testes, epididymis, and spermatic cord of the male, and the vulva, broad ligament, ovary, fallopian tube, and uterus of the female are affected. The worms elicit an immune response; in hypersensitive individuals this may be quite severe, causing an inflammatory reaction in the lymph vessel often accompanied by local heat, redness, swelling, tenderness, and pain and perhaps by constitutional symptoms such as fever and malaise. This is the acute, inflammatory, or early stage of Bancroftian filariasis, and repeated attacks are common. With each attack the lymph vessel is progressively damaged; the vessel becomes dilated, its walls thicken, its valves become damaged, and lymph drainage slows. Eventually, the vessel becomes obstructed by fibrosis and thus lymph drainage stops with resulting permanent accumulations of fluid in surrounding tissue. This is the chronic, obstructive, or late stage of filariasis.

How might fecundity be altered by Bancroftian filariasis? Because the clinical manifestations of the infection do involve the genitals, the disease is presumed to interfere with reproduction (Ayres *et al.* 1976:105). The World Health Organization (1974b:22) has therefore suggested that studies of the effects of filariasis include the patient's reproductive history. Although some authors (e.g., Adadevoh 1974:18) have felt that no definite correlation has been established between filariasis and male infertility, others believe that such a correlation exists (Belsey 1977:12) and some, in fact, have contended that filariasis is the most important cause of male infertility in the tropics (Guest 1978:27). Still others (e.g., Spingarn and Edelman 1965:709), although agreeing that filariasis can cause male, and female, reproductive failure, have felt that the effect is not great enough to be reflected in birthrates. It has been noted, however, that pockets of low fertility often correspond to areas endemic for filariasis (Belsey 1976:333).

What conditions associated with acute filariasis might alter fecundity? One researcher (Spencer 1974:30) claimed that in women bacterial infection secondary to acute pelvic lymphatic filariasis is an important cause of pelvic inflammatory disease (PID). And it is possible that the fevers seen during acute attacks could cause some pregnancy wastage and, even more likely, could interfere with spermatogenesis and cause temporary male infertility (see Eaton and Mucha 1971:456). But it is the chronic stage of filariasis that is most often associated with reproductive dysfunction. Lymph may accumulate in the penis and scrotum of the male and the vulva of the female resulting in genital elephantiasis. In severe cases coitus may be impossible (Lawson 1967b:466; Spingarn and Edelman 1965:709). A hydrocele may also reach a size that makes coitus impossible, though this is rare. More frequently these hydroceles are much smaller; nevertheless, testicular atrophy may be associated with their presence (Spingarn and Edelman 1965:709). Filarial infection may also be associated with the formation of dilated, tortuous veins in the scrotum, a condition called varicocele (Sanjurjo 1970:492), and this too may be a cause of infertility. Also, chronic obstruction of the lymph drainage of the ovaries and fallopian tubes has been mentioned as a cause of dysmenorrhea and sterility (Bloomfield *et al.* 1978:598; Spingarn and Edelman 1965:709). Finally, Nasah and Cox (1978:225ff.) have suggested an association among filariasis, stenotic and obliterative lesions of the testicular blood vessels, and degenerative changes in the seminiferous tubules resulting in oligospermia and azoospermia. In their study of testicular biopsy material from oligospermic men in Cameroon, Nasah and Cox noted ''fibrinoid'' deposits in the small and medium-sized vessels of the testes. The lesions, by diminishing or blocking blood flow in the testis, could have caused the severe degenerative lesions that were noted in the seminiferous tubules (site of sperm production). A number of tests suggested that the vascular lesions were due to the deposition of immune complexes, perhaps from a parasitic infection, on the walls of the vessels. Although the authors found parasitological evidence of genital filariasis in very few of these men, there was evidence in a fair number of late sequelae of filarial infection such as hydrocele or a thickened tunica. Unfortunately the study did not investigate fertile men in the endemic area for similar vascular changes.[1]

Are the lesions associated with acute and chronic filariasis truly ca-

---

[1]A possible correlate to the work of Nasah and Cox (1978) is that of Alexander and of Clarkson in the United States, which suggested, based on experimental work in monkeys, that vasectomized men are more likely to develop artherosclerosis because trapped sperm leak into the bloodstream, eliciting an immune response; the resulting immune complexes injure the artery wall, accelerating the formation of artherosclerotic plaques (*Time* 1981b:63).

pable of causing these (and other) adverse effects on fecundity? If so, who is at risk of suffering such effects? These questions can only be answered by studying the pathophysiology of the disease and examining data collected from areas where filariasis is endemic.

Pathophysiology

The pathophysiology of filariasis is difficult to discuss definitively; as Beaver (1970:187) put it, "From the standpoint of either the biology of the worm or the pathogenesis of the disease, filariasis is probably the least well understood of all the helminthic [worm] infections of medical interest." Denham and Nelson (1976:116) also noted that the pathophysiology of filariasis is especially complicated, and in their review of the subject (1976:116ff) cited the many conflicting hypotheses concerning the genesis of lymphatic lesions. Hence, the exact causes of the early and late lesions, the frequency with which they occur, the reason some individuals are severely affected, some moderately so, and others not at all, and the reason there are variations in clinical manifestations according to geography, sex, socioeconomic status are among the many problems that have not been conclusively resolved. And, most importantly for this discussion, the effects of early and late genital lesions on reproductive potential await clarification. Nevertheless, by analyzing the available data we can draw some conclusions about the potential for this widespread infection to alter individual and population fecundity.

Lymph Supply to the Genital Organs

The human lymphatic system consists of small capillaries that reach into almost every part of the body and larger vessels that connect the capillary beds to the lymph nodes. Degenerating cells and particulate matter from the tissues are carried by the capillaries and vessels to the nodes where the debris is filtered out (Copenhaver 1964:539). Various other substances—normal and abnormal, as in the case of local infection—are removed by the lymph system (Schacher and Sahyoun 1967:241).

The female genital tract is well supplied with lymph vessels. The uterus is particularly well supplied; the lymph vessels are larger and more abundant than in most other organs, probably to drain away the large amounts of water and other substances associated with cyclical changes in the endometrium. All layers of the uterus are laced with lymph vessels except the superficial layer of the endometrium (Copenhaver 1964:539). Lymph vessels are also found in several layers of the fallopian tubes, arising as large vessels in the mucosal folds that line the lumen (Copenhaver 1964:530). The lymph vessels of the internal female genitals—broad ligament, ovary, fallopian tube, uterus—empty into the lumbar lymph nodes (Copenhaver 1964:528, 530), and those that supply the external genitals, specifically the vulva, empty into the inguinal lymph nodes (Lawson 1967b:467).

The male genitals are also well supplied with lymph vessels. In the testis, lymph vessels arise in the interstitial tissue surrounding the tubules where spermatogenesis takes place (Copenhaver 1964:498). The lymphatics of the testis, epididymis, spermatic cord, and tunica vaginalis (the sac enveloping the front and lateral aspects of the testis) all drain into the pre-aortic and juxta-aortic lymph nodes (Lich and Howerton 1970:34; Sanjurjo 1970:491). The lymphatics of the scrotum and penis, like those of the vulva, drain into the inguinal nodes (Lawson 1967b:467).

The developing and adult worms spend their entire lives in the human lymphatic system. Many authors (e.g., Gratama 1969b:256; Jones 1967:187; Lawson 1967b:468) have stated that the worms live in both the vessels and the nodes; others (e.g., Nelson 1979:1136) have claimed it is the lymph vessels that are mainly involved. In either case, worms are frequently found in the lymphatics that drain the genitals.

Response to the Worms

When the filarial parasites enter the human lymphatic system they are infective third-stage larvae. In the host lymphatics they must undergo two molts before becoming adult worms capable of mating and producing microfilariae. Many researchers believe that only adult worms are capable of eliciting a significant immune response in the host and that dead worms may cause a far more serious reaction than live ones. Others believe that pre-adult as well as adult worms can cause a reaction. And the animal studies of Schacher and Sahyoun (1967:241) have suggested that even more factors are involved, to varying degrees. They stated that living and dead third- and fourth-stage larvae, their molting fluids and the cuticles they cast, as well as living and dead adult worms and by-products of reproduction such as uterine mucus and infertile eggs have, as foreign bodies, the potential to elicit an immune response in the host. Only the microfilariae are thought to be normally nonpath-ogenic.[2]

Although much is still unknown about the pathological changes that occur in the lymphatics, the animal studies of Schacher and Sahyoun (1967:241) have done much to clarify the causes and development of lesions in the lymph system. They attribute the variability in observed lesions to differences in the underlying cause (e.g., dead or live worms) and differences in duration. In general, the initial reaction to a live worm is an inflammation of the lymph vessel (lymphangitis) and surrounding tissue. The valves in the lymph vessel are thereby damaged, causing a back flow of lymph and dilatation of the vessel. Lymph fluid and blood plasma leak into the surrounding tissue causing local edema. When the worm dies an even more severe reaction occurs. A granuloma forms around the dead worm, partially or completely obstructing the lumen of the vessel. Eventually the granuloma is replaced by permanent scar-like tissue (Gratama 1969b:256; Iturregui-Pagan *et al.* 1976:209; World Health Organization 1967:188). Each inflammatory attack worsens the condition until the vessels are irreversibly damaged and there is no way, save surgery, to reverse the consequences of lymphatic obstruction. Lymph drainage, originally slowed by dilatation, is now stopped alto-gether because of obstruction.

There are several consequences to the cessation of lymph drainage to a part of the body. The transitory swellings seen during the inflam-matory stage become permanent accumulations of fluid. Thus, a devel-oping hydrocele becomes permanent and scrotal swellings, which once would subside, now persist. In severe cases of genital swelling there is an extensive fibrous thickening of the overlying skin until it resembles that of an elephant, hence the name *elephantiasis*. Some authors (e.g., Hunter *et al.* 1976:500; Jones 1967:188) have claimed that the added ten-sion of chronic edema stimulates this proliferation of fibrous tissue. But Yoffey and Courtice (1956, cited in Schacher and Sahyoun 1967:241) maintained that this extensive fibrous overgrowth is similar to that seen about a neglected or infected wound. It is a response to the stoppage of lymph drainage and the resulting accumulation in the tissue of sub-stances normally removed by the lymph. They claimed that even the epithelium (the cell layer covering the innermost and outermost aspects of the body) may be involved in this fibrosis, hence the thickened skin seen in elephantiasis. Yoffey and Courtice also felt that interrupting the

---

[2]In other types of filariasis (e.g., onchocerciasis) the reverse is true, and it is the microfilariae that cause the serious lesions associated with the infection (Nelson 1979:1136).

lymph drainage to a part makes the tissue strikingly susceptible to infection, especially by streptococci. These two responses—fibrous overgrowth and increased susceptibility to infection—are potentially important to the impact of filariasis on fecundity. If, for example, the lymph drainage of the fallopian tubes is interrupted, could fibrosis occlude the lumen or could the tubes become more susceptible to sterilizing infections? Romiti (1935, cited in Muir and Belsey 1980:920), for example, suggested many years ago that filariasis of the lymphatics draining the broad ligaments weakens tubal tissue and renders it more susceptible to secondary infection.

These and other possible effects of filariasis on human reproductive potential deserve study. At present there are no autopsy studies, and the only biopsy studies of affected tissues we are aware of are the study of Nasah and Cox (1978) and the studies of U.S. troops infected during World War II (see, e.g., Wartman, 1947). And because filarial infections in U.S. troops never reached the chronic stage and are believed to be atypical, not at all representative of the way the disease affects the millions in the tropics (Beaver 1970:184), the usefulness of the latter studies is limited. Thus, definitive evidence of the effects of the disease on reproductive potential awaits additional studies, preferably ones including extensive tissue sections from affected persons. Without such studies, it is instructive to review the progress of the disease, especially in the genital organs, and relate how the symptoms and sequelae of infection might alter male and female reproductive potential in light of what we do know of the tissue pathology associated with filarial infection.

Acute Stage

General

The immediate (and long-term) host response to the presence of filarial parasites is variable (see Figure 5.2). In endemic areas many persons show no parasitological or clinical evidence of being infected, despite an exposure to infective larvae that is roughly equivalent to that of persons with clinically expressed filariasis. In the past these "normals" were thought to be "exposed but not infected" (Ottesen 1980:2). However, a newer immunological assay revealed that about half these persons have circulating immune complexes, which suggests that they may in fact have subclinical, undetectable filariasis (Ottesen 1980:5). Another response to infective larvae is demonstrated by the many persons who show no clinical symptoms at all (Hunter *et al.* 1976:500; Spingarn

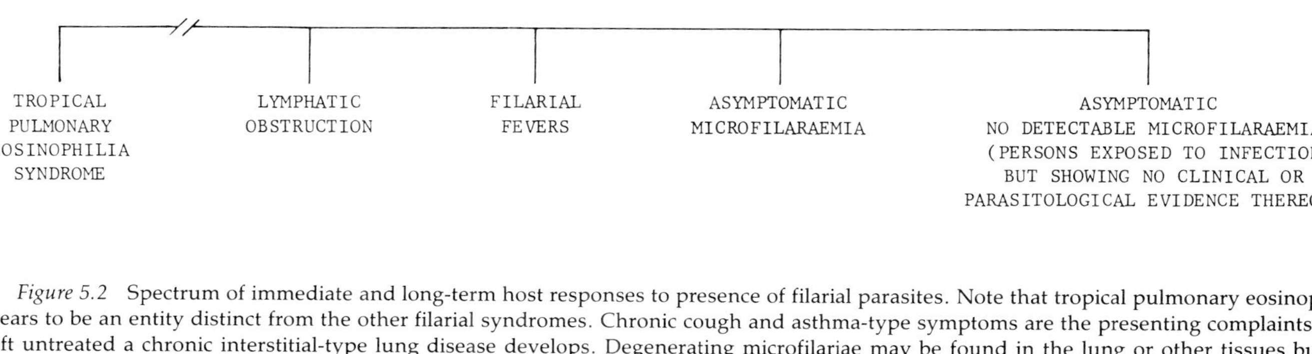

Figure 5.2 Spectrum of immediate and long-term host responses to presence of filarial parasites. Note that tropical pulmonary eosinophilia appears to be an entity distinct from the other filarial syndromes. Chronic cough and asthma-type symptoms are the presenting complaints, and if left untreated a chronic interstitial-type lung disease develops. Degenerating microfilariae may be found in the lung or other tissues but are practially never found in the peripheral circulation (Ottesen 1980:2). Source: Ottesen 1980:8.

and Edelman 1965:709), yet clearly are infected because microfilariae can be demonstrated in the bloodstream. In others the infection is clinically obvious, symptoms appearing as early as 3 months after initial infection. There may be an inflammation of the lymph vessels (lymphangitis), which is visible as a red streak under the skin, or a swelling of the lymph nodes (lymphadenitis). There may be pain, local heat, and edema. Fever is a common symptom, and the entire episode is frequently referred to as filarial fever. These filarial fevers occur two to six times a year, often lasting 1–2 weeks (Iturregui-Pagan *et al.* 1976:208; Ottesen 1980:2; Spencer 1974:26; Spingarn and Edelman 1965:709). Persons with filarial fevers may be microfilaremia-positive or microfilaremia-negative. And although these episodes are more common during the acute stage of the disease, even persons with chronic manifestations such as elephantiasis or hydrocele may have recurrent attacks of filarial fever (Ottesen 1980:2).

The type and severity of any associated symptoms varies greatly among individuals. For example, one person may have no symptoms, another may have no fever but moderate pain, and another may have a very high fever accompanied by acute prostration and great pain. What can account for such variability? Ottesen (1980:2) suggested that differences in clinical manifestations reflect different types of immunological responses among infected individuals. One individual may be only mildly sensitive to the worm, for example, whereas another may be hypersensitive. Some workers (e.g., Schacher and Sahyoun 1967:241) have suggested that hypersensitivity reactions to the different stages of the developing worm may explain the recurrent nature of filarial fevers, but others (e.g., Ottesen 1980:2) have claimed that the exact factors that initiate these febrile episodes are still unknown. Indeed, the fact that filarial fevers can occur in persons with chronic disease seems to argue against a hypersensitivity reaction as a source of the fever, because it is now known that in chronic filariasis the host is *hypo*responsive to filarial antigens. (This sequence of immunological events, from normal immune responsiveness to parasite antigens during the acute stage of the disease to hyporesponsiveness during the chronic stage, is similar to that seen in schistosomiasis [Ottesen 1980:3].) Indeed, the entire question of whether a much greater responsiveness to filarial antigens is the reason some infected persons develop lymphatic inflammation and subsequent obstruction is still not completely resolved. Although studies with Brugian filariasis have supported this hypothesis, earlier studies of patients with Bancroftian filariasis have not. Nevertheless, the implications of the findings with Brugian filariasis are clear and potentially important (Ottesen 1980:4). Although the issue needs to be explored further, the consensus now is that host hypersensitivity is responsible for the acute and chronic manifestations of filarial infection.

Male

The male genitals are frequently the site of inflammatory lesions of filariasis. Inflammation of the spermatic cord (funiculitis), epididymis (epididymitis), and testis (orchitis) are quite common. In fact, in one hospital in an endemic area in Africa recurrent attacks of funiculitis and epididymo–orchitis were one of the commonest causes of male admissions to the hospital (Spencer 1974:27).

Spermatic Cord Funiculitis, inflammation of the spermatic cord, is perhaps the most frequent manifestation of acute filariasis in men (Iturregui-Pagan *et al.* 1976:208). Concomitant involvement of the testis and especially the epididymis may be seen (Boyce and Politano 1970:621). Funiculitis is, by definition, an inflammation of the tissues of the cord *except* the tubule (i.e., the vas deferens). This is an important distinction because involvement of the vas, as in tuberculous or gonorrheal infections of the cord, has a substantially worse fertility prognosis. The vas deferens is thus spared in filarial funiculitis (Iturregui-Pagan *et al.* 1976:208; Wartman 1947:375). Rather, the infection is an inflammation of the lymph vessels of the cord and, to a lesser degree, their surrounding tissue (Wartman 1947:375). Clinical symptoms include severe, sharp pain and swelling of the cord due to edema and/or dilatation of the lymphatics (Boyce and Politano 1970:621; Iturregui-Pagan *et al.* 1976:208).

Although the hydroceles that are associated with repeated attacks of funiculitis over many years are believed to affect fertility adversely, acute attacks of funiculitis themselves are not mentioned as a cause of reproductive dysfunction. Yet the sharp pain experienced by some sufferers is surely great enough to cause temporary coital inability.

Other concomitants of funiculitis may affect conceptive ability. Wartman (1947:344), for example, reported that varicocele, which is frequently cited as an important cause of male infertility (e.g., Amelar *et al.* 1977:57; Clark 1978:70), was seen in 29% of cases of funiculitis, although the etiology was questionable. Wartman (1947:342) also noted that in some cases of funiculitis, even after a limited number of acute attacks, there was a thickening and nodularity of the cord that persisted indefinitely. The significance to reproduction of these two conditions will be discussed in the section ''Varicocele and Other Sequelae,'' for although they may be seen during acute attacks they are more common during the chronic stage of filariasis.

Epididymis   The epididymis, along with the cord, is one of the common sites of adult worms (Gratama 1969b:256), and epididymitis is therefore a common symptom of acute filariasis (Hunter *et al.* 1976:501). As with the cord, the tubule (ductus epididymis) is spared (Wartman 1947:375), and the inflammatory reaction is confined primarily to the lymphatics and their surrounding tissue. Clinically, the epididymis is swollen during an acute attack and small hard nodules may be seen. The swelling is more severe when the cord is also involved (Sanjurjo 1970:494).

Filarial epididymitis is not usually cited as a cause of reproductive dysfunction because the tubules are well preserved. However, one might imagine that, as in the case of funiculitis, severe pain might temporarily curtail coital activity. And if local heat accompanies the inflammation, fertilizing capacity could be temporarily impaired because the tail of the epididymis is a storage area for sperm. If local temperature rises the disintegration of sperm is hastened and temporary oligospermia may result (Glover 1974:243–244).

Testis   Acute filarial orchitis is less common than funiculitis (Itur-regui-Pagan *et al.* 1976:208) or epididymitis (Gratama 1969b:256). And rarely is only the testis involved; usually funiculitis and, especially, epididymitis accompany acute orchitis. The testis is often painful, tender, and swollen (Sanjurjo 1970:494; Wartman 1947:343), and one possible effect on fecundity is temporary coital inability due to the pain that accompanies acute orchitis. Often the swelling involves the interstitial tissue of the testis where testosterone, the hormone that maintains the secondary sexual characteristics and the accessory sexual organs, is produced. At least in one case in which there was substantial involvement of the interstitial tissue no changes in the secondary sexual characteristics were noted (Wartman 1947:363). This is not surprising, however, because this individual had only recently acquired the infection. But in chronic orchitis some changes might be anticipated.

Scrotum and Penis   Acute attacks of filariasis also involve the inguinal lymph nodes and their vessels, which drain the scrotum and penis. These attacks are preliminary to elephantiasis of the male genitals, just as funiculitis, epididymitis, and orchitis are preliminary to the development of hydrocele. The penis is rarely affected and, if so, this is almost always accompanied by scrotal involvement. The scrotum becomes hot, red, edematous, and tender (Sanjurjo 1970:495–496). Fecundity is compromised during an acute attack because coitus may be so painful as to be impossible. Even if it were possible, fertilizing capacity at this time might be severely diminished by the effects of local heat on the spermatozoa.

Fever   Many cases of acute filariasis are accompanied by fever (Barrett-Connor 1978:1905; Sanjurjo 1970:491). Fevers were unusual among U.S. servicemen who contracted filariasis during the Pacific campaign in World War II and, if they did occur, were mild (King 1944:296). But fevers are common among indigenes with well-established cases (Iturregui-Pagan *et al.* 1976:207; King 1944:296), last 1–2 weeks, and may range up to 40°C (104°F) (Hunter *et al.* 1976:501). Often these fevers are confused with malarial fevers (Hunter *et al.* 1976:501; Wijers and McMahon 1976:60). The research of MacLeod and Hotchkiss (1941, cited in Eaton and Mucha 1971:456) indicated that body temperatures of this height and duration are sufficient to raise scrotal temperatures to the point where azoospermia may occur. This is followed by a 1–2 month recovery period of oligospermia. Fertility is subsequently reduced for several months after each episode. The recurrent nature of acute filariasis (2–6 episodes a year) may, therefore, have a very important depressing effect on male fertility.

Female

Very little has been written about acute (or chronic, for that matter) filariasis in women, and much of what has been recorded is unsubstantiated. It is known that the lymph vessels of the broad ligament, ovary, fallopian tube, uterus, and vulva are the sites of filarial worms and therefore of an inflammatory response.

Inflammation of the lymph vessels of the external genitals may influence fecundity. Acute attacks of the lymph vessels of the vulva set the stage for eventual obliteration of lymph drainage and vulval elephantiasis; during an acute attack there is likely some swelling, heat, and tenderness, which would make coitus, if not impossible, at least unwelcome.

It is unlikely that the acute stage of filariasis can cause conceptive failure. Carayon *et al.* (1967, cited in Belsey 1977:12) report that clinical symptoms of acute, subacute, and chronic salpingitis have been attributed to filarial infection. However, Jacobson and Westrom (1969:1096) cautioned that infection of only the lymphatics of the parametrial tissues may mimic those of acute salpingitis. Rather, salpingitis and subsequent sterility probably follow chronic, obstructive disease of the genital lymphatics. This was proposed as early as 1935 by Romiti (1935, cited in Muir and Belsey 1980:920) when he suggested that obstruction of the lymphatics draining the broad ligaments weakens the tubal tissue and renders it more susceptible to infection. Spencer (1974:30) also suggested that pelvic infection, which is so common in the tropics and often of undetermined etiology, may in some cases be "secondary to pelvic lymphatic involvement with filariasis." This hypothesis will be discussed further in the section "Chronic Stage."

Pregnancy wastage may result from filariasis. Some women undoubtedly experience high fevers during acute attacks of filariasis. Although some (e.g., Spingarn and Edelman 1965:709) have felt that filariasis per se is not a cause of pregnancy wastage, it is possible that in the more severe cases the fever would be high enough to cause fetal death (see the section "Pregnancy Loss" in Chapter 4). Because filarial fever is easily confused with malarial fever, some pregnancy wastage attributed to malaria may actually have been caused by filariasis.

Chronic Stage

General

In persons with filariasis of long standing who have suffered repeated acute attacks, damage to the lymphatics gradually becomes permanent and irreversible. Lymph drainage that was slowed is now stopped and many of the symptoms seen during acute attacks, such as swelling, become permanent. Whereas in earlier stages chemotherapy (Nelson 1979:1137) or leaving the endemic area (Wijers and McMahon 1976:62) would have been sufficient to reverse the pathological process, now only surgery can repair the damage. If the lymphatics that drain the superficial aspects of the body have been involved, elephantiasis may occur. The legs and scrotum are usually affected, and less frequently the arms, breasts, or vulva (Hunter *et al.* 1976:502). When the deep lymphatics have been affected, a number of conditions may appear. Among these are chyluria (the appearance of lymph in the urine due to rupture of the lymph vessels draining the kidney) and hydrocele. The latter is the most frequent late sequelae to filarial infection and in some endemic areas affects as many as 80% of adult males (World Health Organization 1981a:1). It is felt that fecundity may be negatively affected by some of the late sequelae of filariasis. Male fecundity is threatened by elephantiasis of the scrotum and penis and by hydrocele, and female fecundity is potentially altered by elephantiasis of the vulva and by obstruction of the lymphatics that drain the internal genitals.

Male

Elephantiasis   Elephantiasis is certainly the most remarkable of all the late sequelae of filariasis and usually the first one to come to mind when the disease is mentioned. Yet it is an infrequent complication made to seem more important simply by its grotesque nature. Of the hundreds of millions of persons at risk of developing elephantiasis, only a small proportion do (Hunter *et al.* 1976:502; Nelson 1979:1136).[3] In highly endemic areas (see Acton and Rao [1930] for classification of endemicity levels) 1–2% of the male population may have elephantiasis, which nearly always involves the legs. In the very worst areas perhaps 5% of the male population has elephantiasis, and again the legs are mainly affected, although there may be more scrotal and arm elephantiasis as well (Wijers and McMahon 1976:60). Elephantiasis is often bilateral (Edeson 1972:62).

Some of the effects on fecundity of elephantiasis are obvious. A greatly enlarged penis or scrotum would, for example, make coitus difficult or impossible. Other effects are more subtle. Surgery of an elephantiasic scrotum reveals that the cord and testis are surrounded by tremendous amounts of a gelatinlike material. This large amount of material, bounded by a thick, inflexible skin, exerts tremendous pressure on the venous circulation (Sanjurjo 1970:496), diminishing its effectiveness in modulating testicular temperatures. The effect is the same as with a varicocele—a reduction in semen quality. (Varicocele is discussed in the "Hydrocele" section.) Indeed, varicocele itself is often seen in cases of scrotal elephantiasis (Sanjurjo 1970:496). It is, therefore, not surprising that testicular biopsies in scrotal elephantiasis reveal degenerative changes in the testis and even the absence of spermatogenesis in some cases (Spingarn and Edelman 1965:709).

Leg elephantiasis has no particular effect on fecundity per se. But close examination of individuals with leg elephantiasis will almost always reveal a hydrocele (Wijers and McMahon 1976:61), and the possible effects on fecundity of that condition will be discussed next. This is an important observation because leg elephantiasis is more common than elephantiasis of the scrotum.

Hydrocele   Hydroceles are the most common genital manifestation of filariasis (Iturregui-Pagan *et al.* 1976:208). They are a much more important complication of filariasis than the infrequently seen elephan-

---

[3]Migrants to endemic areas develop elephantiasis more often and much sooner (sometimes within 1–2 years) than do persons indigenous to endemic areas (World Health Organization 1981b:12).

tiasis. One of the first population-based studies of the relationship between filariasis and hydrocele was that of Jordan (1960) in Tanganyika (now part of the United Republic of Tanzania). Since then many studies have recorded significant rates of hydrocele in filariasis-endemic areas. In the Lango district of Uganda, 25% of the adult males had hydroceles in 1950 (*Uganda Atlas of Disease Distribution* 1968:143), and other populations have recorded prevalence rates of almost 80% among adult males (World Health Organization 1981a:1). A certain proportion of these hydroceles are, undoubtedly, of nonfilarial origin. They may be due to inflammation of the epididymis caused by tuberculosis or gonorrhea, or be the result of a tumor or the generalized edema associated with heart disease (Gratama 1969a:274). And a certain proportion have no known cause. Such hydroceles are seen in approximately 1% of adult males (Gratama 1966:98), and this figure remains constant from one part of the world to another. Thus, in areas where filariasis is endemic the majority of hydroceles are probably due to filariasis. With large hydroceles, filariasis is always suspected. But it should be remembered that small, ordinary-looking hydroceles are also often the only manifestation of a long-standing filarial infection (Iturregui-Pagan *et al.* 1976:208). One possible way of differentiating hydroceles is to examine the tunica vaginalis; thickening of the tunica is far more frequent in hydroceles caused by filariasis (Gratama 1969a:271).

Hydroceles are formed after repeated attacks of funiculitis and epididymo–orchitis.[4] One study (Gratama 1969a:275) suggested that these hydroceles are bilateral in 35% of cases. The fluid in the hydrocele may be absorbed after an acute attack, but generally it persists or increases gradually (Sanjurjo 1970:492–493). Eventually lymph drainage is totally obstructed and the hydrocele becomes permanent. The suspended position of the scrotum, its easy distendability, and the lymph drainage against gravity are all factors favoring the formation of a hydrocele (Gratama 1969b:255).

The effects of a hydrocele on fecundity are twofold. First, it can cause coital inability. Masters and Johnson (1970:184) listed hydrocele as a cause of impotence; and if a hydrocele is large—a unilateral hydrocele containing 2300 cc of fluid has been described (Sanjurjo 1970:492)—coitus may be impossible (Wolfe and Aslamkhan 1972:28). Second, a

---

[4]There are two types of hydroceles caused by filariasis. Most frequently encountered are hydroceles of the testis. But hydroceles of the cord may also follow an acute funiculitis with fluid accumulating between the two leaves of the membrane that covers the cord (this membrane is continuous with the tunica vaginalis, which covers the testis).

hydrocele can diminish or abolish fertilizing capacity (Belsey 1977:12; Spingarn and Edelman 1965:709). In hydroceles of long standing the tunica vaginalis is often thickened (Boyce and Politano 1970:628; Sanjurjo 1970:493)—Gratama (1969a:275) noted in his survey that in 30% of hydroceles the tunica was markedly thickened and in 40% of cases was moderately thickened—and if the tunica vaginalis is thick, greater pressure is exerted on the testis, thereby interfering with testicular circulation (Boyce and Politano 1970:628). The pressure on the testis is also very great if the hydrocele is very large. In both cases atrophy of the testis is said to be not uncommon (Boyce and Politano 1970:628) and is probably due to increased testicular temperature. Testicular biopsies have supported this conclusion (Spingarn and Edelman 1965:709). Interestingly, Belsey (1977:12) has noted that whereas there is a positive correlation between hydrocele and male infertility in areas endemic for filariasis, studies (e.g., Krahn *et al.* 1963) have failed to show such a correlation outside endemic areas. Perhaps this is because the tunica vaginalis is thicker in filarial hydroceles, exerts more pressure on the testis, and therefore poses a greater fertility risk. Infertility is a possible outcome with very large hydroceles for yet another reason. Fuller (1974:13) noted that among the Fulani tribesmen of Uganda there was an inordinate tendency toward hydrocele; if these were very large—some hung down to the knees and weighed up to 60 lbs. (28 kg)—it was necessary to amputate the entire testicle.

Varicocele and Other Sequelae Hydrocele is a well-recognized complication of repeated attacks of funiculitis and epididymo–orchitis. But are there not other changes—perhaps in the cords, epididymides, and testes themselves—that might result from an obstruction of their lymph vessels? One possible effect on fecundity that is rarely mentioned is the association of filarial funiculitis and varicocele. Although not a constant finding, varicocele is noted in some cases of filarial funiculitis and is the result of repeated inflammation of the veins of the cord (Sanjurjo 1970:492). It is believed that dilatation of the cord vein results in higher testicular temperatures because the vein's function of dissipating heat from the testicular artery is interfered with (Boyce and Politano 1970:622). The result may be testicular atrophy (Boyce and Politano 1970:622) and poor semen quality in regard to both the number and the motility of sperm (Davis *et al.* 1967:844).

There are several other possible sequelae to chronic lymphatic obstruction in the genitals. The chronic edema that sometimes accompanies obstruction might compress the genital ducts to the point where they are partially or totally occluded; a similar mechanism of chronic congestion has been forwarded for closure of the fallopian tube in women (Spingarn and Edelman 1965:709). A second mechanism for tubal occlusion is suggested by the work, described earlier, of Yoffey and Courtice (1956, cited in Schacher and Sahyoun 1967:241) who felt that interruption of lymph drainage to a part results in fibrous overgrowth of the layer of tissue beneath the epithelium and, in some cases, overgrowth of the epithelium itself—a sort of scar formation in response to the accumulation of substances the lymphatics would normally remove (Schacher and Sahyoun 1967:241). If this fibrosis should involve the epithelium of the vas or ductus epididymis, partial or complete occlusion could result. King (1944:296) noted, for example, that although acute funiculitis is an inflammation of the lymph vessels of the cord and the vas is spared, repeated attacks could result in severe fibrosis and obstruction of the vas. In addition, because the epithelium of the epididymis secretes substances that aid the survival of spermatozoa (Copenhaver 1964:505), fibrosis of the epithelium of this tissue could result in spermatozoa of questionable vitality. And if the layers below the epithelium—the fibromuscular layers that contract during seminal emission—are involved, ejaculation could be affected. In all these cases, fertilizing capacity would be impaired.

Although inflammation of the interstitial tissue of the testis—the tissue that secretes testosterone—has not been accompanied by changes in the secondary sexual characteristics, might not repeated attacks cause some alteration in hormone levels with resulting changes at the cellular level that cannot be seen by eye? If the testosterone level is lowered (this has not been recorded), the prostrate, seminal vessels, the epithelium of the ducts—all those structures that are maintained by this hormone—may not be functioning at full capacity and fertilizing capacity would be compromised.

A final effect on fecundity was also suggested by Yoffey and Courtice, who remarked that when lymph drainage to a part is interrupted, that part becomes "strikingly susceptible to infection particularly to infection by streptococci" (Yoffey and Courtice 1956, cited in Schacher and Sahyoun 1967:241). Could it then be that gonorrheal and other genital infections are more frequent and more severe in men who experienced funiculitis or epididymo-orchitis?

It should be mentioned that because these possible sequelae as well as hydrocele are the result of repeated attacks of funiculitis and epididymo-orchitis, two or more conditions could coexist. Varicocele and hydrocele are therefore often seen together in endemic areas, each negatively affecting fecundity.

Female

Elephantiasis Elephantiasic changes in the female include enlargement of the extremities, breasts, and external genitals. Vulval elephantiasis, which is usually bilateral, may interfere with coitus if severe enough (Lawson 1967b:466). Pregnancy may be a particularly difficult time for women with elephantiasis. An affected breast may increase in size during pregnancy (Spingarn and Edelman 1965:709) and elephantiasis of the labia and clitoris may cause difficulties during labor (Bloomfield *et al.* 1978:598) and perhaps necessitate a cesarean delivery (Spingarn and Edelman 1965:709–710).

Transplacental Transmission The question of whether or not an infected woman can transmit microfilariae to her offspring transplacentally has been investigated. Although some studies (Bloomfield *et al.* 1978:597; Spitz 1959:243) could not find evidence of fetal involvement, Hawking (1975:14) reported a study (Neves and Scaff 1952) that found microfilariae in the blood of a 3- and a 10-day-old child. However, because the microfilariae of W. *bancrofti* are generally nonpathogenic, their presence in these children should have no implications for future health (or fecundity).

Tubal Occlusion Usually the only reported complications of long-standing chronic filariasis in women are those resulting from obstruction of the superficial lymphatics that drain the breasts, vulva, etc. But because the deep lymphatics that drain the internal genitals are also the site of adult worms and obstruction, it seems possible that there might be late pathogenic changes in these structures also. Filariasis is believed to cause tubal obstruction (Bloomfield *et al.* 1978:598; Spingarn and Edelman 1965:709). It has been stated (Spingarn and Edelman 1965:709) that this obstruction and the resulting dysmenorrhea and sterility are due to ''chronic congestion'' of the tubes and ovaries due to damage in the lymph vessels and nodes of the pelvis. Alternately, the closure of the tubes might be due to intense fibrosis of the tubal epithelium or subepithelium as suggested by Yoffey and Courtice. And because the uterus is so dependent on its lymphatics for removing water and waste products associated with cyclical changes in the endometrium, involvement of this lymph system would probably result in menstrual disorders and an endometrium unsuitable for implantation of a conceptus and maintenance of a pregnancy. In addition, as also suggested by Yoffey and Courtice, the internal genitals become more susceptible to infection when their lymph drainage is interrupted. Thus, gonorrhea and other sterilizing infections are probably more frequent and more severe in women whose genital system is compromised by filarial infection (see also Muir and Belsey 1980:920).

Summary of Pathophysiology

It appears that filariasis infection is capable of adversely affecting male and female fecundity in many ways. Negative effects on coitus and conceptive ability, and perhaps even pregnancy, are experienced during the acute and chronic stages of the infection. In the male acute attacks of funiculitis, epididymo–orchitis, and lymphangitis of the scrotum are accompanied by pain, which is often severe and can make coitus impossible. The local heat associated with epididymitis and lymphangitis of the scrotum can negatively affect semen quality and, therefore, fertilizing capacity. In women acute attacks of the lymph vessels of the vulva are accompanied by tenderness, which could make coitus impossible. In both males and females acute attacks are accompanied by high fever with serious repercussions. In the male spermatogenesis may be affected, and in the female pregnancy may be prematurely terminated.

The effects on fecundity of chronic filariasis are also varied. Elephantiasis of the scrotum or vulva could make coitus impossible. An occasional hydrocele may also be so large as to interfere with coitus. Elephantiasis of the scrotum and hydrocele both may cause a rise in testicular temperature with a negative effect on fertilizing ability. Another important result of long-term filariasis infection is varicocele; it too may reduce fertilizing capacity by raising testicular temperature. A number of hypothetical results have been formulated, including tubal occlusion due to chronic edema or fibrosis. A very important result of long-term lymphatic obstruction is the striking susceptibility to infection of a part whose lymph drainage has been interrupted. This means that if the lymph vessels of the male and female genitals are affected, these tissues are more likely to be the sites of more frequent and more severe infections with pathogens such as gonorrhea and sterility might result.

Variables Affecting the Development
of Filariasis

Once bitten by an infected mosquito individuals may, as noted earlier, respond in many different ways. They may have an inflammatory reaction and/or show microfilariae in the blood and/or eventually develop chronic disease. Or they may show no evidence whatsoever of infection except a positive reaction to an immunologic test that identifies infected persons (i.e., those who have been exposed to adult worms and/or microfilariae).

Next are considered the factors that determine the course that filarial infection takes in an individual and, therefore, the likelihood that reproduction will be impaired—that is, the factors that determine the chances of becoming infected, of experiencing acute attacks, and of developing chronic disease.

Chances of Becoming Infected

Filariasis is distributed throughout the tropical and subtropical world. Yet the areas of infection are usually not expansive; rather, the disease is confined to focal areas of infection. It is not unusual, for example, for a village where nearly all individuals are infected to be surrounded by unaffected areas because filariasis occurs only in those areas where there is a high density of infected mosquito vectors. In fact, it has been estimated that an individual must receive 15,000 infective bites to produce adequate microfilarial densities in the blood to ensure transmission (Hairston and De Meillon 1968, cited in Nelson 1979:1137–1138). In one endemic area outside Calcutta, exposure to mosquitoes was so intense that one individual was bitten 695 times in one night without once awakening (Gubler and Bhattacharya 1974:1027, 1034).

With such intense levels of transmission it is not surprising that immunologic tests (skin tests for microfilarial antigens and serologic tests for antibodies against adult worms) show that most children in endemic areas are infected with filariasis before the age of 6. In fact, many small children give a history of acute lymphatic inflammation. Yet microfilaremia is not seen in such children, appearing only at age 6 or later (Brown 1975:148; Grove *et al.* 1978:977–979). Microfilaremia is not seen even in many infected adults. In the study of Grove and associates (1978:981) in the Philippines, 90% of adult men and women had immunologic evidence of infection but only 37% of men and 17% of women had microfilaremia, even though the more sensitive membrane filtration method of detecting microfilariae was used. Perhaps some cases of microfilaremia were missed because parasite densities were below the level of detection. But it is likely that a good proportion of individuals simply did not have microfilaremia. Either the microfilariae had disappeared from their blood as an infection waned or, though they had been infected once or many times in the past, the requirements of microfilarial mating—a male and female worm in the same place at the same time—were never met. Gubler and Bhattacharya's (1974:1027, 1035) study outside Calcutta found that microfilaremia rates and densities there were not nearly as high as the intense level of transmission would suggest, simply because each infective bite contained few infective larvae and the chances were therefore much reduced that the conditions could be met for mating and production of microfilariae.

Though clearly more people are infected with filariasis than demonstrate microfilaremia, microfilaremia rates are the standard way of expressing infection rates. This practice is more useful anyway because microfilaremia rates, and especially *densities*, are significant epidemiologically: They increase with the number of reinfections (which do not seem to be limited) and are a good barometer of disease rates and severity (Edeson 1972:62; Gratama 1969b:265; World Health Organization 1967:9). In a given endemic area microfilaremia rates will differ among certain population subgroups. Because microfilaremia rates rise with increasing exposure to infection, they are higher in older age groups and among those who work in the most mosquito-infested areas (Grove *et al.* 1978:978, 982). Lower rates among women have been recorded in some studies but not in others (Grove *et al.* 1978:981), and animal studies suggest that any differential may be due to hormonal differences (Edeson 1972:61).

Although microfilariae rates are frequently used as a proxy for infection rates, there are certain groups that, although obviously infected, rarely show microfilaremia. For example, U.S. servicemen in the Pacific who became infected with *W. bancrofti* rarely developed microfilaremia (Wartman 1947:354), even though this was a common feature of the infection in indigenes. At first it was thought that the difference could be explained by the fact that the repeated infections necessary to ensure detectable microfilaremia were not experienced by these men because of their short stay in endemic areas. But Beaver (1970:184) suggested that microfilaremia may also be absent in Europeans and Americans living for many years in endemic areas, that persons not native to endemic areas are not adapted to the parasite, and that filarial infections in them are "biologically aberrant."

Microfilaremia is also not found in persons with chronic disease. It has been suggested that the microfilariae are walled off in obstructed lymph vessels and therefore are not detectable. But it is more likely that they have been eliminated by an immunologic process and the hydrocele or elephantiasis remains as evidence of past infection (Lawson 1967b:468; Nelson 1979:1137). Presumably the immune reaction around the parasite—the same reaction that causes inflammation and eventual obstruction—prevents the parasite from completing its cycle of maturation–mating–egg laying. Thus, the greater the immune reaction to *W. bancrofti*, the greater the clinical disease but the lower the level of microfilaremia (Gratama 1969b:258).

Chances of Developing Disease

An individual's chances of developing acute or chronic filariasis depend on a number of intrinsic and extrinsic factors. Host hypersensitivity to a parasite is the major (intrinsic) factor determining the development of disease. But other factors, both intrinsic (age, sex, etc.) and extrinsic (number of reinfections, number of infective larvae per inoculum, etc.), play a role as well.

Acute Filariasis

Because the symptoms associated with acute filariasis are the result of the host's immune response to the parasite, host hypersensitivity is a major factor. Extrinsic factors such as the size of the worm load, the number of reinfections, and the presence of secondary bacterial invaders can also influence the severity of an acute attack. In persons exposed to repeated infections each acute attack is worse than the previous one because the worm load is increased and present pathological reactions are superimposed on an already damaged lymph system. For example, the severity of attacks of acute funiculitis were noted to increase as the number of reinfections and worm load increased (Sanjurjo 1970:491).

The role of bacteria in acute filariasis is a matter of some controversy. Some authors (e.g., Iturregui-Pagan *et al.* 1976:208) have claimed that the symptoms of acute filariasis are caused by secondary invasion of bacteria into the lymph vessels and have noted that these symptoms frequently disappear with the use of antibiotics. Others (e.g., Brown 1975:148; Hunter *et al.* 1976:500) have taken the more widely held position that the acute stage represents an allergic reaction to the worm, but that bacterial and fungal infection may be superimposed. Although careful study of the acute attacks in U.S. servicemen during World War II showed that bacteria played no role in the observed symptoms (Spencer 1974:26; Wartman 1947:390), some authors (e.g., Spencer 1974:26) felt that secondary bacterial infection is very common among indigenes and is linked to the lack of footwear and minor associated trauma. Belsey (1977:12) summed up the situation by saying that although secondary bacterial infections of the genital lymphatics in both males and females have been described, their frequency and significance have not been established.

An interesting observation is that although children may be infected with filariasis and give a history of acute lymphatic inflammation they rarely show inflammation of the genital lymphatics; genital lymphatic inflammation occurs more frequently after puberty (Sanjurjo 1970:491). A similar situation exists for schistosomiasis, infection of the internal female genitals being more frequent after puberty. And seeding of these organs with the tubercle bacillus is also noted to occur primarily during adolescence. It is thought that in both these cases the increased vascularization of the organs associated with their rapid growth during puberty offers many new avenues of attack for blood-borne pathogens. It is likely that the lymph system of these organs is similarly expanded during puberty, allowing the filarial parasite to enter at that time and cause genital lymphatic inflammation.

Chronic Filariasis

Because chronic disease is the result of the cumulative damage incurred with each acute attack, many of the same factors—hypersensitivity, worm load, bacteria—that play a role in acute attacks also determine the severity of chronic filariasis. Other factors that seem to be influential include age, sex, socioeconomic status, and the strain of parasite and biting habits of the vector.

Hypersensitivity   Just as host hypersensitivity to worms is the primary factor responsible for the symptoms of acute filariasis, it is, by extension, the primary factor responsible for the development of chronic disease. The greater the immune response to the parasite, the greater the inflammation and resulting fibrosis and the greater the disease. However, repeated infections are essential to this formula. Even the most hypersensitive individual, if removed from an endemic area early enough, will not develop chronic filariasis (Wijers and McMahon 1976:62); U.S. servicemen infected during World War II were hypersensitive to *W. bancrofti* (Wartman 1947:392), but their removal from the endemic area prevented the repeated infections necessary for the appearance of chronic sequelae. Thus, hypersensitivity is a necessary but not sufficient factor in the development of filarial disease.

Reinfection and Worm Load   The number of infections is the second most important factor in the etiology of chronic filariasis. Repeated infections mean an ever-increasing worm load and repeated inflammatory reactions in already damaged lymph vessels. In areas where microfilaremia densities are high—indicating high worm loads—filarial disease is not only more common but also more severe (Beaver 1970:187; Edeson 1972:62; World Health Organization 1967:9). It should be noted that this association between microfilaremia densities and disease is true at the population level. However, at the individual level such an association disappears. As mentioned earlier, microfilaremia is often absent in persons with chronic filariasis. Several studies, such as that of Wijers and McMahon (1976:59) in Kenya and Tanzania, that of Grove *et al.* (1978:978) in the Philippines, and that of Wolfe and Aslamkhan (1972:26) in East Pakistan (now Bangladesh), have confirmed this, finding no association in individuals between microfilaremia and obstructive disease. Thus, the greater immune responsiveness of those with chronic filariasis has obliterated most evidence of infection, and thus it is hard to prove by usual laboratory techniques that the lesions were caused by *W. bancrofti* (Gratama 1969b:258).

If repeated infections in hypersensitive individuals are essential to the development of disease, it seems reasonable that persons with chronic filariasis should give a history of repeated acute attacks. Although Spencer (1974:27) reported, to his surprise, that not many patients with hydrocele gave a history of acute recurrent attacks of funiculitis or epididymitis, others (e.g., Grove *et al.* 1978:982) noted that persons with obstructive disease have a longer history of acute inflammatory episodes. The consensus is that hydrocele and elephantiasis are preceded by repeated acute inflammatory attacks (Brown 1975:149; Hunter *et al.* 1976:502; Sanjurjo 1970:492). Sanjurjo (1970:492) felt that a massive initial infection may also be sufficient to cause permanent elephantiasic changes.

Bacteria   Just as the role of bacteria in acute filariasis is a matter of debate, their role in the development of chronic filariasis is viewed in various ways. Some consider bacteria a contributing factor in the development of disease because so many persons are infected but only a few develop complications, but others say bacteria are not important (Sanjurjo 1970:491). Yoffey and Courtice (1956, cited in Schacher and Sahyoun 1967:241) have taken the position that interruption of lymph drainage alone will result in chronic disease but that a superimposed bacterial infection will accelerate the process. In their words, "each attack of local infection simply intensifies what will occur inevitably, but more slowly, if lymph drainage is blocked but infection does not occur" (Yoffey and Courtice 1956, cited in Schacher and Sahyoun 1967:241).

Age   Age differentials in the frequency and severity of disease do exist, obstructive disease being uncommon in persons younger than 30

(Brown 1975:146). Although elephantiasis and fully developed hydroceles may be seen in teenagers in the very worst affected areas, they usually develop much later (Wijers and McMahon 1976:61, 59). A study (see Gratama 1966:67) of the male population of Dar es Salaam found that the prevalence of hydrocele rose steadily with age (age 15–25, 6.1%; age 25–35, 23%; age 35–45, 32.2%; age >45, 40%). The study of Grove and associates (1978:978) in the Philippines noted very low rates of obstructive disease affecting the genitals before age 25, at which time there was a tremendous increase. At age 25 only about 6% were so affected; 10 years later about 22% were affected and by age 45 about 28%.

Increasing disease rates with age are simply a reflection of the fact that repeated attacks are necessary to precipitate permanent changes. Formation of hydroceles, the most frequent late manifestation of filariasis, depends on repeated episodes of funiculitis or epididymo–orchitis, which do not begin until puberty; it is thus not surprising that hydroceles do not appear until the mid-twenties or early thirties. Nevertheless, the data from Dar es Salaam and the Philippines show that a considerable proportion of the male reproductive population have hydroceles or another genital abnormality that could interfere with their fecundity.

Sex The literature on filariasis, particularly as it affects the genitals, is almost exclusively concerned with male disease. Vulval elephantiasis is not a frequent sequela of filariasis (nor, for that matter, is scrotal elephantiasis). Hydrocele is by far the most frequent late manifestation of filariasis. Its counterpart in women is not well defined and has been referred to in vague terms of chronic congestion of the tubes and ovaries due to damage to the pelvic lymphatics (Spingarn and Edelman 1965:709). This and many other instances of obstructive disease in women may be missed altogether because in some societies cultural restrictions allow only examination of the female extremities (Wolfe and Aslamkhan 1972:24), and because the affected female structures lie deep in the pelvis and are not easily palpated (Nelson, personal communication, 1981). Or the greater prevalence of disease in men may simply be a reflection of greater infection rates and densities. Grove and associates (1978:981–982) found that women in their study had lower microfilaremia rates and densities and lower rates of obstructive disease than men. However, the study of Wolfe and Aslamkhan (1972:25–26) found that microfilaremia rates and densities among men and women were similar but that disease rates were remarkably lower in women, 0.2% versus 21% for the men. In general, disease rates are lower for women—though not as low as in the Wolfe and Aslamkhan study—and microfilaremia rates and densities are either lower or comparable to those recorded for males (see Grove *et al.* 1878:981). Where female disease rates are lower than expected, secondary infection may play a role. Lawson (1967b:468) suggested that the vulva is less frequently affected by elephantiasis than the scrotum, not because of male–female differences in susceptibility to infection but because trauma and secondary infection, which predispose to elephantiasic changes, are more likely to occur in men.

Socioeconomic Status Two studies have noted a significant relationship between socioeconomic status and the frequency and severity of obstructive disease. Wijers and McMahon (1976:62) noted that the part of the village where a person lived and the sort of house he occupied were important in determining the severity of disease. Grove and associates (1978:980, 982) noted that men with the lowest socioeconomic index had a significantly higher prevalence of obstructive disease, which was explained by a greater occupational exposure to infected mosquitoes.

Strain of Parasite and Vector Biting Habits Regional differences in the particular strain of parasite and the vector's biting habits (along with differences in endemicity, the species of parasite, host susceptibility, and the like) may help explain regional differences in the clinical picture associated with filariasis (Gubler and Bhattacharya 1974:1035; World Health Organization 1975:9): In some parts of the world chyluria is frequently observed and in other parts it is rare; in some areas leg elephantiasis predominates and in others scrotal elephantiasis does; in some areas hydroceles are preceded by local heat, redness, fever, and pain and in others such symptoms are absent. Wijers and McMahon (1976:62), for instance, proposed that the presence of an attenuated strain of parasite could be responsible for the mild disease they saw in East Africa. And Beaver (1970:187) noted that variations in disease patterns have been attributed to differences in the biting habits of vectors because the anatomical site of entry is important in determining disease manifestation. Thus, in areas where mosquitoes bite the upper half of the body, arm and breast elephantiasis would be common; in areas where mosquitoes bite the lower half, leg and genital elephantiasis would predominate.

Results of Studies

It is clear that various intrinsic and extrinsic factors combine to make each endemic community unique in regard to the impact of filariasis. Thus, each community should be analyzed carefully and individually before estimating the impact of filariasis on factors such as reproduction. Wijers and McMahon (1976:62), for example, felt that lower worm loads explained why the hydroceles on the East African coast were preceded only by pain and local swelling and not by the redness, local heat, and fever that were reported in other study areas. Effects on reproduction would be greater in the latter areas: In the coastal areas coitus might be impaired *during* an acute attack because of the pain, but in the other areas local heat and fever might result in oligospermia *persisting* for 1–2 months after each acute attack. The intensity of transmission is also very important in assessing the effects of disease on fertility. In areas where transmission is intense and attacks frequent, permanent lesions such as hydrocele appear earlier in reproductive life with greater consequences for reproduction.

Studies investigating reproductive performance in filariasis-endemic areas have come to conflicting answers to the question of whether or not fecundity is impaired. Of the three studies we found, two reported an effect on fecundity and the third did not. A study by Modawi (1965, cited in Belsey 1976:333) in the Sudan noted that among 166 men from infertile unions, a great proportion had conditions that could have been caused by filariasis: 11.9% had hydroceles, 4.4% had lymphovaricoceles, 6.6% had epididymo–orchitis, and 7% had testicular atrophy. The significance of these conditions to the observed infertility must be questioned, however, because their rate among fertile men was not recorded.

A study by Ayres and associates (1976:107–108) in Brazil compared the reproduction performance of "filarial patients" and their controls. The results show that there was evidence of "reproductive compensation" among the filarial patients. They had more pregnancies that terminated in an abortion or postnatal death but they had a significantly greater total number of pregnancies, and thus both groups had the same number of children. Unfortunately, the authors did not say what particular manifestation of filariasis their patients were afflicted with or what other conditions they may have had that could have accounted for the greater number of pre- and postnatal deaths. And because persons with filariasis tend to be of a lower socioeconomic level (Grove *et al.* 1978:980) and tend to have poorer health and a greater number of spontaneous abortions, specific attribution of cause is difficult.

A study by Grove and associates (1978:978,980) in the Philippines examined the relationship between obstructive disease and reproductive performance. Of the married men, 9% claimed they had genital swelling that interfered with sexual intercourse; 17% of the women claimed their husbands had such swelling, although in 20% of these cases examination of the husband revealed no abnormality. They found no relationship between obstructive disease in men or women and the number of their live-born children. Nor did they find any relationship between the presence or absence of microfilaremia in men or women and the number of their live-born children. The total number of pregnancies was not stated, and thus some degree of reproductive compensation as suggested by the Ayres *et al.* (1976) study might be involved. In any case, the fact that no relationships were found does not necessarily negate any filariasis–fertility relationship. Because microfilaremia was not associated with either acute or chronic filariasis, its relationship to fertility would appear to be irrelevant. And the finding of no relationship between the presence or absence of obstructive disease and the number of live-born children is not altogether surprising because most persons who suffer acute attacks do not develop obstructive disease and both groups (those with obstructive disease and those who suffer acute attacks) are, we believe, subject to diminished reproductive potential. However, we would have expected somewhat lower fertility in those with obstructive disease as a result of their permanent lesions combined with their longer histories of acute attacks.

Summary of the Role of Filariasis in Reproductive Impairment

We believe that filariasis has a definite negative effect on male reproductive ability. And despite previous reports (see, e.g., Grove *et al.* 1978:982) associating reproductive impairment only with obstructive disease we feel that the acute stage also diminishes fecundity. The effect of the disease on female fecundity is hard to assess because very little has been written on disease consequences in women. If, however, filarial fevers among indigenes are as high as some reports indicate, an acute attack in a pregnant woman could cause fetal loss. And if the only effect of the disease were to make the genital tract of males and females more susceptible to infection, that alone would produce a negative effect on fecundity, considering the magnitude of the venereal disease (VD) problem in the developing world. Because many millions of persons suffer from acute and chronic filariasis the disease could have an important role in population subfecundity. Nevertheless, a definitive answer to the question of whether or not filariasis has a negative effect on population fecundity awaits further study. Preferably studies will be undertaken to determine (1) whether or not oligospermia follows acute attacks in which there is fever and/or local heat, (2) what types of hydroceles in regard to size and duration are associated with testicular atrophy and/or spermatogenic failure, (3) how often such hydroceles are found in men during the reproductive period, (4) the frequency of varicoceles in acute and chronic filariasis and their effect on fertilizing capacity, (5) the effects of filariasis on the internal female genitals, (6) whether persons with filariasis are more often the victims of genital infections such as gonorrhea, etc. Until these and many other questions are answered, it can only be said that the pathophysiological consequences of filariasis clearly show the infection can seriously jeopardize individual fecundity, and that some epidemiological data, which reveal that areas of low fertility coincide with filariasis-endemic areas, make further investigation of filariasis as a population fecundity factor desirable.

Diagnosis

Detection of patent infections consists of demonstrating microfilariae in the peripheral blood. Most population surveys use the thick film method; the finger is pricked at the time of day when microfilaria counts are peaking and a thick smear of blood is examined under the microscope for microfilariae. Parasite densities may also be determined in this way, and the species identified by appropriately staining the preparation (World Health Organization 1967:10). This method is simple and inexpensive but misses those cases where microfilaremia densities are low, as in children and treated adults. A more sensitive, but more expensive, method involves taking a larger sample of blood and passing it through a membrane filter to concentrate the parasites.

Positive confirmation of a diagnosis of filariasis may be difficult in patients with early filariasis or obstructive disease as microfilariae are often absent from the blood. Although there are immunologic tests that are valuable in confirming a diagnosis in persons in whom microfilariae cannot be found (Brown 1975:146), their usefulness is limited by their lack of specificity, as there are always false positive and false negative results (Nelson 1979:1137). Thus, diagnosis in persons without detectable microfilariae is usually based on clinical appearance (many cases of genital filariasis in women may be missed because of reluctance to be examined [Lawson 1967b:468; Wolfe and Aslamkhan 1972:24]) and a medical history of lymph node enlargement, acute lymphatic inflammation, filarial fever, and so on (World Health Organization 1974b:11, 22). Some studies have also used microscopic examination of excised tissue to confirm a diagnosis of filariasis. Gratama (1969a:277), unable to find positive evidence of filariasis in many cases of hydrocele from an area in Liberia where *W. bancrofti* prevalence is high, felt that examination of tissue for lesions characteristic of filariasis would be the only way to confirm the diagnosis. Indeed, in the case of filarial infections among U.S. servicemen there was no detectable microfilaremia in the overwhelming majority of cases and a positive diagnosis was based on clinical findings and microscopic examination of tissue (Wartman 1947).

Most studies do not examine excised tissue, both because it is not available and because of the expense involved. Instead they must rely heavily on clinical appearances. In such instances differential diagnosis is a problem because the symptoms of filariasis may be confused with those of many other diseases. During the acute stage filariasis may be confused with malaria because of the recurring bouts of high fever (Gratama 1969b:259; Hunter *et al.* 1976:501). And tuberculous and gonorrheal epididymitis present a clinical picture similar to that of filarial epididymitis (King 1944:292). The chronic stage of filariasis may be confused with a large number of other disorders. Filarial hydroceles are difficult to differentiate from those found in areas where there is no filariasis. One diagnostic clue is that filarial hydroceles exhibit a thicker tunica vaginalis than nonfilarial hydroceles (Gratama 1969a:274, 271). Similarly, filarial and nonfilarial elephantiases are difficult to distinguish. Because only sophisticated techniques can do this (World Health Organization 1967:8–9), it is difficult to tell if a particular elephantiasic change is due to filariasis or to tuberculosis (Nelson 1979:1137; Spencer 1974:27) or even to chemicals (Nelson 1979:1137). Filarial vulval lymphedema and elephantiasis may be confused with that caused by tuberculosis (Lawson 1967b:467, 469) or lymphogranuloma venereum (Lawson 1967b:467; Spencer 1974:27), and filarial elephantiasis of the scrotum or penis is hard to tell from that caused by gonorrhea or schistosomiasis (*Schistosoma haematobium*) (Gratama 1966:86; Spencer 1974:27). And the lymph node enlargement seen in many cases of filariasis is similar to that caused by tuberculosis, syphilis, and Hodgkin's disease (King 1944:292).

Control

The life cycle of the filarial parasite was understood by the first part of the twentieth century. And even earlier, in the nineteenth century, surgery was being performed to correct some of the consequences of the disease such as elephantiasis. However, it was not until World War

II that effective measures to control filariasis emerged. During this time modern chemistry and the demands of wartime medicine combined to produce two effective weapons against filariasis, powerful insecticides and effective drugs of low toxicity. Although drugs alone could control the disease in some areas and insecticides in others, a combined assault is recommended.

Modern insecticides, specifically the organic phosphates and chlorinated hydrocarbons such as DDT, have been quite effective against the mosquito vectors of filariasis. Residual spraying with DDT to control malaria has had the additional benefit of lowering filariasis rates where the *Anopheles* mosquito is the vector for both diseases. However, many vectors have shown resistance to one or more of the insecticides, primarily DDT and dieldrin (Edeson 1972:64). And in the large endemic areas of India and in many other parts of the world the vector *Culex* has acquired resistance to almost all the available insecticides (Hawking 1975:14; Nelson 1979:1138). This is an unfortunate development because *Culex* is the primary vector in the urban centers where filariasis is becoming an increasingly serious problem.

Other antivector methods have been directed against the larval stage of the mosquito, using herbicides to destroy the water plants used by the larvae. Insect repellents have also been used. One, dimethyl phthalate, is particularly effective because when sprayed on the skin it not only repels the insect but also kills on contact any infective larvae of *W. bancrofti* (Edeson 1972:63–64).

Drugs have also been used, with considerable effectiveness in some instances, to control the spread of filariasis. The aim of these drugs is to interrupt transmission by lowering levels of microfilaremia. The 1940s saw remarkable improvements in treatment with the discovery and testing of the piperazines, especially diethylcarbamazine (DEC; Hetrazan). This drug is relatively nontoxic and can be administered orally. This gives it an advantage over previously used but toxic drugs such as suramin, antimony, and the arsenicals.

But even DEC has disadvantages that make effective treatment of large numbers of people difficult. First, repeated doses are necessary to ensure removal of all parasites from the blood (Benenson 1975:116). In countries like India where the disease is most prevalent, clinic reattendance rates are low and treatment campaigns have therefore been unsuccessful (Nelson 1979:1137). And even with repeated doses some persons remain persistently microfilaria positive (Edeson 1972:63; Mahoney and Kessel 1971:35), usually those with *W. bancrofti* infections and high density microfilaremia (World Health Organization 1974b:10).

Second, most persons involved in mass treatment programs, though harboring microfilariae, feel well and many are reluctant to take a drug that may make them feel quite miserable. Persons with *B. malayi* show a sharp febrile reaction within a few hours after the first dose of DEC. Fever may reach 40°C or higher and last several days; headache, backache, nausea, and vomiting may accompany the fever. The reaction is most severe in persons with high parasite counts (World Health Organization 1974b:10). In persons with Bancroftian filariasis fever may also occur after the first course of DEC treatment (Wijers and McMahon 1976:60), though fevers are neither as severe nor as frequent as with *B. malayi* (Edeson 1972:63; World Health Organization 1974b:11). Headache, dizziness, and nausea may also be seen (Brown 1975:150). Administration of antihistamines or antipyretics may alleviate discomfort (Spingarn and Edelman 1965:710; World Health Organization 1974b:11); the adverse reactions probably represent an allergic shock to the simultaneous death of many microfilariae with the liberation of their proteins (Jones 1967:188; Spingarn and Edelman 1965:710). These febrile reactions may themselves become a threat to fecundity by causing a temporary azoospermia in males. And treatment of pregnant women should be postponed until after delivery (World Health Organization 1974b:11) to avoid possible pregnancy loss. Fortunately, subsequent courses of treatment do not show such severe reactions, even though microfilaria counts may still be quite high. In addition to the "early" febrile reaction to DEC caused by the death of microfilariae—a reaction rarely seen in those with clinical lesions and no microfilariae—there is a "late" reaction that may occur in any infected individual. This reaction is presumably around dead or dying worms and presents as a localized swelling and inflammation of lymph vessels or glands, and again is accompanied by fever (Lawson 1967b:469; World Health Organization 1974b:11).

Because there is little evidence of acquired resistance to reinfection, constant surveillance is needed to see that microfilaremia rates do not increase again after treatment. One way to ensure this is to give regular doses of antifilarial drugs. In Japan this has been accomplished by adding DEC to popular foodstuffs (Edeson 1972:63). It is only because DEC is relatively nontoxic and the parasites have shown no sign of becoming resistant to it that such uncontrolled administration is possible. However, in areas where onchocerciasis coexists with Bancroftian and Malayan filariasis great care must be taken in dispensing DEC because the drug causes severe reactions in persons infected with *O. volvulus* (Duke 1980:6).

Control measures have met with varying degrees of success. Vector control has been attempted in only a few areas and the results are ambiguous. In the Pacific Islands DEC has been administered with good results against *W. bancrofti*, but results with the same parasite in India were disappointing. In those areas where prevalence rates are decreasing (*W. bancrofti*: Cape Verde Islands, Japan, Mauritius, Puerto Rico, Réunion, Sri Lanka, southern Togo, and many of the Pacific Islands; *B. malayi*: the state of Kerala in India, some areas of Indonesia and southern Thailand and Sri Lanka [from which the parasite has disappeared]) the credit is given not only to control efforts but also to improvements in the socioeconomic status of the community and to ecological change. The improved housing and water facilities that accompany such changes lower the number of sites for vector breeding. And as the standard of living and literacy rates rise, people become more aware of health hazards and the means to avoid them, such as the use of mosquito nets and use of treatment facilities and drugs (World Health Organization 1974b:6–8). Yet the overall picture is one of increasing prevalence at a time when many of the more dramatic tropical diseases are disappearing (Nelson 1979:1136). Thus, the best hope for control of filariasis (and many of the other tropical diseases as well) is the discovery of new drugs and especially the development of a vaccine. A WHO Special Program for Research and Training in Tropical Disease aimed at finding new drugs and a vaccine has been formed, and prospects are bright (Nelson 1979:1138).

Treatment

Drugs and surgery are the two tools used in the treatment of filarial disease. In patients with elephantiasis or a fully developed hydrocele drugs can do little more than prevent the disease from becoming worse (World Health Organization 1974b:10), and surgery to create new lymph channels is necessary to correct the damage (Jones 1967:188). In some cases this surgery carries its own risk, at times to reproductive potential. For example, surgical repair of a hydrocele may be followed by atrophy of the testis (Boyce and Politano 1970:630). And a calcified tunica vaginalis should be left alone as surgery only increases the symptoms or the chances that removal of the entire testicle will be necessary (Iturregui-Pagan *et al.* 1976:209).

The drug DEC is used at earlier stages of the disease. Administration of the drug prevents further episodes of fever and inflammation and may result in the regression in size of an early elephantiasis (Nelson 1979:1137; World Health Organization 1974b:10). During an acute attack, antibiotics may be given to control any secondary bacterial infection.

CHAPTER 6

Schistosomiasis

Introduction

Schistosomiasis, which has been called the "unconquered plague" (Weisbrod *et al.* 1973:46), is the third most prevalent disease worldwide, trailing only tuberculosis and malaria. It is estimated that 200 million people are infected with this parasitic disease. The infecting organisms are worms of the genus *Schistosoma*, commonly called blood flukes because they live in the blood vessels of the intestines and bladders of their definitive host, humans. The worms are remarkably fecund and long-lived; a gravid female lays 300–3000 eggs daily over a lifetime of 5 to 10 years (Warren 1978:610). These eggs possess enzymes that allow them to chew their way through the walls of the blood vessels and surrounding tissue until they reach the lumen of the bowel or bladder. They then pass out of the body along with the stools or urine. If deposited in a suitable body of fresh water the eggs liberate ciliated organisms called miracidia, which are capable of infecting certain species of freshwater snails. In the snail host asexual reproduction takes place, one miracidium producing many larvae called cercariae. These larvae pass from the snail into the surrounding water and wait for the human host necessary for the completion of their life cycle. Upon contact, the cercariae penetrate the human skin and migrate to the lung and then to the liver where they undergo sexual maturation and mate. The adult worms then migrate in pairs to the blood vessels that drain the intestines and bladder, and here the female worm begins to lay her eggs.

Distribution and Prevalence

There are three major species of *Schistosoma* that can infect humans, and each has its own characteristic, though not necessarily exclusive, geographical range (see Figure 6.1), species of snail intermediate host, location in the human circulatory system, egg morphology and output, and disease consequences. *Schistosoma japonicum* is the least well characterized of the three. It is found in the Far East, specifically China, Japan, Thailand,[1] the Philippines, and Celebes. The snail intermediate hosts are mollusks of the genus *Oncomelania*. The eggs, which are spheroidal with a small knob, are deposited primarily in the blood vessels of the large intestine. The female of this species is by far the most fecund, producing 3000 eggs daily compared with 300 for the other two species of *Schistosoma*. Because schistosomal disease is dependent on, among other things, the number of eggs produced, *S. japonicum* is a particulary malignant form of the disease. The major disease entity associated with *S. japonicum* is caused by eggs that dislodge from the intestinal vessels and are swept by the blood to the liver where they become lodged in the vessels. The pathological picture of the resulting liver disease is similar to that described in 1904 for *S. mansoni* (Warren 1978:610).

Schistosoma mansoni is the best characterized of the schistosomal diseases. Its geographical range is quite extensive and includes Africa, the Middle East, South America, and some Caribbean islands such as Puerto Rico. The snail intermediate hosts are mollusks of the genus *Biomphalaria*. The eggs of *S. mansoni*, which are ellipsoidal with a lateral spine, are laid at the rate of 300 per day per female worm and are deposited primarily in the blood vessels that drain the large intestine. As with *S. japonicum*, the involvement of the liver is responsible for the major disease associated with this type of schistosomiasis. This serious liver disease is called Symmers' fibrosis after William St. Clair Symmers, who first described the disease in 1904 while working in a Cairo hospital (Warren 1978:610).

Half a century before Symmers' descriptive work on *S. mansoni*, German pathologist Theodore Bilharz discovered *S. haematobium* while performing an autopsy on a young Egyptian male in the same Cairo hospital (Warren 1978:609). This disease, often called bilharziasis, is prevalent in the Middle East and Africa and is particularly rife in the

---

[1]The schistosome species found in the Mekong Delta of Laos and Thailand has been designated *Schistosoma mekongi*, but for most practical purposes can be lumped with *S. japonicum* (Cheever, personal communication, 1980).

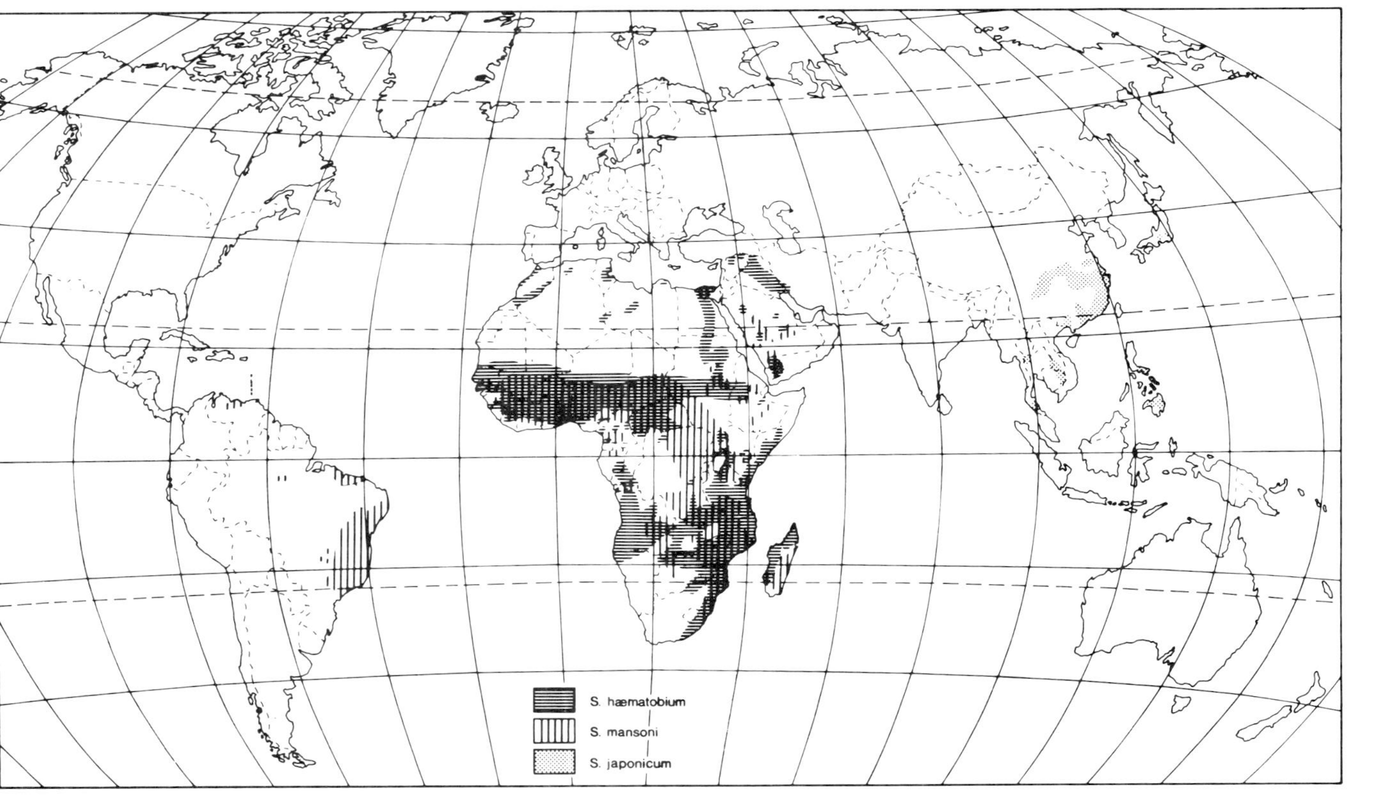

Figure 6.1 Global distribution of the three important forms of schistosomiasis. Source: Rée 1977:19. Reprinted with permission from ''Schistosomiasis.'' In G. Howe (ed.), *A World Geography of Human Diseases*. Copyright Academic Press Inc. (London) Ltd.

Nile Valley, Saudi Arabia, Yemen, Israel, Syria, and Iran (Kazzaz and Salmo 1974:333). Thus, *S. haematobium* coexists in many parts of the world with *S. mansoni*, and in these areas mixed infections are very frequent (Jones 1967:119; Jordan and Webbe 1969:82; Wright 1972:697). The snail intermediate hosts are mollusks of the genus *Bulinus*. The eggs, which are ellipsoidal with a terminal spine, are laid primarily in the vessels draining the urinary tract at the rate of 300 eggs per day per female worm. Although eggs of *S. haematobium* may reach other organs including the liver, lung, and rectum, they rarely produce any disease there, and pathological consequences are thus confined to the bladder and ureters.

Schistosomiasis continues to be a serious problem in over 70 tropical countries, where it is estimated that 200 million people are infected. It is advancing rather than receding in distribution and intensity in almost all African countries. One of the most important reasons for its growth is water resource development, which provides new breeding grounds for the snail intermediate hosts. For example, water projects around Volta Lake, Ghana, resulted in an increase in prevalence in the surrounding population from 10% to nearly 100% within 5 years (World Health Organization, World Bank, and United Nations 1982:6). In only a few areas—Brazil, China, Iran, Saint Lucia, Tunisia, and Venezuela— have noteworthy successes in control been achieved. Because schistosomiasis control is a biosocial–environmental matter and not exclusively a medical problem, effective control demands governmental commitment, interdisciplinary collaboration of political, educational, medical and sociological teams, and constant community involvement at all levels (McCullough 1980:2).

Role of the Schistosome Egg
in Disease

The schistosome egg is the principal factor responsible for schistosomal disease. But the egg itself is not at fault; disease is a consequence of host hypersensitivity to the presence of these eggs (Warren 1978:612). Thus, schistosomiasis may be classified as one of the immunological diseases. Of the hundreds (or thousands) of eggs laid each day by each gravid female, about 40% are excreted from the body (Warren 1978:610), usually via either the intestinal or urinary tract. These eggs cause no harm to the host. Trouble arises from those eggs that persist in host tissue. Because the proteins of the egg are antigenic (i.e., capable of eliciting an immune response in the host),[2] the eggs are soon surrounded by host lymphocytes, macrophages, and other members of the cellular defense team whose task it is to destroy these foreign bodies. This abnormal accumulation of cells is called a granuloma. It is an inflammatory response and is the first step in the development of schistosomal disease. After a few weeks the eggs have either been destroyed or have lost their antigenicity, and the initial inflammatory response is followed by healing, at times with the formation of permanent fibrous scar tissue (Cheever *et al.* 1978:67).

In *S. haematobium* infections the progression is usually to a greatly diminished inflammatory lesion and finally to a small amount of fibrous tissue overlying substantial numbers of dead eggs that have become calcified (Warren 1978:610). The most serious complications are caused either by early, bulky inflammatory granulomas, which may reach a size 100 times that of the egg (Mahmoud 1977:1329) or by the simple accumulation of large numbers of calcified eggs (Cheever *et al.* 1978:69). When urine flow is blocked because these lesions are in critical anatomic sites, such as where the ureters empty into the bladder, serious and sometimes fatal kidney disease may develop (Cheever *et al.* 1978:69–70).

On the other hand, the most serious complications associated with *S. mansoni* infection are caused not by early inflammatory lesions or accumulated eggs, but by the formation of large amounts of fibrous tissue. The serious liver disease seen in *S. mansoni* infections is the result of restricted blood flow caused by massive fibrosis of the tissue surrounding the hepatic vessels. Late in the disease *S. mansoni* eggs may be very difficult to find, as unlike *S. haematobium* eggs they are rapidly destroyed and do not accumulate. Therefore, in persons with mixed infections, although *S. haematobium* eggs may greatly outnumber those of *S. mansoni* in tissues such as those of the liver, intestine, or lung, observable pathology is usually due to *S. mansoni* (Cheever *et al.* 1978:68; Kamel *et al.* 1978:936).

A discussion of the pathophysiology of *S. japonicum* is omitted for two reasons: Not a great deal is known about it, and the role of *S. japonicum* in reproductive ability, which is our main interest, is not treated in the literature.

---

[2]The principal antigens are associated with the embryo, the shell being apparently inert (Cheever, personal communication, 1980).

Variations in Host Response

The most virulent host response to newly laid eggs occurs early after the initial infection (i.e., in the acute stage of the disease). A modulating effect that soon develops suppresses the host response and reduces pathological consequences. Thus, once the infection is established (i.e., chronic) the granulomatous response around newly deposited eggs is much smaller than around eggs laid during the acute stage (Mahmoud 1977:1329). This same modulating effect would hold true for eggs laid by worms resulting from a superinfection. But if one infection runs its course before a subsequent infection takes place, some of this immunosuppression is lost and a return to the more serious tissue reactions and serious pathological consequences is anticipated. In fact, the desirability of curative treatment of schistosomiasis has been questioned because it is feared that a cure might not only destroy any existing immunity to reinfection but also interfere with the suppression of immunopathology that coexists with chronic infection (World Health Organization 1978a:365). However, studies have shown that although reinfection may follow chemotherapy, it is unlikely to precipitate significant pathology ((McCullough 1980:4).[3] Also, reinfection rates in humans after treatment are generally low (World Health Organization 1978a:365). Nevertheless, it is believed to be safer (and more economical) to reduce to a low level the worm load in that minority of severely infected individuals who are at risk of developing serious disease and not to treat the vast majority of persons whose worm load is low and in whom the infection generally remains subclinical and well tolerated (McCullough 1980:2).

Other variable effects on the pathological consequences of schistosomal disease have been noted and are of considerable interest to any population-based survey. It has been noted that serious schistosomal disease tends to run in families (Tachon and Borojevic 1978:605) and therefore a genetic predisposition has been proposed. However, many investigators feel that the observed familial predisposition is linked more to common exposure patterns to infested water than to a common genetic trait. Nevertheless, two genetic traits do seem to be linked to the development of schistosomiasis. First, persons with type A blood are more likely to develop serious disease when infected with *S. mansoni* (Camus *et al.* 1977:182; Kamel *et al.* 1978: 937), whereas those with type O more frequently develop mild disease (Camus *et al.* 1977:182). Sec-

---

[3]This has been confirmed by studies in mice suggesting that the protective effects of schistosomal infection persist after treatment (Warren *et al.* 1977:961).

ond, it has been observed in Brazil that serious liver disease is much more likely to develop in whites than in blacks infected with *S. mansoni* (Kamel *et al.* 1978:937). Others (e.g., Cheever *et al.* 1978:68; Gelfand 1976:178; Jordan and Webbe 1969:68) have also noted racial variability in the degree and type of response to schistosomal infection. Another interesting observation was made by Hiatt and Gebre-Medhin (1977:476), who noted that a past history of malaria seems to be inversely related to the pathological consequences of *S. mansoni* infection. This observation is supported by an animal study in which mice infected with malaria and subsequently infected with *S. mansoni* showed fewer and smaller granulomas around eggs in the lung (Abdel-Wahab *et al.* 1974:915). (This may well have been due to the immunosuppressive effects of malaria.) These preliminary findings suggest that schistosomiasis may be a less serious disease in areas where malaria infections are common.

Several other variables have been mentioned as altering the host response to schistosomal infection, such as the strain of infecting species of *Schistosoma* (Jordan and Webbe 1969:99), viral hepatitis (Spingarn and Edelman 1965:714), and nutritional deficiencies (Jordan 1972:55; Spingarn and Edelman 1965:714; Weisbrod *et al.* 1973:47). Two reports (Cheever *et al.* 1978:72; Kamel *et al.* 1978:937) stated that the intensity of infection (the number of eggs per gram of tissue) is the single most important factor in determining the pathological consequences of infection. This is certainly true for *S. mansoni* infections (Cheever *et al.* 1978:72). But for *S. haematobium* there is an intensity threshold (below which urinary schistosomiasis will not develop) above which the intensity of infection seems to bear little relation to the severity of the disease (Cheever *et al.* 1978:69). Other factors such as the location of lesions may be of greater importance; strategically located lesions, such as those in the ureters or around the site where the ureters empty into the bladder, are more likely to cause serious disease than lesions elsewhere in the bladder (Cheever *et al.* 1978:69). It should also be noted that the correlation between intensity of infection and schistosomal disease, though an invaluable tool from a public health standpoint in evaluating disease probabilities in a population, has much less relevance to schistosomiasis in the individual. This is largely because two individuals may respond very differently to the same intensity of infection (Cheever *et al.* 1978:72).

The interest in this volume is on any adverse effects of schistosomiasis on the reproductive organs. But most studies deal with the pathological consequences of infection in the bladder, bowel, liver, or lungs, and such information cannot always be applied to other organs such as the male and female genitals. This is primarily because the egg concentration–tissue damage relationship is influenced by the anatomic site of egg deposition (Cheever *et al.* 1978:68). Gelfand *et al.* (1970:782), for example, noted a lack of correlation between the number of eggs and the inflammatory reaction present in different male reproductive organs; in certain organs there was a marked response to a few eggs, but in others there was little or no response to many eggs. Thus, the evaluation of the effects of schistosomal infection in a particular organ should include a thorough review of large numbers of tissue specimens, recording both the number of eggs per gram of tissue and the tissue reaction to their presence.

Some time was spent describing the pathophysiology of schistosomiasis to give the reader a better understanding of the complexities of this disease. All the variables discussed here have relevance to the effects of schistosomiasis on the reproductive organs and must be considered when assessing any effects of the disease on population fecundity. Discussed were the diminished response to newly deposited eggs that appears as the duration of infection increases, the positive correlation between intensity of infection and severity of disease, the variable response of different organs to the schistosome egg, differences in the types of lesions produced by *S. haematobium* and *S. mansoni*, and the susceptibility of persons of certain blood and racial groups to more serious forms of the disease.

Effects on Fecundity

The important question of whether schistosomiasis causes pathophysiological changes in the male or female that might diminish reproductive capacity is not easily answered. Scientific understanding of the real impact of schistosomiasis on all of human health has changed radically since the 1970s, making some earlier statements suspect. The once-common notion that schistosomiasis causes "mass chronic invalidism" (Gallagher 1969:97) has been totally discounted. Hiatt and Gebre-Medhin (1977:473) said it well:

> In recent years, population-based studies of *Schistosomiasis mansoni* have begun to provide sound information on the clinical significance and public health impact of this disease. Earlier studies of morbidity based on hospital and clinical patients or other types of selected individuals tended to bias observations toward severe forms of the disease.

Two excellent studies in Latin America—Cook and the Rockefeller group in Saint Lucia and Lehman and the Harvard–Wellcome collaborative project in Brazil—showed that in areas of low to moderate endemicity *S. mansoni* has few overt manifestations except for liver and spleen enlargement in children (Weller 1976:212). And Siongok *et al.* (1976:282) have shown that even in parts of Kenya where *S. mansoni* is hyperendemic, the majority of the population have light or moderate infections with no significant morbidity. Even as early as 1962 Elsdon–Dew (1962:209), in speaking of *S. haematobium*, warned that too many investigators were generalizing from the worst cases of the disease and that the vast majority of cases were so mild they would be missed altogether were it not for small amounts of blood in the urine during the early stages of bladder infection. He reported that "so common is infection that an African mother took her teenage son to the doctor because his 'menses' had not yet appeared" (Elsdon–Dew 1975:76). And the complaints of weakness, diarrhea, and abdominal pain recounted by many persons with schistosomiasis were found not to be due to the disease, except in persons with the very heaviest infections (Gremillion *et al.* 1978:926), because many uninfected persons complained of the same ailments when asked (Warren *et al.* 1974:902). Probably one or more of the other infectious agents so ubiquitous in developing nations were responsible for these discomforts, not schistosomiasis. Thus, there is the tremendous problem of making a differential diagnosis when so many diseases with similar pathological consequences are found in the same place.

Is then schistosomiasis, as one of the most prevalent infections in the developing world, also one of the major etiological factors in the subfecundity there? Again, the answer to this question is difficult because of the two problems just mentioned—the re-evaluation of earlier conclusions on the health consequences of schistosomiasis at the population level and the problem of differential diagnosis in areas of the world where so many diseases with similar clinical pictures coexist. An adequate answer could be had by answering four important questions: (1) Are schistosome eggs found in the genital organs? (2) If they are, are resulting lesions sufficiently severe to affect the functioning of these organs adversely? (3) Are there any secondary sequelae such as secondary infections, toxic by-products of the worms or eggs, or systemic effects such as fever or anemia, that could be of interest? (4) What is the timing and duration of any adverse effects?

Male

Frequency and Intensity of Genital Infection

It is certainly true that in highly endemic areas the genital organs of many men are infected with schistosomiasis. In Rhodesia (now Zimbabwe), Gelfand *et al.* (1970:781) found 77 cases of schistosomiasis, primarily *S. haematobium*, in 100 consecutive male autopsies, and in no fewer than 70 of these men the genital organs were infected. The number of persons with infected genital organs necessarily varies from study to study, consistent with the prevalence of infection in the study population (see discussion in next paragraph). Also important is the species of schistosome in the study area, as *S. mansoni* is much less often found in the genitals than *S. haematobium*. In areas of the world such as South and Central America where *S. mansoni* is the exclusive schistosome, genital infection is extremely rare. After performing over 3000 autopsies and reviewing 78,000 specimens in Puerto Rico, Arean (1956a:1010) found just 10 cases of genital tract involvement. In areas such as Africa where both schistosomes coexist and mixed infections are frequent, *S. mansoni* occasionally finds its way to the genitals with the assistance of *S. haematobium* (Cheever *et al.* 1977:712). Edington *et al.* (1975:153) reported that *S. mansoni* is of little importance in Nigeria, being found in only 4% of all cases of schistosomiasis. But in the Gelfand *et al.* (1970:781) study in Rhodesia, 15.5% of the seminal vesicles and 8% of the vasa deferentia contained eggs of *S. mansoni*. The presence of *S. mansoni* eggs could mean severe fibrotic reactions in these organs, but egg loads were quite low. And, according to Cheever *et al.* (1977:712), most *S. mansoni* eggs in the seminal vesicles are calcified, whereas this is not true at their primary sites of deposition (i.e., the colon and liver). The accumulation of calcified eggs suggests that in these tissues *S. mansoni* eggs were destroyed much more slowly than at their normal sites, and this implies a lesser tissue reaction and thus less tissue pathology.

In a population, the proportion of those infected whose genital organs are infected rises as the prevalence of schistosomiasis in that population rises. For example, Edington *et al.* (1975:153–154), in a study that found schistosomiasis in 22% of males autopsied, observed that of these infected men 35% had infected seminal vesicles and 24% had infected prostate glands. In the study by Gelfand *et al.* (1970:781), where a much higher proportion of autopsied males were positive for schistosomiasis (72.5%), the respective figures for involvement of the seminal vesicles and prostate were 54 and 28%, respectively. The reason for this association is simply that the higher the frequency of infection in a population the higher the average intensity of infection; when an infection is intense and a great number of parasites exist in the body, they often find their normal sites of egg laying too crowded and are forced to move into other vessels, often finding their way to the vessels draining the genital organs (Madgi 1967:418). In addition, the more intense the infection, the greater the number of displaced worms in the genital region and the more severe the disease there. Thus, in areas where schistosomiasis is hyperendemic, not only will more persons have genital infections but schistosomal disease will be more serious in all organs, including the genitals. Thus, because the frequency of schistosomal infection was higher in the Gelfand *et al.* (1970) study, more cases of severe genital infection would be expected than in the Edington *et al.* (1975) series.

Within the male genital tract some organs are more frequently the sites of infection than others, and egg loads vary considerably from organ to organ. The seminal vesicles are by far the most frequently infected of the genital organs, and in one study (Gelfand *et al.* 1970:781) were more often infected than the bladder. Nevertheless, egg loads, though the very highest of any genital organ, are still only 20–25% those seen in the bladder (Cheever *et al.* 1977:709; Edington *et al.* 1975:154; Gelfand *et al.* 1970:787). The next most frequently infected genital organ is usually the prostate gland, but its egg load is substantially below (less than 10%) even that of the seminal vesicles (Cheever *et al.* 1977:709; Gelfand *et al.* 1970:781). The testes and epididymis are infrequently the sites of egg deposition (Edington *et al.* 1975:154) and egg loads are very low (Cheever *et al.* 1977:709; Edington *et al.* 1975:154).

Tissue Reaction and Possible Sequelae to Infection

It has been said that "among the common aetiological factors leading to obstructive azoospermia in Egypt is infestation of the urogenital tract by *Schistosoma haematobium*" (Aal *et al.* 1975:403). And many serious lesions that would undoubtedly cause subfecundity have been reported in the literature (Edington *et al.* 1975:157; Gelfand *et al.* 1970:783–784). Nevertheless, the most recent and reliable studies, which use unselected autopsy material, indicate that male fecundity is rarely affected by schistosomiasis. This is because reactions to the eggs, though not infrequent (Gelfand *et al.* [1970:783] found positive reactions in 31% of infected seminal vesicles and 14% of infected prostate glands, whereas Edington *et al.* [1975:157] found positive reactions around eggs in 37% of infected seminal vesicles and 62% of infected prostates), are usually very mild.[4]

[4]Because a past history of malaria seems to be associated with a lesser tissue reaction to schistosome eggs, persons living in malarious areas such as Zimbabwe and Nigeria, the locations of the two cited autopsy studies, might have less serious lesions than persons from northern Africa and the Middle East where malaria is not found. Other infections that suppress the immune response, such as African sleeping sickness, may also alter the response to schistosomal infection. It would be worthwhile, therefore, to study a population infected with schistosomes but relatively free of malaria or African sleeping sickness to see if the results of the Gelfand *et al.* (1970, 1971) and Edington *et al.* (1975) studies are truly representative.

Although Gelfand *et al.* did not specifically characterize the reactions, saying only that inflammation was seen, Edington *et al.* characterized the lesions in the seminal vesicles as being seldom severe and usually inactive with fibrosis, and said that lesions in the prostate were all inactive.

But is it not possible—in fact, probable—that even mild lesions could cause an imbalance in the intricate complex of biochemical and mechanical events necessary for full reproductive capacity? And just because a lesion is presently characterized as being inactive and insignificant, could it not have been of some significance during the early inflammatory stage? The importance of understanding the past significance of presently healed lesions was emphasized by Cheever *et al.* (1978:69), who noted deformed ureters in men with minimum residual *S. haematobium* pathology. They felt that earlier in the disease, when inflammatory lesions were present, one of two possible events may have occurred: (1) The inflammatory response may have been so great as to cause a narrowing or blockage of the ureter, slowing or stopping urine flow and causing a permanent billowing of the ureter, or (2) the inflammation and fibrosis of the ureteral wall may have caused functional damage, thereby interfering with normal peristaltic motion that moves the urine toward the bladder. They felt that a large part of significant genitourinary pathology was being overlooked simply because autopsy material selected against the young, who were the most likely to have active disease.

What are the implications of this hypothesis for our assessment of the role of schistosomiasis in male fecundity? Could the rather substantial egg loads seen in the seminal vesicles, for example, have been preceded by larger inflammatory lesions that might have diminished the quality or quantity of seminal fluid? Could the inflammation have set the stage for chronic vesiculitis? And although egg loads are usually much lower in the prostate gland and possible inflammatory responses are much reduced, could a heavily infected prostate be adversely affected? Could the quality or quantity of prostatic fluid have been diminished? Could the prostate have been so inflamed that the ejaculatory duct that passes through it was narrowed, resulting in a smaller ejaculate volume? Because schistosome eggs in the prostate are usually associated with the ejaculatory duct (Cheever *et al.* 1978:65), this latter scenario is particularly possible.

Definitive answers to these questions must await further study. This is because our hypothesis depends entirely on the presence of active infection, and most reliable data on the effects of schistosomiasis on male fertility are from autopsy studies in which young persons with active disease are seriously underrepresented. (Active disease with the highest rates of egg excretion is seen in children and adolescents 6–16 years of age [McCullough 1980:4].) Once the infection becomes chronic and early lesions heal, any adverse effects on reproductive ability would be resolved, unless chronic vesiculitis or prostatitis sets in and the role of schistosomiasis in these complications is not yet resolved (Edington *et al.* 1975:157).

But the story does not end here with a proposal that schistosomiasis may more often be a cause of male subfecundity, albeit of a temporary nature, than hitherto accepted. Simply extrapolating back from late cases of the disease can be misleading, especially when dealing with the seminal vesicles. This is the one organ, according to Cheever *et al.* (1977:709), in which the proportion of eggs changes with age. In their study, eggs were rarely found in the seminal vesicles of males less than 15 years of age; in men 20–40, about 4% of all eggs were in the seminal vesicles; and after age 40, 18% could be found there. This substantially reduces the potential impact of schistosomiasis on male fecundity, because seminal vesicle involvement was less during the peak reproductive years. Also, eggs deposited in the seminal vesicle, or any other organ, during the later chronic stage of the disease are known to meet with a much-reduced tissue response compared to eggs deposited during the acute stage (Mahmoud 1977:1329). Also, the results of a study by Azm *et al.* (1977:775) of 40 patients with bilharzial seminal vesiculitis make unlikely any profound effect on reproductive ability from involvement of this organ; the men in this study all had patent ducts and fructose in their ejaculate, and all had fathered two or more children.

Summary of Effects on Male Fecundity

In sum, we must agree with the majority opinion that schistosomiasis is not a frequent cause of genital lesions that can cause male subfecundity. However, the possibility that other factors associated with schistosomal infection might alter fecundity cannot be dismissed. For example, Abdul *et al.* (1974, cited in Ledward 1980:118) suggested that *S. haematobium* infections may cause male infertility because urogenital bilharziasis is thought to enhance the autoimmune response, leading to a higher incidence of antispermal antibodies. Altered immunoresponsiveness is also thought to lead to increased antispermal antibodies in women with cervicovaginal schistosomiasis and to be a cause of sterility (El-Mahgoub 1972:783–784) (see the next section, which discusses effects on female fecundity). Also, hypogonadism has been reported in some persons with severe *S. mansoni* and *S. japonicum* infections. A causal association with schistosomal infection is supported by the fact that all the young adults with this condition have the hepatosplenic form of this disease and respond dramatically to splenectomy (El-Mofty 1962:183; Jordan and Webbe 1969:102).

Female

The effect of schistosomiasis on female fecundity has also been the subject of contradictory opinions. Many workers feel schistosomiasis of the female genital tract is a serious disease inimical to reproduction. Retel-Laurentin (1978:119) claimed that bilharziasis, when serious or chronic, causes multiple miscarriages and sterility. Zinsou *et al.* (1967:281) believed that schistosomiasis is a decisive etiological factor in the female sterility that affects more than 25% of the female population in some parts of Africa. Correa (1969:14) also believed it to be important in female sterility in the Central African Republic. And Gilbert (1943:332) stated that "the peculiarities of the disease as it is encountered in the genital tract rest primarily in the colossal fibrosis which is present."

On the other hand, many researchers (e.g., Edington *et al.* 1975:159–160; Gelfand *et al.* 1971:849) have felt that although the eggs of schistosomiasis (*S. huemulobium* is the usual infecting organism) are distributed throughout the female genital tract, substantial reactions to the eggs are confined to the lower tract (i.e., the vagina and cervix), and therefore any effects on fecundity are minimal. The stand of the WHO study group on infertility (World Health Organization 1975:15) was however, one of uncertainty. They believed that schistosomiasis may play a part in causing male and possibly female infertility, but maintained that this had not yet been well defined.

What is the evidence for any effect on fecundity? Are these women easily identifiable, that is, are there certain symptoms or clinical signs of genital infection? In endemic areas how likely is there to be genital involvement? Which genital organs are most frequently infected? And is schistosomiasis of any of the female genital organs sufficiently severe to cause a dimunition of reproductive capacity? All these questions must be answered before any assessment of the role of female schistosomiasis in population subfecundity can be made.

Symptoms

Some researchers have reported that schistosomiasis of the female genital tract is associated with pain and menstrual disorders. Charlewood (1956:43) stated that menstrual disorders are frequent. And Gilbert (1943:333–334) listed scanty and short menses, dysmenorrhea, and dyspareunia as features of genital schistosomiasis. He further stated that malaise and anorexia are symptoms, as well as general pelvic pain in advanced cases. Delayed menarche and early menopause are also cited as possible responses to ovarian involvement in the fibrotic process.

That schistosomiasis is not usually associated with malaise has already been discussed. And Frost (1975:1203), when questioning uninfected women as well as those with schistosomiasis, found that their menstrual cycles were similar and that the incidence of dysmenorrhea, vaginal discharge, and acute and chronic pain were similar. Again, persons from areas where schistosomiasis is prevalent are often infected with any one of a number of pathogens, and bodily complaints are frequent and difficult to ascribe to any particular infection. It is therefore important to interview those persons not infected with a certain organism as well as infected persons.

Frequency of Genital Infection

Because symptoms are usually absent in female genital schistosomiasis, the number of women so affected in a population is best determined by autopsy studies. Ideally, such studies should be performed in areas where prevalence rates, and thus the average intensity of infection, are high, because genital infection is more likely in those persons with heavier infections (Edington *et al.* 1975:158). Edington *et al.* (1975:155) noted in their study that when bladder infections were severe, 100% of the vaginas and cervices, 66% of the uteri, 33% of the tubes, and 33% of the ovaries were infected. But in the mild bladder infections these figures dropped to 20% of vaginas, 30% of cervices, 10% of uteri, 0% of tubes, and 15% of ovaries. A possible reason for this was forwarded by Magdi (1967:418), who proposed that the terminal vessels at the normal sites of egg laying (bladder and rectum) are so crowded in heavy infections that some parasites are forced to seek other outlets and migrate to the vessels draining the genital organs.

Exact figures on the number of women in a population with genital schistosomiasis were difficult to find because the major autopsy studies selected women positive for schistosomiasis in any of the pelvic organs—bladder, rectum, genitals—and described genital tract involvement among them. Gelfand *et al.* (1971:846) found schistosomiasis of the pelvic organs in 37 of 64 (58%) consecutive autopsies of women in Rhodesia (now Zimbabwe). Of these women, 12 had schistosomiasis of the vagina, 13 of the cervix, 4 of the uterus, 8 of the fallopian tubes, and 7 of the ovaries. Edington *et al.* (1975:153,155) found 34 (16%) of the females autopsied in Nigeria in their study to be positive for schistosomiasis of the bladder. Of these women 15 had infections of the vagina, 14 of the cervix, 6 of the uterus, 3 of the tubes, and 9 of the ovaries. Because many women in these studies had involvement of more than one organ, the overall number with genital schistosomiasis could not be determined. Nevertheless, it is apparent that schistosomiasis of the pelvic organs is fairly common in women in both Zimbabwe and Nigeria, and at least one-third to one-half of these infected women have involvement of one or more genital organs.

Intensity of Infection and Tissue Response

At least 20% of consecutive autopsies in the Gelfand *et al.* (1970) study and at least 7% of those in the Edington *et al.* (1975) study had genital schistosomiasis; thus, it is possible the disease might have a significant impact on the fecundity of such populations if the lesions are severe enough to compromise reproductive ability. As with males, this depends on the egg load and tissue response in each organ. Although one excellent study (Cheever *et al.* 1977:708–709) of an area of high prevalence in Egypt (50% of 400 consecutive persons autopsied were infected with schistosomiasis) concluded that the number of eggs in the females genitals was "insignificant," other studies have found measurable egg loads in some organs and have quantitated the number of eggs in each organ and described any tissue response. The results of these studies follow.

Vulva and Vagina Schistosomal infection of the vulva and vagina is not uncommon and fibrotic reaction to the eggs may be very severe. Large papillomatous masses of the vulva and vagina have been described in populations in Egypt and South Africa (Edington *et al.* 1975:159), and these may be difficult to distinguish macroscopically from cancer or from other chronic granulomatous infections such as tuberculosis (Stewart 1967c:454). Vaginal infection, if severe, may be associated with a fistula to the bladder (Charlewood 1956:40; Gilbert 1943:330; Spingarn and Edelman 1965:715). Ulceration of the vagina and "sandy patches" containing massive numbers of eggs have also been described (Edington *et al.* 1975:159). These however, are extreme cases. In the two cited autopsy studies lesions were usually mild. All the cases of vaginal infection found by Edington *et al.* (1975:159) were inactive with only mild fibrosis despite some cases of what they described as "fairly heavy egg loads." And Gelfand *et al.* (1971:848) found relatively light egg loads in their series and noted only two inflammatory lesions in 12 cases of vaginal schistosomiasis.

Thus, the vulva and vagina, although capable of dramatic tissue reactions to schistosome eggs, usually do not show such reactions even when egg loads are fairly heavy. No effects on reproductive ability would then be anticipated, although coital frequency could be severely restricted in those few women with ulceration or large papillomatous lesions (Magdi 1967:423).

Cervix   Severe reactions of the cervix to schistosomiasis have also been reported. Cervical masses accompanied by ulceration have been described (Charlewood 1956:40; Spingarn and Edelman 1965:715) and these often look a great deal like cervical carcinoma. Other cervical lesions caused by schistosomiasis resemble tuberculosis of the cervix (Charlewood 1956:40) and have been described as "pseudotubercles" (Williams 1967:787). But such severe reactions do not seem to be the rule. Indeed, the cervix may contain a variable number of eggs and still remain normal in appearance (Williams 1967:789). In the two cited autopsy studies cervical reactions were infrequent. Edington *et al.* (1975:159) saw light egg loads and only inactive infections with mild fibrosis. Likewise, Gelfand *et al.* (1971:848) saw inflammatory reactions in only 3 of 13 women with cervical schistosomiasis despite light to moderate egg loads in some cases. Although no effect on reproductive ability would be anticipated from these mild cervical lesions, it is possible that the ability to secrete mucus favorable to sperm survival could be altered, lowering conceptive ability.

Cervicovaginal Schistosomiasis and Antispermal Antibodies   Although most schistosomal lesions of the vagina and cervix are not believed to be sufficiently severe to adversely affect fecundity, certain by-products of these lesions have been so implicated. El-Mahgoub (1972:783–784) believed that cervicovaginal schistosomiasis is associated with the local production of antispermal antibodies detectable in the circulation. He noted that more than 60% of women with cervicovaginal schistosomiasis who were sterile produced serum antibodies that precipitated *any* sample of human spermatozoa. Of sterile women with schistosomiasis at other sites, such as the bladder, 10% or fewer had such serum antibodies. He stated that the unfavorable postcoital tests in most patients with genital schistosomiasis support his theory, but conceded that nonspecific effects of the infection on the sperm, such as toxic products, could not be excluded. (Hostile or insufficient cervical mucus is another possibility; see the discussion in the section "Cervix.") Of his 41 patients with cervicovaginal schistosomiasis, 8 conceived 6 to 18 months after antischistosomal therapy was initiated.

Although the results of this study are potentially very important, the study suffers from the problem of unrepresentativeness. El-Mahgoub did not study all women with cervicovaginal schistosomiasis, but selected only sterile women. Thus, the proportion of all women with cervicovaginal schistosomiasis who are sterile and/or produce antispermal antibodies is not known.

Uterus Whereas schistosomiasis of the lower genital tract is believed to be more common before puberty, the uterus, as well as the tubes and ovaries, are more likely to be infected during adult life when these organs become more highly vascularized (Magdi 1967:419–420). Uterine infections, when noted, are usually of the myometrium, or muscular layer of the uterus; schistosomiasis of the endometrium, or lining of the uterus, is rare (Edington *et al.* 1975:160). Indeed, schistosomal infection of any part of the uterus is considered by some (e.g., Arean 1956b:1047; GIlbert 1943:329) to be unusual. Perhaps, suggested Magdi (1967:424), this is because the venules that drain the uterus twist and turn and the worm has difficulty in reaching the terminal areas of the uterine vessels. Yet Edington *et al.* (1975:155) noted uterine infection in 6 of 34 women with pelvic schistosomiasis and Gelfand *et al.* (1971:848) noted it in 4 of 37 such women. But both groups noted very small egg loads and neither study could find any uterine lesions attributable to the infection (Edington *et al.* 1975:155, 160; Gelfand *et al.* 1971:848).

Thus, reports that uterine schistosomiasis is a cause of spontaneous abortion and premature labor (Charlewood *et al.* 1949, cited in Edington *et al.* 1975:160; Williams 1967:790) describe the rare case. It also seems unlikely that uterine masses, which are frequent in some African populations with high rates of sterility, are due to schistosomiasis, as some researchers feel. In addition, there is no agreement as to whether such masses are even a cause of subfecundity (Adadevoh 1974:18), although some workers (e.g., Potts *et al.* 1977:47) have definitely believed they are. Nevertheless, Correa (1969:14, 16) stated that uterine masses are a common cause of sterility in the Nzakara group in the Central African Republic and suggested that schistosomiasis contributes to this condition.

Transplacental Infection It is agreed that the uterus of an infected woman may contain some eggs; is there any evidence that in pregnant women these eggs could cross the placenta and enter the fetus? Although eggs have been recovered from the placenta (Jordan and Webbe, 1969:81)—in 7 of 21 placentas in one study (Sutherland *et al.* 1965, cited in Edington *et al.* 1975:160)—their ability to cross the placenta is not fully settled (Williams 1967:790). Studies in Japan and Angola (see Williams 1967:790) do, however, suggest that the adult worms can enter the placental blood vessels and infect the fetus. But because mention of such an occurrence is rare in the literature, it must be assumed that transplacental infection is a very unusual event.

Transplacental Antigen Transfer   Perhaps less unusual is the passage of schistosomal antigens (proteins from the worms and/or eggs) across the placenta. The immune system of the fetus thus becomes sensitized to these antigens and such sensitivity may persist for many years after birth. This could modify the individual's resistance to infection or the phenomenon of hypersensitivity to worms and their eggs, which is immensely important to reaction to infection and disease consequences. It is felt that close follow-up of these children is necessary before it can be said with any certainty what the consequences of prenatal sensitization are, but it has been suggested (Tachon and Borojevic 1978:608) that this may be one reason for the previously mentioned phenomenon of the clumping within families of severe cases of the disease.

On the other hand, infection of the fetus early in its development, before it is immunocompetent, may result in immune tolerance. In such a case the fetus is incapable of recognizing the invading organism as "foreign" and does not now, or in the future, mount an immune response to the organism. This would greatly alter sequelae to infections such as schistosomiasis, where host overresponsiveness (hypersensitivity) is responsible for disease manifestations. (For further discussion see Hang *et al.* [1974].)

Fallopian Tubes   The effect of schistosomiasis on the fallopian tubes has perhaps received the most attention. The frequency of tubal involvement in different populations has been recorded at various levels, depending, of course, on the prevalence of schistosomal infection in these populations. One study (Gelfand and Ross 1953, cited in Edington *et al.* 1975:160) found tubal infection in 63% of women with *S. haematobium* of the bladder—a very high figure. Another study (Bland and Gelfand 1970:1025) found far fewer cases, 16%, in women positive for *S. haematobium*. The autopsy study of Edington *et al.* (1975:160) found evidence of tubal infection in only 11% of women with schistosomiasis, whereas that of Gelfand *et al.* (1971:848) found tubal schistosomiasis in 22% of women with pelvic schistosomiasis.

In tubal schistosomiasis the lining (mucosa) of the tubes is not usually affected and therefore the tubes are rarely occluded, except in *S. mansoni* tubal infections, which are rare (Rosen and Kim 1974:413). Rather, the muscle layers are involved in the fibrotic process. Hence, only a few researchers (e.g., Zinsou *et al.* 1967:282) believe that tubal schistosomiasis is a *direct* cause of sterility. (It has been suggested, however, that tubal schistosomiasis is an *indirect* cause of sterility; see following discussion.)

Tubal schistosomiasis is, however, frequently cited for its role in ectopic pregnancy (Frost 1975:1202; Gilbert 1943:328; Magdi 1967:424; Zinsou *et al.* 1967:281). It is felt that the thickened, damaged muscle layers cannot properly perform their function of propelling the fertilized egg through the tube into the uterus, and thus tubal implantation occurs (Arean 1956b:1041).

Is there any documented support for such a hypothesis? A study in Rhodesia (Bland and Gelfand 1970:1026) did find a significant difference between the incidence of tubal pregnancy in women with and without tubal schistosomiasis. However, in 4 of the 6 patients with tubal schistosomiasis and tubal pregnancy there were no inflammatory lesions or structural damage deemed sufficiently great to have caused the ectopic implantation. The study concluded that, except in the less-common case where there is a severe inflammatory response, the presence of schistosome eggs is of little or no consequence in the tubes. And Frost (1975:1201), who also did research in Rhodesia in an area where schistosomiasis is relatively common, found no statistically significant difference in the incidence of tubal schistosomiasis between control women and those with an ectopic pregnancy. Rather, she concluded (1975:1202) that in studies reporting schistosomiasis as a cause of ectopic pregnancy, ''It is likely that schistosomiasis was an incidental finding in their patients and that their condition could more accurately have been described as an association of tubal pregnancy with [schistosomiasis].'' The conclusions of the two autopsy studies (Edington *et al.* 1975:160; Gelfand *et al.* 1971:848) are in agreement with this view. Finding generally light egg loads and mild or negligible lesions in the fallopian tubes they examined, these authors concluded that schistosomiasis was an uncommon cause of ectopic pregnancy, at least in those areas where the studies were conducted.

These two autopsy studies also concluded that schistosomiasis is an uncommon cause of sterility in these areas. Because, as mentioned earlier, the tubal mucosa is spared and tissue response to the eggs is not significant, this conclusion is not surprising. However, it has been suggested (Muir and Belsey 1980:920) that schistosomiasis may be an *indirect* cause of salpingitis and sterility, that schistosome eggs may irritate and weaken the tubal tissues and render them more susceptible to infection. Evidence that schistosomiasis predisposes to salpingitis and subsequent sterility is mixed. Frost (1975:1201) found no statistically significant difference in the incidence of tubal schistosomiasis in control women and those with salpingitis. On the other hand, Bullough (1976) reported a significantly higher rate of *S. haematobium* infection (site unspecified) in women with primary and secondary sterility (41.8% and 38.0%) compared to fertile controls (21.4%). More research is therefore necessary to determine whether or not women with tubal schistosomiasis are more likely to experience pelvic infection.

Ovaries   Ovarian involvement with schistosomiasis has the potential to severely diminish fecundity. Schistosome-infected ovaries with regions of inflammation, abscess formation, or fibrosis have been described (Edington *et al.* 1975:160). Under such conditions, ovulation would likely be suppressed and sterility would result (Gilbert 1943:325). Heavy infection of the ovaries has also been associated with other abnormalities such as dysmenorrhea, delayed menstruation, and premature menopause (Edington *et al.* 1975:160).

Again, reports differ as to the frequency with which the ovaries are involved and the extent of any serious lesions. Magdi (1967:425) reported that bilateral involvement of the ovaries in women with schistosomiasis was not uncommon, but that only the most serious lesions were capable of adversely affecting fecundity. The two cited autopsy studies quantitated such impressions. Gelfand *et al.* (1971:848) found that the ovaries were infected in 7 of 37 (19%) women with pelvic schistosomiasis. Egg loads, which were quite variable, were fairly high in some cases. Nevertheless, no inflammatory lesions were seen. In the series of Edington *et al.* (1975:155, 159) the ovaries were infected in 31% of women positive for schistosomiasis. Egg loads were very light and no microscopic lesions were seen. The conclusion must be that ovarian schistosomiasis is an infrequent cause of reproductive problems.

Most of the studies cited to this point have offered convincing evidence that schistosomal lesions of the female genital tract are usually insignificant and would be expected to have little or no influence on fecundity. Nevertheless, two studies concluded that genital schistosomiasis is an important cause of sterility. Zinsou *et al.* (1967:281–282) believed that female genital schistosomiasis is ''a decisive factor'' in the sterility that affects more than 25% of women in some areas of Africa. The authors examined biopsy material from 325 women in Senegal. Of these women, more than half of whom complained of primary or secondary sterility, 39 had schistosomiasis of the genitals. Lesions of the upper tract were quite severe. Macroscopically, there were nodules in the uterus, irregular thickening of the tubes, and occasionally a sclerotic fibrosis of the ovaries. Microscopic examination of tissue revealed eggs typical of *S. haematobium*, most often found within a granuloma. Unfortunately, Zinsou *et al.* did not specify whether or not the 39 women positive for genital schistosomiasis were in the half of the study group that presented with sterility, although the seriousness of the observed lesions suggests that sterility was likely. However, descriptions of the macroscopic and microscopic lesions is so similar to tuberculosis (TB) that concomitant infection with the tubercle bacillus must be suspected. Macroscopically, tubes infected with schistosomiasis look very much like tubes infected with tuberculosis (Magdi 1967:424). And microscopically, the study's description of instances of "caseous necrosis" strongly suggests a degenerating lesion of tuberculosis. In fact, Gilbert (1943:332) claimed that the presence of caseous material resembling that of TB virtually excludes a diagnosis of schistosomiasis.

An even more cautious appraisal must be made of studies, such as that by Bullough (1976:820–821), that propose a cause and effect relationship between genital schistosomiasis and reproductive failure based on indirect evidence. Bullough selected 138 infertile and 42 fertile women and tested them for schistosomiasis by searching for eggs in the urine or, failing positive results there, in a rectal biopsy. He found a significant difference in the frequency with which the two groups were infected: 41% of the infertile women were infected whereas only 21% of the fertile women were positive for schistosomiasis. The data further showed that the difference was significant for primary sterility but not for secondary sterility, perhaps because other forms of pelvic inflammatory disease were common in these patients. However, this study is flawed. It suffers primarily from a lack of direct evidence for genital tract involvement. Evidence of schistosomal infection of the bladder or rectum is no guarantee of infection of the genital organs and certainly can say nothing about the extent or the severity of any lesions in these organs. He would have been on firmer ground if he had shown that the intensity of infection in the bladder was high because there is a much greater chance of genital involvement in such cases.

Summary of Effects on Female Fecundity

The bulk of direct evidence, that is, evidence from studies using autopsy or biopsy material, shows that although schistosomiasis, particularly *S. haematobium*, is frequently found in female genital tissue it is seldom associated with lesions capable of altering fecundity. But these studies may be slightly flawed in that young persons with active disease are poorly represented and early inflammatory lesions are seldom encountered. Cheever *et al.* (1978:69), as cited earlier, felt that many studies were underestimating "a large part of significant genitourinary pathology" for this very reason. They felt that early lesions in the ureters, which later healed with minimum residual pathology, could have been the cause of permanent ureteral deformities. If this same line of reasoning is applied to the female genital tract, especially the fallopian tubes, the role of schistosomiasis in subfecundity is enhanced, at least in those cases where egg loads in the tubes and host hypersensitivity are fairly high. In such cases bulky inflammatory lesions could cause a temporary stenosis or occlusion of the tubes, with resulting sterility or a predisposition to ectopic pregnancy. Upon resolution of the inflammatory lesions, however, the lumen would again be fully patent and the woman's fecundity should return to normal. But the muscular contractility of the tubes, which is all-important in propelling the fertilized egg toward the uterus, could, like the peristaltic contractions of the ureter, be permanently disrupted by inflammation and minimal fibrosis; a predisposition to ectopic pregnancy might result. However, as discussed earlier, surveys have not established a relationship between tubal schistosomiasis and ectopic pregnancy. Furthermore, the very fact that egg laying in the upper genital tract commences with puberty minimizes any serious reaction, temporary or permanent, to their presence. This is because of the modulating effect that accompanies infections of some duration, and means that there is much less tissue reaction around an egg laid during the chronic stage of infection than around one laid during the acute stage. Because most individuals in endemic areas are infected during childhood, by puberty most infections are chronic and any sequelae to egg deposition is less severe. However, in those persons who escape childhood infection and are first infected with schistosomiasis during or after puberty, both temporary and permanent genital lesions are probably more severe.

It is then possible that the difference between the upper and lower genital tracts in pathological reaction to eggs is not due entirely to inherent differences in the sensitivity of the tissues to the eggs, but also to the overall level of host hypersensitivity as determined by the duration of the infection at the time of tissue involvement. Thus, infections of the lower genital tract, which usually occur before puberty, are more often associated with serious sequelae such as papillomas and ulcers than are infections of the upper genital tract, which usually occur during or after puberty.

It would appear that in the majority of women *S. haematobium* of the genital tract is an infection of little consequence. Few, if any, symptoms are experienced and reproductive potential remains unchanged. The notion that tubal schistosomiasis predisposes to pelvic inflammatory disease (PID) needs to be explored further. Although *S. mansoni* is capable of provoking more serious pathological reactions in the genitals

(Arean 1956a:1010, 1956b:1052; Zinsou *et al.* 1967:281) and thus has the greater potential to render the individual subfecund, the infrequency with which it is found in the female genital tract denies it any significant role in population subfecundity.

Diagnosis

One reason the population impact of schistosomiasis is so difficult to gauge is that accurate assessment of the frequency of infection in a population may be difficult. The egg excretion method is the most widely used diagnostic tool and involves checking urine and stool samples for the presence of eggs. This technique is valuable for the evaluation of disease rates in young populations where active disease—that is, on-going egg laying—predominates. But active disease is less common after age 20 or 30, and egg excretion rates for these persons with inactive disease are generally below the sensitivity level of the technique. Thus, many cases of tremendous egg burdens with severe disease may be missed if only this method is employed (Smith *et al.* 1974:167). It was hoped that serologic tests would offer an easy and accurate way of detecting schistosomal infection. Although these tests are reasonably good and certainly can detect light, active infections (Cheever 1980), they too are of limited value in detecting inactive infections. The most accurate method is probably that prescribed by Mahmoud (1977:1330). He advised checking both the stools and urine for excreted eggs and, if these tests are negative, performing a rectal biopsy to see if eggs are lodged in the tissue there. This should detect most, but certainly not all, infections with any of the schistosomes.

Control and Treatment

The control of schistosomiasis has become an increasingly difficult problem. Irrigation projects, such as the Aswan High Dam in Egypt, have aided the economic development of the less-developed countries by allowing the cultivation of previously arid land. But these irrigation projects have provided the snail intermediate hosts of schistosomiasis with additional breeding grounds. And the migration of the population to these arable lands has increased the number of persons at risk of contracting the disease. Because of these two factors, the snails are undergoing a population explosion and there is a great increase in the prevalence of schistosomiasis in Africa and South America (*British Medical Journal* 1972a:367).

Initial efforts at schistosomiasis control were aimed at eliminating the snail population by the use of molluscicides. Although effective molluscicides are available, there are many technical difficulties associated with their use and the cost is often prohibitive for many of the poorer countries. Therefore, an adequate strategy for their application has yet to be developed (World Health Organization 1973:26). The development of a vaccine was briefly considered, but vaccination was felt to be a two-edged sword—it could produce resistance to natural infection but it could also, in hypersensitive individuals, produce those immunological changes thought to be responsible for the more severe complications of the disease (*British Medical Journal* 1972a:367).

Hopes for the control of schistosomiasis rest on chemotherapy. Although chemotherapy is a curative agent, it is also a major preventive measure because it rapidly suppresses egg production and excretion and thus lowers transmission potential (McCullough 1980:4). Although drugs directed against the adult worm have been available approximately since the 1920s, it has only been since the 1970s that mass chemotherapy has been possible due to the introduction of new compounds with improved efficacy and reduced side effects (Cook *et al.* 1977:890–891).

The compounds most commonly used in large-scale treatment campaigns are metrifonate and oxamniquine. Metrifonate is the drug of choice for *S. haematobium* infection; it is not very effective against the intestinal schistosomes. The drug is inexpensive, the regimen short, and cure rates of 60 to 80% are achieved with very few and minor side effects (McCullough 1980:4). Oxamniquine, which is an oral drug, is now in widespread use for the treatment of *S. mansoni* infections. Cure rates are generally highly satisfactory and side effects are relatively uncommon, mild, and transitory. In areas where mixed infections with *S. haematobium* and *S. mansoni* are common, niridazole has been used with success since 1970. It is a particularly useful drug because it is effective against both vesical and intestinal schistosomiasis. It has several disadvantages, however, including serious side effects and considerable cost (McCullough 1980:4). And there are suspicions, based on animal studies and limited observation of humans, that niridazole has a depressing effect on sperm counts (Ledward 1980:118). Niridazole may soon be supplanted by praziquantel, a newer drug that can be administered in a single oral dose, is free of major toxicity, and is highly effective against *S. haematobium*, *S. mansoni*, and *S. japonicum*. Cost is the only present deterrent to its widespread use in the developing countries.

Eradication of the infection is seldom attainable and it may neither be necessary nor desirable. Persons with light infections will probably suffer no ill effects from the parasites, so control efforts should be aimed only at those areas where transmission is intense and the risk of severe infections high. In general, results with chemotherapy have been extremely encouraging. Mass chemotherapy campaigns in Egypt against *S. haematobium* (Jordan 1972:58) and in Saint Lucia against *S. mansoni* (Cook *et al.* 1977:892) have resulted in fivefold or greater reductions in infection rates at a relatively low cost. It should be noted that antischistosomal drugs are effective only against the adult worms and can do nothing to reduce existing egg loads. The resolution of early inflammatory lesions has been noted following treatment, but the fibrotic lesions associated with chronic infection are resistant to chemotherapy (Bullough 1976:821).

CHAPTER 7

African Sleeping Sickness

Introduction

The African trypanosomiases probably originated in the large grazing animals of Africa, and humans and their domestic animals became new hosts during their prehistoric invasion of the continent (Jones 1967:52, 55). The earliest known records in Africa noted the disease, and the "Negro lethargy" was well known to slave traders (Baker 1974:39). Today the African trypanosomiases rank high on the World Health Organization's list of the top 10 global health problems, as they are diseases of great social and economic importance. In humans infection causes a disease commonly called sleeping sickness because of the protracted lethargy that is one of its symptoms. Sleeping sickness is a cause of serious morbidity and mortality. It can devastate whole villages, and in the early part of the century killed more than 200,000 persons in Uganda alone. In domestic animals the infection causes a disease called nagana. Because the meat of affected animals is flaccid, watery, and inedible, the disease has effectively kept 4 million square miles (10.2 km^2) of otherwise ideal grazing land idle, an area that could support 125 million head of cattle in a protein-starved continent (Jonas 1978:1, 2). Because of the effect of the African trypanosomiases on humans and their domestic animals, one-quarter of the total land area of Africa is barred to agricultural development (Jones 1967:55).

The infectious agents in the African trypanosomiases are protozoa of the genus *Trypanosoma*. They are free-moving, slender organisms, 10–30 μm long and 1–3 μm broad, with one pointed and one blunt end and an undulating membrane that projects beyond one end of the body as a free flagellum (Patel, personal communication, 1981). The two trypanosomes that cause African sleeping sickness are believed by some (e.g., Baker 1974:29) to have evolved independently from the animal trypanosome, *Trypanosoma brucei brucei*. *Trypanosoma brucei gambiense*, which causes Gambian sleeping sickness, has long been established in West Africa; its range was extended east and southeast at the end of the nineteenth century, possibly due to the movements of European settlers. Epidemics accompanied the spread of the disease into previously unaffected areas, and the devastating nineteenth-century epidemic on the north shore of Lake Victoria may have been the result of one of Stanley's expeditions. *Trypanosoma brucei rhodesiense*, which causes Rhodesian sleeping sickness, evolved much more recently, perhaps within the past 100 years. It was first noted in the late nineteenth century in southeastern Botswana and had reached Tanzania by 1910 and southern Kenya by 1930. In 1940 it caused an epidemic on the northeastern shore of Lake Victoria, where 50 years earlier the devastating Gambian epidemic had occurred. Rhodesian sleeping sickness still continues its northward spread (Baker 1974:29, 40).

Fortunately, because of the effects of climate on the survival of the vector of trypanosomiasis, the dreaded tsetse fly, the potential spread of the disease is limited to that area between the two tropics where annual rainfall exceeds 20 inches (50 cm). Scientifically known as *Glossina*, the fly was given the name *tsetse* by the Kalahari Desert people in accurate imitation of its buzz (Jonas 1978:3). Gambian sleeping sickness is transmitted by *Glossina palpalis* and Rhodesian sleeping sickness by *Glossina morsitans*, although these vectors are interchangeable (Basson *et al.* 1977:453). Both types of sleeping sickness are rural diseases because population densities greater than 200 persons/square mile (80 persons/km^2) are associated with human activities (farming, housing, etc.) on such a scale that tsetse habitats are destroyed. However, the denser the population within the limits of tsetse survival the greater human–fly contact will be, with a resulting increase in prevalence of the disease (Scott 1970:625–626).

Glossina palpalis inhabits the forested banks of rivers and other wet places and is therefore known as the riverine tsetse. Thus Gambian disease is usually acquired at village watering and washing places and where rivers and streams are forded. Because all villagers—men, women, and children—frequent such places, Gambian sleeping sickness is found equally in both sexes, at all ages (Baker 1974:34). The epidemiology of Rhodesian sleeping sickness is considerably different: Triple contact between human, fly, and game is necessary because *G. morsitans* prefers to feed on game animals. Thus, humans expose themselves to infection only when they venture into the bush to hunt, gather honey, or the like. Because these are primarily male activities Rhodesian sleeping sickness is usually seen in men (Baker 1974:36); its appearance in women or children signals that an outbreak is occurring (Apted 1970b:653).

Life Cycle

Although the life cycle of Gambian sleeping sickness is a human–fly–human cycle and that of Rhodesian sleeping sickness is a human–fly–game cycle, parasite development in both cycles is essentially the same. When a tsetse fly feeds on an infected person (or animal) trypanosomes are ingested. These forms migrate from the insect's gut to its proboscis and/or salivary glands where, within 3 to 5 weeks, they develop into metatrypanosomes that are infective for humans and animals. The development of the parasite in the tsetse fly is so complex that even under maximal laboratory conditions less than 10% of flies ingesting trypanosomes eventually produce metatrypanosomes and therefore become infectious. And in natural populations of *Glossina* the infection rate is rarely greater than 1/100th of this figure (Baker 1974:30). For this reason persons can live for many years, or even a lifetime, in a tsetse area yet never develop sleeping sickness.

The part of the life cycle that takes place in the mammalian host is not very well understood. In humans, at the site where metatrypanosomes are introduced a characteristic chancre may appear 4–10 days after the fly bite. From this chancre the parasites spill over into the bloodstream where they are transformed into trypanosomes, which are probably the largest organisms that can infect human blood. Early in the disease trypanosomes can also be found in the lymph (especially in the enlarged lymph nodes of the neck that often appear) and in the tissues.

The trypanosomes multiply rapidly, but exactly where is a matter of some disagreement. Hoare (see Boreham *et al.* 1970:814) believes multiplication occurs primarily in the blood, but Goodwin (1970:800–801) feels that connective tissue is the favored site of trypanosome multiplication. The most satisfying explanation (World Health Organization 1969:25) is that multiplication of trypanosomes proceeds independently in the general circulation and tissues, but profusely in the tissues. When the trypanosomes overflow from the tissues into the blood, the number there is raised to a microscopically detectable level and this causes the onset of fever. Successive waves of parasitemia occur, each time accompanied by fever. And each time the trypanosome alters its surface proteins so that host antibodies produced in the past are useless against the new antigenic variant.

The appearance of trypanosomes in the nervous system marks the beginning of the second stage of sleeping sickness and the onset of the neurological disorders that are the trademarks of the disease. But the presence of the trypanosomes in the general circulation is most important for the parasite's life cycle because it is here that they are accessible to the tsetse when it feeds on an infected person, thus continuing the cycle.

Prevalence

African sleeping sickness is endemic throughout the part of Africa lying between 15° north latitude and 30° south latitude (see Figure 7.1), an area as large as the United States. Gambian sleeping sickness is found in the western half of Africa, in Senegal, Gambia, Guinea, Sierra Leone, Liberia, Ivory Coast, Upper Volta, Ghana, Togo, Benin, Nigeria, southern Chad, Cameroon, Central African Republic, Zaire, Gabon, Congo Republic, and northern Angola (Baker 1974:30–31). Rhodesian sleeping sickness is prevalent in the eastern third of Africa, in Ethiopia, Kenya, Tanzania, Burundi, Rwanda, Mozambique, Zambia, Malawi, Angola, Zimbawbe (formerly Rhodesia), and Botswana (Buyst 1973a:110). In some areas, such as Uganda, the two types coexist (Apted 1970a:682). But neither Gambian nor Rhodesian sleeping sickness is found at elevations greater than 7000 feet (2.1 km) above sea level.

African sleeping sickness is a threat to 45 million persons in 38 countries in Africa (World Health Organization, World Bank, and United Nations 1982:7). There are approximately 10,000 new cases of sleeping sickness reported each year (Jonas 1978:1), Gambian disease accounting for the vast majority (Apted 1970b:645). Although the number of persons stricken is small when compared with tuberculosis, malaria, and the like, the impact on affected populations is great because, if untreated, sleeping sickness is almost invariably fatal, having the highest case–fatality rate of any communicable disease except rabies (Duggan 1973:162). And such numbers do not reflect the magnitude of past epidemics that depopulated large parts of Africa. Nor do they reveal that the present situation of controlled endemicity remains vulnerable to epidemic outbreaks. In the 1970s disastrous outbreaks occurred in Zaire, Sudan, Cameroon, and Uganda because normal surveillance was ne-

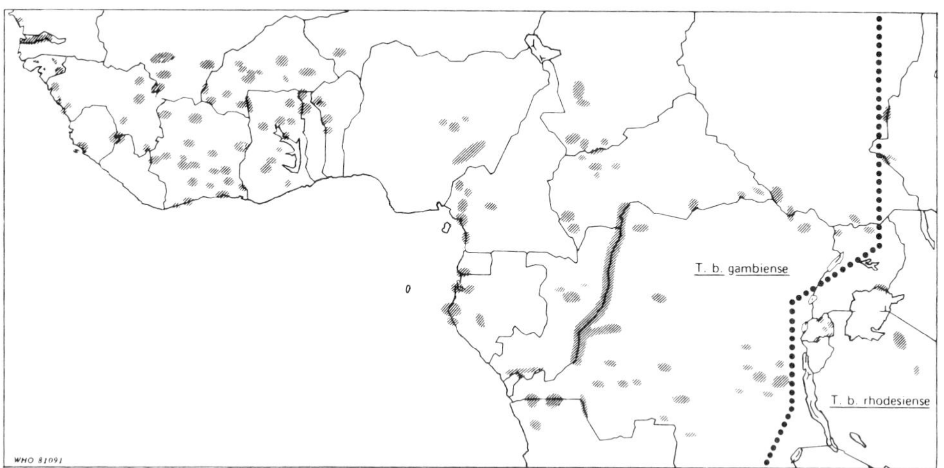

Figure 7.1 Distribution of African sleeping sickness. Source: World Health Organization 1982:822.

glected (World Health Organization, World Bank, and United Nations 1982:7) (see subsequent discussion). And certainly these numbers seriously underestimate the true number of cases of African sleeping sickness because of the limitations of present diagnostic methods and the limited skills and services of rural health services (DeRaadt 1976:114). Buyst (1977b:201) stated that even in hospitalized patients the diagnosis is missed more often than not. The usual method of determining the incidence of infection in a population may also be a factor in the underestimation of the number of cases. For example, three population surveys in an endemic area revealed an average infection rate of .6%. But hospital and census data for the same time period revealed that some of the investigated villages had annual infection rates of 2.9%, 3.7%, and even 16.5% (Buyst 1976:455).

Thus, it is believed (e.g., Schultz 1977:1259) that no one can even estimate the number of cases each year. And certainly detailed infection rates by sex, age, etc., are simply nonexistent (Scott 1970:619). All that can be said with certainty is that within a given locale the incidence of infection does not vary much from year to year. In some areas rates are always high, in others moderate, and in still others they are low or the disease is absent altogether (Scott 1970:635).

The stability of the present situation is due in large part to the surveillance and treatment methods that are continuously in force. But an interruption of these control measures can have disastrous consequences. In Zaire, for example, the incidence of infection was 0.02% in 1958. But in 1964, following a period of political turmoil during which control measures were interrupted, that figure had surged to 15%. Under similar circumstances a recrudescence occurred in the Sudan (*British Medical Journal* 1976a:1298). Thus, political disturbances and economic difficulties favor focal epidemics of African sleeping sickness, even where the disease is fairly well controlled (Poltera *et al.* 1977:249). Other causes of epidemics include travel of individuals carrying more virulent strains, movement of populations into tsetse areas without accompanying control measures, and increased human–fly contact due to environmental changes that force flies to concentrate on humans as a source of food (DeRaadt 1976:114).

Although Rhodesian sleeping sickness is more virulent and rapidly fatal, epidemics of *T.brucei rhodesiense*, though devastating, are self-limiting. Humans are not good hosts for the parasite. Although parasitemia is high, rapidly progressing ill health forces victims to retreat to bed where soon they will die. Victims and their many circulating trypanosomes are thereby not available to the tsetse, and the parasite's ability to continue its life cycle is seriously jeopardized (Baker 1974:36). Hence, a human–fly–human cycle can be maintained for only a limited period of time in Rhodesian sleeping sickness (see the section ''Altered Response''). The reservoir of infection will therefore remain with the large grazing animals, in whom levels of parasitemia are not harmful but yet are sufficiently high to ensure parasite survival.

Thus, Gambian sleeping sickness has been responsible for most of the major epidemics. Humans are the reservoir of infection for *T.brucei gambiense* and a human–fly–human cycle is favored. There have been two major epidemics of Gambian sleeping sickness since 1900. The first occurred in Uganda between 1900 and 1920 and killed more than 200,000 people. The second major epidemic began about 1915 in the Congo basin and spread throughout central and western Africa for over 25 years. As the epidemics receded focal areas of infection remained, and these are the permanent homes of the trypanosomes. Any future epidemics will be initiated from these residual endemic foci. And when an epidemic does occur these foci will be the hardest hit, rates of infection decreasing steadily as distance from the foci increases. Thus, during an epidemic in Ghana the infection rate at the focal point was 30.7%, 1–2 miles (1.6–3.2 km) away it was only 11.75%, 3–5 miles (4.8–8.0 km) away it was 3.6%, and more than 5 miles (8.0 km) away it was 1.53% (Scott 1970:637). So those very areas where sleeping sickness is always a feature of life will be hardest hit when there is an epidemic. It has been noted (e.g., Adadevoh 1974:18) that these endemic areas are also those in which infertility and subfertility have been reported. Because African sleeping sickness is thought to cause many forms of reproductive dysfunction from impotence to menstrual disorders to abortion, it certainly deserves close scrutiny to determine what impact it might have on individual and population fecundity.

Pathophysiology

General

An understanding of the pathophysiology of a disease is necessary in order to evaluate its importance as a subfecundity factor. Unfortunately, as with many of the tropical diseases, little is known about the pathology of the trypanosomiases. Description of the pathological changes in the tissues has developed little since the turn of the century (Ormerod 1970:599), and even the cause of death in sleeping sickness is still obscure (Goodwin 1974:108). The important book, *The African Trypanosomiases* (Mulligan and Potts 1970), was criticized by one of its editors, Mulligan, (see Boreham *et al.* 1970:813) for the weakness of the two chapters dealing with pathology, a weakness attributed to the lack of information on the subject. Mulligan had at one time collected many tissues from people and animals with trypanosomiasis, but they were lost before he could follow through with an analysis. He felt that ''it would be rewarding to undertake detailed histological studies at all stages of infection with different species of pathogenic trypanosomes in different hosts'' (Boreham *et al.* 1970:814). Other researchers (see Boreham *et al.* 1970:817) have also felt that the time has arrived for a reinvestigation by modern methods of the histopathology of trypanosomiasis. We could find only one investigation of the tissue pathology associated with African sleeping sickness (see Poltera *et al.* 1977), and the number of cases (14) was limited.

So little of certainty is known that it is hard to accept unquestioningly the assertion that disorders of male and female reproduction are caused by the disease. We shall give an overview of what is known about the pathology of African sleeping sickness and relate this to the myriad reproductive dysfunctions that have been noted among sufferers. Last, we shall evaluate the importance of the disease to the population fecundity of affected areas.

African sleeping sickness is a two-stage disease: The first stage begins following the bite of a tsetse carrying an infective dose of metatrypanosomes and ends when the cerebrospinal fluid is invaded by trypanosomes. Once the trypanosomes are found in the nervous system the second or advanced stage of the disease has begun. One of the most salient distinctions between Gambian and Rhodesian disease is in the length of the total disease process and of each of the two stages. The first or early stage of Rhodesian disease lasts only about 1 month; this stage in Gambian disease usually lasts several months, and occasionally 4 years or even longer (Duggan 1973:162). Similarly, the advanced stage of Rhodesian disease lasts only several months, whereas that of Gambian disease may last up to several years (Hoare 1970:47). Despite these differences the basic pathology in each stage is quite similar in the two types of sleeping sickness (Ormerod 1970:588).

First Stage

The first stage of African sleeping sickness is a generalized disease, parasites moving from the site of inoculation via the blood and lymph to invade the skin, heart, liver, kidneys, adrenals, and other organs (Duggan 1973:162), as well as the reticuloendothelial system (Apted 1970a:661; Poltera *et al.* 1977:262).[1] The trypanosomes multiply in these tissues and in the general circulation, though more profusely in the former. When the trypanosomes overflow from the tissues into the blood the levels in the blood are raised to microscopically detectable levels and fever is initiated. Although the host is able to produce large quantities of antibody, particularly immunoglobulin M (IgM), in response to the infection, few of the antibodies are specific for the antigenic surface components of the trypanosome (Goodwin 1970:810). In addition, the chameleonlike trypanosome can alter its antigenic profile, so even when appropriate host antibodies destroy one population of trypanosomes another population with a distinctly different antigenic makeup appears (Mansfield 1978:204). Successive waves of parasitemia thus occur, each accompanied by a febrile episode. Other constitutional symptoms include rigors, malaise, headache, dizziness, weight loss, and general itching (World Health Organization 1979:31). Enlarged lymph glands are common (Apted 1970a:665; DeRaadt 1974:199; Ormerod 1970:592; World Health Organization 1979:31), and needle puncture of these glands often reveals large numbers of parasites. Edema is seen (World Health Organization 1979:31), often about the face and eyelids (Apted 1970a:665). The reflexes may be overresponsive and minor blows to the body may be followed by exquisite deep pain (Apted 1970a:665; World Health Or-

---

[1]The reticuloendothelial system includes all the highly phagocytic cells (cells that are able to engulf other cells or particles) except leucocytes. These cells are found in the liver, lymph system, spleen, bone marrow, adrenals, and pituitary (Copenhaver 1964:88–89).

ganization 1979:31), the latter symptom being a helpful diagnostic clue. Anemia appears early in the disease (Basson *et al.* 1977:457; World Health Organization 1979:36) and is accompanied by splenic enlargement (Apted 1970a:665; Ormerod 1970:593; Woodruff *et al.* 1973:336), although there is no "big spleen disease" as earlier thought (Poltera *et al.* 1977:262).

Although there is a tendency for affected tissues to recover from the effects of trypanosome invasion (Goodwin 1970:801), inflammatory lesions of the heart and skeletal muscle may be followed by permanent degenerative changes. The fibers of the skeletal muscles suffer and this may be an important cause of the muscular wasting characteristic of chronic trypanosomiasis (Goodwin 1970:807). And pathological changes in heart muscle are accompanied by abnormalities in heart rate and rhythm, heart murmurs, and low blood pressure (World Health Organization 1969:31).

Second Stage

The second stage of the disease is initiated by trypanosomal invasion of the nervous system. Trypanosomes enter the cerebrospinal fluid via the lymph nodes in the neck (Ormerod 1970:597). This breech is confirmable by the finding of IgM antibodies, or the parasites themselves, in the cerebrospinal fluid. Later other indicators—elevated protein levels and a high leucocyte count—will appear there (World Health Organization 1969:23). Although these events mark the beginning of the second or advanced stage of sleeping sickness, it should be remembered that they can occur quite early in the course of an infection, 3–4 weeks after the bite in the case of Rhodesian sleeping sickness. It should also be noted that many of the features of the first stage of the disease may be seen in the second stage as well. Edema (DeRaadt 1974:199) and anemia (DeRaadt 1974:199; Ormerod 1970:596; World Health Organization 1979:36), for example, continue into the second stage and may become more severe as the disease progresses.

But it is the neurological involvement that is the hallmark of African sleeping sickness. Although the central nervous system, peripheral nervous system, and autonomic nervous system are all reported to be affected (Poltera *et al.* 1977:262), the central nervous system is the primary target of the trypanosome (World Health Organization 1969:28), and the predominant pathology is a diffuse meningoencephalitis (i.e., an inflammation of the meninges, the membrane that covers the brain and spinal cord, and of the brain itself) (Apted 1970a:668, DeRaadt 1974:199). Because actual tissue destruction occurs in the brain and meninges (Goodwin 1970:808), if treatment is not initiated before the infection becomes more chronic and the inflammatory process more intense and widespread, irreversible brain damage will result (Ormerod 1970:597) (see the section ''Altered Response'').

The base of the brain, where the infected cerebrospinal fluid is most abundant, is the most severely affected (Apted 1970a:668; Ormerod 1970:597). Thus, lesions are distributed primarily in the diencephalon and hypothalamus, which accounts for the important symptoms of the disease such as misbehavior, instinctive behavior, heightened sensitivity to stimuli, damage to the systems that control muscle tone, and, most importantly for reproductive ability, endocrine disorders (World Health Organization 1969:29). Interestingly, because of the rapidity with which it kills, signs of advanced-stage nervous system damage are not seen, or only rarely seen, in Rhodesian sleeping sickness (see the section ''Altered Response''). Rather, classical sleeping sickness with its increasing sleepiness and muscle wasting is primarily a feature of Gambian sleeping sickness (Apted 1970a:669; Manson-Bahr 1966:99). Similarly, endocrine disturbances are also not usually a feature of Rhodesian sleeping sickness unless the disease is prolonged, as with unsuccessful treatment, for example, with tryparsamide before the advent of the newer drugs (Apted 1970a:669–670). This is an important fact to remember when considering the influence of each disease on reproductive ability.

If untreated, Rhodesian sleeping sickness is often fatal within a year, heart failure being a common cause of death (Apted 1970c:709). This may be due to peripheral and lung edema and low blood pressure (World Health Organization 1979:31), or perhaps to inflammatory changes in the heart initiated by the trypanosomes (World Health Organization 1969:27). Gambian sleeping sickness takes a more chronic course, death coming slowly after 2 or more years. Death is usually caused by pneumonia or another intercurrent infection (Apted 1970a:669) because the body's immune system, exhausted by its attempts to repel the successive waves of parasites, is no longer able to mount a sufficient response to any infection (Goodwin 1974:109) (see the section ''Altered Response''). Malaria is particularly serious in sleeping sickness patients, and resembles more the clinical picture as seen in nonimmunes or in semi-immune children (Buyst 1975:98).

Altered Response

Although Rhodesian sleeping sickness is usually characterized as following an acute, rapidly fatal course, this is not true in all cases. Buyst (1975, 1977a, 1977b, personal communication, 1981) noted that the ability to resist *T. rhodesiense* infection or, once infected, to survive the infection varies with ancestry. European and Nilotic people, whose ancestors had little or no experience with African sleeping sickness, typically develop severe disease. But in the Bantu-speaking people, who have for centuries been exposed to sleeping sickness, the disease runs a subacute course, and in their villages *annual* infection rates of 12–16% have been recorded, indicating that a human-fly-human cycle is being maintained. Generally the disease is milder in the eastern and southern *G. moristans* belts (i.e., eastern Tanzania, Mozambique, Malawi, Zambia, Zimbabwe, and Botswana). Here many persons are not ill in the early stages of the disease and defer treatment until the more advanced stages. As in Gambian sleeping sickness, these persons show exhaustion of the immune system upon admission—pneumonia, severe malaria, and enteritis are common causes of death. But, unlike the case with Gambian disease, central nervous system involvement does not result in irreversible brain damage.

The altered response to *T. rhodesiense* suggests that the impact on fecundity might also be altered. For instance, because the early stage of the disease is reportedly so mild, accompanying fevers might not be high enough to affect fecundity adversely. On the other hand, the protracted course of the disease means that endocrine dysfunction is present. And the fact that in many of these areas *T. rhodesiense* is a constant feature of life affords the organism a greater impact on fecundity than it has in areas where it appears only sporadically.

Causes of Pathology

Many causes have been forwarded for the tissue pathology (primarily in the brain, heart, and skeletal muscles) associated with African sleeping sickness. Three of these, which have been discussed by Goodwin (1970:809), are concerned with cell damage caused either by toxic substances produced by the parasites or by their movement in and about the tissues. Although toxic substances liberated by the parasite could be at fault, no toxic substances have yet been discovered. Because the parasites are motile they are theoretically capable of damaging tissue by mechanical means. But this too is unlikely because the tissues are accustomed to movement; migrating leucocytes and wandering macrophages move about freely in the tissue spaces causing no ill effects. Third, the growth of the parasite places considerable demand on the host to provide certain nutrients, most notably carbohydrates, and this too could possibly have a negative effect. In fact, it is felt that in a person supporting a large number of trypanosomes the continuous demand for glucose by the parasites may result in a condition resembling diabetes (Goodwin 1974:109). However, because the pathological process advances as the number of trypanosomes decreases it seems likely that the pathology is not the result of a direct action, chemical or mechanical, of the parasites themselves. Rather, damage is probably due to the immune response of the host to the parasites.

Although the immune response of the host has emerged as the most likely etiological factor in the pathogenesis of trypanosomiasis, exactly which features of the immune response are responsible is undetermined. Kinins, substances released during an antigen–antibody reaction, may be an important factor. Kinins increase the permeability of blood vessels causing hemostasis, local inflammation, edema, and tissue anoxia (Goodwin 1970:805, 806, 1974:112), and this may account for the tissue changes that occur in sleeping sickness (Ormerod 1970:601). Red blood cell destruction is enhanced in sleeping sickness via an immune mechanism (Basson *et al.* 1977:457; Woodruff *et al.* 1979:1057; World Health Organization 1979:36), and the resulting anemia may contribute to tissue damage in the central nervous system, heart, muscles, and liver (World Health Organization 1979:36). Autoimmunity, where the body erroneously begins to make antibodies against itself, has also been proposed as a possible, though not very important, cause of the tissue pathology (Goodwin 1974:113). Various other mechanisms have been proposed including allergic reaction to the continual destruction of trypanosomes (Ormerod 1970:600) and damage to normal cells resulting from the unleashing of large numbers of defender cells such as monocytes and phagocytes (Goodwin 1970:808, 810). Immunosuppression is yet another result of the host's immune response to trypanosomal invasion (Goodwin 1974:109; Voller 1974:181), and although a state of immunosuppression is not a cause of tissue damage, the host's well-being may be severely compromised, as immunosuppression may predispose to other infections and/or increase their severity (Goodwin 1970:804, 1974:109; Poltera *et al.* 1977:262). All these responses—kinins, anemia, autoimmunity, etc.—are results of the host's frantic yet ineffective self-defense efforts against successive waves of antigenically diverse trypanosomes. Goodwin (1970:810) put it well: "It's all rather like a Tom and Jerry cartoon, with a monstrously inept cat pulling the place down in his efforts to pulverize a diminutive, agile and highly resourceful mouse."

Effects on Fecundity

Given what we do know about the pathology associated with African sleeping sickness, can the reported effects on reproductive potential be substantiated? Can the menstrual disorders, pregnancy wastage, perinatal and infant mortality, prematurity, impotence, and feminization reported among sufferers be attributed to the disease? The answer is yes, but not always for the reason usually cited, that is, direct effects of the trypanosomes on the male reproductive organs and on the pituitary gland of males and females (see Ikede 1974:89). It seems likely that the fevers and anemia associated with the disease may also be responsible for some of these reproductive dysfunctions. Most cases of African sleeping sickness are detected and treated before involvement of the nervous system and, by extension, the pituitary; therefore, the effect of sleeping sickness on population subfecundity may currently be limited to those conditions such as fever that are seen early in the disease.

Fever

The first febrile episode in African sleeping sickness occurs within a few days of the appearance of the chancre, when trypanosomes that have been multiplying rapidly in the tissues overflow into the bloodstream (World Health Organization 1969:25). The initial fever may last for 1 to 7 days, and is often accompanied by headache and vomiting (Apted 1970a:663). A succession of parasitemic waves follows, each wave accompanied by fever (DeRaadt 1974:201). In one individual a succession of 19 peaks of parasitemia were noted at 3 to 4 day intervals, each accompanied by fever (Goodwin 1970:803). The fevers associated with African sleeping sickness may be high (Mackie *et al.* 1954:356; Ormerod 1970:595), often reaching 103–104° F (39.4–40° C) (Mackie *et al.* 1954:356), and occasionally peaking at hyperpyrexial levels of 106.6° F (41.4° C) (Manson-Bahr 1966:84).

Because the fever level is directly related to the level of parasitemia, fever height varies with those factors that affect parasite density, such as the duration of illness, the subspecies of trypanosome, the virulence of a particular strain of parasite, and host susceptibility. For instance, as the disease progresses the parasitemic waves not only occur at longer intervals, but the number of organisms decreases also (DeRaadt 1974:201). Thus, fevers should be most severe at the onset of illness and become more mild as the disease becomes more chronic. The subspecies and strain of trypanosome are particularly important in determining parasitemia levels and, therefore, fever levels. The Rhodesian subspecies is associated with higher levels of parasitemia than the Gambian subspecies (Baker 1974:34; DeRaadt 1974:201), and fevers are therefore higher in the former (Baker 1974:29). Strain differences may account for unusual degrees of virulence (Apted 1970a:671; Scott 1970:629), as in the terrible epidemic of Rhodesian disease in Nyasaland (now Malawi) and Tanganyika early in the twentieth century where fevers were observed to be very high (Apted 1970a:663), although this is not proven (World Health Organization 1969:31).

Host susceptibility also plays an important role in modulating fever levels. It is likely that persons receive some degree of protection by being exposed fairly regularly to the nonpathogenic trypanosomes such as *Trypanosoma vivax* and *T. congolense* (Apted 1970b:654). And persons living in tsetse areas also acquire a degree of immunity to local variants by receiving subinfective doses of pathogenic trypanosomes (Apted 1970b:657; Buyst 1973a:110; Ormerod 1970:558). Thus the disease is more severe when first introduced into communities that were previously untouched (Apted 1970a:672). Rhodesian sleeping sickness, for example, is always more severe and fevers higher when the disease is breaking new ground and there is no existing acquired immunity in the population (Apted 1970a:663; Baker 1974:41). Substantial differences have also been noted in the reactions of Europeans and Africans to African sleeping sickness, the disease being much more severe in Europeans during the early stages. Whether this difference is due to an innate racial difference in susceptibility or whether it merely reflects differences between Europeans and Africans in levels of acquired immunity is difficult to say; however, although high fevers and great constitutional upset are certainly features of both Gambian and Rhodesian sleeping sickness in Europeans, in Africans only Rhodesian sleeping sickness produces severe illness in the early stages, Gambian disease often going unnoticed at this point (Apted 1970a:663).

Thus, in Europeans and those Africans with Rhodesian sleeping sickness episodes of fever lasting several days are seen early in the disease; fevers often reach 103–104° F (39.4–40° C) and hyperpyrexial levels of 106.6° F (41.4° C) in some cases. These fevers are especially high in areas where the strain of parasite is particularly virulent or the disease is breaking new ground. The severity of the fevers and their repetitive nature may suggest malaria (Mackie *et al.* 1954:357). As noted in the chapter on malaria (Chapter 4), fevers of this intensity and duration may adversely affect fecundity. Male reproductive ability is lowered because body temperatures this high are sufficient to elevate testicular temperatures to the point where azoospermia occurs, followed by a 1–2 month recovery period of oligospermia (Eaton and Mucha 1971:456). Female reproductive ability may also be compromised, as such fevers may cause spontaneous abortion.

Low sperm count in men with sleeping sickness has not been investigated. But pregnancy wastage in affected women is a common feature of the disease, some of which is probably due to high fevers during the early stages of the disease. But Gambian sleeping sickness is very mild in the early stages in Africans and Rhodesian sleeping sickness is a much rarer disease and is usually seen in men and only infrequently in women, mostly during epidemics; therefore, the total effect on population fecundity of the fevers associated with African sleeping sickness should be low under normal endemic conditions.

Anemia

Anemia is also a common feature of African sleeping sickness (Goodwin 1974:114; Woodruff *et al.* 1973:336). It appears during the first stage of the disease and continues into the advanced stage (World Health Organization 1979:36). This anemia has been characterized both as severe (Woodruff *et al.* 1979:1055) and as moderate (Goodwin 1974:114). In a study of several individuals with Rhodesian sleeping sickness, Woodruff and his associates (1973:330) noted the exact level of anemia in patients with trypanosomiasis before treatment was initiated. Four given hemoglobin levels were 4.8 g/100 ml, 7.6 g/100 ml, 9.7 g/100 ml, and 10.4 g/100 ml. Hemoglobin levels less than 9.2 g/100 ml are believed to increase prematurity rates by 50% (McFee 1973:159), and levels less than 8.7g/100 ml seriously impair both maternal and fetal prognosis (Lawson 1967a:73). Hemoglobin levels under 6.5 g/100 ml are considered severe and cause greatly increased rates of abortion and stillbirth (Lawson 1967d:66), as well as prematurity and perinatal mortality (Lawson 1967a:86). Even moderate levels of anemia (<10 g/100 ml) are reported to cause a twofold increase in intrauterine growth retardation (Fleming 1973:317; Harrison 1974:229; McFee 1973:158), which greatly increases the risk of perinatal death. Thus, if the figures of Woodruff *et al.* (1973) are fairly representative, substantial numbers of pregnant women with sleeping sickness would be at risk of an unfavorable termination. In addition, anemic women are predisposed to postpartum infections with the risk of subsequent sterility (Lawson 1967a:86).

Endocrine Dysfunction

In 1953 Ridet proposed that the reproductive problems seen in women with African sleeping sickness were due to incomplete uterine development secondary to defective secretions by the pituitary gland and ovary (see Ikede 1974:87–88). This view that endocrine dysfunction is responsible for reproductive failure has received widespread support (e.g., Apted 1970a:667; Spingarn and Edelman 1965:696; World Health

Organization 1969:29, 1979:32), and has been bolstered by animal studies showing that the pituitary gland is directly invaded by trypanosomes and that severe degenerative and inflammatory lesions develop. A mechanism similar to this has been proposed for humans (Ikede 1974:88). Although involvement of the pituitary in humans has not been documented, the gland may well be affected as it is located near the base of the brain where lesions are most abundant. An adjacent part of the brain, the hypothalamus, is definitely affected (World Health Organization 1969:29), and because the hypothalamus directs pituitary activity, hypothalamic involvement alone is sufficient to alter reproductive function.

It is unlikely, however, that any observable hypothalamic lesions are due to direct invasion by trypanosomes, as they are in animals. Rather, in humans the lesions are believed to be caused by the host's immune response because the lesions become more numerous and more severe as the number of parasites declines (Ormerod 1970:600). Thus, endocrine dysfunction should be more pronounced as the disease becomes more chronic. In fact, endocrine disorders, and many of the characteristic neurological sequelae of the disease as well, are not usually seen in Rhodesian sleeping sickness unless the disease is prolonged, as with unsuccessful treatment (Apted 1970a:669–670) (see the section "Altered Response"). Endocrine dysfunction is, therefore, primarily a feature of Gambian sleeping sickness and even then is more likely to appear as the disease becomes more chronic. For example, it has been observed that although the menses may be arrested soon after the onset of illness, this is more common later (Apted 1970a:667). Given current control measures, many cases of Gambian sleeping sickness are probably detected and treated before endocrine dysfunction is evident. Thus, reproductive failure secondary to endocrine dysfunction is probably far less important in endemic areas today than in the past.

Altered pituitary function can adversely affect fecundity in myriad ways. The secretions of the pituitary—the body's master gland—direct thyroid function, estrogen secretion by the ovary, growth and maturation of the ovarian follicle, ovulation, secretion of testosterone by the testis, spermatogenesis, and so forth (Copenhaver 1964:567–568). Interference with ovulation can cause infertility in women, and altered hormone secretion can jeopardize proper maintenance of a pregnancy. Menstrual disorders, including amenorrhea, are frequently observed in women with sleeping sickness (Connor *et al.* 1976:254; Ikede 1974:87; World Health Organization 1979:32). In one study of women with sleeping sickness, 25% had menstrual disorders, the incidence increasing as the disease became more chronic (Apted 1970a:667).

It is felt, therefore, that many affected women are probably unable to conceive (see Apted 1970a:667), and women already pregnant before the onset of endocrine dysfunction are likely to experience a premature termination of the pregnancy. In fact, it is rare in African sleeping sickness for a pregnancy to proceed uneventfully (Traub *et al.* 1978:479). High abortion rates have been noted among affected women (Connor *et al.* 1976:254; Ikede 1974:87; Spingarn and Edelman 1965:696). Abortion rates in infected areas may reach 32% of pregnancies, compared to 7% in uninfected areas (Apted 1970a:667; Manson-Bahr 1966:85; World Health Organization 1979:32). And higher rates of stillbirth, prematurity, and perinatal mortality have been noted (Apted 1970a:667; Ikede 1974:87). However, some perinatal mortality may not be due to endocrine dysfunction, but may be the result of severe maternal illness (Buyst 1973b:20–21). And the higher rates of infant mortality that have been recorded (see Ikede 1974:87)—50% in infected areas versus 29% in uninfected areas (Manson-Bahr 1966:85)—are almost certainly not due to endocrine dysfunction but rather to a lack of maternal care (Ikede 1974:88). Buyst (1977b:201) noted that children of sleeping sickness patients are frequently the victims of protein–calorie malnutrition, and that during outbreaks of sleeping sickness the nutritional status and health of all children in the affected community is greatly impaired.

In men the observed impotence (Apted 1970a:667; Ikede 1974:87; World Health Organization 1979:32) and feminization (breast development and feminine distribution of fat) (Apted 1970a:667; Ikede 1974:88) are probably due to abnormal testosterone secretion because this hormone is responsible for potency and the maintenance of the secondary sexual characteristics. Trypanosomes have been found in hydrocele fluid (Ormerod 1970:593); thus, it is possible that the male reproductive organs are directly invaded by trypanosomes and that lesions in the testis, not in the hypothalamus and/or pituitary, cause the impotence and feminization. Perhaps the orchitis that was frequently seen in the first year of the Rhodesian sleeping sickness outbreak in Nyasaland (now Malawi) early in the twentieth century (Apted 1970a:667) was due to direct invasion. In animals trypanosomes are localized and multiply in the hydrocele fluid, tunica vaginalis, and epididymis and their presence is accompanied by testicular degeneration and inflammation, periorchitis, and epididymitis (Ikede 1974:88). And in rhesus monkeys trypanosomal infection is accompanied by edematous thickening of the scrotal wall (Sadun *et al.* 1973:327). What significance these findings have for humans is difficult to determine because in many instances trypanosomiasis in animal models does not mimic the situation in humans (see, e.g., Ormerod 1970:589).

Congenital Infection

The notion that trypanosomal infection of the placenta and, by extension, of the fetus could result in reproductive dysfunction has not been adequately tested. Buyst (1973b:20–21) suggested that because the tissues are the primary site of trypanosomal infection in humans heavy infection of the placenta could cause abortion and premature birth, but this has not been systematically investigated. Intrauterine (congenital) infection as a cause of abortion, stillbirth, prematurity, and neonatal mortality has received mixed reviews, with some researchers saying it is a factor, others saying it is not (see Ikede 1974:88). Again, a systematic investigation of fetal material for evidence of trypanosomal infection has not been undertaken. There are occasional reports of congenital transmission, but well-documented cases are few, allowing the possibility that some reported cases were due to infection during the birth process or were contracted after birth by fly contact (Traub *et al.* 1978:477, 479). In general, it is felt that although congenital infection can occur it is unusual (Apted 1970a:673; Manson-Bahr 1966:79). Indeed, it may be unusual simply because infertility is so common a sequel to trypanosomal infection (Spingarn and Edelman 1965:696). (It was reported early in the twentieth century that trypanosomes could be transmitted via breast milk, but this was later denied [Ormerod 1970:590].)

Conclusions

Although the endocrine dysfunction associated with African sleeping sickness is usually cited as the cause of the observed reproductive failures, it is likely that the fevers and anemia seen in the disease are responsible for a portion of this subfecundity. Indeed, endocrine dysfunction is not usually a feature of Rhodesian sleeping sickness, and in Gambian sleeping sickness appears only as the disease becomes more chronic. But the fevers and anemia are seen early in the disease and therefore may be more important in most endemic areas today, because widespread control measures detect and treat most cases of the disease before there is nervous system or pituitary involvement. However, in Africans fevers are sufficiently high to affect male and female fecundity adversely only in Rhodesian sleeping sickness, which accounts for less than one in five cases of sleeping sickness. And although Gambian disease is found in equal proportions of men and women, Rhodesian disease and any negative effects thereof are usually limited to men because infection is acquired during trips into the bush. Therefore, the negative effects of fever on fecundity are effectively limited to the effects on males with Rhodesian sleeping sickness.

The impact of anemia on the fecundity of men and women with Rhodesian or Gambian sleeping sickness is not well defined. Anemia appears to be an important subfecundity factor in women only, but whether the anemia is more severe in one type of sleeping sickness than in another has not been stated. But because this anemia is due to an immune mechanism and is not dependent, as are fevers, on the number of parasites, it may be equally severe in both types of African sleeping sickness. In pregnant women this hemolytic anemia may be complicated by a second type of anemia, megaloblastic anemia, which is caused by a deficiency of folic acid (a nutrient essential to the manufacture of red blood cells). Pregnant women are at greater risk of developing this type of anemia because they must provide folic acid for the manufacture of large numbers of red blood cells—adult red cells to replace those destroyed by the hemolytic anemia plus red cells for the developing fetus. In West Africa, where Gambian sleeping sickness is prevalent, the situation is particularly serious because diets are very poor in folic acid (Lawson 1967a:77). Therefore, in pregnant women with African sleeping sickness, especially those living in West Africa, anemia may be quite severe and can compromise maternal and fetal well-being.

Thus, under normal, nonepidemic conditions, the negative effects of trypanosomiasis on fecundity are due to fevers in men with Rhodesian sleeping sickness and to anemia in pregnant women. Lower fertilizing ability in men and increased rates of pregnancy wastage in women are the most common reproductive outcomes. Of course, when normal disease patterns are altered, as when an epidemic breaks out or a particularly virulent new strain of trypanosome is introduced into an area, the pattern of reproductive dysfunction changes also. For example, during an epidemic of Rhodesian sleeping sickness women, and increasing numbers of men, become infected and subject to the negative effects of high fevers. And because epidemics of Gambian sleeping sickness usually reflect an interruption of normal control measures, victims will probably remain untreated longer, and thus endocrine dysfunction will be an increasingly important factor in both men and women.

Yet another negative effect on fecundity could arise from the immunosuppression that accompanies trypanosomal infection, which has been sustantiated in persons from one endemic focus of *T.brucei gambiense* in West Africa (Goodwin 1974:113). Because infected persons are at a greater risk of intercurrent bacterial, viral, or parasitic infection, African sleeping sickness could render infected persons more susceptible to other diseases that cause subfecundity, including sterilizing genital infections such as gonorrhea. And there may be synergistic effects. For example, as noted earlier, anemic women are more susceptible to postpartum infections. Thus, in a pregnant woman with African sleeping sickness anemia weighs against a favorable pregnancy outcome and the anemia plus the immunosuppression ensures that postpartum infection is not only more likely but could be more severe as well.

In sum, we believe that African sleeping sickness, if untreated, is an important cause of individual subfecundity. Treatment, especially if initiated early in the course of the disease, will often allow reproductive function to return to normal. But, although cured, the individual has little immunity and reinfection is possible. The number of reported cases of African sleeping sickness, 10,000 per year, suggests that the disease is not an important subfecundity factor at the population level. However, it is believed that many cases go unreported, and it is these very unreported and untreated cases that have the greatest effect on fecundity. Thus, although control measures have been adequate to keep this rural disease generally in check, there are undoubtedly some remote areas where health services are insufficient, where the disease goes undetected and untreated, and disease rates reach levels at which the fecundity and fertility of a locale is affected. Adadevoh (1974:18) has noted that areas endemic for African sleeping sickness often correspond to those with low fertility, and it may be that in some endemic foci population fecundity and fertility may be lower because of African sleeping sickness. The importance of African sleeping sickness as a population subfecundity factor is also increased considerably when the usual state of controlled endemicity is disturbed, such as occurred during the outbreak in Ghana cited earlier in which infection rates rose to 30.7% (Scott 1970:637). Finally, as Buyst (personal communication, 1981) suggested, the greatest impact of sleeping sickness during the reproductive period may be the adult deaths. He felt these deaths may occur in great numbers without medical authorities being aware of them because sleeping sickness patients often tend to believe that hospital medicine is more suitable for diseases with a different symptomatology.

Diagnosis

A positive diagnosis of African sleeping sickness is not easily made because demonstration of the parasites is often very difficult and clinical appearance is similar to many other endemic diseases. Indeed, Buyst (1977b:201) suggested that in persons who come to the hospital for treatment the diagnosis is probably more often missed than correctly made. The usual method of diagnosing African sleeping sickness is direct demonstration of the parasite. Whether the trypanosome is sought at the inoculation site or in the peripheral blood, lymph nodes, or cerebrospinal fluid depends on the stage of the disease (Poltera *et al.* 1977:259). Early in disease examination of the blood for trypanosomes is the most common method. A drop of blood from the finger or earlobe is placed on a slide and examined under a microscope. A thick film of blood is examined to determine whether or not trypanosomes are present, and a thin film is used to identify the species (Baker 1970:68–69). Because trypanosomes are often scanty in the blood, it is best to repeat the test over several days. Chances of a positive result are further enhanced if the blood is taken at the onset of fever (Apted 1970a:675).

In general, demonstration of trypanosomes is much easier in Rhodesian sleeping sickness than Gambian because parasitemia levels are higher, but even with Rhodesian sleeping sickness a negative blood smear does not rule out the diagnosis. If making a diagnosis is difficult, it is better to concentrate the parasites by centrifugation or filtration techniques; these are 100 to 1000 times more sensitive than the straight blood smears. Immunoglobulin M levels are also a useful tool in the diagnosis of trypanosomiasis: Greatly elevated levels strongly suggest that diagnosis whereas normal IgM levels exclude it (Basson *et al.* 1977:456–457). Other more sophisticated methods, such as animal inoculation or immunofluorescence studies, are available if necessary. As the disease progresses the number of trypanosomes declines; thus in advanced cases demonstration of parasites in the blood or in the now-involved cerebrospinal fluid may be very difficult. However, diagnosis may now be made with a fair degree of confidence if examination of the cerebrospinal fluid reveals an elevated protein concentration and cell count.

The clinical appearance of African sleeping sickness suggests so many other endemic diseases that a diagnosis based on symptoms alone is extremely difficult. There are three symptoms specific to African sleeping sickness—a characteristic chancre and rash and heightened sensitivity to pain—but these are not found in all victims, and the other symptoms such as fever, headache, and splenic enlargement are seen in many other disorders (Apted 1970a:673–674). The fevers may suggest such disorders as malaria, relapsing fever, typhoid fever, brucellosis, kala-azar, Hodgkin's disease, mononucleosis, and influenza (see Apted 1970a:680; Buyst 1973a:110; DeRaadt 1974:201). The enlarged lymph glands may suggest Hodgkin's disease or one of the other lymphomas, tuberculosis, or mononucleosis (see Apted 1970a:680; Buyst 1973a:110). The nervous disorders are reminiscent of syphilis or of meningitis caused by the tubercle bacillus, a virus, or one of the pyogenic bacteria (see Apted 1970a:680; Buyst 1973a:110; Ormerod 1970:598). Finally, the wasting associated with advanced sleeping sickness may be confused with hookworm disease (see Apted 1970a:681; Buyst 1973a:110). The similarities between sleeping sickness and other diseases endemic to Africa and the difficulties of demonstrating infection by microscopic or other means are two reasons the prevalence of the disease is underestimated. In Zambia, for example, increased awareness of these problems led to a fourfold increase in the number of diagnosed cases of *T.brucei rhodesiense* (Buyst 1973a:110).

Treatment

There have been reports that some persons may be infected with the pathogenic trypanosomes for indefinite periods of time without signs of disease. This symptomless carrier state is believed to occur frequently among the people of Malawi, for example (Manson-Bahr 1966:99). However, other reports (e.g., Scott 1970:622) have indicated that there is no definite proof of such "healthy carriers." The idea of spontaneous cure has also been debated. Although the disease is believed to be almost invariably fatal if untreated, spontaneous cure is reported to occur in the early stage of some cases of Gambian sleeping sickness (Manson-Bahr 1966:85), though this is very exceptional with Rhodesian disease (Apted 1970c:709). Thus, treatment should be initiated promptly in all cases of African sleeping sickness. Unfortunately, the available drugs, though effective, are rather toxic; there have been no advancements in the treatment of the disease since the introduction of the arsenicals 35 years ago. Working against the introduction of new drugs are the increased cost of drug development, the small drug budgets of developing countries, and the widespread evolution of drug resistance (Williamson 1976:117). One advancement in treatment has been the recognition that secondary infections are often the cause of death and that the use of antibiotics along with antitrypanosomal drugs is desirable (Goodwin 1970:116). And more recent studies have suggested that the routine administration of antimalarial drugs may be even more useful than antibiotics in reducing mortality rates during sleeping sickness treatment (Buyst 1975, 1977a).

In the early stages of African sleeping sickness pentamidine is effective against Gambian disease and suramin against Rhodesian disease. After the nervous system is involved the arsenicals and nitrofurans must be used (Apted 1970c:684; Basson *et al.* 1977:457; Newton 1974:285). These drugs are also effective in the early stages but are too toxic for their use at that point to be justified. In fact, they may be one of the causes of high mortality in endemic areas (Basson *et al.* 1977:457). The drugs used in the early stages are ineffective against late disease, so the cerebrospinal fluid should be examined to see if there is evidence of involvement before treatment is begun (Apted 1970c:704).

If the disease is detected and treated before the nervous system is involved the cure rate is 100%. But as the disease advances and indicators (such as protein levels in the cerebrospinal fluid) rise, the prognosis becomes progressively less favorable, though never hopeless. Similarly, if the disease is treated early there are no residua of infection. But if the disease is far advanced there may be some irreversible brain damage in Gambian sleeping sickness (Apted 1970c:708, 710). In infected women with menstrual disorders and sterility, these conditions often return to normal after treatment (Apted 1970a:667, 1970c:710). Although the influence of the antitrypanosomal drugs on fetal development is unknown their use is recommended during pregnancy, as early treatment may prevent an abortion or stillbirth. However, pentamidine is not safe enough for chemoprophylaxis in pregnant women as it may cause abortion (Spingarn and Edelman 1965:697).

In addition to the serious side effects of the antitrypanosomal drugs—the arsenicals are associated with a high incidence of optic atrophy (Apted 1970a:668; Ormerod 1970:595; Spingarn and Edelman 1965:697) and with life-threatening reactive encephalopathies (Buyst 1975:97)—there are increasing numbers of reports of drug resistance, especially to the widely used pentamidine (Basson *et al.* 1977:457; Williamson 1976:117). This makes it even more imperative that new drugs be found. Perhaps the new drugs will capitalize on the trypanosome's "metabolic vulnerability" (*Lancet* 1978b:1190); nutritional studies have begun to reveal metabolic deficiencies in the parasite that could be exploited for drug action (Newton 1974:298). But it is estimated that development of a new drug will cost more than 40 million dollars (*Lancet* 1978b:1190) This is far too large a sum for the affected countries to expend and, according to Goodwin (1974:116), "the pharmaceutical industry does not find the difficult search for new drugs for a disease that affects a limited number of impoverished Africans an attractive financial proposition."

Control

Just as the available curative drugs could be improved upon, so too could the prophylactic drugs and methods of fly control. Intramuscular injections of pentamidine or propamidine will keep the blood free of trypanosomes for 4 to 6 months but have serious side effects ranging from low blood sugar and increased pulse rate to toxic encephalitis and sudden death. And, as noted earlier, pentamidine may be an abortifacient. Furthermore, in *T. rhodesiense* areas prophylaxis given at yearly intervals may in some cases mask the early stage of the disease. Diagnosis is therefore delayed until a much more advanced stage of the disease when treatment carries a higher risk of serious reactions (Buyst, personal communication, 1981). Present methods of tsetse control concentrate on the widespread use of insecticides such as DDT and endosulfan. Resistance to insecticides is always a threat and future control measures will probably use genetic control methods such a sterile insect release or tsetse attractants such as sex pheromones. Fortunately, an earlier method of tsetse control, the eradication of game animals, has been abandoned (Jordan 1976:128–129).

Through the use of a combination of mass treatment (curative and prophylactic) and tsetse control, Gambian sleeping sickness has been under control and eradication has even been achieved in some parts of Africa. Eradication is not presently possible with Rhodesian sleeping sickness because of the large reservoir of infection in game animals, and control of this disease therefore requires the continuous application of drugs and fly control (Jones 1967:56). Such continuous efforts require a great deal of money. Relaxation of control methods for Gambian and Rhodesian disease can have disastrous effects on the existing state of controlled endemicity, as in Zaire where rates soared from 0.02% to 15% between 1958 and 1964 (*British Medical Journal* 1976a:1298). In 1976 Zaire still had the highest number of sleeping sickness patients (DeRaadt 1976:116).

A vaccine remains the single best hope for control of African sleeping sickness, although there are significant obstacles to the development of such a vaccine. At first it was thought that a vaccine could not be produced because the trypanosome is repeatedly changing the surface proteins (antigens) to which the vaccine would be made (Jonas 1978:2). But reports (World Health Organization 1979:38) have revealed this obstacle may be surmountable because the antigenic repertoires of the trypanosomes are not unlimited and there are similaries in the repertoires of parasites from a given geographical area. However, several vaccines would probably be required. Repeated vaccination might be necessary because even with a natural infection there is little protection against reinfection (see Gray 1976:119; Mackie *et al.* 1954:355; Ormerod 1970:594). And there are fears that if not 100% effective the vaccine could mask the early stages of the disease (Buyst, personal communication, 1981).

Despite these problems and reservations, the search for a vaccine continues. A breakthrough has been accomplished by two scientists working at Nairobi's International Laboratory for Research on Animal Disease. They have succeeded in growing the trypanosome in culture (*Intercom* 1977b:13), a necessary first step in the production of a vaccine against this dread disease.

CHAPTER 8

Chagas' Disease

Introduction

American trypanosomiasis, more commonly known as Chagas' disease after its discoverer, Carlos Chagas, is a major public health problem in Central and South America. By one conservative estimate (World Health Organization, World Bank, and United Nations 1982:7) 24 million persons are chronically infected by the parasite *Trypanosoma cruzi*, which causes the disease, and 65 million persons are at risk. The hardest-hit areas are Brazil, Argentina, Chile, and Venezuela (Marsden 1971:98) (see Figure 8.1).

American trypanosomiasis was originally an infection of the wild mammals of the American continent. Humans became hosts when the insect vectors of *T. cruzi* became adapted to their dwellings. Because of the peculiar evolutive nature of Chagas' disease, the disease went unrecognized until 1909 when Carlos Chagas, a doctor working in Brazil, did some sophisticated sleuthing. He first noted that bugs of the family Reduviidae harbored trypanosomes in their intestines, and he later found the parasites in wild mammals and human autopsy material. He knew that the trypanosomes were agents of disease in Africa and reasoned that they could be the cause of a yet-unrecognized disease in South America (Jones 1967:50). At first comparatively few cases of Chagas' disease were reported, but by 1936 the wider use of serological diagnosis (detection of antibodies) and awareness of the disease's late clinicopathological effects led to a recognition of its importance and extensive distribution (World Health Organization 1969:6). Thus, the prevalence of Chagas' disease, especially in South America, is far greater than originally supposed.

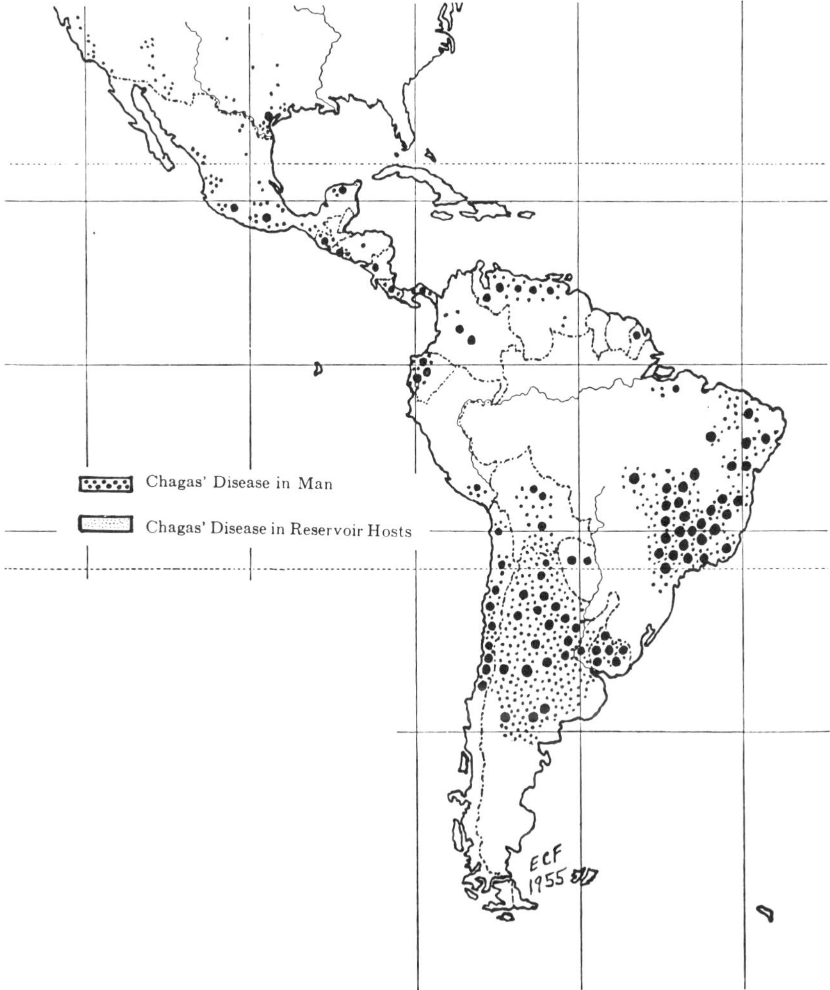

Figure 8.1 Distribution of Chagas' disease. Source: Faust and Russell 1964:148.

Life Cycle

The causative organism in Chagas' disease, like that in African trypanosomiasis, is a trypanosome, *T. cruzi*. Like the Rhodesian type of
African trypanosomiasis, American trypanosomiasis is a zoonosis. That
is, it is a disease of animals that may secondarily be transferred to man.

The disease is found in armadillos and other mammals, both wild and domestic. A survey of dogs and cats in Brazil and Chile found infection rates of 10–20% (Neghme and Schenone 1960, cited in Zeledon 1974:66). Guinea pigs, rats, and other peridomestic animals are also frequent reservoirs of infection. Adult trypanosomes circulate in the blood of infected individuals and are thus accessible to blood-sucking insects of the family Reduviidae, subfamily Triatominae, which are vectors of the disease. Although there are a large number of insects in this classification, only a dozen are epidemiologically important as vectors of Chagas' disease (Zeledon 1974:51). Called by scientists reduviid bugs or triatomes, the bugs have been given more descriptive names by the inhabitants of affected areas such as "kissing bug" because of their predilection for biting victims about the face. Other common names are "cone-nosed bug" and "assassin bug" (Marsden 1974:12).

Upon biting an infected animal or man, the bug ingests adult trypomastigotes. In the insect's foregut these are transformed into parasite forms called amastigotes. In the midgut they become epimastigotes and in the hindgut metatrypanosomes (Teixeira 1977:244). The entire process takes only 8–10 days (Arean 1976:443; Manson-Bahr 1966:101), and the bug remains infective for life, which may be several years (Edgcomb and Johnson 1976:245). The infective metatrypanosomes, which accumulate in the rectum, are discharged in the feces. If defecation occurs about the time the bug is feeding, the parasites may gain access to the victim's body via the puncture wound (Jones 1967:50). At the point of inoculation the metatrypanosomes parasitize macrophages and other local tissues (Teixeira 1977:246). A lesion called a chagoma, which is a local inflammatory swelling of the skin and surrounding tissue, may appear at the inoculation site in response to rapid parasite multiplication (Arean 1976:443; Manson-Bahr 1966:102). If the conjunctiva of the eye is the site of entry a unilateral swelling of the eye may appear. This is called Romaña's sign and was considered quite characteristic of chagasic infection. However, this swelling may occur in some persons even when the reduviid bug is not infected with *T. cruzi*, and in these cases probably represents an allergic reaction to irritating substances in the insect's saliva.

Once infected the cell becomes a factory for the manufacture of parasites. Inside the cell the metatrypanosomes are transformed into amastigotes. These multiply by binary fission to produce large numbers of parasites that fill the cell and distend its membrane, transforming it into a "pseudocyst" (Arean 1976:443). Some amastigotes are transformed into epimastigotes and then into trypomastigotes, which are liberated when the pseudocyst ruptures (Dvorak 1977:4; Edgcomb and Johnson 1976:248; Teixeira 1977:246). The released trypomastigotes can now invade cells in the immediate area, or they can be ingested by host defender cells (the first step in specific antigenic stimulation and subsequent production of an immune response), or they can make their way to the blood and be carried to the other tissues of the body (Dvorak 1977:4).

Any tissue or cell type can be parasitized, but preferred sites of attack are cardiac muscle, skeletal muscle, smooth muscle, cells of the reticuloendothelial system, and neuroglia (Arean 1976:443; Teixeira 1977:246; World Health Organization 1969:22). Favored organs are the heart, brain, esophagus, and colon (Edgcomb and Johnson 1976:244). The greatest number of intracellular parasite forms (i.e., amastigotes) are found in the skeletal muscle and in the muscle fibers of the heart, esophagus, and intestine; fewer are seen in the brain except in congenital infections. Smaller numbers are seen in other tissues such as the adrenals, testis, spleen, lymph nodes, skin, fat, stomach, and placenta (Edgcomb and Johnson 1976:245; Marsden 1971:104; World Health Organization 1969:22).

The entire reproductive cycle, which takes 3–6 days in the human host (World Health Organization 1969:22), is repeated several times, a febrile episode accompanying each release of parasites into the blood. After a few weeks or more parasite multiplication is suppressed as host defenses rise; parasites become scanty in the blood and in the tissues as well (Marsden 1971:104). The acute stage has run its course. In children the acute stage may be quite severe with high fevers and substantial mortality from severe inflammatory changes in the heart and brain, whereas in the majority of adults the acute stage is often so mild as to go unnoticed. But once infected an individual remains so for life (Marsden 1974:13). The infection may remain latent for a lifetime or after 10 or 20 years of latency the signs and symptoms of chronic Chagas' disease, such as heart failure, may appear. Throughout the latent and chronic stages the trypanosomes continue to multiply and provoke an inflammatory response (Marsden 1974:14; World Health Organization 1969:22), but the nature of the reproductive cycle during these stages is not well understood (World Health Organization 1969:22). Therefore, parasites, although scanty after the acute stage has subsided, may usually be demonstrated in persons with latent and chronic Chagas' disease, though often with great difficulty. Thus, feeding reduviid bugs may ingest trypanosomes upon biting persons in any stage of the disease, thereby continuing the life cycle of *T. cruzi*.

Clinical Features

Chagas' disease existed for an indefinite period in Latin America before Carlos Chagas identified it early in the twentieth century. One important reason for this oversight is that Chagas' disease is indistinguishable in its early and chronic stages from many other diseases. Because clinical features are rarely sufficient to substantiate a diagnosis, examination of the blood and/or tissues for parasites and immunologic tests are usually necessary. Nevertheless, the disease does evolve in a fairly uniform, though peculiar, way; for the uninitiated it will be useful to review briefly the clinical features of Chagas' disease.

The acute stage of the disease begins when *T. cruzi* penetrates the human host. Multiplication of the parasites at the inoculation site may produce characteristic inflammatory swellings such as Romaña's sign or a chagoma. During the acute stage parasites, which are easily detectable in the blood, actively invade body tissues. This stage, which lasts 6–12 weeks, often passes unnoticed or with little in the way of symptoms save a mild febrile illness (Marsden 1974:13). But a certain proportion of infected persons develop acute Chagas' disease, primarily infants and children (Marsden 1974:14; Spingarn and Edelman 1965:698). Acute Chagas' disease is characterized by high fever up to 104° F (40° C), loss of appetite, vomiting, diarrhea, edema, and enlargement of lymph nodes, the liver, and spleen. There may be tremors or convulsions if the brain and meninges (the covering of the brain and spinal cord) are involved. There may be weakness and a pulse so rapid as to suggest involvement of the heart, and this can often be confirmed by an electrocardiogram (Arean 1976:445–446; Edgcomb and Johnson 1976:247; Marsden 1974:13). Of those with acute Chagas' disease, 5–10% die of myocarditis (inflammation of the muscular walls of the heart), meningoencephalitis (inflammation of the meninges and brain), or intercurrent infection (Jones 1967:52; Marsden 1974:13; Teixeira 1977:248). In the 90–95% who survive, the disease subsides spontaneously in a few months (Teixeira 1977:248) and parasites become scanty in the blood and tissues. But any infected person, whether experiencing acute Chagas' disease or essentially asymptomatic, will harbor the parasites for life.

Once the acute stage subsides the latent or indeterminate stage begins. This stage may last for several decades and, in fact, many infected persons remain in the latent stage all their lives, never showing any evidence of Chagas' disease (Marsden 1974:14). But 10–20 years (or even longer) after the initial infection, a significant but undetermined proportion of infected persons show signs of chronic Chagas' disease. Although some authors (e.g., Zeledon 1974:52) have stated that only 1% of infected persons have clinically obvious symptoms of chronic Chagas' disease others (e.g., Marsden 1974:14) have felt that 5–15% show significant heart or gut damage, and still others (e.g., Cerisola 1977:35) have felt this figure may be as high as 20–30%. Regional differences in the prevalence and severity of Chagas' disease could account for these disparate views of the disease's importance.

Heart disease is the principal manifestation of chronic Chagas' disease. The muscles of the heart are frequently damaged and clinical symptoms range from racing of the heart (tachycardia) to progressive heart failure (Arean 1976:446; Edgcomb and Johnson 1976:248; Jones 1967:50). In some areas heart disease secondary to Chagas' disease is a major cause of death. In an urban area in Brazil 13% of all deaths in persons aged 15–74 were reportedly due to Chagas' disease, as were 29% of all male deaths and 22% of all female deaths in the 25–44-year age group (Zeledon 1974:52).

The so-called megasyndromes, principally megacolon and megaesophagus, are the second most common manifestations of chronic Chagas' disease. These may be observed both in persons with and without chagasic heart disease. Because any hollow organ may be affected, in addition to the colon and esophagus a greatly enlarged bronchus, ureter, duodenum, and stomach have been observed (Edgcomb and Johnson 1976:248). Normal function of these organs is disrupted due to damage to the nerves that supply them. For example, the peristaltic movements of the esophagus and colon may be impaired, and the victim will be unable to swallow or will become severely constipated. At first the association of the megasyndromes with *T. cruzi* infections was questioned. But immunologic tests have shown that 86% of persons with megaesophagus have been infected with *T. cruzi*. And involvement of these organs (esophagus and colon) may be even more widespread than previously thought. Abnormal esophageal function, for example, was noted in fully 35% of patients with chronic Chagas' disease (Arean 1976:446–447). The megasyndromes are not found in all endemic areas. They are absent in Venezuela, Colombia, and Central America, yet are frequently encountered in Brazil, Chile, and Argentina (Edgcomb and Johnson 1976:248). Such geographical differences could be attributable to differences in local strains of *T. cruzi* (World Health Organization 1969:30).

Other late manifestations of Chagas' disease have been reported, although there is some doubt as to their importance. Although it has been stated (Spingarn and Edelman 1965:698) that spastic paralysis and mental deterioration are late sequelae, others (e.g., Edgcomb and Johnson 1976:251) feel this is not true. Hypothyroidism was once regarded as secondary to chagasic infection because this disorder was prevalent in some endemic areas. But although there are documented cases of thyroiditis caused by *T. cruzi,* most cases of hypothyroidism are unrelated to Chagas' disease (Arean 1976:447; Mackie *et al.* 1954:369).

Prevalence

The distribution of Chagas' disease is limited to those areas where the vector, the reduviid bug, is found. Thus, the disease may be found between 42° north latitude (northern California and Maryland) and 43° south latitude (southern Argentina and Chile) (Edgcomb and Johnson 1976:244; Teixeira 1977:244). It is present in all Central and South American countries. Although once believed to be rare in Mexico (see Edgcomb and Johnson 1976:244), studies (e.g., Goldsmith *et al.* 1978:249) have shown that it may be of considerable importance in some areas. The Caribbean islands remain free of *T. cruzi,* with the exception of Aruba, Trinidad, Jamaica, and Curaçao (Edgcomb and Johnson 1976:244). On these four islands the vector is present and wild animals are infected, but the disease is rare in humans and is, therefore, not a serious public health problem (Petana 1978:49–50). Although human infections have been known to occur in the United States, they are exceedingly rare (Marsden 1974:12).

Despite its potentially extensive geographical range, Chagas' disease is actually quite restricted in its distribution, affecting large numbers of people in certain circumscribed areas (Spingarn and Edelman 1965:697). Most victims live in Brazil, Argentina, Venezuela, or Chile where the vectors are peridomestic (Marsden 1974:12). In Brazil alone, up to 5 million people are probably infected (Bittencourt 1976a:97; Jones 1967:52). The vast majority of victims live in rural areas (Hanson 1977:22; Schultz 1977:1259; Van den Bossche 1978:626; Zeledon 1974:62), for it is here that the reduviid bugs have left their sylvan habitats to invade the primitive homes and outbuildings of the poor. They have found the cracks and holes in the mud walls and floors of primitive homes most hospitable places to live and breed. And a source of food is never a problem. The domestic animals such as chickens, pigs, goats, and cattle that are kept in or near the house are ready sources of blood, as are the guinea pigs that are raised in the house as a food source. One survey found 25–60% of the latter to be infected with *T. cruzi* (Zeledon 1974:63). During the night bugs living in the house can descend and feed on the sleeping inhabitants (Arean 1976:443; Zeledon 1974:62). Thus, the disease is essentially one of poverty and ignorance (Marsden 1974:12), and any successful control program will have to include sweeping economic and sanitary improvements (Van den Bossche 1978:626). But even simple measures, such as denying the bugs a hiding place by filling the holes and cracks in the house with a mixture of sand and cow dung (a cement used for centuries by South American oven birds), have reduced transmission rates (Jones 1967:52).

In 1980 an estimated 65 million persons were at risk of contracting Chagas' disease and another 24 million were believed infected (World Health Organization, World Bank, and United Nations 1982:7). The latter figure can only be a very rough estimate because of the difficulty in diagnosing infected persons, the expense of extensive surveys, and the insidious nature of chronic Chagas' disease (Edgcomb and Johnson 1976:244). Where careful surveys have been conducted, the results have shown much higher rates of infection than previously reported. In the Mexican state of Oaxaca, for example, Goldsmith and associates (1978:249) found that 16% of the general population and 35% of those over 20 years of age were infected with *T. cruzi*—in a country where Chagas' disease had been only recently said to be rare (see Edgcomb and Johnson 1976:244).

Because the distribution of vectors and the occurrence of *T. cruzi* in animals is more widespread than the extent of human infection (World Health Organization 1969:6), the potential for the spread of Chagas' disease is great; there are indications that this has already happened. What was once a strictly rural disease has appeared in the cities due to the migration of infected persons from rural areas (Bittencourt 1976a:97). (As noted earlier, a substantial proportion of deaths in an urban area of Brazil were reportedly due to Chagas' disease [Zeledon 1974:52].) As persons from endemic areas move into the cities or development areas they frequently transfer the infestation of infected reduviid bugs from one residence to another (Miles 1976:521). This adaptable creature is able to live in buildings in large cities and, in fact, has even been found on long distance passenger trains (Zeledon 1974:62). Large-scale infestation of the cities would expose many millions more to the risk of infection and would elevate what has already been considered by some (e.g., Koberle 1974:151) the most severe and important medical–social problem in Latin America to disastrous proportions.

Modes of Transmission

Although the reduviid bugs are the primary transmitters of Chagas' disease—whether by their bite or by general contamination of the area with their parasite-laden feces, which then come into contact with the victim's eyes, mouth, or food (Zeledon 1974:58, 65)—other means of transmitting the disease do exist and are becoming increasingly important. In 1936 workers in Argentina called attention to the fact that a person could become infected if transfused with the blood of an infected donor. Later surveys showed that 2–6% of potential blood donors in major South American cities gave positive serological reactions to *T. cruzi* antigen (Zeledon 1974:64). Infection is easily achieved by blood transfusion and affected blood should be treated with gentian violet or a similar compound for 24 hours just prior to its use to kill the trypanosomes (Marsden 1974:14; Zeledon 1974:64). Unfortunately, this procedure gives the blood a blue color that is often not acceptable to the recipient, so in many cases blood suspected of containing trypanosomes is thrown away (Ciba Foundation Symposium 1974:338).

Infection with *T. cruzi* may occur in the laboratory due to contact with infected blood or cultures (Edgcomb and Johnson 1976:245). Transmission of *T. cruzi* through breast milk has been reported in humans (see Bittencourt 1976a:97; World Health Organization 1969:17; Zeledon 1974:65), and although some workers (e.g., Zeledon 1974:65) have felt this possibility deserved further study, others (e.g., Bittencourt 1976a:97) have described this mode of transmission as "questionable."

One of the more disturbing aspects of Chagas' disease is that it can be transmitted across the placenta, resulting in pregnancy loss or a congenitally infected infant. The magnitude of the problem of transplacental transmission may be substantial and, by extension, so too may its effects on population fecundity. Does the pathophysiology of Chagas' disease suggest that many or few opportunities exist for transplacental transmission? During which stage or stages of the disease can transmission occur? Are there other aspects of the disease in men and/or women that could lower reproductive ability? These questions can only be answered by understanding the pathophysiology of the disease.

Pathophysiology

The pathophysiology of Chagas' disease has been extensively studied, yet many questions remain regarding the mechanisms by which the local effects of the parasite are produced (World Health Organization

1969:26). That is, what are the possible causes of the inflammatory reaction observed during the acute stage of the disease and the tissue destruction seen in the chagasic heart and gut?

Acute Stage

The most constant feature of the acute stage of Chagas' disease is parasitemia. Whether the victim is with or without clinical symptoms, parasitemia is present (Arean 1976:446). Some (e.g., Cerisola 1977:35) have claimed the parasitemia during this stage is high and constant, but others (e.g., Edgcomb and Johnson 1976:245) have characterized it as low grade. It is generally agreed, however, that the acute stage and its concomitants, parasitemia and the resulting fever, are more severe in children (Manson-Bahr 1966:101). Similarly, in children the inflammatory reactions are more severe, many more children than adults dying of myocarditis or meningoencephalitis.

These inflammatory reactions are usually believed to be a direct response to the presence of parasites. When the parasites are still within the pseudocyst there is little or no inflammatory response, but upon rupture of the cell with release of the parasites and their subsequent digestion by host defender cells a severe inflammatory response is seen (Arean 1976:444; Edgcomb and Johnson 1976:248; Koberle 1974:152). Whether this is due to the action of a toxic product of parasite degeneration (Arean 1976:444) is not known, but as yet no specific toxin has been identified (World Health Organization 1969:26, 28). Some workers (e.g., Hanson 1977:22; Teixeira 1977:254) have believed the tissue pathology associated with acute Chagas' disease is more probably due to immunologic reaction, noting that there are inflammatory reactions in which parasites are not seen. And still others (see World Health Organization 1969:26) have felt that some enzymatic factors may be responsible.

Latent and Chronic Stages

After the acute stage has subsided, parasites are much less numerous. Parasitemia is now easily measured only during an occasional febrile episode, and it becomes increasingly difficult to detect parasites in the tissues. Yet parasites are believed to be present. Even in chronic Chagas' disease approximately 50% of cases show parasites in the blood and/or tissues. And it is believed that more rigorous searches and more sensitive methods would reveal even more positive cases. Thus parasites, though scanty, persist throughout the latent stage and even into the chronic stage of Chagas's disease. What is not known is whether the tissue destruction seen in chronic Chagas' disease is the result of events occurring in the acute stage, in the latent stage, or in both. Is the appearance of chronic Chagas' disease the result solely of damage that occurred during the acute stage, acute inflammation becoming chronic with eventual healing and replacement of normal tissue with fibrotic connective tissue? Some workers (e.g., Edgcomb and Johnson 1976:250; Koberle 1974:152) have believed this is true. In this framework the heavy, enlarged heart whose muscle has been replaced by fibrous tissue is perceived to be the consequence of severe myocarditis (Edgcomb and Johnson 1976:250) and the megasyndromes are felt to be the result of acute stage damage to the nerves that direct peristaltic movement (Marsden 1974:14). But because few patients with chronic Chagas' disease give a history indicating a significant acute infection (Edgcomb and Johnson 1976:248; Marsden 1974:13), severe early disease is not a prerequisite for later development of chronic Chagas' disease. Some workers have concluded that the tissue degeneration observed in chronic disease is the result of an ongoing host reaction to the parasites, which continues through the latent state. Several other causes of chronic Chagas' disease have been forwarded. Antiheart antibodies were found in infections with *T. cruzi* (Ormerod 1970:601; World Health Organization 1969:31), and it was felt, therefore, that autoimmunity could be causing the pathological changes in the heart. But others (e.g., Teixeira 1977:254) have believed that such autoantibodies are the consequence, not the cause, of heart cell destruction. One interesting hypothesis is that heart cells share a common antigen with *T. cruzi* and thus host defender cells, primed to attack *T. cruzi*, attack heart cells as well (Teixeira 1977:254). All these hypotheses are incomplete, however, and further research is necessary to clarify the mechanisms involved in the pathophysiology of Chagas' disease.

Variations in Host Response

Another unanswered question regarding the pathology of Chagas' disease is why some persons infected with *T. cruzi* develop serious heart and/or gut disease and others develop only a mild subclinical disease or are completely unaffected. The answer may, according to Marsden (1974:14), lie with various host or parasite factors. Perhaps the most important host factor is the individual's immunologic state. Teixeira (1977:254) believed, for example, that chronic disease is most likely to appear in those who are hypersensitive (i.e., allergic) to the parasite. Others (e.g., Arean 1976:444) have also believed that the severity of the inflammatory reaction is conditioned by the host's immunologic state. Reports (see Teixeira 1977:253) have indicated that cell-mediated immunity (immunity in which phagocytic cells predominate, as opposed to humoral immunity in which the importance of circulating antibodies predominates),[1] which has the important role of limiting *T. cruzi* infections, seems to have a secondary effect (i.e., an allergic component) that may cause the tissue damage in chronic Chagas' disease.

Zeledon (1974:69) believed that hormonal, nutritional, and climatic factors may also be important in the pathology of Chagas' disease, and these factors have been explored by other workers. Goble (1970:607), for example, stated that Chagas' disease probably has a greater incidence and severity in males, and this could be due to hormonal differences (see Hanson 1977:22). However, others (e.g., Arean 1976:443) have felt there is no evidence of a differential distribution of Chagas' disease between the sexes. Nutrition may be important in the pathology of Chagas' disease (Hanson 1977:22), and it has been noted (Spingarn and Edelman 1965:699) that a diet high in vitamins is important in combating the disease. Climate, because of its effects on the distribution of vectors and on the rate of growth of parasites within the vectors, may also influence the degree of pathological change (Zeledon 1974:51).

The parasite itself is also very important in determining the severity of Chagas' disease. Strain differences in the virulence of parasites are the major factor. Strain differences are probably also responsible for geographical differences in responses to *T. cruzi* infection. They probably explain why megacolon is frequent in southern South America but is absent in northern South America and Central America (World Health Organization 1969:30) and why treatment with the drug Lampit gives excellent results in parts of Argentina but is met with failure in some areas of Brazil (Peters 1974:311).

Summary of Pathophysiology

In sum, the pathophysiology of Chagas' disease is still being explored. In the acute stage affected organs may show inflammatory

---

[1]Although humans have no innate immunity to *T. cruzi*, immunity may be acquired by exposure to infection. During the acute stage, when parasitemia is high, antibody titers are high. Nevertheless, these antibodies have no direct lytic effect on trypanosomes and it seems that cell-mediated immunity has the more important role in resistance to *T. cruzi* (Teixeira 1977:250, 251, 253).

changes in response to the parasites, and there is accompanying edema. Parasitemia is high and fever is common. All these signs and symptoms are more severe in young children, in whom there is considerable mortality because of myocarditis and meningoencephalitis. As the acute stage subsides parasites become less numerous in the blood and tissues, and there is a tendency for the inflammatory lesions to heal. The long latent period, which may or may not terminate with the appearance of chronic Chagas' disease, then begins. If chronic Chagas' disease does develop it is usually characterized by destruction of muscular and nervous tissue, primarily in the heart and gut. Chronic disease may appear regardless of the seriousness of the acute stage. Indeed, in most cases of chronic Chagas' disease no recollection of an acute illness can be elicited. It seems more likely, therefore, that the tissue destruction seen in chronic disease is the result of continuing host response to the parasites throughout the latent stage, rather than the result solely of damage occurring during the acute attack.

A number of host and parasite factors affect the severity of chronic Chagas' disease, the most important being the immunologic state of the host; those who are allergic to the parasite display the most severe disease. Hormonal, nutritional, and climatic effects on the severity of disease have also been proposed. And strain differences in the parasite may account for differences in the severity of disease as well as regional differences in disease manifestations, drug susceptibility, and the like.

Effects on Fecundity

Transplacental Transmission
(Congenital Chagas' Disease)

The idea that *T. cruzi* can cross the placenta and infect the developing fetus was first proposed in 1911 by Carlos Chagas. By 1921 transplacental transmission was confirmed experimentally in animals, and by 1949 congenital infection in humans was noted. But not until 1962 were the clinical, epidemiological, and pathological features characterized (Howard 1976:212; Zeledon 1974:64–65), and much remains unknown. Many workers (e.g., Hoff *et al.* 1978:250; Howard 1976:214; Pan American Health Organization 1976:221) have felt that current epidemiological methods register only those cases in the middle of the spectrum of disease, missing cases at either extreme—subclinical disease in newborns, which though mild may cause considerable disability later in life, and the most severe cases, which probably end as a spontaneous abortion.

Spectrum of Disease Manifestations

In a typical case of congenital Chagas' disease the infant is small; in one study birth weights were less than 2000 g in 80% of cases. In most cases the infant is premature, but a minority of infected infants are full term (Howard 1976:212). The clinical presentation is identical to that seen in acute Chagas' disease (Edgcomb and Johnson 1976:250). There may be myocarditis (Spingarn and Edelman 1965:698). Meningoencephalitis, often with tremors or convulsions, is common (Bittencourt 1976b:218; Howard 1976:213; Spingarn and Edelman 1965:698). The digestive tract is severely involved in most cases (Bittencourt 1976b:218), and the liver and spleen are often enlarged (Arean 1976:446; Bittencourt 1976b:218; Howard 1976:212; Spingarn and Edelman 1965:698). A high susceptibility to bacterial infection is observed. Death from encephalitis or intercurrent infection is common. In one series (Bittencourt 1976a:99) 8% of 66 live-born infants with congenital Chagas' disease died on the first day of life, 35% died before 4 months, and 14% died between 4 and 24 months. For those infants who survive, the long-term prognosis is poor. Physical development is retarded and there are often severe neurological sequelae such as mental deficiency or behavioral or learning problems. Only in a minority of cases does the child recover and become asymptomatic (Howard 1976:213).

Infants with mild disease may be asymptomatic at birth, clinical disease developing days or months later (Howard 1976:212). And there are indications that many children may harbor *T. cruzi* for many years without developing clinical disease, as in the case of cytomegalovirus inclusion disease (Hoff *et al.* 1978:250). However, some of these children may eventually show learning or behavioral problems (Pan American Health Organization 1976:221).

On the other hand, some congenital infections are so severe that the pregnancy is prematurely terminated. It is believed that congenital Chagas' disease can be an important cause of abortion (Edgcomb and Johnson 1976:250; Zeledon 1974:64). In one study in Brazil 1% of abortuses had congenital Chagas' disease (see Bittencourt 1976a:97), and an estimated 10% of spontaneous abortions in Brazil and Chile may have been due to transplacental transmission of *T. cruzi* (Edgcomb and Johnson 1976:248). Stillbirth is another frequent outcome of congenital infection (Bittencourt 1976b:216; Edgcomb and Johnson 1976:250). The actual frequency of each outcome of transplacental transmission—abortion, stillbirth, neonatal death, and extended survival with and without serious late sequelae—is not yet determined, and pleas have been made (see Pan American Health Organization 1976:221; Zeledon 1974:65) to perform extensive surveys examining placental and fetal tissue in order to make a more accurate estimate of the frequency of the various outcomes.

There are numerous reasons the frequency of congenital Chagas' disease is so difficult to assess. One reason is that the disease suggests several other serious congenital infections and differential diagnosis often requires laboratory analyses not usually available to the rural poor. Another reason is that when infection ends as a spontaneous abortion efforts are rarely made to determine the cause of death. Also, if the disease is mild in the newborn it is likely to be overlooked because the mother is almost always apparently healthy and asymptomatic, giving the physician no reason to suspect that the infant may be congenitally infected with *T. cruzi* (Bittencourt 1976a:216; Howard 1976:214). Yet in one survey in a surburban area in Brazil, where reduviid bugs were not observed and transmission rates would presumably be low, 16.5% of almost 300 women tested showed antibodies against *T. cruzi*. Placentas from 17 seropositive women were examined and one was positive; in this case congenitally infected twins were born (Hoff *et al.* 1978:247). The numbers in this study were too small to estimate the rate of congenital transmission, yet this and similar surveys indicate that the problem is more common than previously assumed (Hoff *et al.* 1978:249).

Factors Promoting Transplacental Transmission

One critical question is what factors promote transplacental transmission. Maternal parasitemia during gestation is a prerequisite of congenital infection, as the fetus becomes infected when the trypomastigotes that are in the maternal circulation penetrate the placental villi and enter the fetal circulation (Bittencourt 1976a:97). Although parasitemia is more intense during the acute stage, intermittent parasitemia is present throughout the course of Chagas' disease and transmission may, therefore, occur at any stage. Many women then undoubtedly have parasitemia during their pregnancies yet never transmit the infection (Bittencourt 1976a:98). Chances that they will transmit the infection are greater, however, when parasitemia is high—that is, during the acute stage. But because the acute stage is so short, only about 5% of all documented cases of congenital Chagas' disease occurred in women with acute disease (Bittencourt 1976a:97–98).[2]

[2]A person is identified as being in the acute stage of Chagas' disease if there is parasitemia but antibodies are not yet detectable.

One factor that was thought to promote congenital transmission is damage to the placenta (Arean 1976:443; Zeledon 1974:64). But placental damage is no longer viewed as a necessary prerequisite because it has been noted that *T. cruzi* can actively penetrate the cells lining the placental villi (Bittencourt 1976b:216). Thus, trypanosomes that are circulating in the maternal compartments of the placenta (intervillous spaces) actively penetrate the villi. Here they multiply and are then liberated into the fetal circulation. Microscopically the placenta shows focal or diffuse areas of inflammation and necrosis, frequently with many parasites within the placental villi; macroscopically it is much larger than normal, pale, and yellowish (Bittencourt 1976a:216, 219; Howard 1976:214). The affected fetal organs show the same inflammatory changes noted in acute Chagas' disease. Although maternal antibodies are transmitted transplacentally as well they offer no protection to the fetus, as it has been noted that circulating antibodies are unable to destroy *T. cruzi* (Teixeira 1977:251). Thus, unlike the case with malaria, substantial levels of maternal immunity do not protect the fetus when parasites also cross the placenta.

Yet another factor that possibly could promote congenital transmission is the particular strain of parasite. Perhaps the more virulent strains with their higher levels of parasitemia carry a greater risk of congenital infection. But animal studies indicate this is probably not so. The strains associated with lower levels of parasitemia and lower rates of mortality in experimentally infected animals are the same strains that are associated with more congenital infections in humans (Bittencourt 1976a:98). Of course, what relevance these animal studies have to human infections is questionable.

Thus, the factors that promote congenital infection and determine its severity are unknown. The integrity of the placenta, the immune status of the mother, and the strain of parasite are all unsatisfactory explanations. However, the later in pregnancy that placental and fetal infection occurs the less severe fetal involvement will be. In fact, infected placentas have been noted where the fetus is spared, and it is felt that in these cases the placental infection was recent and parasites had not yet spread to the fetus (Bittencourt 1976a:98).

Diagnosis and Treatment

Until factors promoting congenital transmission are known, all women who live in endemic areas and all seropositive women who have lived in such areas should be considered at risk of bearing a congenitally infected child, the risk being greatest for women who become seropositive during pregnancy. Although no drug prophylaxis has been attempted on seropositive pregnant women or those known to have parasitemia (Bittencourt 1976a:102), it is believed that such treatment will prevent congenital Chagas' disease (Howard 1976:215). However, some workers (e.g., Bittencourt, personal communication, 1981) have felt it is unwise to treat infected pregnant women until more is learned about the collateral effects of these drugs on the fetus.

Treatment of the congenitally infected infant has improved and increasing numbers are being cured, although no drug can reverse the existing neurological damage (Howard 1976:213, 214). But before treatment can be initiated the disease must be correctly diagnosed. This means ruling out congenital diseases that present a similar clinical picture, such as syphilis, fetal erythroblastosis, cytomegalovirus inclusion disease, and herpes simplex infection (Bittencourt 1976a:98; Howard 1976:213). Several means of diagnosis are available. Demonstration of the parasite by direct examination of the blood or by xenodiagnosis (see the section "Diagnosis") is the best proof of infection (Bittencourt 1976a:102). Although parasitemia is always present in congenitally infected infants it may be low on the first day of life, but it will increase afterward, always being present 10–20 days after birth (Bittencourt 1976a:99; Howard 1976:213). It has been noted (Bittencourt 1976a:99) that there is a negative correlation between the level of parasitemia and prognosis; if on the third day of life there are more than 10 trypanosomes/mm^3 of blood the child will not survive.

In most cases of congenital Chagas' disease parasitemia is high enough at birth or 1–2 weeks later to yield a positive blood smear (Bittencourt, personal communication, 1981). Serologic tests such as the complement fixation test (CFT) or immunofluorescent antibody test (IFAT) are less useful because an infant can give a positive reaction to these tests but not be infected due to transplacental passage of maternal antibodies. The lab may, however, perform a CFT or IFAT specific for fetal immunoglobulin M (IgM) versus maternal immunoglobulin G (IgG) antibodies. Unfortunately, reports (Hoff *et al.* 1978:249) have indicated that although a positive IgM test is confirmatory of congenital infection, negative test results may be seen in some cases of congenital disease. Thus, serologic test results should always be confirmed, if possible, by results of parasitologic tests.

Other Effects on Fecundity

Aside from transplacental transmission of *T. cruzi*, which results in pregnancy loss, Chagas' disease does not appear to have any other negative effects on fecundity. Coital ability is not affected by the disease, although coital frequency is probably reduced in those men and women disabled by severe late sequelae such as heart failure. Although the fevers that accompany acute Chagas' disease may reach levels (104° F; 40° C) that could adversely affect male and female fecundity, high fevers are usually experienced only by children. Parasitization of the testis has been reported and inflammatory and degenerative changes in this tissue would have a severe negative impact on male fertility. But the number of parasites in this tissue is scanty (Marsden 1971:104), and it is therefore unlikely that serious lesions would be seen.[3]

Summary of Effects on Fecundity

Better means of diagnosing Chagas' disease and a better understanding of its peculiar evolutive behavior led to a recognition of its importance as a major public health threat in Latin America; so too, we believe, better means of diagnosis and extensive surveys of placental and fetal material will lead to the conclusion that transplacental transmission of *T. cruzi* is a moderately important cause of pregnancy loss (and neonatal mortality and morbidity) in endemic areas. The prior notions that congenital Chagas' disease is "rare" (Marsden 1971:103), "uncommon" (Edgcomb and Johnson 1976:248), or "occurs to a limited degree" (Spingarn and Edelman 1965:698) have already been replaced by ideas that congenital Chagas' disease is more prevalent than generally suspected (Arean 1976:446) and that milder forms of the disease may commonly occur (Hoff *et al.* 1978:250; Howard 1976:214)

Diagnosis

Diagnosis of Chagas' disease cannot be made solely on clinical grounds. There is nothing distinctive about the acute stage unless a characteristic chagoma or Romaña's sign is present. And chronic disease, primarily cardiopathy, may be confused with heart disease that is due to other causes. Thus, a positive diagnosis of Chagas' disease must use parasitological and immunologic methods (Cerisola 1977:35). There are several available diagnostic techniques in both these categories.

---

[3]Studies in mice have shown parasitization with *T. cruzi* of the male and female genitals, the semen, and the male germ cells (Zeledon 1974:66). Parasites have been reported in the human testis (Marsden 1971:104), but no widespread involvement of the human reproductive organs, male or female, has been noted.

The simplest type of parasitological diagnosis is to take a sample of the patient's blood and examine it under the microscope for trypanosomes. If parasite densities are low, as they often are after the acute stage has subsided, three more sensitive methods may be used: culture of the patient's blood in blood agar medium, inoculation of a small amount of blood into a susceptible animal such as a white mouse or guinea pig, or xenodiagnosis (Marsden 1974:13). The latter method consists of allowing clean, laboratory-bred reduviid bugs to feed on the patient and checking the bug's feces for parasites 30 days later. The procedure is cumbersome and examining the fecal matter for parasites is extremely time consuming. And chances of getting a positive result, especially after the acute stage, depend very much on the number of bugs used. If, for example, 5 bugs are used only 25–30% of sero-reactors will give a positive result, but if 42 bugs are used this percentage jumps to 50% (Marsden 1974:14). Occasionally parasites will be sought in the tissues. Biopsy material from the deltoid muscle is commonly examined because skeletal muscle is a favored site of parasite multiplication. Also, parasites may be found in samples of cerebrospinal fluid, spleen, bone marrow, or enlarged lymph glands (Manson-Bahr 1966:104).

Several immunologic tests have been developed for the detection of Chagas' disease. In general, an immunologic diagnosis is only presumptive or indicative of past infection (Lumsden 1976:122). Yet a positive immunologic test for Chagas' disease is usually interpreted (e.g., Marsden 1974:14) as meaning that living *T. cruzi* are still in the body. This is consistent with the observation that there are no spontaneous cures (Goble 1970:601) and that existing drugs cannot eradicate intracellular parasites (Edgcomb and Johnson 1976:247). However, others (e.g., Maekelt 1970:557) have disagreed, feeling that antibodies persist in individuals who harbor no parasites. The two most commonly used immunologic tests are the CFT and IFAT. At times immunologic tests may be misleading; false negative reactions have been noted with the CFT, for example. Also, this test requires a lab specializing in the procedure. In addition, results are often not uniform because of a lack of standardized test antigen. Thus, the IFAT is preferable (Marsden 1974:14).

Which tests should be performed depends primarily on the stage of the disease. During the acute stage, if the patient is severely ill the immunologic tests are useless because the victim does not become seropositive for some weeks after infection and may die before the seroconversion occurs. Xenodiagnosis is also contraindicated under such conditions because the results take 3 weeks or more, and again treatment must be initiated earlier or the patient may die. Thus, the best way to diagnose acute Chagas' disease is to examine a drop of blood under the microscope for trypomastigotes (Edgcomb and Johnson 1976:247). If the disease is taking a more benign course, as is usually the case, xenodiagnosis, animal inoculation, and culture on blood agar medium are all acceptable and sensitive methods of diagnosing Chagas' disease during the acute stage.

After the acute stage has passed, parasites are scanty and can only be demonstrated by xenodiagnosis (Cerisola 1977:35), and then in only about 30% of cases (Marsden 1974:15). Thus, immunologic methods offer the most practical way of detecting infected persons, and are especially useful for large population surveys wishing to identify those with latent or chronic Chagas' disease. But for any individual suspected of having chronic Chagas' disease the diagnosis is best based on a combination of clinical findings, CFT and IFAT results, and the demonstration of parasites whenever possible (Edgcomb and Johnson 1976:248).

Treatment

Perhaps the best-known fact about Chagas' disease is that no effective drugs exist for its treatment. In the first 70 years since the disease was discovered, only 8 basic chemical structures had been found that showed sufficiently high activity against *T. cruzi* to warrant extensive clinical testing. Only 3 of these, the nitrofurans (e.g., Lampit), the 8-aminoquinolines (e.g., Primaquine), and the 2-nitroimidazoles (e.g., RO-7-1051) are still under consideration (Gutteridge 1976:123). Of these, Lampit is the most widely used. It is very effective in clearing the blood of parasites, but there are doubts about its ability to eradicate intracellular parasites; one might be ''cured'' of acute Chagas' disease but still develop chronic disease (Edgcomb and Johnson 1976:247). Nevertheless, a cure rate of 90% is claimed if the drug is administered under optimum conditions. The therapeutic course is long—120 days—and close medical supervision is necessary during the last 40 days because of potentially serious side effects (Gutteridge 1976:123). Unfortunately, there is also concern over the mutagenicity and carcinogenicity of all nitro compounds. If this proves true, only the 8-aminoquinolines will remain as potentially acceptable chemotherapeutic agents (Gutteridge 1976:124). Until a conclusion is reached, Lampit should be used only with great caution in pregnant women, and then only in those cases of acute Chagas' disease during pregnancy (Bittencourt, personal communication, 1981).

The initiation of treatment early in the disease when it is most curable is important because there are probably no spontaneous cures (Goble 1970:601). However, some workers (see Ciba Foundation Symposium 1974:339) have believed it is better to withhold treatment. They believe that all the damage observed in chronic Chagas' disease occurs during the acute stage and, therefore, treatment is unwise if the patient is returning to an endemic area, for resistance to reinfection is low following treatment and it is likely that the dangerous acute stage will be repeated. However, the fact that most patients with chronic Chagas' disease are subclinical during the acute stage suggests that much of the damage occurs later (see, for e.g., Edgcomb and Johnson 1976:248; Marsden 1974:13), and treatment early in the disease is recommended.

The drugs that are effective early in Chagas' disease are useless later. Once heart or gut lesions appear little can be done. Symptomatic treatment of heart disease with digitalis, diuretics, etc. is employed, but often the patient will not respond well. Half the patients with heart failure are dead within 1 year after the onset of the failure. Megasyndromes such as megacolon can be treated only by surgery because there is no curative treatment of peristaltic dysfunction (Marsden 1974:15).

The threat, therefore, of a debilitating, incurable condition (and of a congenitally infected child) hangs over the head of every person who has been infected with *T. cruzi*, unless the disease was detected and treated in the early stages (few are) with drugs of high toxicity and perhaps questionable efficacy. The need for new drugs is, therefore, great, especially ones effective against the intracellular parasites. But when the host and parasite are in such intimate contact, development of compounds with selective toxicity against the pathogenic organism is quite difficult (Peters 1974:324). Only three major pharmaceutical companies routinely test new compounds for activity against Chagas' disease. If the compounds of current interest are not successful and if the companies do not return to this area of research, the prospects for effective chemotherapy are bleak (Gutteridge 1976:124). And despite the magnitude of the problem, Chagas' disease is not considered by those who control research funds to be of sufficient public health or economic importance to merit an all-out effort (Peters 1974:311).

Control

The control of Chagas' disease will, therefore, have to depend on something more than chemotherapy. Vector control, host control, environmental changes, and development of a vaccine all have been considered. Vector control to this point has hinged on the use of insecticides. The use of DDT in antimalarial campaigns has had the secondary effect of controlling Chagas' disease in some parts of Mexico (Goldsmith *et al.* 1978:249). Benzene hexachloride and dieldrin have also been sprayed on the walls of affected homes (Marsden 1974:16). But the use of insecticides is rarely a long-term solution because resistance so frequently develops. Therefore, other types of vector control such as interference with the bug's genetic or hormonal mechanisms must be considered. Release of sterile bugs and the use of pheromones to attract and trap bugs are two such mechanisms.

Host control is very problematic. Because 100 species of wild and domestic animals can be infected with *T. cruzi,* eradicating the infection by eliminating all nonhuman hosts would be extremely difficult (Teixeira 1977:243). Social change offers one of the best methods of lowering transmission rates. Better housing would eliminate many of the hiding places of the reduviid bugs, for example. And a better standard of living would probably put a stop to the practice of keeping animals in and close to the house.

But because sweeping social change in the affected areas is unlikely host and vector control are difficult, and chemotherapy is deficient, control will probably best be achieved by immunization (Lumsden 1976:122). Prospects for the development of an effective vaccine seem good because unlike the African trypanosomes *T. cruzi* has not shown antigenic variation. In addition, cross-protection among strains appears to exist (Lumsden 1976:122). And, although in the past it was stated that the live organisms necessary to produce effective protection were inevitably risky (Marsden 1974:16), vaccines using live but nonreproducing organisms have already given promising results (Lumsden 1976:122).

Sexually Transmitted Diseases

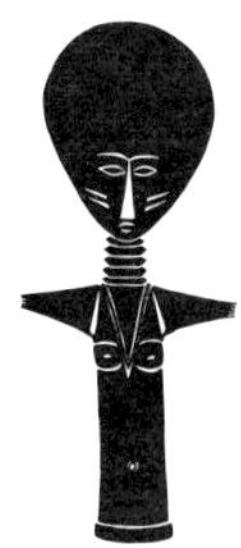

CHAPTER 9

Overview

Introduction

As noted in Chapter 1, the important causes of population subfecundity fall into five broad categories: nutritional deficiencies, psychopathology, genetic factors, environmental factors, and disease. Yet the first four of these sets of subfecundity causes have largely been ignored by population scientists because their roles as subfecundity factors were unproven and/or because they were felt to be not prevalent enough. Almost by default disease became the only factor receiving much attention in the population literature. The sexually transmitted diseases (STDs), particularly syphilis and gonorrhea, were known to be quite prevalent in many low-fertility societies, and their proven association with reproductive failure provided a ready explanation for the fertility impairment. But this handy explanation diminished the incentive to investigate other causes of subfecundity. The deficiencies of this limited approach were also compounded by the fact that critical assessments of the actual contribution to subfecundity of even these diseases were often absent. For example, the statement that only a minority of pregnancies in a syphilitic woman will end with the birth of a normal, full-term infant is frequently encountered in the population literature, even though the disease as it affects reproduction is self-limiting and a woman with untreated syphilis of more than 2 or 3 years duration will almost always bear an unaffected child.

These criticisms are meant only as precautions and to urge a more

careful assessment of the contribution of the STDs to population subfecundity. There can be no doubt that these diseases are important subfecundity factors and are important explanatory variables for fertility
levels, especially in the developing world. The question is how important they are.

There are 21 pathogens for which sexual transmission is a major
means of spread. These pathogens include bacteria, viruses, fungi, protozoa, and parasites. Table 9.1 shows the more important organisms and
the diseases they cause. Gonorrhea, syphilis, chancroid, lymphogranuloma venereum (LGV), and granuloma inguinale are considered the
classical venereal diseases. Of these gonorrhea and syphilis, the major
venereal diseases, are the most important, both in the developing and
the developed worlds. Syphilis (which is discussed in Chapter 11) is an

Table 9.1
Sexually Transmitted Diseases

Pathogen	*Disease*
Bacteria	
Treponema pallidum	Syphilis
Neisseria gonorrhoeae	Gonorrhea
Chlamydia trachomatis (serotypes D–K)	Chlamydial urethritis, cervicitis, etc.
Chlamydia trachomatis (serotypes L_1, L_2, L_3)	Lymphogranuloma venereum
Mycoplasma hominis and *Ureaplasma urealyticum (T-myco- plasma)*	Genital mycoplasma
Haemophilus ducreyi	Chancroid
Calymmatobacterium granulomatis	Granuloma inguinale
Viruses	
Herpes simplex virus type 2	Genital herpes
Cytomegalovirus	Cytomegalovirus inclusion disease
Hepatitis B virus	Hepatitis
Genital wart virus	Anogenital warts
Fungi	
Candida albicans	Moniliasis
Protozoa	
Trichomonas vaginalis	Trichomoniasis
Parasites	
Phthirus pubis	Pubic lice
Sarcoptes scabiei	Scabies

important subfecundity factor only in women, in whom it causes pregnancy loss. Gonorrhea, on the other hand, is an important cause of subfecundity in men and women. In men, a gonorrheal infection that spreads beyond the anterior urethra to the posterior urethra, vas deferens, epididymis, and/or to the prostate and seminal vesicles may result in urethral strictures, obstructive azoospermia and sterility, and perhaps seminal fluid abnormalities capable of reducing fertilizing capacity. In women acute salpingitis, also called acute pelvic inflammatory disease (PID), is the most frequent complication of gonococcal infection and may result in tubal occlusion and sterility. If the tube is only partially occluded an ectopic pregnancy may occur because the tiny spermatozoa can pass a partially blocked section of tube whereas the much larger fertilized ovum cannot. Studies in the developing world have shown that oligo–azoospermia and tubal occlusion are very prevalent in infertile men and women (Edstrom 1978:31; Gray 1977:240; Guest 1978:27; World Health Organization 1975:15), underscoring the potential importance of gonorrhea as a major cause of population subfecundity there.

In recent years increasing numbers of cases of salpingitis and urethritis have yielded no gonococci on culture, and subsequent studies have shown that sexually transmitted pathogens such as *Chlamydia trachomatis* and the genital mycoplasmas *Mycoplasma hominis* and *Ureaplasma urealyticum* are responsible for a large proportion of these cases. These nongonococcal infections are, however, probably less important in those countries where gonorrhea is still rampant. Thus, whereas nongonoccal infections are frequent in the developed world they are likely to be much less frequent in the developing world where gonorrhea is widespread and uncontrolled.

The minor venereal diseases—chancroid, LGV, and granuloma inguinale—though rare in the developed world may be quite common in parts of the developing world, and the similarity of many of their symptoms to those of gonorrhea and syphilis makes a differential diagnosis difficult.

Although it is not one of the classical venereal diseases, genital herpes has since the 1970s become one of the most widespread and most feared of the venereal diseases. Although its importance in the developing world has not been evaluated, it is highly prevalent in the developed world. In the United States, for example, 5–20 million persons had this incurable disease by the late 1970s, with another .5 million new infections occuring each year (Brody 1980:C1; Raeburn 1981:E14; Subak-Sharpe 1978:155; *Time* 1980a:76).

Sexually Transmitted Diseases
in the Developing World

Factors Favoring Spread

The STDs are a particularly serious problem in developing countries because not only are there more venereal diseases in the developing world, but their incidence is many times that in most developed countries and is on the increase. The social upheaval occurring in many of these areas has been accompanied by frequent population movement, increasing urbanization, family disruption, and abandonment of tribal norms, all of which favor the spread of STDs. Prostitution is an important source of genital infection in poor urban areas and in one series (Taha *et al.* 1979:314) was the source in half the men with VD. The patterns of sexual behavior in some areas, such as those noted by Grech *et al.* (1973:124, 126) in Uganda (young age at first sexual experience, young age at marriage, multiple sexual partners, widespread polygamy, and frequent extramarital relationships for both men and women), are also very favorable to the spread of sexually transmitted diseases. And because fertility is so desirable in most developing societies, an infertile union is frequently dissolved and additional wives taken, further encouraging the spread of VD.

The rapid spread of VD in the developing world cannot be contained by the inadequate health services. Public health measures such as contact tracing and casefinding, which have been important in controlling STD rates in developed countries, are woefully inadequate in developing countries. There are few lab facilities to diagnose VD accurately and clinical criteria alone often must suffice; the result is that most genital sores are diagnosed as syphilis and treated accordingly, and most urethral discharges are labeled gonorrhea and so treated. And when treatment is initiated it is often inadequate because of improper treatment regimens prescribed by undertrained medical personnel, a shortage of drugs, or the patient defaulting on treatment because of ignorance or a lack of money. Self-treatment is often the rule. In rural areas traditional remedies are popular, and in urban areas antibiotics may be bought at the pharmacy and pills at the marketplace.

As a result of such practices, resistant strains of organisms are becoming increasingly important. Of the gonorrhea strains now seen in developing countries, 80% are relatively resistant to penicillin. Another result of inadequate treatment is an increase in complications such as salpingitis and epididymitis that can cause sterility.

Hence, in the developing world there exists a socioeconomic climate favoring the spread of venereal infections, increases in the number of antibiotic-resistant organisms, and increases in complication rates. The STD problem in the developing world has been further exacerbated by what was originally a medical success story. The successful eradication in many tropical areas of yaws, caused by *Treponema pertenue*, has resulted in loss of protective cross-immunity against *Treponema pallidum*, the treponeme that causes syphilis. Thus, in yaws-endemic areas where previously there had been little or no syphilis the disease began to appear and in some localities has become highly prevalent.

Prevalence

Problems with National Statistics

The incidence of STDs in developing countries is unknown. Arya and Lawson (1977:54–55) noted that in tropical areas 80% of the population receives its primary care at peripheral medical units, most of which have no lab facilities, meaning that a diagnosis is made on clinical grounds only. An accurate diagnosis is often impossible under such circumstances, even for the best clinician, and gonorrhea and syphilis tend to be overdiagnosed. That the STDs are overdiagnosed was supported by Taha *et al.* (1979:313), who noted that 51% of persons referred to a venereal disease clinic in Khartoum Province, Sudan, did not have an STD.

On the other hand, Muir and Belsey (1980:915) felt that national statistics of reported cases represent minimal estimates because of underreporting. The degree of underreporting can be illustrated by comparing reported rates from developed and developing countries. Reported rates of gonorrhea per 100,000 population in 1967 were 142.4 for New Zealand and only 108.3 for Vietnam, despite the fact that several years earlier U.S. medical authorities in Vietnam had estimated that there were 40,000 new cases of gonorrhea each *week* among the civilian population. And it seems reasonable that in the absence of contact tracing and casefinding many mild and asymptomatic cases are missed altogether. Willcox (1980b:279) further cautioned that reports of increases in the number of reported cases do not necessarily indicate a real increase in prevalence but can reflect improved detection and reporting of cases. Thus, national statistics on STDs must be considered inaccurate and more reliable information must be sought elsewhere, such as in population surveys.

Problems with Population Surveys

Incidence rates cited by population surveys must, however, also be viewed with some skepticism. Many problems are associated with the generation and interpretation of data, whether such data are of a clinical, laboratory, or personal nature.

Unrepresentativeness of the Study Population   Often the study population is unrepresentative of the population as a whole. This is the case when the study population is a group of infertile men or women, individuals attending a VD clinic, or persons living in low-fertility areas. Even for these population subgroups the data may not be representative. Henin (1969:189), for example, cautioned that although VD was noted in 40% of women examined in his study of nomads in the Sudan, a low-fertility population, these women were not representative of the total nomadic population because only women with fertility problems presented for examination.

Inaccuracy of Self-assessments   Individuals are frequently asked if they have ever experienced symptoms suggestive of VD. Although helpful to the investigator, such self-assessments should not be the sole basis of any conclusion regarding the importance of VD. Howell's (1979) assessment of the demographic impact of VD on the fertility of the !Kung has been criticized (see Dyson 1980:412) for relying too heavily on the proportion of women who merely reported having had a venereal disease. Whether such self-assessments result in over- or underestimations of STD is unknown and probably varies by population. Some studies (e.g., Henin 1969:188) have suggested that overestimates are a problem because minor diseases are frequently interpreted by some persons as being serious venereal diseases. On the other hand, Arya *et al.* (1973:592) noted that more than 50% of Teso (Uganda) men with gonorrhea were not aware of a urethral discharge or any other symptom. And the asymptomatic nature of gonorrhea in the female is well appreciated. Scragg (1957:90, 79) further noted that a discharge and even a substantial degree of discomfort, such as that associated with salpingitis, is often ignored by native men and women, and only when debility occurs or an ulcer appears does the individual seek medical attention. Thus, self-assessments may over- or underestimate the importance of the STDs. And, as noted earlier, even physicians frequently miss the mark if their diagnosis must rely solely on clinical impressions.

Inaccuracy of Pregnancy Histories   A woman's pregnancy history—the number of pregnancies, abortions, stillbirths, and live births—is very important to investigators. Frequently there is no documentation of such events and they must rely on patient recall. Inaccuracies are common both because of faulty memory and a desire to withhold some types of information. In some societies abortion or miscarriage is considered a shameful event or the consequence of a breach of a sexual taboo and is kept secret (Nag 1968:138). And in many parts of Africa there is a reluctance to mention children who have died, meaning that the investigator must check birth registrations (if they exist) to determine the number of children born. But in cases of neonatal death it is likely that neither the birth nor the death was registered (Romaniuk 1968:317, 315). To circumvent these problems some investigators have installed checks in their studies. Scragg (1957), for example, noting that spontaneous abortion was rarely reported among women in New Ireland, confirmed the absence of prior pregnancy among childless women by examining the cervix. He also noted that even after several years of observing hospital admittances in New Ireland he saw few miscarriages.

Limitations of Diagnostic Tests Good studies should, therefore, rely less on subjective information and more on the results of specific diagnostic tests. In the developing world performance of such tests is difficult for many reasons. Insufficient resources of monies and trained personnel limit the numbers and types of tests that can be performed. Lab facilities are often many miles from rural examining rooms, meaning that labile samples must be transported considerable distances under unfavorable circumstances such as extreme heat. An accurate diagnosis of syphilis is particularly difficult in tropical areas because there is currently no way to differentiate the treponeme of syphilis from the treponeme of the tropical disease yaws.

Even when sophisticated diagnostic techniques are available, their accuracy must be evaluated. Edstrom (1978:32) assessed the relative value of the three major techniques of diagnosing tubal occlusion—tubal insufflation, laparoscopy, and hysterosalpingography—and concluded that ideally both laparoscopy and hysterosalpingography should be used as they give complementary information. In the event that only one technique is available this should be laparoscopy, as it has the added advantage of identifying those cases that are most likely to benefit from surgery. Curran (1979:174) noted, however, that laparoscopy could miss those cases where the pathology is confined to the tubal mucosa. Edstrom (1978:31) further cautioned that tubal insufflation, though the easiest to use of the three methods, gives the least information and is the least accurate (see also Carty and Chatfield, 1972). Thus studies that rely solely on tubal insufflation must be evaluated with this in mind.

The ability of the individual physician to evaluate the results of tests may also vary. Scragg (1957) performed hysterosalpingography on infertile women in his series and found a large number of cases of bilateral occlusion. He did repeat exams in those cases where the X-ray pictures showed that the occlusion was in that part of the tube closest to the uterus (cornual end). This concerned him because his working hypothesis was that the occlusion was the result of gonococcal salpingitis, but gonorrhea most frequently produces occlusion at the other end of the tube (fimbriated end), filling defects at the cornual end being more suggestive of tubal spasms caused by the procedure. Thus, he was very familiar with the procedure and knew how to interpret the results correctly.

Erroneous Assignment of Causality   No matter what test is used, assignment of causality is difficult. Certainly Scragg's findings on hysterosalpingography, when coupled with his other data (see Scragg 1957), are highly suggestive of tubal occlusion and sterility caused by gonorrhea. But they are not irrefutable proof of a gonococcal etiology. Palpatory findings are frequently misused to establish a diagnosis of infertility due to gonorrhea. But epididymal thickening or pelvic masses may be due to infection with the tubercle bacillus as well as with *Neisseria gonorrhoeae* and other STDs. Furthermore, according to studies in Sweden, palpatory findings are frequently inaccurate. Jacobson and Westrom (1969:1096) reported that 25% of women thought to have pelvic swelling or masses were normal by laparoscopy.

Even histopathological examination of excised tubes often cannot establish a diagnosis. If a tubercle is found in a tube with evidence of inflammation (and much searching must often be done to find one) a diagnosis of tuberculous salpingitis can be made. In the absence of such a finding, the etiology of salpingitis will probably remain indeterminate. Was it gonococcal or nongonococcal? Was the infection the result of an STD or did it follow an abortion or childbirth? During the active stages of disease more of these questions can be answered. Examination of the patient can determine if there is genital trauma consistent with recent childbirth or abortion, and culture of material from the tubes and/or cul-de-sac as well as from the cervix may permit identification of the microbes involved.

Absence of Standard Values   Another problem in evaluating study data is determining whether results are truly indicative of pathology in that particular population. Ledward (1980:118) found that in a group of infertile women in Saudi Arabia, many of whom were not ovulating, serum prolactin levels were elevated, at least by European standards. The author treated these women accordingly with bromocriptine but noted that because the average prolactin level of fertile women in this population was not known, it was indeterminate whether the levels found in infertile women were the cause of ovulatory failure. Similarly, though Chukudebelu (1978:239) found that 93% of men from infertile unions in his series in Nigeria had sperm counts <60 million/ml, which he felt was significant, the true significance of these results cannot be assessed because the values for fertile men in this environment is not known. For example, in another study in Nigeria (Ladipo 1980:788) where mean sperm counts for men in fertile as well as infertile unions were determined (fertile, 71.2 million/ml; infertile, 46.8 million/ml), it was noted that even the fertile men had a mean sperm count considerably lower than the means for fertile men published in the literature, which were anywhere from 79 to 137 million/ml.

Because the baseline values for many variables used to evaluate reproductive function may vary by population, determination of these values for the fertile as well as the infertile members of a given population is very important. But it is difficult to get large numbers of persons to submit to unpleasant or even painful tests when the results will not directly benefit them. Scragg (1957:98) wanted to get semen samples from fertile men in New Ireland to see whether the very low semen volumes he observed in infertile men were a sign of pathology, were due to faulty collection methods, or were normal for this population. But the fertile men were unwilling to cooperate and he noted (1957:99) ''they declined as they knew they were fertile and the matter must affront even the mind of the sterile native.'' In some areas the task of examining the genitals and obtaining specimens, even blood samples, may be particularly difficult because of cultural taboos and suspicions (Arya *et al.* 1973:587).

Sexually Transmitted Diseases in the Developed World

In the developed world VD is a serious public health problem, though not of the magnitude experienced by the developing nations. The first recorded VD epidemic swept Europe late in the fifteenth century—hence the notion that Columbus's voyagers had brought VD back from the New World. More likely both gonorrhea and syphilis had been around for some time. It is thought that cases of leprosy described in the Bible were really a venereal disease and that historical figures such as Henry VIII, Cellini, Napolean, and Goethe were probably victims of gonorrhea or syphilis.

The causative organism of gonorrhea was demonstrated in 1886 and that of syphilis in 1905. By 1909 arsenic was found to be effective against syphilis and by the 1930s a prolonged course of arsenotherapy effective in curing infectious syphilis was introduced. But the treatment was not widely employed because it was long, painful and dangerous. Sulfonamides were used to treat gonorrhea during the 1930s and 1940s and were effective in reducing complication rates. But it was not until the late 1940s with the widespread use of penicillin, to which gonorrhea and syphilis are exquisitely sensitive, that substantial reductions in morbidity and mortality were recorded. This trend continued until the late 1950s, at which time both diseases began a worldwide resurgence that has been attributed in part to greater promiscuity and the abandonment of barrier methods of contraception in favor of the pill.

The post-1957 increase in syphilis has not been of the magnitude of the increase in gonorrhea, and by the 1970s syphilis was found primarily in homosexual men (see, for example, Wiesner and Holmes 1975:21; Wilcox 1977:215–216). The rate of increase of gonorrhea has been leveling off, but nongonococcal infections are becoming increasingly more important. Although gonococcal urethritis (GCU) is about equally as common as nongonococcal urethritis (NGU) in the United States, several European countries have reported that NGU and nongonococcal cervicitis and their complications are far more important (Felman and Nikitas 1981:381; Mardh *et al.* 1981:127). In the United States a preponderance of nongonococcal infections exists among certain population subgroups. For example, among higher socioeconomic groups such as college students cases of NGU far outnumber cases of GCU (Bowie 1980:19; Felman and Nikitas 1981:381; Wang *et al.* 1975:40; Weisner and Holmes 1975:22). In the developing world this same GCU–NGU breakdown exists by social class. Meheus *et al.* (1980:244) noted that whereas a urethral discharge meant gonorrhea in 80 to 90% of patients in Rwanda, Kenya, Malaysia, and Swaziland, among men of high social class studied in Ibadan, Nigeria, only 33% of urethritis cases were gonococcal.

One of the most dramatic features of the current VD picture in the developed world is the phenomenal increase in the prevalence of genital herpes. Rarely seen before the 1970s, by the 1980s genital herpes had become among the most important of the STDs in the United States, trailing only GCU and NGU. Its recurrent nature is the cause of much misery, and unlike syphilis and gonorrhea it is incurable. Its association with cervical carcinoma and its devastating effect on the newborn have created a climate of fear that will probably do much to encourage a more discriminating choice of sexual partners and the use of protective measures during intercourse, actions which will slow the rate of increase.

The minor venereal diseases—chancroid, LGV, and granuloma in-guinale—are rare in the developed world, except in port cities that are in direct communication with endemic areas.

The resurgence of the venereal diseases has stimulated a great deal of research into their pathogenesis and treatment. Herpes research is very active in the United States, and both American and Scandinavian researchers have done a great deal of important work on gonococcal and nongonococcal infections and their complications. They have illustrated the inaccuracy of a clinical diagnosis of pelvic inflammatory disease (PID) and the usefulness of laparoscopy. Finding in recent years fewer cases of PID where the gonococcus could be isolated from the cervix, they searched for other organisms and established the importance of *C. trachomatis*. They have also performed experimental infections in grivet monkeys to determine if *C. trachomatis* and *M. hominis* are capable of causing tubal pathology. They have followed large numbers of women treated for salpingitis to determine the effect on subsequent fertility. They have further defined the risk of PID by showing that fertility is jeopardized more by nongonococcal than gonococcal infections and that repeated episodes of PID greatly increase sterility rates. In all, in both the United States and Europe the effects of the STDs on reproductive potential have been extensively studied and such studies are continu-ing. The results of these studies form the basis of this assessment of the impact of the sexually transmitted diseases on human reproductive po-tential.

Because gonococcal and nongonococcal infections, syphilis, and genital herpes are the most prevalent of the STDs and all may affect fecundity, we decided to focus our attention on these diseases in Part III.

CHAPTER 10

Gonococcal and Nongonococcal Infections and Their Complications

Uncomplicated Gonorrhea in the Male and Female

Introduction

Gonorrhea is a specific inflammation of the mucous membrane of the genitourinary tract caused by the bacterium *Neisseria gonorrhoeae,* a gram-negative diplococcus. Its role in genital infections was first demonstrated in 1886 by a Swedish physician, Frans Wistermark, who isolated the gonococcus from exudates of infected fallopian tubes. Since that time gonorrhea has been found to also cause urethritis, cervicitis, endometritis, and peritonitis in women and urethritis, epididymitis, prostatitis, and seminal vesiculitis in men. An inflammatory response is elicited as the gonococci penetrate and multiply within the epithelial and subepithelial cells of these tissues. This is followed by a denuding of the epithelium and fibrosis upon healing. The genital ducts may be narrowed or obliterated as a result of extensive fibrosis, peritubal adhesions may cause kinking of the fallopian tubes, and normal cellular functions such as secretion and ciliary movement may be altered. Such structural and functional changes often result in the dimunition or loss of reproductive ability.

Prevalence

Gonorrhea is a disease of young adults; in the United States the highest age-specific case rates are from ages 20 to 24 (Wiesner and Holmes 1975:17). The incidence of the disease increased more than threefold between 1958 and 1974 (Wiesner and Holmes 1975:16), largely as a result of increased sexual activity. The pill has been important in the spread of gonorrhea, not only because it supplanted the barrier contraceptives, such as the condom and diaphragm, which protect against transmission, but also because the hormones in the pill increase the pH of the vagina, creating an alkaline environment particularly favorable to the gonococcus. Whereas one act of unprotected intercourse with an infected male normally carries a 40% risk of infection, that risk in pill users is almost 100%.

Because private physicians in the United States usually do not report cases of gonorrhea—a 1968 survey of 250,000 U.S. doctors revealed that about 80% of all cases of gonorrhea were treated by private physicians and these physicians failed to report 90% of their cases (Wiesner and Holmes 1975:15–16)—incidence rates in the United States are estimates. Hager and Wiesner (1977:47) reported that in the United Kingdom and Sweden, where reporting is more complete than in the United States, incidence rates among the highest-risk group, 20–24 year olds, are quite high—451/100,000 for the United Kingdom and 1,538/100,000 for Sweden.

Incidence rates for the developing world are, as noted earlier (see Muir and Belsey 1980:915), completely unreliable. Nevertheless, results of population surveys suggest that gonorrhea is very common in much of the developing world. Hager and Wiesner (1977:47) cited the results of a number of studies from Africa: In Nigeria gonorrhea was found in 3.5% of asymptomatic women; in Nairobi, Kenya, it was found in 17.5% of women attending a family planning clinic; and in Uganda 18% of women tested were gonorrhea-positive.

Factors Affecting the Risk of Becoming Infected

The risk of becoming infected with *N. gonorrhoeae* is not evenly distributed throughout the population, but is dependent on certain environmental, host, and organism variables. Age, sex, race, number of sexual partners, the health care system, and even blood type may influence the likelihood of becoming infected.

Environmental Variables

Sexual contact is the almost exclusive means of transmission of gonorrhea, although in wet tropical areas the gonococcus may remain infective for at least 3 to 4 hours outside the body and can be transmitted to children who share clothing, bed linens, or towels with an infected adult (Alausa and Osoba 1980:241). The greater the number of sexual contacts the greater the risk of infection. Also, transmission is much more likely to occur when no barrier contraceptive such as the diaphragm or condom is used. And use of the pill may actually enhance transmission rates, increases in the vaginal pH caused by the pill creating an environment particularly favorable to gonococcal growth and reproduction.

The risk of infection probably also varies with inoculum size—contact with an individual with a profuse exudate with many organisms constituting a greater risk—and with whether or not the contact is already colonized with bacteria that have an antigonoccocal activity (Holmes 1975:83).

Host Variables

In addition to these environmental variables, there are host variables—primarily sex, age, and race—that influence the risk of infection.

Sex The risk of becoming infected following one act of coitus with an infected partner is substantially greater for women than for men. Whereas most studies (e.g., Grimble 1972:615; Holmes 1975:83) have estimated that a man runs a 20–30% risk after one or two acts of coitus with an infected partner, this risk is placed at 50 to 70% or greater for women (Pariser 1972:1127; Wigfield 1972:672). Wigfield (1972:672) suggested the woman is at greater risk because she has infectious organisms ''thrust'' upon an appropriate culture medium (the cervix) but the male is exposed only to seepage from the cervix. And whereas simply voiding or washing after coitus will often rid the male of many organisms, douching is required for the female to accomplish the same result.

Age Verzin (1975:164) has stated that young girls are more susceptible to infection with *N. gonorrhoeae* because the vaginal epithelium is thin and unprotected before puberty. Gibbons (1977:403–404) has speculated that the epithelial cells have certain receptors that interact with bacteria and that age can alter these receptors and thereby alter susceptibility to infection.

Race There are several bits of evidence suggesting racial differences in susceptibility to infection with *N. gonorrhoeae*. Foster and Labrum (1976:329–330) reported that a disproportionate number of the 584 black women in their study with blood type B had gonorrhea; whereas 14% of women with blood type A and 22% of those with blood type O had gonorrhea, 32% of women with blood type B were gonorrhea-positive. This study and one by Gibbons (1977:403) suggest that there may be an immunological basis for blood group differences in susceptibility to *N. gonorrhoeae* infection. And because Mourant *et al.* (1958, cited in Hager and Wiesner 1977:49) have noted that the frequency of blood group B is much higher in blacks than whites, it might be concluded that the greater incidence of gonorrhea among blacks is due in part to nonsociological factors.

Disease and Nutritional Status If an individual suffers from numerous diseases and dietary deficiencies, his or her immunological defenses are exhausted and the ability to resist infections such as gonorrhea is greatly diminished. This is particularly true with certain diseases such as malaria and African sleeping sickness. In the latter, immune exhaustion is common and the patient often dies—not of sleeping sickness but of an intercurrent infection such as pneumonia. It has also been noted that persons with anemia are more susceptible to infection (Lawson 1967a: 86–87; Stewart 1967a:243). However, two qualifiers must be placed on this statement: (1) According to McFee (1973:157–158), the anemia must be severe ($<8g\%$ Hgb); (2) according to Masawe *et al.* (1974:314) only a hemolytic or megaloblastic type of anemia increases susceptibility to bacterial infection. (Iron-deficiency anemia, for example, does not increase susceptibility to bacterial infection but does increase susceptibility to malaria, a parasitic infection.) Hence, persons with a severe hemolytic or megaloblastic anemia, those with African sleeping sickness or malaria, and those suffering from numerous diseases and dietary deficiencies are more susceptible to bacterial infections such as gonorrhea.

Organism Variables

It is known that different strains of gonorrhea differ in their virulence, some strains causing higher rates of PID than others (Mosher and Aral 1983:17), for example. Whether this is associated with their infectivity is uncertain, though possible (Holmes 1975:83). It is likely that infectivity and virulence are linked because studies have shown that virulent gonococcal colony types (T_1 and T_2) have organisms with threadlike projections (pili) extending from their surface, whereas organisms in the nonvirulent colony types (T_3, T_4, and T_5) do not.[1] Each cervico-vaginal cell has 10^4 receptors for these pili, and although the nonpilated organisms can attach to these cells they do so with less avidity than the T_1 and T_2 organisms (Danielsson 1975:31–32; Ronda *et al.* 1980:252). Thus, the more virulent organisms are also more likely to initiate an infection.

Repeat Infection

Environmental, host, and organism factors are therefore important in determining gonorrhea transmission rates. In areas where these factors impact negatively on a significant proportion of the population, rates can reach very high levels. Because infection offers little or no resistance to reinfection (Danielsson 1975:32), except for short periods of time and then only against the same immunotype of gonococcus (Eschenbach 1980:144S), persons at high risk are infected again and again. Epidemiologists believe that a core of frequently infected, highly active, and effective transmitters does exist (Yorke *et al.* 1978:56). A study (Brooks *et al.* 1978:163) in Marion County, Indiana, reported that 22% of gonorrhea cases during the study period were among repeaters. The authors (1978:167) concluded that "gonorrhea repeaters constituted an extremely small segment of the population [0.06%] but yielded a very large proportion of the morbidity due to gonorrhea [22%]." Similarly, Brown *et al.* (1970:65) noted that "morbidity statistics for syphilis represent different persons with disease, whereas gonorrhea statistics reflect a count of infections, *many of which occur in the same patient more than once* [emphasis added]." Thus, in viewing gonorrhea rates for a population and attempting to assess from them the impact of the disease in that population, it must be remembered that risk of infection is not evenly distributed throughout the population. Although some individuals are infected over and over again, others are never infected.

---

[1]Five distinct colony morphology types were demonstrated by culturing the gonococcus on a specially prepared medium. T_1 and T_2 colonies were smaller and were found on the culture of pus prepared from fresh clinical infections. These types were able to be subcultured by using selective culture methods. The other colony types (T_3, T_4, and T_5) were larger and developed on unselected subculture. These represent the laboratory variant of the gonococcus. Experimental infection of male volunteers showed that the virulence of the gonococcus was associated mainly with colony types T_1 and T_2 which had been subcultured for a long time, and not with the other colony types (Danielsson 1975:31; Ronda *et al.* 1980:252).

Effect on Fecundity

It is generally felt that gonorrhea does not have a negative impact on fecundity unless complications such as pelvic inflammatory disease (PID) or epididymitis develop. However, some workers feel that this view is too restrictive. Sweeney (1968:241, 243), for example, felt that gonococcal cervicitis and vaginitis may affect fecundity. He cited the study by Matthews and Buxton (1951, cited in Sweeney 1968:241) that showed that *Escherichia coli* and other bacteria are spermicidal and he suggested that an endocervical infection could cause infertility by creating an environment in the cervical mucus that is hostile to spermatozoa. Behrman and Kistner (1968:8) noted also that certain bacteria may affect the fertilizing capacity of spermatozoa without affecting sperm count, morphology, or motility. Hence, gonococcal infections in men or women may result in a temporary reduction in fecundity, which returns to normal once the infection is gone.

Symptoms

Symptoms of uncomplicated male gonorrhea include frequent and painful urination (dysuria) and a urethral discharge which may first be mucoid but later is a purulent yellow-green. The most frequent symptom in females is dysuria, although there may be an increased yellow vaginal discharge which in severe cases is bloodstained. Prolonged menstrual bleeding may also be seen. These symptoms are caused by a patchy destruction of the mucosa (urethral or cervical) with an accumulation of gonococci and pus cells (Danielsson 1975:31). In both sexes these symptoms can appear as soon as 3–7 days post exposure, and usually within 2 to 4 weeks.

However, a large proportion of infections in both men and women are asymptomatic, that is, no signs or symptoms are detected by the patient or the physician and a diagnosis is made solely on the basis of lab tests (Pariser 1972:1127). It has been reported (Akerlund *et al.* 1975:172; Catterall 1975:7; Curran *et al.* 1975:195; Hansson and Juhlin 1975:75) that 50–90% of women with gonorrhea are asymptomatic. Although it was once believed that fewer than 10% of men with gonorrhea were asymptomatic (see Catterall 1975:7; Pariser 1972:1130), studies of men in the community at large (as opposed to men presenting at treatment centers) and studies of contacts of infected women have revealed that 40–75% of men are asymptomatic (Bowie 1980:20; Handsfield *et al.*

1974:117; *Journal of the American Medical Association* 1981:609; Portnoy *et al.* 1974:169). The asymptomatic carrier state may last for many years (Portnoy *et al.* 1974:169–170) and is a danger to both the infected individual and any sexual contacts as the infection may produce serious later complications in some of the carriers and, if transmitted, may produce a symptomatic infection in the contact (Pariser 1972:1127).

Diagnosis

A diagnosis of gonorrhea depends on identification of the gonococcus in exudates from the urethra or cervix. (The rectum or pharynx may also yield organisms.) The easiest method is to Gram stain a urethral or cervical smear and look under the microscope for the typical gram-negative intracellular, equal-size diplococci that characterize a gonococcal infection. A superior method is to culture the sample on Thayer–Martin medium. This medium, which is selective for *N. gonorrhoeae* and *N. meningitides* only, has been available since 1962 and was improved in 1966. Its sensitivity is high, one culture yielding positive results in 85% of cases. An even more recent development is Stuart's transport medium, which maintains the sample during transport from the examining room to the laboratory, further enhancing the sensitivity of the technique.

Diagnosis in men is relatively simple. During the acute stage of the disease urethral pus is easy to obtain and intracellular gonococci are usually found by Gram stain (Hansson and Juhlin 1975:73). When the Gram stain indicates gonorrhea, culturing is unnecessary because a characteristic Gram stain correlates with isolation by culture in 98% of men (Bowie 1980:21). However, in 15% of men with urethritis[2] the Gram stain is not diagnostic and the investigator must do a culture to distinguish gonococcal from nongonococcal infections (Swartz 1977:16).

The diagnosis of gonorrhea in women is more difficult. Gram staining is useful only as an adjunct to Thayer–Martin medium because 60% or fewer women with gonorrhea give a characteristic Gram stain (Bowie 1980:24; Hansson and Juhlin 1975:74). And even if the Gram stain in-

[2]An inflammatory condition such as urethritis can be confirmed by a number of methods. The simplest is to express fluid from the structure and look under the microscope for cell types associated with an inflammatory response, namely polymorphonuclear leucocytes (PMNs). According to Felman and Nikitas (1981:383–384) ≥ 5 PMNs observable in a high-power field (HPF) indicate inflammation; Swartz (1977:17) applied the stricter criterion of ≥ 10 PMNs/HPF. Eliasson (1975:117–118) noted that a technique called exfoliative cytology can confirm a diagnosis of inflammation even when there are no demonstrable PMNs, cells from the affected area showing degenerative changes.

dicates gonorrhea a diagnosis must be made with caution because in women the Gram stain gives false-positive as well as false-negative results (de Leon 1973:194), due to the frequent presence of other gram-negative cocci in the female urogenital tract. Thus, in most, if not all, cases a culture should also be done (Bowie 1980:24; Curran 1979:175; Grimble 1972:620; Hansson and Juhlin 1975:74) and, if possible, repeated; up to 30% of cases may be missed if only one investigation is performed (Schofield and Shanks 1971:259). Seeking organisms at more than one site will also increase the number of positive cases because, for example, 10% of women with gonorrhea have a positive rectal culture only (Brown *et al.* 1970:93).

In developing areas of the world the percentage of gonorrhea cases that can be positively diagnosed is often limited by resources. The availability and proximity of lab facilities stocked with Thayer–Martin medium (which should be freshly made), the availability of Stuart's transport medium for the examining room, the number of sites cultured, the number of cultures done per sample, and the number of times samples are taken are all limiting factors. One research group (Carty *et al.* 1972:376) felt that the number of cases of gonorrhea would have been higher in their Nairobi study if multiple attempts had been made to obtain and culture exudates.

One of the most recent developments in the diagnosis of gonorrhea, and one that will greatly improve the accuracy of studies that seek to correlate infertility with a history of gonorrhea, is the gonococcal pilar antibody test. This test, which is both sensitive and specific, detects antibodies to the pili that project from the surface of the gonococcus. These antibodies persist for years even in patients treated for gonorrhea. If the titer is high a recent infection is indicated; a low titer means a past infection (Mardh *et al.* 1981:127). Prior studies inferred an association between gonorrhea and infertility from comparisons made on a *community* basis of such indices as prevalence rates of gonorrhea in population surveys, rates of reported gonorrhea and urethritis, and urethral stricture rates with such indicators of fertility as the childlessness rate, the general fertility rate, and total fertility (see World Health Organization 1975:13); however, this test will allow comparison on an *individual* basis.

Treatment

Once diagnosed, the treatment of uncomplicated gonorrhea is usually quite straightforward. In the past, penicillin or similar drugs such as amoxicillin or ampicillin were the most widely used. But because chlamydial infections now so frequently coexist with gonorrheal infections, tetracycline, to which both *N. gonorrhoeae* and *Chlamydia trachomatis* are sensitive, has come into favor. Recommended, but still untested as to efficacy and side effects, is a combined regimen of amoxicillin or ampicillin (or penicillin) and tetracycline (Centers for Disease Control 1982:3–7). Treatment failures under these regimens strongly suggest the presence of a penicillin–resistant strain of *N. gonorrhoeae*, and additional therapy with spectinomycin should be initiated.

Follow-up is important because even with the best of recommended treatment schedules there are some failures to cure. Although gonorrhea spontaneously heals even without treatment, the time between exposure and spontaneous recovery is long (Yorke *et al.* 1978:51). Therefore, therapy is important in shortening the period of infection and reducing the frequency of complications and their sequelae.

In many parts of the world treatment may be more difficult because strains of gonococci are present that are relatively or, in some cases, completely resistant to penicillin and other antibiotics. The ineffectual use of prescribed antibiotics results in low serum levels, which in turn favors the selection of penicillin-resistant strains (Sparling 1972:1137). Strains showing the greatest resistance are found in Africa and the Far East, particularly Thailand, Vietnam, Japan, and the Philippines. (In some tropical areas more than 80% of gonococcal strains are now relatively resistant to penicillin [Arya and Lawson 1977:54], and in some areas such as Swaziland a substantial proportion of strains have a highly diminished sensitivity to penicillin [Meheus *et al.* 1980:243–244].) Strains of intermediate resistance are found in the United States, Canada, and India, and strains with the least resistance are seen in England, Scandinavia, and Northern Europe (Sparling 1972:1135). In the United States, the West Coast cities of San Francisco and Seattle are notable for the frequency of strains relatively resistant to penicillin and tetracycline (Sparling 1972:1136). These strains were probably imported by U.S. servicemen stationed in Southeast Asia (Wiesner and Holmes 1975:17). A strain of penicillin-resistant gonorrhea also resistant to spectinomycin, the newer second-line defense against the disease, was seen in the United States in a serviceman who had been stationed in the Philippines.

Despite the sensitivity of most strains of *N. gonorrhoeae* to penicillin and other antibiotics, gonorrhea continues to be a difficult disease to control. Its short incubation period and frequently asymptomatic nature allow transmission to occur before treatment is initiated. And once the patient completes treatment, reinfection is possible as soon as the antibiotics are excreted. Infection itself offers only a very transitory immunity and then only against gonococcal strains of the same immunotype. Because this bacterium can alter its cell wall proteins with such great facility, each infection represents a new immunotype against which any prior antibodies are virtually useless. Even the same strain passed back and forth in a couple may repeatedly cause reinfection (ping-pong infection) because passage through only one other person can cause antigenic changes sufficient to produce a new immunotype (Grimble 1972:616).

Because of the transitory nature of antigonococcal antibodies and the constantly changing antigenicity of the gonococcus, development of a vaccine has been difficult. However, a University of Pittsburgh research team has developed a vaccine slated for field trial on U.S. troops (Greve 1982:4A).

Complications of Gonorrhea in the Female: Gonococcal Pelvic Inflammatory Disease

Introduction

In some women gonorrhea does not remain confined to the urethra and cervix, but spreads upward to involve the uterus, fallopian tubes, and perhaps the peritoneal cavity. (Complications in the male are discussed in the section "Complications in the Male".) Such supracervical infections are called acute pelvic inflammatory disease (PID), a term frequently used synonymously with acute salpingitis. When a diagnosis of PID is made and the gonococcus is recovered from the cervix it is called gonococcal PID; otherwise it is called nongonococcal PID. The search for etiologic agents in nongonococcal PID has intensified and later discussions in the section "Complications of Nongonococcal Infections in the Female" will cover the importance of these organisms to the overall problem of PID and its sequelae.

Aided perhaps by the reflux of menstrual blood the gonococcus reaches the uterus where it causes a transitory endometritis, which heals spontaneously leaving no residua. The gonococcus continues to spread along the mucosal surface and, less frequently, within the submucosal lymphatics, entering both fallopian tubes and causing an endosalpin-gitis (Monif 1974:103–105). At this point symptoms may be absent or mild and laparoscopy may reveal tubes that appear normal (Thompson and Hager 1977:108). If unchecked, the gonococcal infection now spreads in two directions: (1) along the mucosal surface toward the abdominal (fimbriated) end of the tube, pus eventually dripping out the fimbriated end into the peritoneal cavity, and (2) across the wall of the tube, involving first the muscularis and then the serosa (the membrane covering the tubes, which is continuous with the lining of the peritoneal cavity). In either instance there will be peritoneal inflammation. The ovary or bowel may be infected. In 25% of women with PID there will be a palpable swelling representing tubal inflammation and edema or a tubo-ovarian abscess (Eschenbach and Holmes 1975:40–41). At this stage laparoscopy will reveal tubes that are swollen and red and perhaps distended with purulent material. Pus may be dripping from the open fimbriated end. Involvement of the peritoneum, ovary, bowel, etc. will be apparent.

Residua are almost always present, even after only one episode of gonococcal PID (Monif 1974:105). The healing process has replaced normal tissue with nonfunctional fibrous tissue. The epithelial cells of the tubal mucosa have lost their ciliary motility and the tubal lumen is narrowed by the buildup of fibrous tissue in the mucosal folds. Peritubal adhesions, bands of fibrous tissue that fasten the tube to adjacent pelvic structures, may be present. More significant sequelae include closure of the fimbriated end of the tube, which, if bilateral, means absolute sterility (Eschenbach and Holmes 1975:40; Monif 1974:105; Monif 1980:159S). The infection has left behind an anatomically distorted pelvic structure with an altered blood supply and diminished ability to respond to infection, meaning that subsequent infections will probably be even more serious (Monif 1974:106).

Although one episode of gonococcal PID may result in a poor prognosis for future fertility, this is more likely following a second- or higher-order episode. Combining cases of gonococcal and nongonococcal PID, Westrom (1975:707) stated that one episode of PID results in tubal occlusion in 12.8% of cases, two episodes in 35.5% of cases, and three or more episodes in 75% of cases. With one infection the risk of tubal occlusion varies with severity; a mild episode carries a 4% risk, a moderately severe episode a 14% risk, and a severe episode a 33% risk (Westrom and Mardh 1978:21). (See discussion in the section ''Conceptive Failure'' for criteria for assessing the severity of infection.) And even if the tube remains patent there is no certainty that fertility is normal. The loss of ciliary movement, narrowing of the lumen, and kinking of the tube because of peritubal adhesions can all result in improper movement of the germ cells and/or fertilized ovum with sterility or ectopic pregnancy resulting.

Factors Affecting the Risk
of Developing Pelvic Inflammatory Disease

Certainly not every woman with cervical gonorrhea develops PID. Just as the risk of becoming infected after exposure to a source harboring *N. gonorrhoeae* depends on certain environmental, host, and organism factors, so too does the risk of developing PID depend on these factors.

Environmental Variables

One environmental variable that profoundly influences the risk of PID in a woman with gonorrhea is the type of contraception used. The risk of developing PID is several times higher in IUD users than in non-users, and this risk is higher yet if the woman has never been pregnant. The mechanism of the increased risk is unknown. One theory is that bacteria ascend the tail of the IUD via a wicking action. Another is that the more prolonged and heavier menstrual flow associated with IUD use facilitates movement of bacteria to the upper genital tract. On the other hand, the decreased volume of menstrual flow observed in pill users is one of the proposed reasons for the considerably lower rates of PID in women taking oral contraceptives (*Family Planning Perspectives* 1982:33). (See following section "Host Variables" and Chapter 17 for more detailed discussions of these points.)

The risk of developing PID is probably also greater in women with gonorrhea who have just experienced abortion or childbirth; such events are likely to aid the ascent of bacteria to the upper genital tract. Muir and Belsey (1980:916), in fact, felt that gonorrhea and other sexually transmitted diseases (STDs) play an important role in the etiology of postabortal and postpartum infections. They cited the work of Nasah and Eyang (in press, cited in Muir and Belsey 1980:916), which showed that in Cameroon *N. gonorrhoeae* can be isolated twice as frequently from women with postpartum sepsis as from nonseptic patients postpartum. Although such data do not firmly establish a cause-and-effect relationship they do suggest a role for *N. gonorrhoeae* in postpartum infections. Data from the developed world also suggest an association between gonorrhea and postpartum sepsis. Charles *et al.* (1970:598) noted postpartum fever in 28% of women with gonorrhea, a figure similar to the 32% rate reported by Bernstein and Bland (1948, cited in Charles *et al.* 1970:598). Because the overall PID rate in women with gonorrhea is 15–20%, these figures suggest that childbirth or abortion increases the risk of PID in infected women by 50 to 100%.

Another important environmental variable is the presence of a good health care system capable of finding, diagnosing, and treating cases of lower genital tract infections before they have the opportunity to ascend. Case finding and contact tracing are very important in identifying persons who may be infected with *N. gonorrhoeae* but have not presented for treatment either because they are asymptomatic or because they are unaware of the implications of their symptoms. They are especially important in discovering cases of female gonorrhea because so many women are asymptomatic. In the developed world, even with such public health measures in force, the average length of infection before treatment is 100 days for women, ten times that for men (10 days) (Yorke *et al.* 1978:52). In the developing world, where such public health measures are not normally in effect, many women will go untreated for even longer periods, perhaps until the infection spontaneously subsides, and therefore will be at an even greater risk of developing PID.

Once a case of suspected gonorrhea is identified a positive diagnosis must be made. The diagnosis of gonorrhea in men is fairly easy; the clinical picture is usually quite characteristic and a simple Gram stain of a urethral smear confirms the diagnosis. In women a diagnosis is more difficult; the clinical picture is variable and asymptomatic infections are frequent. Gram staining is unreliable and a positive diagnosis requires isolation of *N. gonorrhoeae* by bacteriologic methods. Until the 1960s the growth and identification of *N. gonorrhoeae* by bacteriologic methods was difficult and time consuming. But in 1962 Thayer and Martin introduced a culture medium of great specificity and sensitivity, which streamlined gonorrhea diagnosis and allowed the identification of more cases. In the developed world most suspected cases of gonorrhea are quickly diagnosed and treated. But in the developing world, where the health services for a large proportion of the population do not include laboratory facilities, a diagnosis on clinical grounds alone must suffice. Some infections in men and many infections in women undoubtedly go untreated in these areas.

Effective treatment of gonorrhea preceded its easy and reliable diagnosis by a decade or so, and was central to the decrease in prevalence recorded in the 1950s. In the late 1930s the effectiveness of the various sulfonamide preparations was demonstrated, and they readily gained favor over all other forms of therapy. But the gonococcus quickly developed resistance to the sulfa drugs and by the middle years of World War II it was obvious that the sulfonamides were no longer effective in many gonorrhea cases (Brown *et al.* 1970:83). In some respects the sulfonamides were not ideal drugs anyway. Pelouze (1939:160) reported toxic reactions in about 50% of cases and considered "watchful waiting" the best course. Sulfa drugs are particularly toxic to persons (usually of African, Sicilian, or Greek ancestry) whose red cells lack the enzyme glucose-6-phosphate dehydrogenase (G6PD). In these persons sulfa drugs may cause a severe and sometimes fatal hemolytic anemia. An estimated 10–14% of U.S. blacks have G6PD deficiency and are at risk of such a severe reaction (Nass *et al.* 1981:494).

Fortunately, penicillin, an antibiotic that produces almost miraculous cures and does not have the serious problems of the sulfa drugs, came into use in the late 1940s and dramatically altered the treatment of gonorrhea. For the first time prevalence rates began to decline.

Before the sulfa drugs and antibiotics, gonorrhea therapy was haphazard. Urethral irrigation, gonococcal vaccines, antitoxins, and fever therapy each had their advocates. So ineffective were these treatments that one eminent researcher (Stokes 1935:178) was prompted to say that the only thing that kept gonorrhea from becoming a practically universal disease was its tendency to cure itself. Some researchers (e.g., Brown *et al.* 1970:83) felt that such therapies may actually have contributed to complications of the disease. Rendtorff (1975:235) suggested that in past years the urethral strictures that followed male gonorrhea may have been largely due to treatment. And Adler (1980:208) noted that urethral irrigation with potassium permanganate, as routinely performed in the United Kingdom after World War I *always* led to epididymitis because the vessel containing the potassium permanganate was elevated so high that the solution entered the infected urethra with such force that the gonococci were swept posteriorly.

Hence, prior to the introduction of effective chemotherapy gonococcal cervicitis and gonococcal urethritis were essentially untreatable and complications were frequent. Indeed, such complications as posterior urethritis and epididymitis were probably more likely to occur in treated than untreated individuals. In the developed world effective antibiotic therapy now keeps complication rates relatively low. But in the developing world, in areas where antibiotics are not available or are used incorrectly, complication rates are much higher.

Host Variables

Host differences in susceptibility to complications may exist. It is possible that there is a host-dependent variable, probably physiologic or immunologic, that determines whether or not PID will develop. Westrom and Mardh (1978:9), for example, suggested that some women may be more likely to develop PID because of innate physiological factors such as an inadequate closure mechanism of the uterotubal junction. And Eschenbach and Holmes (1975:39) suggested that gonococcal PID develops in women who experience a failure of the normally effective local defense mechanisms. But once an episode of PID does occur, for whatever reason, subsequent episodes are far more likely because of residual tubal damage.

Because attacks of acute gonococcal salpingitis are so frequently correlated with the menses—47–66% of cases occur within 7 days of the onset of the menstrual period (Eschenbach 1980:142S)—individual differences in the frequency, duration, and/or volume of the menstrual flow could affect the risk of developing PID. In menstruating women one of the prime mechanical barriers to ascending infection, the cervical mucus plug, is lost. Other factors related to the onset of menses that have been proposed as aiding the multiplication and ascent of the gonococcus are the stimulation of gonococcal multiplication by other bacteria that proliferate late in the menstrual cycle and the accessibility of the normally protected lymph channels under the endometrium when this barrier sloughs off. Access to the tubes is also greater at this time due to the reflux of menstrual blood through the fallopian tubes (Eschenbach and Holmes 1975:39–40; Eschenbach 1980:142S; Monif 1974:104).

The absence of menses is probably an important factor in the rarity of PID in premenstrual girls and postmenopausal women. The protection the pill offers against PID has been attributed to a reduction in the duration and volume of the menstrual flow in pill users (Osser *et al.* 1980, cited in *Family Planning Perspectives* 1980b:207). And the increased risk of developing PID associated with the intrauterine device (IUD) may be due in part to the increased duration and volume of menstrual flow in IUD users. (See Chapter 17, on IUD use, for a more detailed discussion of this point.) It is also possible that in the developing world, where severely undernourished women may experience amenorrhea and moderately undernourished women may experience delayed menarche, premature menopause, and irregular menstrual cycles, there is a reduced tendency to develop PID. But because nutritional deficiencies, especially of protein, are associated with a greater susceptibility to infection, these two forces probably counterbalance each other. In countries where extended breast-feeding is widely practiced, lactational amenorrhea could offer women a period of lower risk of developing gonococcal PID. Of course, in those societies that do not permit intercourse during breast-feeding (some because they fear the sperm could reach the milk and harm the baby) the protection offered by amenorrhea is secondary.

Organism Variables

It is possible that the risk of developing PID varies with the virulence of *N. gonorrhoeae*. One worker (Grimble 1972:617) believed that the gonococcus has become less virulent than in the pre-antibiotic era, probably as a result of the use of antibiotics. He argued that whereas severe infections in the past were accompanied by malaise, fever, headache, weight loss, and occasionally vomiting and joint pains, this toxic reaction has become uncommon in recent years and is evidence of a change in virulence. He also drew attention to the fact that gonococcal opthalmia in newborns, even when diagnosis and treatment are delayed, now results in little or no serious damage, in striking contrast to the prognosis in the past. Whether or not extant gonococcal organisms differ in their ability to produce complications is debated, but Wiesner and Holmes (1975:24) could find no difference in gonococci recovered from women with PID and those recovered from women with uncomplicated gonorrhea.

Rates of Pelvic Inflammatory Disease in Women with Gonorrhea

It has been shown in the preceding discussion that a number of environmental, host, and organism variables impact on the proportion of cases of cervical gonorrhea that progress to gonococcal PID. What are the reported rates of PID in women with gonorrhea? And how can differences in reported rates be attributed to differences in environmental, host, and organism factors?

There are few reports of salpingitis rates prior to effective chemotherapy. A number of texts in human sexuality (e.g., Crooks and Baur 1980:345; Hyde 1979:444; Nass *et al.* 1981:478), each seemingly citing the same unidentified source, reported that 50% of women with untreated gonorrhea develop salpingitis. This is a much higher figure than the one most frequently cited in the medical literature, which is based on a Finnish study conducted between 1924 and 1952. In this study 14% of women with gonorrhea developed salpingitis in the presulfonamide, preantibiotic era, whereas only 2% did so after effective chemotherapy became available (see Rees and Annels 1969:206). However, these rates are lower than we would have anticipated, considering that current complication rates frequently exceed both these figures and that current rates are computed from a total number of gonorrhea cases including many asymptomatic and mild cases that would have gone unnoticed and unreported in the past.

Current complication rates are recorded at anywhere from 1 to 20% of cases. Although Belsey (1976:327) cited studies recording complication rates of 1 to 10% and Grimble (1972:621) reported salpingitis in only 4% of women with gonorrhea in his area of southeastern London, many more recent studies have reported substantially higher rates. Ronda *et al.* (1980:252) reported rates of 10 to 15%, Danielsson *et al.* (1975:151) a rate of 14%, Bowie (1980:21) a rate of 10%, Marano (1971:101) a rate of 20%, and Westrom (1975:707) a rate of 21.2%. Eschenbach (1980:142S) cited rates of 10 to 17%, concluding that these are low estimates because asymptomatic carriers are overrepresented in most series. Juhlin and Wallin (1972:12) reported that 15% of gonorrhea cases in Uppsala, Sweden, are followed by salpingitis and felt that complications are more frequent than before. But Westrom and Mardh (1978:1) reported that complications following gonorrhea have decreased substantially in Lund, Sweden, in recent years; a 20% salpingitis rate was recorded between 1960 and 1964, but only a 10% rate was recorded between 1970 and 1974. Data reveal very high complication rates in the United States. Wiesner and Holmes (1975:19) cited a 19.6% rate, and Urquhart (1979:467) cited a 17% estimate by the U.S. Centers for Disease Control. The actual number of women in the United States who get gonococcal PID has been estimated at about 250,000 per year (De Lora *et al.* 1981:245). If all types of PID, gonococcal and nongonococcal, are considered, the figure increases to 500,000, meaning that 15% of U.S. women of reproductive age are in a post-PID state (*Family Planning Perspectives* 1980b:206).

Data suggest that the resurgence in gonorrhea that began in the late 1950s was accompanied by an increase in complication rates. It must then be asked why this is so. At first one might speculate that increasing use of the IUD, which predisposes to pelvic infection, might have been a factor. But oral contraceptive use has grown even faster, and the pill has been shown to protect against the development of PID. Perhaps more resistant strains of *N. gonorrhoeae* have appeared, and thus formerly effective treatment methods failed to cure in some cases. Or perhaps more very young women were being affected, a group that has traditionally delayed seeking treatment. Or, as suggested in an article in the *British Medical Journal* (1975:501), the increase may have been due in part to improved methods of diagnosis. Fortunately, complication rates leveled off in the United States in the mid-1970s and perhaps have begun to decrease.

Effect on Fecundity

Pelvic inflammatory disease, which affects both tubes in more than 90% of cases (Eschenbach and Holmes 1975:42), has a tendency to heal spontaneously (Eschenbach and Holmes 1975:46; Thompson and Hager 1977:108; Wright and Laemmle 1968:986). But this healing process, as much as the infection itself, produces damage in the fallopian tubes (Westrom and Mardh 1978:20). So although therapy can shorten the period of infection and reduce the number of extent of sequelae, it cannot eliminate them altogether. Thus, rates of tubal occlusion, sterility, and other sequelae, though undoubtedly lower with effective chemotherapy, are still substantial.

The following sections report on the sequelae of PID as recorded by a number of studies. Because the importance of nongonococcal PID has only recently been appreciated—such infections probably constituted only a small fraction of PID cases in the past anyway—most studies, with the exception of Falk's (1965) study, do not differentiate between gonococcal and nongonococcal PID. More recent studies (e.g., Jacobson and Westrom 1969:1095; Westrom and Mardh 1977:89) have shown that nongonococcal PID has about a twofold greater negative impact on fertility (which may be the result of suboptimal treatment of nongonococcal PID, not greater virulence, because Westrom [1975:712] noted that before the use of penicillin fertility was reduced more by gonococcal than nongonococcal salpingitis); if these studies had reported the sequelae of gonococcal and nongonococcal infections separately, we would anticipate rates of negative sequelae following gonococcal PID to be lower than the cumulative average. But Falk's study, which did report separate figures for the two types of infection, noted no difference in subsequent pregnancy and tubal abnormality rates following gonococcal and nongonococcal cases of PID. This only further illustrates how very difficult it is to evaluate studies. In the following discussion the term *PID* will refer to all cases, gonococcal and nongonococcal, unless otherwise stated.

Coital Inability

Coital pain (dyspareunia) is experienced by some women following salpingitis because of chronic PID or pelvic adhesions (Crooks and Baur 1980:346; Masters and Johnson 1970:285). Extensive pelvic adhesions are undoubtedly more frequent in those cases where the infection has become chronic, either because it did not respond to normally effective treatment regimens or because it was improperly treated or left un-treated. In the developing world, where lack of treatment and improper treatment are more frequent, chronic PID and its sequelae such as dys-pareunia are more common.

Conceptive Failure

Although it is frequently stated that before the use of chemotherapy pregnancy was exceptional following bilateral gonococcal salpingitis (see Hedberg 1965:125; Kraus 1972:1119; Scragg 1957:90), Holtz (1930) re-ported that pregnancy occurred in 30% of such cases. And Westrom and Mardh (1975:162) stated that pregnancy occurred in at most 43% of women following untreated PID. Thompson and Hager (1977:108) took the position that although adverse reproductive sequelae were certainly frequent before the use of antibiotics, they were most pronounced in women with repeated infections, which has continued to be the case. These data suggest that sterility was not inevitable following untreated PID but occurred in about 60 to 70% of cases.

The fertility prognosis following PID has improved markedly since the introduction of antibiotics. The prognosis has also improved over time, probably as a result of better application of these drugs. Thus, whereas a 1958 study (Hedberg and Spetz, 1958) reported at 37% sterility rate, a 1965 study (Falk, 1965) reported sterility in only 15% of cases. Although Jacobson and Westrom's 1969 study (1969:1098) reported an 8% sterility rate following PID, they felt this was rather low and reflected a disproportionate number of cases with early diagnosis. Most of the more recent studies (e.g., Mardh *et al.* 1977:1379) report about a 20% sterility rate. And the American Social Health Association (undated) es-timated that an even greater proportion of PID cases—at least 25%—result in permanent sterility.

Sterility rates for any one series exceed tubal occlusion rates because some tubes, though patent, may be kinked or partially occluded, or may have suffered functional damage. The abnormality may not lie with the tube at all, but with the ovary; the ovarian capsule may have been thick-ened by the infection so that the egg cannot break free. Sweeney (1968:251–252) felt that this perioophoritis is generally overlooked as a cause of sterility, and indeed we encountered few references to ovarian failure as a cause of post-PID sterility. Decker and Loebl (1978:96) did mention this association and cited PID as a ''serious'' and ''frequent'' cause of ovarian failure. Another possibility is that even though the tubes and ovaries are normal, the pelvic structures have been so distorted by a peritonitis that sterility follows. Sweeney (1968:252) noted, for example, that adhesions may isolate the ovary and prevent normal tubal pickup of the ovum.

That sterility rates exceed bilateral tubal occlusion rates has been revealed by a number of studies. Hedberg and Spetz (1958) showed only a 20% bilateral occlusion rate by hysterosalpingography but a 37% sterility rate, and Falk (1965) showed that more women were sterile than had abnormal tubes. More recently, rates of tubal occlusion have been reported at 3% (Jacobson and Westrom 1969:1095), 5.5% (Belsey 1976:329), and 6.1% (Westrom and Mardh 1977:89) following gonococcal PID. (The rates following nongonococcal PID in these studies are 7%, 16.6%, and 17.3%, respectively).

Sterility rates following PID have thus shown a remarkable improvement since 1930, although contrasting the results of studies done at the beginning and the end of this period is risky because of differences in diagnostic techniques, patient selection, and so forth. Nevertheless, the trend is clear. Although the sterility rate was 60–70% before the use of antibiotics and 40% in the early days of penicillin, by the mid-1960s the rate was only 15–20%. Nevertheless, in the United States alone, according to the American Social Health Association (1981), 100,000 women become sterile *each year* due to gonococcal PID.

Fertility prognosis depends greatly on the severity of the infection at the time of diagnosis. Falk (1965) noted tubal abnormalities in only 3% of women without pelvic masses before treatment, but in 33% of women whose disease had progressed to that point. Similarly, Westrom and Mardh (1978:21) noted sterility in 4% of women who presented with a mild tubal infection, in 14% of those with a moderately severe infection, and in 33% of those with a severe infection. (Westrom [1975:707–708] defined an infection as being mild if the tubes are red and swollen and covered with a purulent material but are free to move despite adhesions and are open. In a moderately severe infection the changes in the tube are similar but more marked; the tube is not freely moveable and the patency of the tube is questionable. A severe infection is characterized by pelvic peritonitis and/or abscess formation with closure of the tubes at their fimbriated end.) Repeated espisodes of PID are the greatest threat to reproductive potential. Describing the sequelae of PID (gonococcal and nongonococcal), Westrom (1975:707) showed tubal occlusion rates increased from 12.8% after one episode to 35.5% after two episodes and to 75% after three or more episodes.

Pregnancy Loss

Ectopic Pregnancy   Ectopic pregnancy is another possible consequence of gonococcal salpingitis. In fact, many workers have regarded
previous gonococcal salpingitis as a major predisposing factor in tubal
pregnancies. Rendtorff (1975:236) made the conservative estimate that
50% of the ectopic pregnancies in his study group were the result of
previous gonococcal infection. Hager and Wiesner (1977:49) noted that
examination of the tubes following an ectopic pregnancy will reveal
pathologic changes consistent with prior salpingitis—cause unspecified—in 42 to 53% of cases. The cause of the salpingitis—gonococcal,
nongonococcal, tuberculous, or the result of a postpartum or postabortal
infection—is difficult to determine and often remains unknown. The
woman's medical history and/or the differential frequency of the various
causes in the study population may, however, strongly suggest one etiology over another.

A comparison of data from the pre- and postantibiotic eras does not
indicate that effective chemotherapy has had a beneficial effect on ectopic pregnancy rates. But data from the preantibiotic era are so sparse—
only one study, that of Holtz (1930, cited in Eschenbach and Holmes
1975:52), providing adequate data—that definitive conclusions cannot
be drawn. The Holtz study noted that about 1 in 50 pregnancies were
ectopic following salpingitis. Figures from the postantibiotic era actually
show a higher rate of 1 in 24 pregnancies (Westrom and Mardh 1978:21).
It is likely that in some cases antibiotics are able to stop the infection
before the tubes become occluded, but not before there is functional or
structural damage that favors an ectopic implantation. Hence, use of
antibiotics has resulted in a tremendous improvement in tubal occlusion
and sterility rates, but a negligible improvement, if any, in ectopic pregnancy rates. Improper use of antibiotics exacerbates the problem. Thus,
in developing countries where antibiotics are often improperly used ectopic pregnancy is a major problem. In some tropical countries a ruptured tubal pregnancy is the most common surgical emergency among
women (Stewart 1967b:371).

Ectopic pregnancy is not only a cause of pregnancy loss, but may
also contribute to future conceptive failure because the tube is often so
badly damaged by an ectopic pregnancy that it must be removed. If the
tube is not visibly damaged, it may be left in place and allowed to heal.
Hysterosalpingography is then done to determine if there are any abnormalities that would predispose to a second ectopic implantation and
therefore necessitate removal. Such conservative treatment, though

common in the developed world, is impractical for the developing world, so removal of an ectopic pregnancy there also means removal of the tube in most cases. Also, in the developing world, because of delays in seeking and/or receiving medical care, ruptured tubal pregnancy is much more common, and in this instance the tube cannot be saved.

Septic Abortion   Despite its association with infertility, gonorrhea is not uncommon in pregnant women. The incidence among pregnant women in the developed world is reported at anywhere from 0.4 to 7.3% (cf. Charles *et al.* 1970:595–596; Handsfield *et al.* 1973:701; Nickerson 1973:816; Sarrel and Pruett 1968:672; Spence 1973:225), differences in reported incidence rates reflecting for the most part differences among studies in the women's socioeconomic status (Spence 1973:225). Reports from the developing world also show vastly different rates. Weissenberger *et al.* (1977, cited in Muir and Belsey 1980:919) isolated *N. gonorrhoeae* from 2% of pregnant women in Zimbawbe and Osoba *et al.* (1973, cited in Muir and Belsey 1980:919) from 3.4% of asymptomatic pregnant women in Nigeria, but Nasah and Eyang (in press, cited in Muir and Belsey 1980:919) found gonorrhea in 13.6% of asymptomatic pregnant women and 15.2% of symptomatic pregnant women in Cameroon. In a number of African studies gonorrhea rates have been even higher in pregnant than nonpregnant women. Arya *et al.* (1973:591) found gonorrhea to be twice as common in pregnant as nonpregnant Teso (Uganda) women (40.0% vs. 19.8%). And Nasah and Eyang's study in Cameroon found asymptomatic gonorrhea in seven times as many pregnant as nonpregnant women (13.6% vs. 1.9%)—a difference that did not hold, however, in the case of symptomatic gonorrhea, where rates for both pregnant and nonpregnant women were approximately equal (15.2% vs. 21.0%).

Gonorrhea in a pregnant woman is a hazard not only to the woman herself, but also to her child. Pregnancy increases the risk of disseminated infections such as gonococcal septicemia and arthritis (Handsfield *et al.* 1973:697; Nicol 1971b:383). And a newborn child that has just passed through an infected birth canal is at risk of developing a severe conjunctivitis with the potential to cause blindness. Legislative measures requiring the use of prophylactic drugs in the eyes of newborns has virtually eliminated gonococcal ophthalmia neonatorum in most parts of the world. In the United States the percentage of students in a school for the blind whose condition was caused by a neonatal infection (usually gonococcal) dropped from 28.2% in 1907 to 0.1% in 1955 (Brown *et al.* 1970:130). It would seem that because gonorrhea is a major source of congenital blindness in untreated populations with a high prevalence of gonorrhea, such populations should show significant rates of congenital blindness. It would be interesting to examine rates, if available, for black Americans in the early part of this century to see if they generally support or refute the ''VD hypothesis.''

Gonorrhea may also cause salpingitis in a pregnant woman, although such infections are generally believed to be uncommon and confined to the first trimester of pregnancy because of the protective effect later in pregnancy of the cervical mucus plug and intact membranes (Acosta *et al.* 1971:284; Monif 1974:106; Nickerson 1973:816; Thompson and Hager 1977:108). But cases of gonococcal PID have been recorded after the first trimester and are probably the result of vascular or lymphatic spread from the endocervix or a flare-up of pre-existing pelvic disease (Nickerson 1973:816; Thompson and Hager 1977:108). Acosta *et al.* (1971:284) believed that gonococcal PID during pregnancy may be more common than generally believed due to the problems associated with culturing *N. gonorrhoeae* and establishing a differential diagnosis; thus some cases of infected abortion may actually be the result of gonococcal PID. In their study of 35 pregnant women with gonorrhea, Sarrel and Pruett (1968:670) noted 2 cases of first trimester salpingitis and 13 septic abortions. However, other studies of pregnant women with gonorrhea (e.g., Charles *et al.* 1970:598; Handsfield *et al.* 1973:697), though recording elevated rates of maternal and fetal morbidity, did not reveal findings of the gravity or magnitude of the Sarrel and Pruett study.

In sum, there does exist the possibility of an ascending gonococcal infection during pregnancy, resulting in salpingitis and pregnancy loss. However, this risk has not been quantitated. In the United States and other developed countries where most women receive good antenatal care, gonorrhea is detected early and treated. But in the developing world where antenatal care is virtually nonexistent the possibility of an ascending infection during pregnancy is much greater. Indeed, the much-greater frequency of infected spontaneous abortions in the developing world (*Population Reports* 1980a:121; Rendle-Short and Stewart 1967:401) may as much reflect more cases of infection (probably gonorrhea) *causing* spontaneous abortion as it does more cases of infection *following* spontaneous abortion.

There are also indications that gonorrhea in pregnant women may be associated with prematurity and premature rupture of the membranes (Handsfield *et al.* 1973:697; Sarrel and Pruett 1968:670).

Diagnosis

One of the more difficult problems encountered in the practice of gynecology is determining whether or not a patient has PID. Reliance on the usual clinical criteria—pain, fever, irregular bleeding, tenderness at examination—will frequently lead to an incorrect diagnosis. Although Wright and Laemmle (1968:980) felt that an elevated ($\geq$ 99.8° F; 37.7° C) oral temperature is a necessary concomitant of PID, Eschenbach and Holmes (1975:42) reported an elevated temperature in only 33% of salpingitis cases confirmed by laparoscopy. Similarly, abnormal bleeding occurs in only 35 to 40% of women with acute salpingitis (Eschenbach and Holmes 1975:42) and is found with equal frequency in women with and without pelvic infection (Eschenbach 1980:148S). Lab tests such as an ESR (erythrocyte sedimentation rate) or WBC (white blood cell count) are usually not helpful in establishing a diagnosis (Westrom and Mardh 1978:17). Lower abdominal pain is the most reliable of all the associated symptoms, being found in more than 90% of patients (Eschenbach 1980:148S), although its exact character—unilateral or bilateral, intermittent or constant, mild or severe—is quite variable (Thompson and Hager 1977:109). It has been observed (Curran 1979:174; Jacobson and Westrom 1969:1092; Westrom and Mardh 1978:1) that a diagnosis based on clinical criteria is more likely to be correct if the salpingitis is the result of *N. gonorrhoeae* because gonococcal salpingitis is more often associated with an elevated temperature and is more multisymptomatic than nongonococcal salpingitis.

Because diagnoses based on clinical criteria alone are often incorrect, some gynecologists will perform a laparoscopy, which allows direct visualization of the pelvic organs. Jacobson and Westrom's classic study in 1969 showed that of 814 cases where the clinical diagnosis was PID, this diagnosis could be confirmed by laparoscopy in only 65% of cases; in 23% of cases the pelvis was visually normal and in 12% of cases another disorder was observed. Eschenbach (1980:148S) compiled data from three studies of laparoscopic examination of patients with a clinical diagnosis of PID. The diagnosis was confirmed on average in only 62% of cases; 22% were normal, and ovarian cysts accounted for 5%, ectopic pregnancies for 4%, appendicitis for 3%, endometriosis for 1%, and other causes for 3%. (The ''normal'' cases may, suggested some researchers [e.g., Jacobson and Westrom 1969:1096; Westrom and Mardh 1978:16], represent infections of the lower genital tract or of the endometrium, which mimic PID.)

Laparoscopy has been criticized, however, in that it could miss some early cases of PID where the infection is still confined to the endosalpinx, classifying these as visually normal. However, of the 184 patients in Jacobson and Westrom's 1969 study who were normal at first laparoscopy, only 1 later developed acute salpingitis (Westrom and Mardh 1975:162).

Clinical diagnosis of PID is associated not only with a high false-positive rate (~35%), as noted earlier, but with a high false-negative rate as well (Eschenbach 1980:147S). According to Jacobson and Westrom (1969:1097), "fully developed inflammatory reaction of the tubes may be consistent with scarcity of symptoms." Indeed, in their study these authors noted that 91 women with other preoperative diagnoses were found upon laparoscopy to have PID. Cases that are mild or asymptomatic are a particular threat to future fertility because of delays in diagnosis and treatment (Rees and Annels 1969:207).

When a diagnosis of PID is made, an attempt is made to identify the causative organisms. Material from the cervix, and perhaps from the cul-de-sac and tubes as well, is cultured on Thayer–Martin medium, which is specific for *N. gonorrhoeae*. Special McCoy's cells are used to isolate *C. trachomatis*, and various other culture media and techniques may be employed to identify the genital mycoplasmas and other aerobic and anaerobic organisms that may cause PID (see the following section on nongonococcal PID). Determining the organisms involved is very important because drug sensitivity varies greatly and optimal treatment is impossible without a firm diagnosis.

Treatment

Treatment of choice in PID has not been established because it is often impossible to establish the exact etiologic agent (*N. gonorrhoeae*, *C. trachomatis*, *Mycoplasma hominis*, etc.). A combination of intravenous doxycycline and cefoxitin over 4 days provides optimal coverage for *N. gonorrhoreae* and *C. trachomatis*, although perhaps not for certain anaerobes or in the case of a pelvic mass or IUD-associated PID. In such instances other antibiotics such as clindamycin or gentamicin may need to be employed (Centers for Disease Control 1982:9–11). And not infrequently there is a pelvic abscess that antibiotics cannot reach and surgical drainage is required.

The effective management of PID when no gonococci can be isolated is more difficult. Nongonococcal infections respond more slowly and are more likely to require pelvic surgery regardless of which antibiotic regimens are used (Curran 1979:177). Tetracycline has been extensively used with nongonococcal infections in the United Kingdom and a cure rate of 65 to 75% has been observed. But experience has shown that the longer and more careful the follow-up the higher the relapse rate (Catterall 1975:12). Secondary invaders are a particular problem with nongonococcal salpingitis, being more common than after gonococcal salpingitis (Eschenbach 1980:143S). Fortunately, even without treatment the overwhelming majority of PID cases resolve spontaneously (Eschenbach and Holmes 1975:46), though taking a greater toll on health and fecundity than if the course of the infection had been arrested by proper treatment. If the tubes have been badly scarred surgical reconstruction may be attempted, but this is successful in only about one-third of cases (Witters and Jones-Witters 1980:331).

Complications of Nongonococcal Infections in the Female: Nongonococcal Pelvic Inflammatory Disease

Introduction

Most cases of spontaneously occurring PID in developed countries are the consequence of sexually transmitted pathogens. *N. gonorrhoeae* was the preeminent cause for many years, but its position as number one eroded considerably during the 1970s. In the mid-1970s Swedish physicians noted that although the number of cases of PID had increased during the 1960s and 1970s, the proportion of cases from which gonococci could be isolated had decreased (Mardh *et al.* 1977:1378; Westrom and Mardh 1975:159). Similar decreases were noted elsewhere, though usually not of the magnitude of the Swedish experience. In general, Sweden had the lowest gonococcal PID rate (less than 10% of cases) in the late 1970s, whereas the United States had the highest rate and Europe held an intermediate position (Mardh *et al.* 1981:127).

The increase in the number of PID cases from which gonococci could not be isolated, so-called nongonococcal PID, was an ominous development because tubal occlusion and sterility rates were double those of gonococcal PID. Perhaps the etiological agents were not sensitive to penicillin, which was routinely used to treat PID. Or perhaps the organisms responsible were simply more virulent. In either case, it seemed imperative to identify the organisms involved, examine the pathophysiology of tubal infections with these organisms and their effect on fertility, determine drug sensitivities, and institute public health measures to control spread.

Identification of Organisms

Traditionally the causative agent of PID was sought in the endocervix. If *N. gonorrhoeae* were isolated the PID was attributed to this known pathogen. Of course, this did not really prove that the gonococcus was the pathogen for that particular infection. Therefore, more recent studies have cultured material aspirated from the cul-de-sac (also called the pouch of Douglas, this is the portion of the pelvic cavity posterior to the vagina and anterior to the rectum), anticipating that organisms involved in a tubal infection will often spill out of the fimbriated end of the tube into the pouch of Douglas. During laparoscopy samples have been isolated from the tube itself.

These studies have shown the presence of a wide variety of organisms: sexually transmitted organisms such as *N. gonorrhoeae, C. trachomatis* and the genital mycoplasmas, as well as aerobic and anaerobic enteric bacteria which, though found in the lower genital tract of about 50% of healthy women, are potential pathogens (Akerlund *et al.* 1975:172). Correlation of recovery from the cervix with recovery from the tubes and cul-de-sac varies widely among studies. Curran (1979:175) reported that when the cervix yields gonococci, *N. gonorrhoeae* can be found in the tubes or peritoneal cavity in anywhere from 8 to 70% of cases.[3] Mardh *et al.* (1977:1379) reported only a 10% correlation rate for *N. gonorrhoeae* but an 85% rate for *C. trachomatis.* Again, finding a particular organism even in the tubes or peritoneal cavity is not proof that the organism caused the infection. Perhaps the organism is just an opportunistic pathogen, moving into the tube only after damage has already occurred.

The pathogenic potential of *N. gonorrhoeae* is known to be considerable; thus many workers (e.g., Curran 1979:175; Danielsson *et al.* 1975:155) have believed that if the gonococcus is found in the cervix of a woman with PID it can be said to be the primary cause of the inflam-

---

[3]The likelihood of finding *N. gonorrhoeae* in the tubes or peritoneal cavity decreases with time. Monif (1980:156S) believed that superinfection with anaerobic bacteria frequently follows gonococcal infection and that these anaerobes create an environment unfavorable to the gonococcus, ultimately leading to its elimination from the tubes and cul-de-sac; thus microbial studies instituted after the earliest stages of the infection will be negative for *N. gonorrhoeae.*

matory reaction. (We say "primary" cause because it is known that an infection with anaerobic bacteria may be superimposed on a gonococcal salpingitis, intensifying the inflammation.) Two other sexually transmitted organisms, *C. trachomatis* and *M. hominis,* have been isolated from cervical, tubal, and peritoneal material. These organisms have pathogenic potential and are believed to cause the majority of cases of nongonococcal PID. (These two organisms have also been implicated in other types of human reproductive dysfunction, and more detailed discussion of both appears in Chapters 13 and 14.) In some cases of PID no sexually transmitted organism can be isolated and the infection is believed to be caused by endogenous vaginal organisms.

Chlamydia

Chlamydia trachomatis was an unmeasured factor in human genital infections until relatively recently because of difficulties in clinical and laboratory diagnosis. Distinctive clinical signs and symptoms of genital chlamydia infection (cervicitis and salpingitis in women, urethritis and epididymitis in men) may be absent (Paavonen *et al.* 1979:301) or may mimic those of gonorrhea (Bowie 1980:18). Although similar to a bacterium in most respects and classified as such, this organism, like a virus, requires living cells for its growth and reproduction (Felman and Nikitas 1981:381–382). Hence, routine culture methods for bacterial organisms are inadequate for the isolation of *C. trachomatis,* irradiated or cyclohexamide- treated McCoy cells being the growth medium of choice. As of 1980, techniques for culturing chlamydia were not widely available (Bowie 1980:27). Reports (Mardh *et al.* 1981:128) have noted that sampling time is another critical detail because high antibody titers may result in a negative culture. But when good diagnostic facilities are available they show that *C. trachomatis* is a frequent genitourinary pathogen. It is estimated that in the developed world the frequency of *C. trachomatis* in men and women equals and probably exceeds that of *N. gonorrhoeae* (Berger *et al.* 1978:304; Bowie 1980:24; Holmes and Puziss 1980:640; Mardh *et al.* 1977:1377).

There is a considerable body of evidence supporting a role for *C. trachomatis* in PID. First, rates of isolation of chlamydia are higher in PID cases (20–36%) than in control populations (3–13%) (Eschenbach 1980:143S). Mardh *et al.* (1977:1377) reported that although *C. trachomatis* was not found in women who had no genital tract infection, it could be isolated from the cervix of 36% of women with acute salpingitis and 6% of women with a lower genital tract infection. And in PID cases where the cervix is chlamydia-positive there is an excellent chance of finding chlamydia in tubal cultures. Mardh *et al.* (1977:1379) reported that tubal material contained *C. trachomatis* in 6 of 7 PID cases where the cervix was positive.

Second, results from serologic investigations support a role for *C. trachomatis* in pelvic infections because PID is frequently accompanied by a significant rise in antichlamydial antibodies (Eschenbach 1980: 143S). Using serologic and clinical criteria, Treharne and associates (1979:26) determined that two-thirds of their PID cases were the result of *C. trachomatis.* And some cases of chlamydial PID may be missed altogether because it has been observed (Henry-Suchet and Loffredo 1980:539) that this organism can silently ascend to the upper genital tract and cause an asymptomatic chronic inflammation with adhesions and progressive obliteration of the tubal lumen.

The third piece of evidence supporting a role for chlamydia in PID is the work of Moller and Mardh (1980:107ff) showing that grivet monkeys develop salpingitis following inoculation of organisms onto the cervix or into the uterus. The salpingitis was confirmed by gross pathology (the tubes were red and swollen and covered with exudate) and by histopathology (there were inflammatory infiltrates in the tubal epithelium and subepithelial tissues, thickening of the tubal mucosa, and adhesions between mucosal folds). In two of the four monkeys with salpingitis partial tubal occlusion persisted 2 months postinfection. Although in one additional case there was a lesion in the uterine endometrium and the infection spread via the lymphatics and blood vessels to produce a peritonitis, the four cases of salpingitis involved contiguous surface spread from the cervix to the endosalpinx in the same manner as an ascending gonorrhea infection.

Bowie (1980:21) estimated that chlamydial cervicitis progresses to PID as frequently as does gonococcal cervicitis. Occlusion rates for nongonococcal PID, much of which is probably chlamydial, are placed at 7 to 17.3% (Belsey 1976:329; Jacobson and Westrom 1969:1095; Westrom and Mardh 1977:89). And Falk (1965) reported a 21% sterility rate following nongonococcal PID. These studies were conducted before the importance of *C. trachomatis* in PID was widely appreciated and treatment with antichlamydial drugs such as tetracycline and erythromycin routinely employed; thus, reported rates of occlusion and sterility are probably higher than those that will follow optimally treated infections. But an 8–10 year period of observing pregnancy rates following properly treated chlamydial PID is necessary to determine how many of these women have maintained adequate tubal function.

Genital Mycoplasmas

Within the Mycoplasmataceae are two bacteria commonly isolated from the genital mucosa of sexually active adults—*Ureaplasma urealyticum* and *Mycoplasma hominis*. Both organisms have been studied for their effects on various aspects of reproduction and the results of these studies are discussed in Chapter 13. Whether or not the genital mycoplasmas can cause PID is not firmly established, although a role for *M. hominis* appears more likely than one for *U. urealyticum*.

Ureaplasma urealyticum Colonization of the cervix with ureaplasmas is common, being seen in 49–83% of women studied (Desai *et al.* 1980:470); because there is usually no correlation with disease, most workers (e.g., Shepard 1970:1338) have concluded that women are primarily asymptomatic carriers of *U. urealyticum*. There is some evidence that the ureaplasmas can cause an endometritis, however, and these organisms are isolated significantly more frequently from the endometria of infertile patients (50%) than controls (7%) (Desai *et al.* 1980:470).

Although an antibody response to *U. urealyticum* has been noted in patients with PID and the organism has been isolated from the tubes and from pelvic abscesses in PID patients, there is no evidence that ureaplasmas are capable of causing the pathological changes recognized as PID (Monif 1974:157–158; Taylor-Robinson and McCormack 1980a:1008). Infection of organ cultures of fallopian tubes with *U. urealyticum*, for example, produces no obvious damage. However, because organ cultures are not affected by the immunological response of the host, which plays a role in inflammatory reactions, these experiments cannot be considered conclusive (Taylor-Robinson and McCormack 1980a:1008).

In sum, because of the frequency with which ureaplasmas are isolated from the cervices of healthy women, most workers believe that their recovery from the lower genital tract of women with pelvic infection is of no particular diagnostic significance. Recovery from the endometrium or tubes may be more meaningful, although more study is necessary before conclusions can be drawn.

Mycoplasma hominis Epidemiological evidence suggests that *M. hominis* plays a role in lower genital tract infections because the organism can be isolated significantly more frequently from women with signs of inflammation (50%) than from controls (5%) (Mardh *et al.* 1975:56). However, *M. hominis* is often isolated in association with other pathogens such as *Haemophilus vaginalis*, making it difficult to determine which organism caused the infection and which is there simply because the infection produced environmental changes advantageous to its growth (Taylor-Robinson and McCormack 1980a:1007). Reports on whether eradication of *M. hominis* results in cure are mixed (cf. Mardh *et al.* 1975:56; Taylor-Robinson and McCormack 1980a:1007), so although a role in lower genital tract infections is likely it is unproved.

Evidence for a role in PID is quite strong and some workers (e.g., Urquhart 1979:467; Westrom and Mardh 1975:161) believe it is the etiological agent in a not-negligible proportion of salpingitis cases. In one study (Westrom and Mardh 1975:161), *M. hominis* was not isolable from the tubes of healthy women but was isolated in 4 of 50 women with salpingitis, and concomitant with its presence in the infected tube there was a significant rise in antibody titers to the organism, indicating an active role in the infection. Organ cultures of fallopian tubes infected with *M. hominis* support growth of the organism and produce swelling of the cilia observable under the electron microscope (Westrom and Mardh 1975:161; Taylor-Robinson and McCormack 1980a:1008). And Moller *et al.* (1978:248ff) produced a self-limiting salpingitis and parametritis—structures were normal 4–5 weeks postinfection—by introducing *M. hominis* into the tubes of grivet monkeys.

From these experiments it appears that *M. hominis* can produce a salpingitis. However, the effect on reproductive potential is probably not as great as for *C. trachomatis* or *N. gonorrhoeae* because only the muscularis and serosa are involved, the mucosa remaining intact. However, the involvement of the muscle layer could, if severe, compromise fecundity. As yet there are no studies of tubal occlusion, sterility, and ectopic pregnancy rates in women following salpingitis in which *M. hominis* was the isolate.

Endogenous Nonvenereal Pelvic Inflammatory Disease

In a certain proportion of women with PID there is no recent history of childbirth, abortion, or of any diagnostic or surgical procedure involving the genital tract, nor can any sexually transmitted pathogen such as *N. gonorrhoeae*, *C. trachomatis*, or *M. hominis* be isolated. But in a large proportion of these cases culdocentesis or laparoscopy will yield aerobic and anaerobic bacteria, particularly the *Bacteroides* species, peptococci, peptostreptococci, and gram-negative bacilli, which are endogenous to the bowel but are frequently found in the vagina (Eschenbach *et al.* 1975:168; Gall *et al.* 1981:51). In these cases of what Westrom and Mardh (1978:13) called endogenous nonvenereal PID, the current infection is believed to be initiated by these endogenous organisms. This is not to be confused with the role of these same organisms as secondary invaders following close on the heels of an initial gonococcal or chlamydial salpingitis. (Research shows that secondary invaders are more likely to follow a nongonococcal salpingitis—Eschenbach [1980:143S] stated that in the United States they are found in only 14 to 31% of cases of gonococcal PID but in 46 to 90% of cases of nongonococcal PID—and appear to be more often associated with severe cases [Westrom and Mardh 1975:161]. Curran [1979:177] noted, for example, that pelvic abscesses, from which anaerobes are frequently isolated, are found in less than 1% of cases of gonococcal PID but in 12% of cases of nongonococcal PID.)

Because about 50% of healthy women harbor these potential pathogens in the vagina (Akerlund *et al.* 1975:172), what are the factors favoring their occasional spread to the upper genital tract? Eschenbach (1980:143S) has proposed that sexual activity could cause a nonspecific anaerobic vaginitis and that the resulting proliferation of bowel organisms in the vagina would predispose to PID. Akerlund *et al.* (1975:170) have also suggested that coitus might mean trauma to the vulva, urethra, and vagina, thereby increasing the risk of infection. (Some type of mechanism associated with sexual activity is always sought in PID cases because pelvic infections are rarely seen in premenstrual and postmenopausal women and women who are not sexually active, such as nuns [Eschenbach and Holmes 1975:39; Wright and Laemmle 1968:980].) Westrom and Mardh (1978:13) have noted that these cases of endogenous nonvenereal PID occur more frequently in older women and they suggest that these women may have anatomic changes induced by pregnancy and delivery that allow the bowel flora to reach the vagina more easily. They also noted that pelvic infections with these endogenous aerobic and anaerobic organisms are more frequent in women who have had a prior episode of PID and suggested that resulting tubal damage renders the genital tract more vulnerable to infection with the endogenous flora.

This last hypothesis is the most attractive. Thus Ronda *et al.* (1980:256) suggested that initial episodes of PID are related to infection with gonorrhea and that this predisposes to future invasion of the endosalpinx with endogenous aerobes and anaerobes. Curran (1980:848) took this a step further, stating that initial episodes of PID are associated with gonorrhea and other sexually transmitted organisms and subsequent episodes are less frequently associated with these organisms; rather, by implication, they are associated with endogenous organisms. Thus, we believe that the sexually transmitted organisms, particularly *N. gonorrhoeae* and *C. trachomatis*, are important primary pathogens of high virulence capable of initiating an infection on healthy pelvic structures, whereas the nonsexually transmitted organisms (i.e., the endogenous aerobic and anaerobic bacteria) are less virulent and are able to initiate an infection only if there is a functional or structural abnormality of the pelvic organs such as those resulting from a prior tubal infection.

It is important to note that the initial episode of PID may go undetected, and thus a first recorded episode may not be associated with a sexually transmitted organism. Eschenbach (1980:144S) noted that women with PID were more likely to have had a prior uncomplicated gonorrhea infection, which he suspected may have actually been a subclinical tubal infection. Similarly, Wiesner and Holmes (1975:24) asked women with nongonococcal PID (undoubtedly some of this was chlamydial) if they had experienced pain during a first or previous episode of gonorrhea. Many said yes, indicating they had an undetected, untreated, and unrecorded episode of gonococcal salpingitis. We do not mean to say that all pelvic infections with endogenous aerobic and anaerobic organisms must follow a prior infection with a sexually transmitted organism, just that most do. And it may be that the higher sterility rate following nongonococcal PID reflects the fact that a subset of nongonococcal PID (i.e., endogenous nonvenereal PID) usually represents second- or higher-order infections, which carry a much more gloomy fertility prognosis.

The gonococcal PID–nongonococcal PID dichotomy in the literature is thus confusing when one is trying to understand the etiology of PID because within the nongonococcal group are both sexually transmitted organisms and endogenous organisms, which behave very differently from each other. Some workers have already replaced the term *nongonococcal PID* with *nongonococcal, nonchlamydial PID*, thereby elevating chlamydial PID to its rightful position as a separate category. As research continues and more of the organisms causing PID are identified it will become less necessary to describe an infection by what it is not, rather than by what it is.

The Pelvic Inflammatory
Disease Problem

Introduction

Muir and Belsey (1980) have presented two models (reproduced here as Figures 10.1 and 10.2) of PID and its consequences as experienced in the developed and the developing worlds. The models show that gonococcal and nongonococcal infections of the lower genital tract

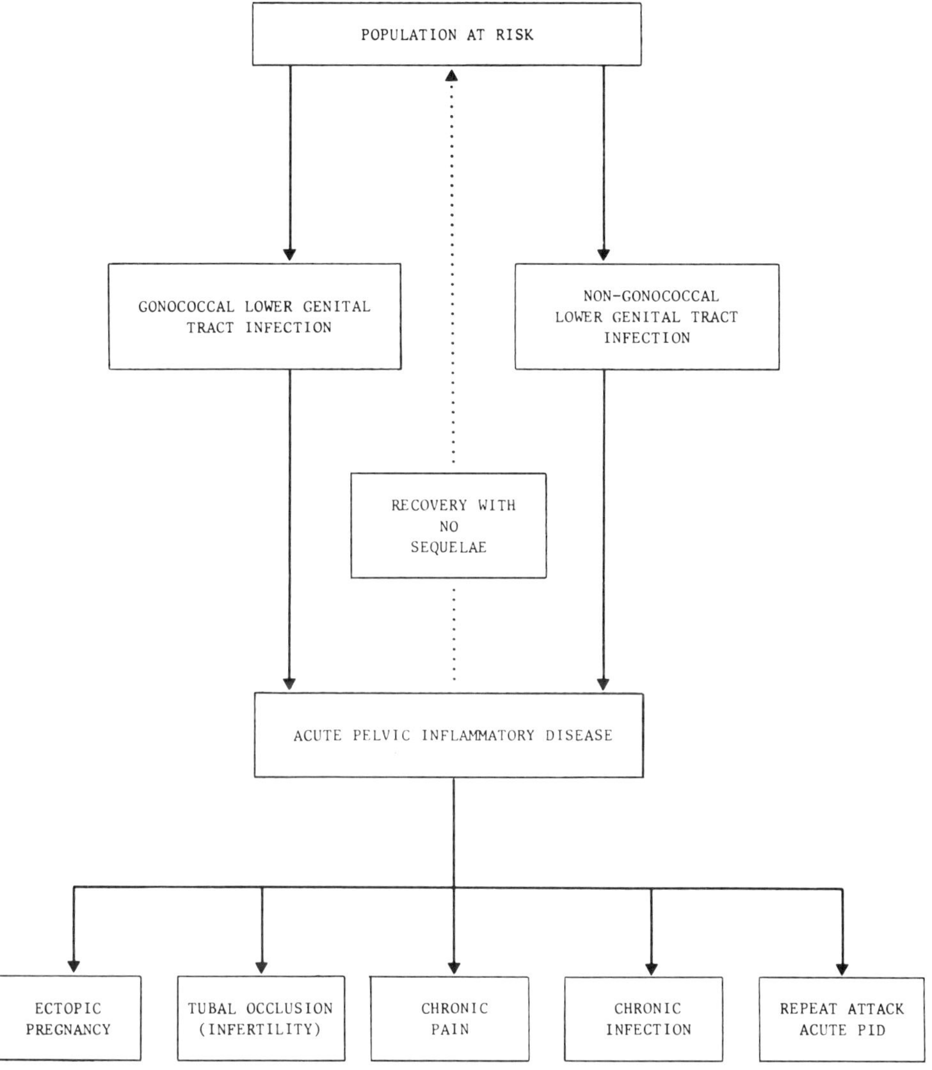

Figure 10.1 A simplified model of pelvic inflammatory disease (PID) in developed countries. Source: D. Muir and M. Belsey, 1980. Pelvic inflammatory disease and its consequences in the developing world. *American Journal of Obstetrics and Gynecology,* **138,** 914.

are important contributory factors to PID in both developed and developing countries. The most important difference between the two models is the additional contribution to PID in the developing world of postpartum and postabortal infections, genital tuberculosis, and, possibly,

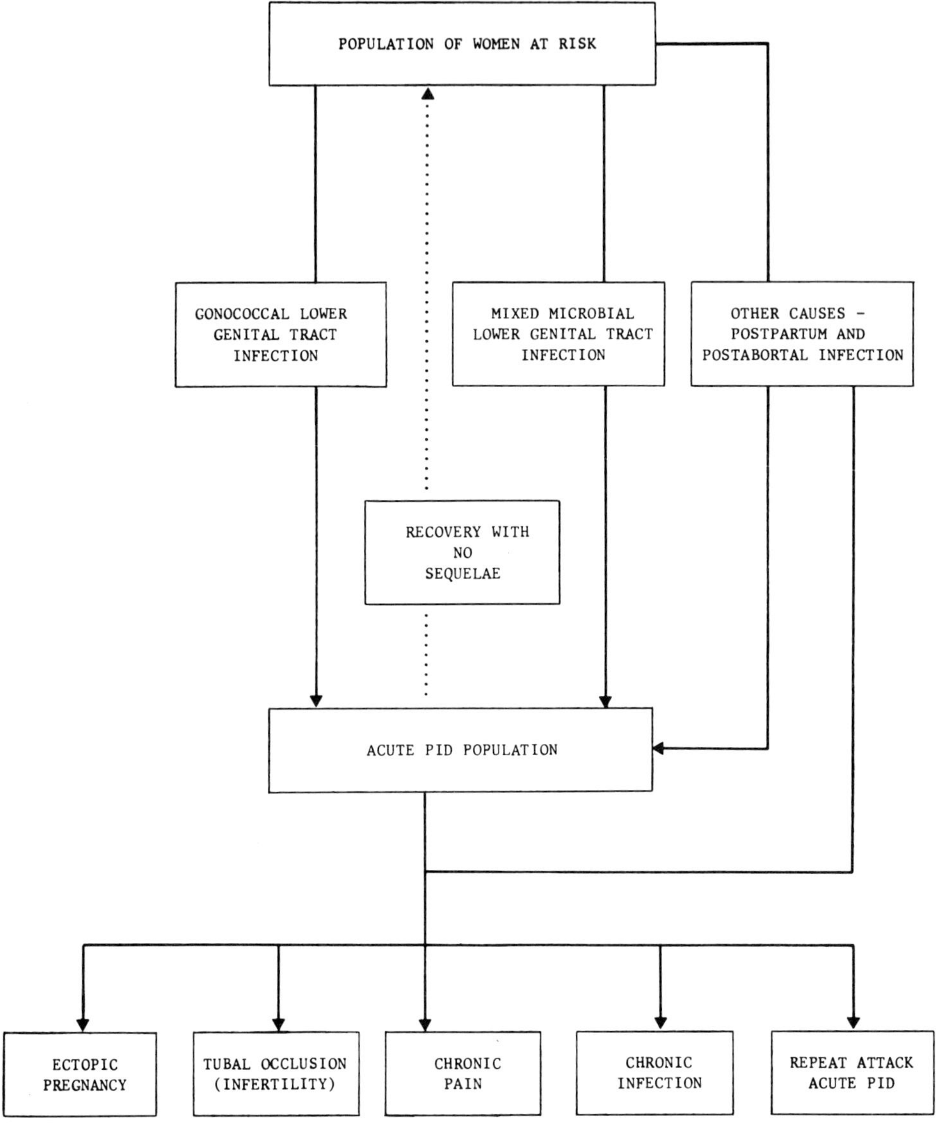

Figure 10.2 An etiologic model of acute pelvic inflammatory disease (PID) and its sequelae in developing countries. Source: D. Muir and M. Belsey, 1980. Pelvic inflammatory disease and its consequences in the developing world. *American Journal of Obstetrics and Gynecology,* **138,** 915.

schistosomiasis and filariasis. Because reproductive outlook varies according to the etiology of the PID (e.g., postabortal infections are a greater threat to fecundity than gonococcal PID, as noted in the following section on PID in the developed world) and is influenced by the availability and use of good health facilities, PID in the developed world and PID in the developing world are discussed separately.

Pelvic Inflammatory Disease in the Developed World

Jacobson and Westrom (1969:1094) reported that in Sweden in the 1960s 14% of PID cases were preceded by events such as childbirth, abortion, curettage, IUD insertion, or hysterosalpingography, which can cause or spread an infection by opening the cervical canal or introducing foreign material into the uterine cavity. But PID following such events, except IUD insertion, has become increasingly less common. However, when PID does follow childbirth, abortion, or diagnostic or surgical intervention in the upper genital tract, the infection takes a more serious course and sterility rates are much higher than following most other pelvic infections. Westrom (1975:711) noted that tubal occlusion rates following such events were 27% versus 6–17% for other types of PID.

In the developed world today PID is usually the result of sexually transmitted pathogens; gonorrhea and chlamydia account for most of the infections, although their relative contribution is extremely variable depending on geographic and socioeconomic factors. But in a substantial number of women no sexually transmitted organism can be isolated nor has there been a recent predisposing event such as abortion or curettage. These cases of PID are initiated by aerobic and anaerobic bowel organisms, which are frequent inhabitants of the vagina. Such endogenous nonvenereal infections are more frequently seen in older women, in women with prior uncomplicated gonorrhea, and in women with a history of PID.

The relative contribution of these causes of PID to the total PID rate has been estimated for the U.S. (*Family Planning Perspectives* 1980b:206–207). According to this estimate, each year 500,000 U.S. women of childbearing age experience their first episode of PID. Of these, 5,000 are postabortal infections and 100,000 are IUD-related. The remaining 395,000 are spontaneously occurring cases of gonococcal and nongonococcal salpingitis in about equal numbers. The number of U.S. women who become sterile each year can be calculated by multiplying these incidence figures by the estimated sterility rates for various types of PID. Westrom and Mardh (1975:163) estimated that about 13% of women become sterile after their first episode of PID (gonococcal or nongonococcal), whereas Westrom (1975:711) noted that at least 27% of women were sterile following first episodes of PID if these episodes were preceded by a predisposing event such as childbirth, abortion, or dilatation and curettage. And Dreifus (1980:8) suggested that sterility occurs in 20% of cases of pelvic infection that follow IUD insertion. Using these figures it can be calculated that 51,350 (395,000 × .13) women become sterile because of gonococcal and nongonococcal PID, 20,000 (100,000 × .20) become sterile because of IUD-associated PID, and 1,350 (5,000 × .27) become sterile following an abortion, for a total of 72,700 women per year. This must be considered a minimum estimate because it covers only women with their first episode of PID. Yet women with repeat infections represent about 20% of all PID cases (Westrom and Mardh 1978:8) and sterility rates are considerably higher after a second- or third- or higher-order infection (Westrom and Mardh 1975:163).

Pelvic Inflammatory Disease
in the Developing World

As serious as the PID problem is in the developed world, it is a far greater problem in the developing world. Not only are all the causes of PID found in the developed world more prevalent, but there is the added problem of genital tuberculosis and, according to some workers, PID precipitated by genital schistosomiasis and filariasis. In addition, availability and use of health services is limited in most developing areas so fewer persons are treated promptly and adequately, resulting in more complications and more chronic infections.

In many areas gonorrhea is a serious problem and is believed to be a cause of high rates of sterility and ectopic pregnancy. Scragg's 1957 study of the causes of depopulation in New Ireland was one of the earliest to attribute high rates of sterility to widespread PID caused by gonorrhea. Many studies followed—Chatfield *et al.* (1970) in Kenya, Carty *et al.* (1972) in Kenya, Arya *et al.* (1973) in Uganda, Grech *et al.* (1973) in Uganda, to name just a few—and they have also concluded that gonorrhea is a major cause of tubal occlusion and sterility. Indeed, the International Planned Parenthood Federation felt that gonorrhea was the primary cause of infertility in Central Africa where birth rates are low (*New York Times* 1978:8). Many researchers feel that gonococcal salpingitis is the most important factor predisposing to ectopic pregnancy. Carty *et al.* (1972:378) found ectopic pregnancy to be the commonest surgical emergency for women in Kenyatta National Hospital and believed this was the result of widespread gonococcal salpingitis. The higher ectopic pregnancy rates in developing countries reflect the greater PID problem: whereas the ratio of ectopic pregnancies to intrauterine pregnancies was 1:133 for Sweden, this figure for Kampala, Uganda, was 1:91 and for Benin, Nigeria, 1:88 (Muir and Belsey 1980:923).

The importance of nongonococcal PID in developing countries is unmeasured. However, nongonococcal urethritis (NGU) has begun to attract attention, and where NGU is important, nongonococcal PID is probably also important.

Postabortal and postpartum infections are important causes of PID in the developing world. Grech and associates (1973:126) noted that in some areas septic abortion is a more important cause of PID than gonorrhea. A study by Smith *et al.* (1976:640, 642) indicated that Kinshasa, Zaire, may be one such area. Their autopsy data revealed that 95% of all obstetric deaths in Kinshasa were due to hemorrhagic or septic complications of induced abortion. In addition, PID appeared to be very common in this study population, being found in 20% of all women over age 10. The importance of postpartum and postabortal infections is so great that we have devoted individual chapters (Chapters 15 and 16) to their discussion.

Muir and Belsey (1980:918) and others (e.g., Nasah *et al.* 1974:75) have pointed to the importance of genital tuberculosis (TB) in the developing world. A cause of sterility, particularly primary sterility, genital TB is often overlooked because it is a silent disease and even if suspected is difficult to diagnose, especially when the endometrium is not involved. We believe that genital TB is an important cause of sterility in highly tuberculous populations and have devoted a chapter (Chapter 3) to its consideration.

Muir and Belsey (1980:920) have also suggested that genital schistosomiasis and genital filariasis may contribute to the PID problem in the developing world, in that such infections may irritate or weaken the tubes and thereby render them more susceptible to infection. We have also devoted a chapter to each of these diseases and discuss how they affect all aspects of human reproduction (Chapters 5 and 6).

Muir and Belsey (1980:913) have emphasized that although PID is an important problem in much of the developing world, the exact etiology of the PID varies greatly among countries. Thus, although genital TB appears to be an important cause of PID in India, it is an insignificant part of the PID problem in South Africa and Uganda. Conversely, PID due to sexually transmitted organisms is much less important in India than in these two African countries (Muir and Belsey 1980:918). Each area then has its own unique mix of PID factors. In assessing the impact of PID on reproductive potential, this particular mixture of causality must be determined. Some types of PID, such as that caused by TB, usually cause primary sterility whereas others such as postpartum and postabortal infections are associated with secondary sterility. Gonococcal salpingitis may be associated with either primary or secondary sterility. Also, the risk of sterility following a pelvic infection varies with etiology, gonococcal salpingitis having the best prognosis, postpartum and postabortal infections having the worst prognosis, and nongonococcal salpingitis somewhere in between.

The impact PID will have on any given population also varies with the quality and availability of health services. Where health services are of high quality and are accessible to and frequently used by the populace complications are less common and the impact of PID on reproductive potential is minimized. Where facilities are poor misdiagnosis and inadequate treatment are frequent, leading to more complications and more chronic infections. Often victims choose to treat themselves with native remedies, with pills sold at the marketplace, or with antibiotics that are readily available without prescription at the pharmacy. And in some outlying areas no professional help is available and most pelvic infections run their course. It has been suggested that complication rates in the developing world today approach those experienced in the industrial world prior to the introduction of effective chemotherapy.

Complications of Gonorrhea in the Male:Posterior Urethritis, Prostatitis, Seminal Vesiculitis, Epididymitis, and Orchitis

Introduction

Most of the environmental, host, and organism factors discussed earlier with regard to the risk in women of developing complications of gonorrhea also apply to men. One notable difference is that because fewer men are asymptomatic, contact tracing and case finding, though important, are not quite as important; more men are aware they are infected and seek treatment. But if diagnostic procedures are below par many cases of gonococcal urethritis will be misdiagnosed and some will be missed altogether, permitting the infection to progress to involve the posterior urethra, accessory glands, vas deferens, and epididymis.

Studies have shown that a purulent urethral discharge, the classical sign of gonorrhea, is not always present in gonococcal urethritis (Watson 1979:785). Thus, reliance on physical findings is unreliable in some instances and a diagnosis of gonococcal urethritis cannot be dismissed unless a urethral swab is negative by culture.

Proper treatment is also essential in preventing and/or limiting complications. As described earlier, urethral irrigation with various chemicals was the favored method of treatment prior to the introduction of the sulfa drugs and antibiotics. Adler (1980:208) noted that urethral irrigation with potassium permanganate solution, as it was performed after World War I in the United Kingdom, invariably led to epididymitis because the irrigating solution was elevated too high above the pelvis and it entered the urethra with such force that gonococci were swept to the posterior. And Rendtorff (1975:235) suggested that uretheal stricture, which was a considerable problem as a complication in the male in past years, may have largely been caused by faulty treatment.

The sulfonamides were the first really effective treatment for gonorrhea, and these drugs gained rapidly in popularity after their introduction in the late 1930s. But the gonococcus soon developed resistance, and within several years of their introduction the sulfonamides were ineffective against many cases of gonorrhea. Pelouze (1939:160) noted that toxic reactions to the sulfa drugs occurred in a substantial proportion of cases and urged watchful waiting as the most prudent course. (Among these toxic reactions to sulfa drugs is the severe and sometimes fatal hemolytic anemia experienced by persons who lack the enzyme G6PD. About 10–14% of black Americans are G6PD deficient.) Penicillin changed all this, revolutionizing the treatment of gonorrhea by producing cures in what was then considered almost miraculous fashion without significant toxic reactions.

Today in the developed world penicillin is still effective against most gonorrhea strains although higher doses are needed to effect a cure than in the past. (Concomitant treatment with tetracycline is recommended to cure any coexisting chlamydial infection.) Thus, complications are seen primarily in men who delay treatment or in asymptomatic men who evade contact tracing and case finding programs. In the developing world the situation is very different because of inadequate health services and a high frequency of penicillin-resistant strains. Complications such as urethral strictures and obstruction of the genital duct are believed to be quite common and partly responsible for the low fertility rates seen in some areas, especially where studies show azoospermia to be an important contributing factor in male infertility. It has been suggested that the present situation in developing countries may be analogous to that in the developed countries prior to the introduction of the sulfa drugs and antibiotics. On the other hand, if Adler (1980:208) and Rendtorff (1975:235) were correct in saying that many cases of urethral stricture and epididymitis in the era before sulfa drugs and antibiotics were the result of early treatment methods, then untreated persons in the past (and now) could be expected to have lower complication rates than those cited by most early studies, which report mostly treated cases.

Complication Rates before and after Effective Chemotherapy

According to Kraus (1972:1115), before antibiotics gonorrhea progressed to prostatitis in 15% of cases and epididymitis in 17%. Pelouze (1939:240) cited a similar figure of 20% for epididymitis. Hofer (1954, cited in Ambrose 1964:233), on the other hand, cited much higher complication rates. He estimated that in the 1930s, before either sulfa drugs or penicillin were available, gonorrhea was complicated by chronic prostatitis in 87% of cases and by epididymitis in 6 to 58% of cases. Lachman (1973:52–55) did not give any figures but stated that before antibiotics urethral strictures, sequelae of posterior urethritis, were common. He further noted that prostatitis, seminal vesiculitis, and epididymitis were frequently seen. Similarly, Fair (1977:56) noted that epididymitis was a common complication of gonococcal urethritis before the advent of chemotherapy. All workers have cited a dramatic reduction in complication rates following the introduction of effective chemotherapeutic agents, especially penicillin (see Table 10.1).

Thus, in the absence of treatment or with improper or inadequate treatment a substantial proportion of cases of gonococcal urethritis will develop complications. An inflammatory response is elicited as the gonococci penetrate and multiply within the epithelial and subepithelial cells. This is followed by a denuding of the epithelium and fibrosis subsequent to healing. Narrowing or obliteration of the genital tract may occur as a result of extensive fibrosis. Urethral stricture is the classic example of fibrous obstruction subsequent to gonorrhea, but the ejaculatory duct, vas deferens, and epididymis may also be involved. Although a narrowing of the duct is possible in the relatively wide urethra, fibrosis in the tiny ejaculatory duct, vas, or epididymis frequently means complete obstruction resulting in azoospermia and sterility (Greenberg 1979:317–318). Data on the proportion of cases of epididymitis that lead to sterility is extremely limited and largely impressionistic. Hence, whereas Pelouze (1939:240), writing in the pre-antibiotic era, reported

Table 10.1

Complication Rates before and after Effective Chemotherapy

Disease	Before chemotherapy (%)	After chemotherapy[a] (%)
Posterior urethritis	—	76 (S); 62 (P)[d]
Prostatitis	15[b]	3[b]
	<2[c]	—
	87[d]	50 (S); 30 (P)[d]
Epididymitis	17[b]	2[b]
	20[c]	—
	6–58[d]	6.6 (S); 5.8 (P)[d]
Seminal vesiculitis	<2[c]	—
Orchitis	<2[c]	—

[a]S, sulfonamides; P, penicillin.
[b]Source: Kraus (1972:1115).
[c]Source: Pelouze (1939:240).
[d]Source: Hofer (1954, cited in Ambrose 1964:233).

that sterility follows about one-third of cases of epididymitis, Davis (1970:1041), writing at a time when many effective antibiotics were available, estimated the sterility rate at 50 to 80% if there is extensive involvement.

More recent studies have indicated that complications of gonorrhea may be more common than generally believed. For example, although it is felt that in the developed world epididymitis is now a rare complication of gonorrheal infection causing less than 5% of all cases of epididymitis (Fair 1977:56; Watson 1979:785), Watson (1979:786) pointed out that a diagnosis of gonococcal epididymitis is often missed because gonococcal epididymitis is indistinguishable from nonspecific, traumatic, or other bacterial epididymitides by patient history or physical findings such as fever, discharge, and site and size of epididymal inflammation. In his series of 88 consecutive patients with acute epididymitis 16% had gonorrhea; the real figure is probably higher because about one-third of the men were taking antibiotics before admission, obscuring a microbial diagnosis. In 50% of these men there was no discharge and neither the physical findings nor the patient's history gave reliable clues as to etiology. But culture of a urethral swab yielded *N. gonorrhoeae*. Because gonococcal epididymitis is apparently such a serious threat to fecundity, accurate diagnosis of all cases of epididymitis is imperative so appropriate therapy can be initiated.

Accessory Gland Involvement and Subfecundity

Most studies of the effects of gonorrhea on male reproductive potential have cited epididymitis with subsequent obstructive azoospermia as the most important complication. Involvement of the accessory glands such as the prostate and seminal vesicles has been mentioned but frequently dismissed as being no more than an inconvenience (Kraus 1972:1115) with no notable effect on fecundity. This is largely because most analyses of semen are concerned only with the number, motility, and morphology of sperm, parameters that are affected primarily by abnormalities in the testes and ducts. Because no correlation has been found between sperm count and morphology and the relative activities or concentrations in the semen of substances secreted by the seminal vesicles or prostate (see Table 10.2), it has been concluded that these substances have no effect on fertility. Yet, as discussed by Eliasson (1975:113ff), these substances are important to the functional properties of sperm such as motility, viability, and metabolism, and may well affect fertilizing capacity. Prostatic fluid, for example, is of great importance for initiating sperm motility and for coating the sperm with factors that increase their viability.

Secretory dysfunction of the prostate and seminal vesicles is not an uncommon occurrence, because up to 60% of cases of urethritis progress to involve the accessory glands. In some instances the secretory dysfunction can be permanent. This is particularly true of infections involving the seminal vesicles, which tend to cause permanent damage to the secretory epithelium. Such infections can be present without

Table 10.2

Some Compounds Specific for the Secretion
from the Various Male Accessory Genital Glands[a]

Organ	Compound
Prostate	Acid phosphatase
	Citric acid
	Zinc
	Magnesium
Seminal vesicles	Fructose
	Prostaglandins
Bulbo-urethral glands	?
Urethral glands	?
Epididymis	Free ℓ-carnitine

[a]Source: Eliasson (1975:114; personal communication, 1983).

causing subjective signs and symptoms and palpatory findings may be normal. However, cytological examination of expressed fluid reveals a frank inflammatory reaction. Greenberg (1979:318) has noted that sperm agglutination and poor semen quality are seminal aberrations of importance to reproduction that are generally ascribed to infection or inflammation. It seems reasonable to assume that altered secretions from an infected prostate and/or the seminal vesicles are responsible.

Seminal Vesiculitis

Seminal vesiculitis may be asymptomatic or give only slight and transitory symptoms resembling those of a bladder infection. Low fructose levels accompany the infection and may, in some cases, persist after resolution of the infection, as there may be permanent damage to the secretory epithelium. Most patients with a low fructose level have or have had vesiculitis. But although a low fructose level may not be normal, there is as yet no evidence that it is a cause of subfecundity (Eliasson 1975:115–116).

Prostatitis

Neisseria gonorrhoeae is capable of causing severe inflammatory changes in the prostate (Amelar and Dubin 1977:84). However, in some cases the infection is completely asymptomatic and must be diagnosed using the two-glass test (Swartz 1977:16–17)[4] or by performing a transperineal prostatic biopsy (Fair 1977:57). Prostatitis may affect fertilizing capacity in a number of ways. When an acute prostatitis is severe and the gland is grossly enlarged, the adjacent ejaculatory duct may be pressed closed (Eliasson 1975:115), producing a temporary azoospermia. And the decreased zinc levels associated with prostatitis are associated with reduced sperm motility. Greenberg (1979:318) believed it possible that infections of the prostate, low zinc levels, and male infertility are related and felt that further investigation into this possible association is warranted.

Prostatitis and seminal vesiculitis are, therefore, possible causes of infertility. Nevertheless, a final conclusion is not possible until appropriate, well-controlled prospective studies are done. Comhaire *et al.* (1980:33) remarked that existing studies of whether infection of the accessory glands can cause infertility are flawed by a disagreement over what constitutes infection. Some workers make a diagnosis of infection

---

[4]Urine is collected in two consecutive glasses. Turbidity in the first glass indicates a urethritis, in the second glass a prostatitis.

once any pathogenic bacteria are detected; others consider the number of bacteria present central to a diagnosis. Still others rely on cytological evaluation of expressed seminal fluid. Until some agreement is reached (for interested readers Comhaire and associates [1980] have presented what they judge to be reliable indices for a diagnosis of accessory gland infection) the literature will remain difficult to interpret.

Summary

Gonorrhea in the male is a serious threat to fertilizing capacity if the infection moves to the posterior urethra and beyond. Strictures in the posterior urethra are a frequent sequela of such infection. Occlusion of the ejaculatory duct, vas deferens, and epididymis are not uncommon and are accompanied by sterility. Involvement of the accessory glands such as the prostate and seminal vesicles may also have a negative impact on fertility because they secrete substances essential to the proper functioning of spermatozoa and perhaps for full fertilizing capacity as well. Such secretory dysfunction may persist even after resolution of the infection. Although sperm motility may be affected by accessory gland infection, the two other criteria routinely used in evaluating semen quality—sperm count and morphology—will be unaffected and the importance of any accessory gland involvement perhaps overlooked.

In the developing world, where health services are frequently poor, more complications would be expected. In the developed world fewer cases of gonococcal urethritis go untreated, so complication rates are much lower. Nevertheless, men with asymptomatic or mild urethritis who delay treatment are at risk of developing serious complications. A better understanding of the vagaries of the clinical picture of male gonorrhea—in some cases the classic symptom of urethral discharge is absent and only a culture of urethral material will reveal the gonococcus—has enabled more recent researchers to attribute many more cases of idiopathic epididymitis to gonorrhea.

Nongonococcal Urethritis
and Its Complications in the Male

Introduction

In more than one-third of men treated for an initial episode of gonococcal urethritis (GCU), symptoms reappear after apparent cure. Over 50% of these cases of postgonococcal urethritis are due not to a recurrence of gonorrhea but to a nongonococcal urethritis (NGU) acquired at the same time but that took longer to incubate (Galton 1980:16). And in many cases NGU occurs in isolation, that is, in the absence of a recent attack of gonorrhea. Improved diagnostic techniques have shown that NGU is usually due to either *C. trachomatis* or *U. urealyticum*.

Prevalence

The most common STD in the developed world is NGU; its frequency increased more rapidly in the 25 years from 1950 to 1975 than that of any other STD (*British Medical Journal* 1979:161). According to the United States Public Health Service 2.5 million cases of NGU are reported each year. The relative frequency of GCU and NGU varies by country and by social class. Whereas there are twice as many cases of NGU as GCU in Great Britain, the U.S. Centers for Disease Control estimated that in the United States NGU and GCU occur in approximately equal numbers (Felman and Nikitas 1981:381). It appears that NGU is more prevalent than GCU among higher socioeconomic groups (Felman and Nikitas 1981:381); whereas NGU accounts for 50 to 66% of urethritis cases treated in STD clinics, it claims 80–92% of the total among college students (Bowie 1980:19; Wiesner and Holmes 1975:22).

The importance of NGU in the developing world has yet to be quantified, but indications are that its importance may be underestimated because of poor diagnostic facilities and a preoccupation with gonorrhea (Arya and Lawson 1977:51). Studies in the developing world among men of higher socioeconomic status have shown that cases of NGU outnumber those of GCU 2:1 (Meheus *et al.* 1980:244). And, according to Arya and Lawson (1977:51), NGU is reported to be common in both East and West Africa. Nevertheless, the majority of urethritis cases in the developing world are believed due to *N. gonorrhoeae*. Meheus and associates (1980:243) estimated the minimal annual incidence of urethritis in Africa to be 3,750/100,000, of which 80% is caused by gonorrhea. They cited studies showing that a urethral discharge is caused by gonorrhea in 90% of cases in Rwanda, 95% in Kenya, 81% in Malaysia, and 82% in Swaziland. Their own study in Swaziland found *N. gonorrhoeae* in 93% of patients with a urethral discharge or other signs of urethritis.

Causes of Nongonococcal Urethritis

Chlamydia

Many workers (e.g., Felman and Nikitas 1981:382; Greenberg 1979:317; Melo 1979:520; Oriel 1977b:38; Wiesner and Holmes 1975:22) have reported that *C. trachomatis* can be isolated in 40 to 50% of cases of NGU. An etiological role for chlamydia in NGU is, according to Bowie (1980:19), convincing and, according to Felman and Nikitas (1981:381), proved. It has been hypothesized (Richmond and Clarke 1977:44–45) that genital chlamydia exists as a latent infection that becomes active (culture-positive) only when the urethra is inflamed, which then prolongs and exacerbates the inflammation. This hypothesis may apply to cases of postgonococcal urethritis from which *C. trachomatis* can be isolated, but chlamydia-positive NGU often occurs in isolation, supporting the notion that *C. trachomatis* can be a primary pathogen initiating an infection (Willcox 1977:222).

Numerous factors support a role for *C. trachomatis* in NGU. Chlamydial organisms are seen in a large number of NGU patients (Felman and Nikitas 1981:382). In North America and Europe *C. trachomatis* is found in 30 to 60% of men with NGU, in 4 to 35% of men with gonorrhea, and in only 0 to 7% of men with no urethritis (Bowie 1980:19). Also, seroconversion is noted in cases of chlamydia-positive NGU within 10 days after onset of illness (Felman and Nikitas 1981:382), indicating that the organism has an active role in the infection. Also, drugs that eliminate chlamydia frequently eliminate NGU (Felman and Nikitas 1981:382).

Meheus and associates (1980:244) warned against relying on serology to diagnose genital chlamydia in developing countries where other *C. trachomatis* organisms such as trachoma and lymphogranuloma venereum exist. However, because each of these diseases has a unique serotype—types A, B, and C for trachoma, types L_1, L_2, and L_3 for lymphogranuloma venereum, and types D–K for genital chlamydia—serology is useful if type-specific antigen is available to distinguish among the various infections.

Genital Mycoplasmas

The role of the genital mycoplasmas in NGU has also been extensively studied. After reviewing these studies Taylor-Robinson and McCormack (1980a:1005) concluded that the classical mycoplasma, *M. hominis,* is not a cause of NGU. *Mycoplasma hominis* occurs with equal frequency in controls as in NGU patients. Furthermore, erythromycin, which is effective in treating NGU, is not effective against *M. hominis* (Shepard 1970:1335).

Evidence for involvement of *U. urealyticum* in NGU has been characterized as "circumstantial" (Bowie *et al.* 1977:27), "good" (Greenberg 1979:317), and "strong" (Shepard 1970:1340). One reason for skepticism is that the ureaplasmas are found so frequently in controls. But whereas 21–48% of controls are positive for *U. urealyticum*, the organism is found about three times more frequently in urethritis patients (Shepard 1970:1337). In addition, NGU is cured by drugs effective against *U. urealyticum*. (Because the ureaplasmas and chlamydiae are sensitive to the same drugs, one must always account for the presence of *C. trachomatis*.) And two workers with negative urethral cultures who inoculated themselves with *U. urealyticum* developed urethritis, which then disappeared with tetracycline treatment (Taylor-Robinson and McCormack 1980a:1005–1006).

Other Causes

If *C. trachomatis* accounts for 40 to 50% of NGU cases and *U. urealyticum* for perhaps 5%, what causes the remaining cases? A large number of microbes have been isolated from NGU patients who are negative for chlamydia and mycoplasma. These include *T. vaginalis, Herpes simplex type 2, H. vaginalis, Streptococcus viridans, Staphylococcus epidermidis,* diphtheroids, *Candida* species, and a number of anaerobic bacteria including *Bacteroides* species and *Clostridium difficile* (Melo 1979:520–521). Whereas Hovelius *et al.* (1979:369) estimated that together *H. hominis, C. albicans,* and *T. vaginalis* may account for 10% of NGU cases, Felman and Nikitas (1981:383) felt that these organisms are rarely a cause of NGU. In a fair number of NGU cases neither *C. trachomatis, U. urealyticum,* nor any other pathogen can be isolated and the etiology cannot be ascertained.

Complications of Nongonococcal Urethritis

The clinical course of NGU is well known: a period of urethral irritation and discharge that usually resolves without treatment after a period of weeks to months. But in a small proportion of cases the infection progresses to involve other genital structures. Late sequelae such as urethral strictures have been noted following complicated NGU (Galton 1980:16). Obstruction at other sites and changes in the secretory function of the accessory glands have not been documented but are likely because NGU can be complicated not only by posterior urethritis but by acute or chronic prostatitis, vasitis, and epididymitis as well (Greenberg 1979:317). The generally asymptomatic or mild nature of NGU means delay in treatment and an increased risk of complications.

Prostatitis was reported by Catterall (1975:11) to be the most common complication of NGU, occurring in a high, but unspecified, percentage of infected men. Though frequently symptomless, it may reveal itself months or years later in a variety of ways. Eliasson (1975:115–116), for example, noted definite pathophysiological conditions in the genital glands of apparently healthy men who had a history of NGU.

The second most common complication of NGU is epididymitis, which occurs in an estimated 4% of cases (Catterall 1975:11). In a study in Seattle in men with idiopathic epididymitis, *C. trachomatis* was isolated from 11 of 13 men under age 35 and endogenous bowel organisms were isolated from 8 of 10 men over age 35 (Berger *et al.* 1978:301–302). These data, and those cited earlier of Watson (1979) showing that many cases of gonococcal epididymitis are misdiagnosed as idiopathic because the clinical picture is atypical and cultures are not done, suggest that idiopathic epididymitis, which comprised 50–100% of epididymitis cases in some studies (cf. Berger *et al.* 1978:301; Fair 1977:56), may in many cases be caused by a sexually transmitted organism. Reflux of sterile urine down the vas deferens caused by straining with a full bladder, a probable cause cited in many cases of idiopathic epididymitis, is relatively unimportant, according to Berger and associates (1978:303). These authors also noted that epididymitis is rare in prepubertal boys, which further supports an STD etiology.

Finally, it is interesting that the etiological agents in epididymitis and those in PID exhibit the same STD–non-STD variability with age. Thus, whereas sexually transmitted organisms such as chlamydia and gonorrhea cause the majority of epididymitis and PID cases in younger men and women, endogenous nonvenereal infections with bowel organisms predominate when these complications occur in older patients.

Diagnosis

Nongonococcal urethritis is bound to become increasingly important in the developed and the developing world because of difficulties in diagnosis and treatment. A proper diagnosis, as described by Felman and Nikitas (1981:383–384), may involve three or four steps. First, the diagnosis of urethritis should be confirmed by examining a Gram-stained urethral smear under the microscope to determine if there are at least 5 PMNs per HPF (see footnote 2). If this criterion for inflammation is met, the physician should examine the smear for gonococci. If typical Gram-negative intracellular diplococci (which are specifically diagnostic for *N. gonorrhoeae* in 98% of cases) are not present, a culture of urethral material on Thayer–Martin medium is necessary to definitely rule out gonococcal urethritis. If the culture is negative, then a diagnosis of NGU can be made. Culturing for *C. trachomatis* and *U. urealyticum*, the two most common causes of NGU, should then be done.

In the developing world there are few medical facilities prepared to perform all these tests, and even in the United States there is a tendency, especially among doctors in private practice, to overdiagnose gonococcal urethritis rather than differentiate GCU and NGU (Wiesner and Holmes 1975:22). Thus, even in the developed world many cases of NGU are concealed under a diagnosis of gonorrhea (*British Medical Journal* 1979:161). Many physicians rely on clinical criteria rather than lab tests to differentiate GCU and NGU. NGU is more often associated with mild dysuria and/or a scant or moderate discharge (penile stripping may be necessary to express the discharge) that is clear or white and mucoid, whereas GCU is more often associated with a spontaneous, profuse, purulent discharge. Thus, a low-grade urethritis is characteristic of NGU while a more severe urethritis is typical of GCU (Felman and Nikitas 1981:381). However, because NGU may present with a severe or mild urethritis (*British Medical Journal* 1979:161), and, as noted earlier, a urethral discharge may not be present in some cases of gonorrhea, a diagnosis that relies solely on clinical criteria may be wrong.

Treatment

As long as cases of NGU are being misdiagnosed as GCU, the disease will remain largely unchecked because the two primary causes of NGU, chlamydia and the ureaplasmas, are resistant to penicillin and spectinomycin. Tetracycline and erythromycin must be used to treat these infections properly (Felman and Nikitas 1981:382, 384; Galton 1980:16). In some instances *U. urealyticum* may present a special problem because some of its strains, and possibly some strains of *C. trachomatis*, are resistant even to these drugs (Felman and Nikitas 1981:384). And some public clinics dismiss NGU as a trivial infection and do not treat it at all (Holmes and Hobson 1977:2). In general, men in the United States are now being properly treated. But all too often the infection is viewed as a urological condition and its sexually transmitted nature ignored. Sexual partners are not contacted, and an infected woman, who is usually asymptomatic, goes untreated and serves as an infectious source (*Time* 1978a:73). Spread is further encouraged by the tendency of NGU to recur within 6 weeks after initiation of treatment, a phenomenon that is more common with chlamydia-negative than chlamydia-positive cases (Bowie 1980:21; Catterall 1975:11). Whether such recurrences represent reinfections or the extension of a chronic prostatitis or other condition is unknown (Oriel 1977b:41).

Summary

Nongonococcal urethritis is an infection of great importance. It is the most common STD in much of the developed world and is important in the developing world among men of higher socioeconomic status. The tendency in many countries, both developed and developing, is to misdiagnose NGU, frequently as GCU, or to make a proper diagnosis but withhold treatment because the infection is viewed as trivial. Thus, NGU is frequently improperly treated or not treated at all. And the mild, often asymptomatic nature of NGU results in delayed treatment. It is not surprising then that complications are frequently reported. An estimated 4% of men with NGU develop epididymitis and even more develop an acute or chronic prostatitis, meaning that obstruction of the seminal tract and/or secretory dysfunction of the accessory glands that produce substances vital to sperm function are possible sequelae in a not-insignificant proportion of men with NGU. And these estimates may be low, as evidence is accumulating that many cases of idiopathic epididymitis in younger men are due to nongonococcal organisms, particularly *C. trachomatis*. As more sophisticated techniques for obtaining specimens—Berger *et al.* (1978:302–303) aspirated the epididymis and this provided some chlamydia-positive material in cases with negative urethral cultures—and culturing *C. trachomatis* become more widely available, the true impact of this infection on male reproductive potential will become obvious. Experimental studies on grivet monkeys indicate that *C. trachomatis* has the same biological potential as *N. gonorrhoeae* in the female genital tract. Whether this is also true in the male genital tract seems likely, but remains unproved.

It is noteworthy that although *C. trachomatis* has been implicated in epididymitis and prostatitis, *U. urealyticum* has not been associated with either complication (Taylor-Robinson and McCormack 1980a:1006–1007). It appears that *U. urealyticum* is a self-limiting infection in men, capable of producing a urethritis but unlikely to affect more posterior structures.

CHAPTER 11

Syphilis

Introduction

Syphilis is a sexually transmitted disease (STD) caused by the bacterium *Treponema pallidum*. Its name comes from a poem by the Italian pathologist Hieronymus Fracastorius, in which the mythical shepherd Syphilus is afflicted with the disease as punishment for cursing the gods. Syphilis is undoubtedly the most dreaded of all the venereal diseases because it can disfigure, disable, and kill. In an adult the relatively benign early stage of syphilis, whose major symptoms are a chancre and skin rashes, is followed by a long period of latency, which may be shattered by blindness, insanity, crippling, aortic insufficiency, and/or death. If an infected pregnant woman transmits the disease to the fetus the child may be spontaneously aborted, stillborn, or born alive but suffer from congenital syphilis.

Although syphilitic infection can now be completely cured by penicillin, the disease is still feared by millions, and with good reason. In some cases the infection goes unnoticed, and therefore untreated, until late sequelae appear. Although penicillin can cure the infection even at this point, and thereby prevent the disease from progressing further, it cannot reverse existing damage. In the developed world routine serologic testing at various points in life (e.g., premarital testing before issuance of a marriage license, prenatal testing, etc.) uncovers many silent infections and prevents such tragedies. But in the developing world few such testing programs exist. In addition, health facilities are simply not available in some parts of the developing world, and in these areas even obvious infections must go untreated.

History

Syphilis made its first recognized appearance in the fifteenth century in Europe. Each country blamed this new affliction on its enemies: The Italians called it the Spanish or French disease, the French called it the Italian disease, and the English called it the French disease. The French were generally held most culpable, and for centuries syphilis was referred to as *morbus gallicus.*

Whether syphilis existed before the fifteenth century is a matter of debate. Its precipitous appearance in Europe at that time has led some medical historians to speculate that Columbus's voyagers brought the disease back from somewhere in the New World, probably Haiti. These proponents of the Columbian theory of the origin of syphilis are opposed by the pre-Columbians who believe that syphilis existed in Europe before the fifteenth century. And whereas the pre-Columbians argue that remains of pre-fifteenth-century Europeans show signs of syphilitic deterioration, other scholars say there is no evidence of such pathological changes. Brown *et al.* (1970:7) believed that syphilis as we know it first appeared in Europe in the fifteenth century, but they were not certain as to whether this new disease was the result of a spontaneous mutation in a spirochetal disease already infecting Europeans or whether it was introduced from the outside, possibly from the Americas. The issue remains unresolved.

Prevalence

It is difficult to make a positive diagnosis of syphilis without modern microscopic and serologic techniques. Hence, no one knows for sure how many Europeans were afflicted with syphilis when the first wave of infections hit and clinical impressions alone were the basis of a diagnosis. Syphilis is known as the "great imitator" and may be confused clinically with psoriasis, chickenpox, leprosy, yaws, infectious mononucleosis, other venereal infections (such as scabies, lymphogranuloma venereum, granuloma inguinale, and herpes simplex type 2), and a host of other infections (Brown *et al.* 1970:3; U.S. Public Health Service 1968:53–55, 66–69). In all, the skin and mucous membrane lesions of primary syphilis resemble those of 23 other diseases, and the lesions of secondary syphilis may be confused with at least 40 other disorders (Cave *et al.* 1971:947).

Syphilis undoubtedly became more prevalent as time passed. As the disease became a familiar one, earlier feelings of horror and repulsion were followed by acceptance. Thus, although infection with syphilis carried a terrible stigma at the end of the fifteenth century—banishment or branding of syphilitics was advocated—by the seventeenth century European gentlemen who had not experienced the "great pox" were considered ungentlemanly, and perhaps unmanly (Gallagher 1969:157).

The magnitude of the syphilis problem first became quantifiable in 1906 when Auguste von Wasserman and Carl Bruck developed a blood test for the disease. Although this and other early serologic tests lacked specificity and therefore tended to overestimate the number of cases, they did reveal that alarming numbers of persons were infected with *T. pallidum*. Adler (1980:207) recounted that serologic surveys in 1914 in London showed that up to 12% of men and 7% of women had syphilis. Reports from Paris at the same time revealed a 15% syphilis rate, and from Berlin a 12% rate. Rates in Russia were even higher. Ninety-five percent of the population in northwestern Russia suffered from syphilis early in this century according to one study (Gantt 1926). Adler felt that even though tests at that time lacked specificity and tended to overestimate the number of cases, the true rates were nevertheless probably very high. And in the United States, extrapolation of data from serologic tests of armed service recruits revealed that during the first half of the twentieth century about 2.5% of the population had syphilis (McFalls 1973:4).

Immediately after Wasserman's discovery of a serologic test for syphilis came Paul Ehrlich's discovery of a cure. In 1907 Ehrlich discovered arsphenamine, an arsenic compound effective against the treponeme of syphilis that quickly supplanted less-effective and highly toxic mercury treatments. However, Ehrlich's hope that one injection of arsphenamine would effect a cure was unrealized. Rather, a series of painful injections over 70 weeks was necessary to cure, and in some cases relapses were noted following cessation of treatment. If the drug was not properly administered poisoning would occur, causing internal bleeding, aplastic anemia, etc. Thus, of those who began arsenotherapy only 20–30% persevered with the treatment to the point where their infections were arrested. No further advances in the chemotherapy of syphilis appeared until the early 1940s. Hence, prevalence rates did not change much in the early decades of the twentieth century. Data for the United States, for example, showed approximately the same infection rates before World War II as before World War I (McFalls 1973:4).

An effective short-term (5–10 days) arsenotherapy regimen was developed just prior to World War II by Harry Eagle. In 1943, Rapid Treatment Centers using Eagle's method were established. Also in 1943, John Mahoney, working in a U.S. Public Health Service hospital on Staten Island, New York, demonstrated that penicillin was effective against syphilis. By June 1944 penicillin was made available to the Rapid Treatment Centers and soon became the only treatment for syphilis. At first closely spaced injections over several days made penicillin practical only on an inpatient basis. But soon delayed absorption preparations made outpatient treatment feasible, and by 1953 single-injection treatment for syphilis became a reality.

In response to these developments, the prevalence of syphilis began a precipitous decline worldwide in 1950. But by 1957 syphilis rates began creeping upward, and by the late 1960s there were 30–50 million reported cases according to World Health Organization (WHO) statistics (Gallagher 1969:163). Three important reasons for this reversal in the syphilis trend are (1) greater promiscuity; (2) complacency about the seriousness of syphilis—Gallagher (1969:162) noted that respect for syphilis, painfully learned during months of heavy metal therapy, was lost when penicillin made the cure painless and swift; and (3) the more discriminate use of penicillin by physicians that followed recognition of adverse effects such as allergic reactions and the emergence of penicillin-resistant organisms. Indeed, some sources (e.g., U.S. Public Health Service 1968:15) have felt that the frequent nonspecific use of penicillin for nearly every condition during the late 1940s and early 1950s led to many "accidental" cures and that this was the most important reason for the dramatic drop in national syphilis morbidity in the post–World War II years.

Developed World

Accurate figures on current rates of syphilis in the developed world are frequently hard to find. In the United States, for example, the overwhelming majority of syphilis cases are treated by private physicians, and these physicians report only one in five cases to health authorities. Thus, the true annual incidence of early syphilis is at least four times the number of reported cases. It was estimated that in 1962 in North America there were 64 new cases of syphilis per 100,000 population (Willcox 1977:211).

A national survey was conducted in the United States in the early 1960s to generate data about the epidemiology of disease that were not biased by the reporting system. This 1962 National Health Examination Survey showed that 4.4% of men and 3.6% of women had a positive serologic test for syphilis, indicating present or past infection (Brown *et al.* 1970:77). These figures indicate that approximately as many women as men are infected, suggesting that the great preponderance of men among reported cases is simply an artifact reflecting the fact that early syphilis, particularly primary syphilis, is more obvious in men (Lucas 1972:1078). It has been estimated (Stokes 1919:64; Victor 1981:34), for example, that whereas 40% of men are unaware of the chancre of primary syphilis, 60–90% of women do not notice the lesion because it commonly forms on the inner labia, in the vagina, or on the cervix. Similarly, although syphilis rates for blacks are substantially higher than for whites, this excess is, according to the National Health Examination Survey, ninefold—not the frequently cited elevenfold or greater excess in reported cases that only reflects the fact that many more whites see private physicians who usually do not report their cases to health authorities (Lucas 1972:1078; McFalls 1973:5).

One demographic fact about the incidence of syphilis that has never been disputed is that syphilis is a disease contracted by young adults. Persons aged 20–24 are at the greatest risk of acquiring syphilis, and it is in this age group that 25% of all cases of early syphilis are found. The age group 25–29 is the second most frequently infected, and the 15–19-year age group is the third most frequently infected and accounts for 17% of all cases of early syphilis (Brown *et al.* 1970:78). Studies in the 1920s (Frazier and Hung-Chuing 1948:32) and in the 1960s (Brown *et al.* 1970:79) have indicated that nonwhites acquire syphilis at a somewhat earlier age than whites, and females of any race at a somewhat earlier age than males (see Table 11.1). Frazier and Hung-Chuing (1948:32) em-

Table 11.1

Percentage Distribution of Reported Cases of Primary and Secondary Syphilis by Age, Race, and Sex: United States, 1966[a]

	White		Nonwhite	
Age	*Male*	*Female*	*Male*	*Female*
0–14	.2	.7	.7	2.3
15–19	7.4	19.4	15.3	26.1
20–24	23.1	27.8	28.3	30.3
25–29	20.2	18.5	22.3	17.8
30–39	28.1	20.8	21.9	16.5
40–49	13.8	9.5	8.3	5.3
50+	7.2	3.4	3.2	1.8
Total	100.0	100.0	100.0	100.0

[a]Source: Brown *et al.* (1970:79). From *Syphilis and other venereal diseases,* published by the Harvard University Press. Reprinted by permission.

phasized that syphilis is a disease of adulthood, not of youth. Looking at age of initial infection for blacks, whites, and Chinese, they found that syphilis was not usually acquired until age 25 or thereafter (see Table 11.2).

Today in many developed countries many, if not most, syphilis cases occur in homosexual men, among whom rates are extraordinarily high. The large numbers of sexual contacts of many homosexual men—some report 50–60 contacts per month—place them at a greatly increased risk of acquiring any STD. In Great Britain in 1972, 42.4% of early syphilis cases were homosexually acquired. The overwhelming majority of such cases were in London; there were few cases of homosexually acquired syphilis in Wales or Scotland (Willcox 1977:215–216). Data from large U.S. cities have revealed that most syphilis cases there are seen in male homosexuals. In Seattle the incidence of syphilis was higher in men and 81% of these men were homosexual or bisexual (Wiesner and Holmes 1975:21). In the state of Pennsylvania—excluding Philadelphia, its largest city—81% of infectious syphilis cases were in men, 51% of whom were homosexual. Health officials estimated that if Philadelphia were included in this statistic, the latter figure would rise to 80% (*Philadelphia Bulletin* 1980:A2). It seems probable that the increase in the 1970s in the number of practicing homosexuals has contributed significantly to the increase in recent years in the syphilis rate in developed countries. Nonetheless, in most countries this increase has been only slight to moderate.

Another relatively recent development in the epidemiology of syphilis is the big risk factor associated with urban residence, syphilis rates in large cities being 5–10 times those in smaller cities and towns (Millar 1973:111). This was not always so. From the 1930s until 1960 place of residence did not play nearly so large a role as today's rates would indicate (Lucas 1972:1078).

Table 11.2

Mean Age and Standard Deviation of Initial Infection by Sex and Race[a]

	Black	White	Chinese
Male	25.1 ± 0.4	29.5 ± 0.6	29 ± 0.4
Female	22.3 ± 1.4	25.6 ± 1.6	26.7 ± 0.9

[a]Source: C. Frazier and L. Hung-Chuing (1948). From *Racial variations in immunity to syphilis,* published by The University of Chicago. © 1948 by The University of Chicago.

Developing World

Accurate syphilis rates for developing countries are simply not available. Because, according to Arya and Lawson (1977:54), the tendency in the tropics is to diagnose almost all genital sores as syphilis, one might suspect that syphilis rates for the developing world are overestimated. Where yaws and syphilis coexist this would be particularly true because clinically and serologically the two diseases are indistinguishable. But counterbalancing this are the many cases that are not reported to the authorities—Muir and Belsey (1980:915) believed underreporting to be a serious problem in the developing world—and the many cases that are never brought to the attention of a physician because health services are simply not available. Most data on the prevalence of syphilis in the developing world come, therefore, not from national statistics but from population surveys.

Asia and the Western Pacific

In Asia and the western Pacific increases in syphilis rates, following an initial post–World War II decline, have been noted in Australia, New Zealand, Fiji, Malaysia, Korea, and Japan, whereas decreases have been noted in Hong Kong, the Philippines, Singapore, Papua New Guinea, New Caledonia, and Western Samoa. The syphilis problem is very heterogeneous in this area, serologic testing of pregnant women during the late 1960s revealing vastly different rates from a low of 0.08% in the Philippines to a high of 10.3% in Thailand (Willcox 1977:211–213) (see Table 11.3). Songhaprasert *et al.* (1972:555) also found high rates in Thailand, reporting that 7.1% of outpatients in a Bangkok hospital gave a positive serologic test for syphilis. In addition to Thailand, high rates of syphilis have been noted in some parts of India, particularly around Bombay (Willcox 1977:211). And Kiraly (1973:121) reported that 20% of men in Papua had mixed infections of both syphilis and gonorrhea following a 1971 outbreak along the Highland Highway. In Papua New Guinea, as well as in other parts of the western Pacific, syphilis was rarely seen until yaws disappeared. And although the syphilis rate is declining in Papua New Guinea, there have been outbreaks along the road across the Highlands. The outbreaks have been traced to prostitutes and truck drivers, and the seriousness of the problem is stated to be in direct proportion to the promiscuousness of the local population (Willcox 1977:212–213).

Table 11.3

Percentage Seropositivity for Pregnant
Women in Selected Areas[a]

Area	Year	%
Korea	1966	6.9
Taipei	1967	6.6
Vietnam	1967	6.4
Taiwan	1967	3.0
New Caledonia	1967	1.5
Japan	1967	1.1
Hong Kong	1967	.3
Singapore	1967	.3
Philippines	1966	.08
Sri Lanka	1970	2.0
Thailand	1969	10.3

[a]Source: Willcox (1977:213). Reprinted with
permission from G. Howe (ed.), *A world geography of human diseases.* © Academic Press Inc.
(London) Ltd.

Africa

Willcox (1977:210–211) reported that syphilis is common throughout
Africa and is particularly prevalent in Ethiopia where in some areas 40%
of the population is seropositive. He also cited reports from Uganda of
a 7–16% seropositivity rate among blood donors and from Morocco of
a threefold increase in early syphilis between 1960 and 1968. Eisenberg
(1973:2181, 2184) studied the change in the seropositivity rate among
the Bantu of Soweto (South Africa) between 1949 and 1971. The rates
for pregnant women, which he believed most closely reflected rates for
the general population, are given in Table 11.4; they show an initially
high syphilis rate, which declined substantially following the routine
use of penicillin in 1955. Dogliotti, working in a dermatology clinic also
serving the Bantu of Soweto, found a 16.82% rate of early syphilis in
one study (1971:9) and a 19.23% rate in a later study (1975:267). Of
course, syphilis is overrepresented among dermatology patients because syphilitic lesions are a compelling reason to seek advice from a
dermatologist. Nevertheless, Dogliotti felt that these rates were very
high compared to those recorded in other countries. Workers in Lagos
(Daramola and Oyediran 1971, cited in Belsey 1976:330), for example,
found syphilis in only 5 of 362 patients (1.4%) with venereological complaints who were in a general hospital and dermatology clinic population.

The magnitude of the syphilis problem in Africa is difficult to gauge,

Table 11.4

Percentage Seropositivity for Pregnant
Bantu Women: Soweto, 1949–1971[a]

Year	%
1949	21
1950	19
1951	22
1952	22
1953	21
1954	18
1955	16
1956	9
1957	10
1958	8
1959	9
1960	10
1961	8
1962	7
1963	7
1964	11
1965	12
1966	10
1967	11
1968	10
1969	10
1970	12
1971	11

[a]Source: Eisenberg (1973:2183).

and there is some reason to believe that although some particular populations (as discussed earlier) and some population subgroups (such as soldiers, prostitutes, and homosexuals) may have very high rates, rates for the general population may be overstated. Belsey (1976:330) cited studies in Uganda that revealed high rates of syphilis (or yaws) in soldiers (9.4%) and bar girls (33%), but low rates among outpatients at a community health center (.01%). And although Bwibo (1971:185) found that 2.6% of children less than 10 years old in Kampala, Uganda, were seropositive, he cautioned that some of these children could have been infected with yaws. And Smith *et al.* (1976:640) found syphilis to be the cause of death in only 1% of 300 consecutive autopsies in Kinshasa, Zaire. Interestingly, in their classic book *Obstetrics and Gynaecology in the Tropics* Lawson and Stewart (1967) discussed tuberculosis (TB), leprosy, smallpox, gonorrhea, malaria, schistosomiasis, lymphogranuloma venereum (LGV), and other diseases and their effect on reproduction, but did not discuss syphilis.

Pathophysiology

Within the order Spirochaetales, family Treponemataceae, are three genera of delicate, spiral-shaped microorganisms important to humans. Within the genus *Borrelia* is the etiologic agent of relapsing fever; the genus *Leptospira* includes organisms responsible for a number of febrile illnesses. The genus *Treponema* is the best known and contains three species pathogenic to man: *T. pallidum*, which causes venereal syphilis and endemic syphilis; *T. pertenue*, which causes yaws; and *T. carateum*, which causes pinta. These four diseases are known collectively as the treponematoses. All are antigenically similar and therefore evoke indistinguishable antibodies. They may, however, be separated antigenically from nonpathogenic species such as *T. microdentium*, which is found in the mouths of normal, healthy individuals. All three pathogenic species are also morphologically similar and all move with similar rotary and undulating motions. In addition, all three pathogenic species may evoke a similar clinical picture. Hence, in areas where two or more treponematoses coexist, a differential diagnosis can be very difficult to make.

Syphilis is characterized by a primary lesion (chancre), a secondary skin eruption, and a long period of latency that may be terminated by late (tertiary) syphilis, that is, by late lesions of the skin, bone, or viscera called gummas, or by lesions of the cardiovascular or nervous systems. Although the gummas are usually not fatal, lesions of the cardiovascular and nervous systems are a cause of aortic insufficiency, blindness, crippling, and insanity, and may be followed by death.

Each stage of syphilis is marked by specific clinical, serological, and pathological changes. Each stage is also marked by a specific distribution of organisms that determines its infectiousness. It is this feature of the disease that is most important to population students, who are interested primarily in the possibility of fetal infection with subsequent pregnancy loss.

Primary Syphilis

Primary syphilis commences with the penetration of abraded skin or the mucous membrane by *T. pallidum*. Within a few hours following exposure spirochetes are carried throughout the body in the blood (spirochetemia) and lymph, although clinical and serologic signs of infection are lacking for a time. Many spirochetes leave the vessels and set up metastatic foci throughout the body.

The first clinical sign of infection is the appearance of a hard chancre at the site of penetration about 3 weeks postexposure. The chancre, which is teeming with spirochetes, is usually solitary, although multiple chancres may be seen. The most frequent sites for a chancre are the penis and cervix, although inspection of the mouth not infrequently reveals these lesions. The lymph nodes near the chancre will often be enlarged and needle biopsy of these nodes will reveal large numbers of spirochetes.

It is not uncommon for primary syphilis to pass unnoticed. Infection without chancre is frequent (Benenson 1975:314). And often the chancre is hidden. This is particularly true in women because the chancre commonly forms on the inner labia, in the vagina, or on the cervix (Victor 1981:34). It has been estimated that 60–90% of women and 40% of men are unaware they have primary syphilis (Stokes 1919:64; Victor 1981:34). In addition, a syphilitic chancre resembles 25 other skin lesions (Cave *et al.* 1971:947), so neither the victim nor the physician may be able to pinpoint the disease by simple examination. Serology is frequently negative because detectable levels of antibody are not present when the chancre first appears, although in most cases detectable levels are achieved after the lesion has been present for 1 month. A positive diagnosis may be made at this stage, however, if the lesion (or nearby lymph node) yields living pathogenic organisms. For observation of live spirochetes a special type of microscopy called dark-field microscopy is used, allowing high-resolution visualization of living organisms. This allows the observer not only to see the treponemes but also to differentiate by their characteristic motility pathogenic treponemes, such as *T. pallidum*, from morphologically identical nonpathogenic treponemes frequently found in the mouth (*T. microdentium, T. macrodentium*) and genitals (*T. genitalis*) of healthy individuals.

Primary syphilis is highly infectious to both contacts and the fetus. Large numbers of organisms are found in the chancre. Spirochetes are also circulating in the blood at this time and leak into other body fluids such as saliva, semen, and vaginal discharges. Their presence in the blood introduces the possibility of placental transfer and presents a hazard to the fetus, and their presence in other body fluids and in the chancre places any close contact at risk.

Secondary Syphilis

Secondary syphilis is extremely variable in its onset, duration, and clinical manifestations. Although many organs such as the eye, liver, and kidney may be involved, a diagnosis is suspected primarily on the basis of skin and mucous membrane lesions. These lesions may appear 6 weeks or 6 months postexposure. They may be apparent before the chancre has healed, but more frequently follow the chancre by several weeks. The skin rash usually heals within 2 to 6 weeks, although it may persist for as long as a year. The rash of secondary syphilis may be flat or raised. The lesions are usually dry, although moist lesions may be found wherever moisture accumulates, such as between the toes, in the mouth, or on the genitals. These moist lesions are extraordinarily infectious.

Secondary syphilis, like primary syphilis, may not be noticed by the victim. The skin rash is often difficult to see. Sometimes the skin is entirely spared and the lesions confined to the mucous membrane surfaces of the mouth or genitals (Cave *et al.* 1971:947). And because secondary lesions resemble those of 40 other skin disorders (Cave *et al.* 1971:947), it is very difficult to make a diagnosis on clinical grounds alone. However, at this time blood tests are strongly seropositive, confirming the diagnosis. As with primary syphilis, dark-field examination of material from lesions should reveal characteristic pathogenic treponemes.

Secondary syphilis is highly infectious. Because spirochetes are present in the blood, in the secondary lesions, and in body fluids and secretions such as saliva, semen, and vaginal discharges, the fetus is at risk, as is any close contact. Although one would suspect that nonsexual contact could lead to infection because of the numerous skin lesions that are teeming with spirochetes, this is not so because the majority of skin lesions are dry and only contact with moist lesions, such as those in the genital region, presents a real hazard. Despite spirochetes in the saliva, children who are kissed and fondled by infectious adults are rarely infected (Benenson 1975:315). Contact during sexual activity is by far the most frequent mode of transmission. But even sexual contact with an infectious individual does not invariably lead to infection; it has been estimated that only about 10–50% of persons having sexual contact with persons with primary or secondary syphilis become infected (Benenson 1975:316; Cannefax 1965:261). Fetal infection is also not invariable in the presence of spirochetemia. Holder and Knox (1972:1152) noted that there are reports of twin births in which one child was congenitally infected and the other was not. This is explained on the basis of separate placentas because identical twins, who share a single placenta, are either both infected or both uninfected.

Early Latency

When the skin rash of secondary syphilis disappears latency begins. This is a period when there are no clinical signs or symptoms of disease. The treponemes have disappeared from the skin and mucous surfaces, having entrenched themselves in the deeper tissues. Hence, there are no apparent, accessible lesions from which organisms can be demonstrated. However, a diagnosis of syphilis may be made on the basis of a positive serologic test.

Occasionally the early months of latency are interrupted by relapses to secondary syphilis. A skin rash may appear that is dark-field-positive. Spirochetes have obviously emerged from the deeper tissues and spread via the blood to the superficial tissues of the body, namely the skin and mucous membranes. The patient is therefore once again infectious to contacts and to the fetus.

The Boeck–Bruusgaard study of untreated syphilitics in Oslo, Norway, showed that only 25% of persons suffer a secondary relapse, about one-fourth of these suffering multiple relapses (Brown *et al.* 1970:19; Kampmeier 1974:1350). Although all relapses were noted within the first 5 years of illness, most occurred in the first year and almost all (97%) occurred within the first 2 years. Therefore, early latency—the period of latency that is potentially infectious—may for all practical purposes be defined as syphilis of less than 2 years' duration. Nevertheless, some health agencies and researchers still prefer to define early latency as syphilis of less than 4 years' duration for statistical purposes.

Because the lesions of secondary relapses, like those of secondary syphilis, may be difficult to see or may appear only on the mucous membranes of the mouth or genitals, some relapses may have been overlooked in the Boeck–Bruusgaard study. Perhaps more than 25% of patients relapsed and more than 3% of these relapses occurred more than 2 years after infection. It seems unlikely, however, that increases in these figures would be significant enough to force a reassessment of the epidemiology of infectious syphilis. Indeed, many health departments in the United States have compressed the period designated as early latency, maintaining that only syphilis of less than 1 year's duration is significantly infectious to be of epidemiological importance (see Brown *et al.* 1970:25; U.S. Public Health Service 1968:23).

During the first 2 years of infection, from shortly after exposure until the end of early latency, individuals with syphilis are potentially infectious. Both close contacts (most especially sexual contacts) and the fetus are at risk of acquiring the infection. But it does not appear that humans transmit the disease as readily as experimental studies might indicate. Although studies in rabbits and humans have indicated that only a small number of organisms are necessary to infect (Cannefax 1965:271), it is estimated that under natural conditions only 10–50% of persons exposed to infectious syphilis become infected (Benenson 1975:316; Cannefax 1965:261). This variable response is due to a variety of factors including host resistance (see the section ''Immunity''), degree of exposure, and stage of the disease, the moist lesions of secondary syphilis being the most infectious.

Late Latency

Late latency begins 1–4 years following infection, depending on the definition used. At this time secondary relapses are so rare as to be inconsequential on the population level. The patient is dark-field-negative and seropositive, titers falling slowly as the disease becomes more chronic. The spirochetes have now retreated permanently to the deeper tissues. Spirochetemia is absent.[1] Because spirochetes are no longer circulating in the blood, they are consequently absent from the skin, mucous membranes, saliva, semen, vaginal discharges, etc. Thus, neither the fetus nor contacts can be infected.

Nevertheless, many sources—even highly reliable, authoritative ones such as Brown *et al.* (1970:26–27), authors of *Syphilis and Other Venereal Diseases*, the U.S. Public Health Service (1968:74–75) publication, *Syphilis, A Synopsis*, and Cave *et al.* (1971:947), authors of the *Encyclopaedia Britannica* article on syphilis—have stated that syphilis of more than 4 years' duration is rarely communicable except in the case of a pregnant woman who may transmit the disease to the fetus regardless of the duration of her disease. Two of these sources (Brown *et al.* 1970:26; U.S. Public Health Service 1968:75) have stated that even *late* syphilis is infectious for the fetus. And Brown *et al.* (1970:26) noted that an untreated syphilitic woman (duration of infection unspecified) has only a slight chance of giving birth to a healthy, uninfected baby.

Nevertheless, it is unreasonable to suggest that the fetus can be infected when contacts are not at risk. If spirochetes are in the blood, a necessary condition for fetal infection, they should also be found in the skin, mucous membranes, saliva, semen, vaginal discharges, or elsewhere so that contacts are also at risk, although this may be a somewhat

---

[1]Cannefax (1965:271) cited a study in which organisms were isolated from the lymph node of one patient with latent syphilis and the semen of another patient with latent syphilis. The latter was undoubtedly infectious to sexual contacts and should be considered to be suffering from a secondary relapse. Whether a syphilis-positive lymph node indicates a secondary relapse and, therefore, infectiousness, is unknown. Because the lymph and blood systems are interconnected it is easy for organisms in one to gain entrance to the other. But if the studies in filariasis can be applied to syphilis—microfilariae are absent from the blood despite their presence in the lymphatics if antifilarial antibody titers are high (Ottesen 1980:4)—then untreated syphilitics with significant antibody levels may be expected to remain blood-negative even though spirochetes are found in the lymph nodes.

lower risk. Thus, if late latency is not infectious for contacts it should not be infectious for the fetus. This alternative position is taken by a number of equally reliable and authoritative sources (e.g., Kissane and Smith 1967:58). The entire issue of fetal infection is discussed in more detail in the section "Pregnancy Loss."

We believe that the situation of when syphilis is infectious and to whom is closely analogous to that seen with hepatitis B, formerly known as serum hepatitis. When tests indicate the presence of hepatitis B virus particles in an individual's blood, that individual is considered infectious. Although the infection is most easily transmitted through the exchange of blood or blood products containing infectious virus (fetal infection is possible), the semen, saliva, etc. also may contain virus and thus close personal, and especially sexual, contacts are at risk of being infected. But once the virus has disappeared from the blood neither it nor the body secretions are infectious and transmission is not possible (Benenson 1975:144–147; Corsaro and Korzeniowsky 1980:44–51).

Late Syphilis

After 5 to 20 years or more of latency, symptomatic syphilis may appear as gummas of the skin, bone, or viscera (late benign syphilis) and/or as lesions of the cardiovascular or nervous systems. Late syphilis develops in about 28% of persons (30% of men and 26% of women) with untreated syphilis. About half of all persons with late syphilis will be incapacitated or killed and half will develop only benign disease (Cave *et al.* 1971:947; Termini and Music 1972:243).

The gummas of late syphilis are believed due to a hyperimmune (i.e., allergic) phenomenon and rarely contain parasites. These gummas are the essential lesions of late benign syphilis. The term *benign* is used because these lesions are rarely incapacitating or life-threatening. Nevertheless, when vital organs such as the brain are involved, the situation is far from benign. Usually, however, the skin or bone is involved. Bone lesions, which usually involve the cranial bones, tibia, or clavicle, are associated with bony tumor, pain, and swelling. Destructive skin lesions are frequently encountered. These may be very disfiguring and often resemble carcinoma (U.S. Public Health Service 1968:83, 85).

The lesions of cardiovascular syphilis and neurosyphilis are caused by inflammatory changes in blood vessels, which are excited by the presence of spirochetes. The lumen of the vessel becomes narrowed, perhaps completely obliterated, and the surrounding tissue develops inflammatory and necrotic changes. Hence, syphilis is a vascular disease from beginning to end (U.S. Public Health Service 1968:75). Spirochetes can be demonstrated in late lesions of the cardiovascular or nervous systems if special stains are used (U.S. Public Health Service 1968:31). Serologic tests are usually reactive, and high titers are frequently present in persons with late benign syphilis or a type of neurosyphilis known as paresis (U.S. Public Health Service 1968:75). Late syphilis is not infectious to contacts. Whether the fetus is in jeopardy is a matter of dispute, as mentioned earlier.

Cardiovascular syphilis and neurosyphilis are the most feared sequelae of infection with *T. pallidum* because they may totally incapacitate or kill their victims. Cardiovascular syphilis affects the aorta, the great vessel that leaves the heart, and is usually rapidly fatal. Neurosyphilis may take many forms depending on which part of the nervous system is affected. Involvement of the optic nerve leads to blindness; involvement of the brain results in a condition known as paresis, a type of insanity that until recently accounted for a significant number of admissions to mental hospitals. And if the spinal cord is involved, a crippling disease known as tabes dorsalis or locomotor ataxia occurs. The categories of late syphilis are not mutually exclusive and a patient may have more than one type of involvement; late benign syphilis may coexist with cardiovascular or neurosyphilis, and some patients have both cardiovascular syphilis and neurosyphilis (U.S. Public Health Service 1968:76).

Interestingly, there are dramatic race and sex differences in the type of syphilis that will occur. Cardiovascular syphilis is twice as frequent in blacks as in whites, whereas white rates of neurosyphilis are three times those seen in blacks. And women, who are somewhat less likely to develop late syphilis, are also less likely to develop severe sequelae such as cardiovascular syphilis or neurosyphilis, thereby accounting for their significantly lower syphilis mortality rates.

Immunity

Are all persons equally susceptible to infection with *T. pallidum*? Are superinfection and reinfection possible? How does treatment affect susceptibility? These are important questions because their answers determine how many times an individual can experience the early stages of syphilis and therefore be infectious to contacts and to the fetus.

Cannefax (1965:260), in his review of immunity in syphilis, remarks that ''the subject is fraught with numerous divergencies of opinion and interpretations of experimental data. There are those who are convinced that true immunity in syphilis does not exist and there are others who are equally convinced that immunity does occur in certain circumstances." With these difficulties in mind, the subject of immunity in syphilis—natural immunity, acquired immunity, and cross-immunity— will be explored.

Natural Immunity

That not all persons exposed to primary and secondary syphilis become infected—figures of 10% (Benenson 1975:316) and 50% (von Werssowetz 1948, cited in Cannefax 1965:261) have been cited—suggests that some natural immunity could exist. However, as noted by Cannefax (1965:261), there are other factors that could account for the variable response such as degree and duration of contact, numbers of organisms present at the contact site, relative virulence of the organisms, and the role of physical and systemic factors, and these factors are impossible to measure. Cannefax believed that man does not possess any significant innate resistance or immunity to infection, and that the principal defense against syphilitic infection is an intact skin and mucous membrane. Although he noted that differences exist in the course of the disease and in clinical manifestations and could be associated with immunity phenomena, they could just as well be associated with environmental and physiological factors. Nevertheless, there are records of many contacts who have been repeatedly exposed to the lesions of syphilis but who never develop clinical or serological signs of infection (Brown *et al.* 1970:22), and for these few individuals a natural immunity is probable.

Acquired Immunity

The question of whether or not acquired immunity exists in syphilis is much debated. The participants in this debate are divided into two groups. One group maintains that individuals can resist infection only if they maintain an infection, that is, if they harbor live spirochetes, and that adequate treatment allows reinfection. In short, they believe that reinfection is possible but that superinfection is not. The second group maintains that resistance to infection can exist in the absence of current infection, but that the level of this resistance is directly related to the duration of disease prior to its termination by adequate treatment (Cannefax 1965:262).

The views of the second group are more widely accepted, and resistance to reinfection apparently does exist under certain circumstances. Possible variables in the determination of the degree of resistance are (1) the duration of the infection, (2) the number of organisms in the challenge inoculum, (3) whether or not the challenge is by an homologous or heterologous strain of *T. pallidum*, (4) whether or not the infection has been treated or left untreated, and (5) its duration before treatment.

Duration of Infection

Infection with *T. pallidum* leads to gradually developing resistance, but this resistance is not absolute and can be overcome under certain conditions. For example, experiments in humans have shown that resistance wanes with time and thus superinfection is possible in late syphilis, producing an asymptomatic infection. (Asymptomatic infections are those in which the patient shows no signs or symptoms of disease, but antibody titers rise and transfer to an animal of lymph node material that was previously negative results in a syphilitic infection.)

Inoculum Size–Strain Homology

Animal studies suggest that resistance can also be overcome if the challenge inoculum contains a large number of organisms. Animal experiments have also shown that syphilitic infection results in good immunity to the homologous (identical) strain of syphilis, but only partial immunity to heterologous (different) strains. However, some workers have questioned just how frequently these conditions—challenge with a large number of organisms and exposure to a heterologous strain of *T. pallidum*—are encountered in nature and result in superinfection in humans. Indeed, Cannefax (1965:264) has urged a reevaluation of certain ideas about immunity in syphilis because many of the animal experiments upon which these ideas are based are seriously flawed, frequently because they used unnaturally high numbers of organisms to challenge. For example, those studies that show only partial immunity to heterologous strains have used challenge inocula containing hundreds or even thousands of times the number of organisms necessary to initiate an infection. Because only very high levels of immunity could overcome such a challenge, the ability of the animal to resist infections with heterologous strains under natural conditions of doze size may be underestimated. Indeed, early experiments in humans by Eberson (1921, cited in Cannefax 1965:270–271) have shown that if antitreponemal antibody exists in a patient's serum, this antibody is effective against all challenge strains, preventing infection in all cases. These results have been confirmed by the more recent animal studies of Turner and Hollander (1957, cited in Cannefax 1965:266), which showed that 3 of 17 natural strains of syphilis gave some degree of protection against inoculation with the laboratory (Nichol's) strain and the remaining 14 strains appeared to be antigenically identical to the laboratory strain (and, by extension, with each other), granting complete immunity. Furthermore, it would be difficult to explain why infection with a heterologous strain of *T. pallidum* would not produce a good level of protective immunity, yet infection with a completely different species, such as *T. pertenue*, does produce good protection (see the section "Cross-Immunity"). For all practical purposes, then, an untreated person is resistant to superinfection.

Treatment Status

If persons with syphilis are treated, their ability to resist reinfection depends on the adequacy of treatment and when it was initiated. Magnuson *et al.* (1956:74) observed that resistance to reinfection is greatest among persons with the highest antibody titers and that titers are a reliable prognosticator of the ability to resist infection.[2] In adequately treated cases of primary syphilis, antibody titers should become nonreactive 6–12 months after treatment; with secondary syphilis seronegativity is reached in 12 to 18 months. Treatment of a late latent or late infection usually has little or no effect on titer, whereas treatment of an early latent infection may produce a titer response characteristic of either treated secondary syphilis or treated late latent syphilis (U.S. Public Health Service 1968:99–100). Thus, most persons cured of syphilis during the earliest stages quickly become susceptible to reinfection. (Often such reinfections are diagnosed as relapses because there is no way to differentiate the two.) But only about half of persons treated for syphilis during latency are susceptible to reinfection, susceptibility varying inversely with the duration of infection before treatment.

If an infection is inadequately treated during the early stages of the disease when antibodies are developing, an antibody titer intermediate to that attained by treated and untreated patients develops. Animal studies show that inadequate treatment early in the course of the disease diminishes the rate of development of immunity to one-sixth that of an untreated infection. This lower antibody level accounts for the frequency of relapses in cases treated early but inadequately. Superinfections are probably also possible in such persons.

[2]On the other hand, Fiumara (1974:1120) has stated that neither reagin nor the antitreponemal antibodies detected by the usual serologic tests are responsible for the observed protection, because reinfection may occur in their presence.

The study conducted in the early 1950s by the U.S. Public Health Service (Magnuson *et al.* 1956) offers the best data on the risk of infection in persons who have had syphilis and controls. Sixty-two prisoners at Sing Sing Prison volunteered to be inoculated with syphilis; 54 had verified histories of syphilis and 8 had no history or evidence of infection. The challenge inoculum was a rather severe one, 2000 times that needed to produce an infection in 50% of susceptible persons. Persons with no history of syphilis showed no resistance to infection. Previously treated syphilitics showed a wide spectrum of reactions to the challenge of reinfection, resistance being directly related to the time between acquiring syphilis and receiving treatment. Thus, all persons who had been treated for early syphilis were reinfected, but only 38% of those treated for late latent syphilis were reinfected. Most importantly, those persons "with untreated latent syphilis showed no clinical or serologic response to challenge and are presumed to have been resistant to reinfection" (Magnuson *et al.* 1956:79). The level of antibody titer was of primary importance in this case; resistance to infection was greatest among persons with the highest titers. Among treated syphilitics, titers (and resistance to reinfection) decreased as the time between infection and treatment became shorter. Titers were highest among untreated syphilitics.

Cross-Immunity

Cannefax (1965:265) noted that, historically, clinicians having experience with both syphilis and yaws have generally concluded that infection with one protects against infection with the other. Epidemiological data support this observation, yaws-endemic areas experiencing little syphilis; the inference is that having yaws in childhood protects the adult against syphilis. In those areas of Papua New Guinea that had 99.5% of the yaws cases only 1.2% of all syphilis cases were found. Conversely, where 98.8% of syphilis cases were encountered only 0.5% of yaws cases were reported (Willcox 1980b:280–281). This cross-immunity appears to exist among all four of the treponematoses—syphilis, endemic syphilis, pinta, and yaws. Wherever one is prevalent there is apparently strong resistance to infection with any of the others (Brown *et al.* 1970:143).

Curative treatment of one of these diseases will, however, jeopardize this resistance. As shown by Medina (1964, cited in Cannefax 1965:267), the duration of the disease prior to treatment is directly correlated to the ability to resist infection. One reason frequently cited for the increase in syphilis in the tropics is the loss of protective cross-immunity following the eradication of yaws (Arya and Lawson 1977:51; Harahap 1980:282; Kiraly 1973:120). Serologic surveys in areas with yaws showed that a large proportion (61.2%) of children younger than 14 years old had antibodies capable of immobilizing *T. pallidum*, but in areas where successful yaws campaigns had been conducted less than 1% of children had these antibodies (Willcox 1980b:280).

Summary of Pathophysiology and Immunity

Syphilis is transmissible to contacts and the fetus only when spirochetes are circulating in the blood. During this time highly infectious lesions of the skin or mucous membrane may appear, and body fluids, such as the semen, saliva, or vaginal discharges, may also contain infectious organisms.

The primary and secondary stages of syphilis are infectious. The latent stage is infectious in only a minority of cases, about 25% of infected persons experiencing one or more secondary relapses during the early years of latency. Thus, 75% of persons are no longer infectious after the secondary stage subsides, which is usually within 1 year of exposure, and most of the 25% who do have an extended period of infectiousness are no longer infectious 2 years postexposure.

There is little evidence for the existence of innate immunity and, therefore, all persons should be considered susceptible to infection with *T. pallidum*. Acquired immunity is a more complex situation. It is usually stated that an untreated syphilitic infection produces good immunity to identical strains of *T. pallidum* but only partial immunity to other strains, and that this immunity is not absolute and may be overcome by challenge with a large number of organisms. However, some studies have shown that there is good cross-immunity among different strains of venereal syphilis. And the studies that have concluded that large numbers of organisms can overcome immunity, although correct, have often used thousands of times the numbers of organisms necessary to initiate an infection, creating an artificial situation that does not reflect the doses encountered in nature, thereby underestimating the protective value of acquired levels of immunity. It can be concluded, therefore, that the evidence supports the idea that a syphilitic infection, if untreated, produces immunity levels adequate to prevent superinfection under normal (as opposed to laboratory) conditions. Acquired immunity does wane with the passage of time, however, and superinfection is possible in late syphilis.

If syphilis is treated in the primary or secondary stage, there is not sufficient time for adequate immunity to develop and reinfection is possible. The general rule is that the greater the duration of infection before treatment the greater the immunity to reinfection. The study of Magnuson *et al.* (1956) clearly illustrates this point, showing that all volunteers with previously treated early syphilis were susceptible to reinfection whereas only 38% of those treated for late latent syphilis could be reinfected. Thus, persons treated early in the disease may be reinfected at some later date and, therefore, be infectious to others once again. Those treated later in the disease are less likely to be reinfected. Untreated persons are, for all practical purposes, resistant to infection and can never again transmit the disease to others. Inadequate treatment presents a different set of responses. Inadequate treatment early in disease does not cure but does interfere with antibody production, so relapses and superinfections are possible. Inadequate treatment later in disease has no effect on immunity levels, the individual remaining resistant to infection.

There are extremely important concepts when trying to determine the impact of syphilis on reproductive potential, for they indicate that even before a cure was known, or in those contemporary societies where treatment is unavailable, the adverse effects of syphilis on pregnancy are rather limited. A woman will usually transmit the disease to her unborn child only during the first 2 years following infection. Untreated, she develops a good immunity and can never again be infected or infect anyone else.

In areas where childhood infection with one of the other treponematoses is common, cross-immunity offers protection against syphilis. Curative treatment early in the course of one of these diseases prevents the development of adequate levels of immunity and the individual is at risk of being infected with syphilis. In tropical areas where successful campaigns against yaws were conducted in the 1950s and early 1960s, populations who were theretofore resistant to syphilis became susceptible; syphilis rates are high in some of these areas.

Effects on Fecundity

Syphilis has frequently been mentioned in the literature as a cause of depopulation. Declines in population size in New Hebrides, Borneo, and Africa were attributed to syphilis, but in many cases later workers found that other diseases such as yaws and LGV had been misdiagnosed as syphilis (Scragg 1957:92–93). Whether syphilis can cause depopulation has been discussed by Belsey (1976), Romaniuk (1967), and Scragg (1957). Because syphilis has little or no direct effect on coital or conceptive ability (see following discussions), any effect on fertility levels must be the result of increased rates of pregnancy loss. And because as the infection becomes more chronic it becomes increasingly more likely that a live, unaffected child will be born, syphilis is a self-limiting factor in pregnancy loss (Belsey 1976:329). Therefore, a temporary decline in births due to high rates of pregnancy loss could be anticipated following the introduction of syphilis into a susceptible population, but with time a more normal pattern of births should be reestablished. Therefore, syphilis does not appear to be an important cause of depopulation.

Retel-Laurentin (1974) felt that this view is too restrictive and does not account for the fact that a spontaneous abortion, perhaps caused by syphilis, may be followed by a sterilizing genital infection. In her study of the Nzakara of central Africa, Retel-Laurentin (1974:69ff) found a low general fertility rate and a very high (40%) childlessness rate. She also found that 35% of the pregnancies were not carried to term and were often followed by sterility. Her research in the area, which included serologic testing, led her to conclude that the sterilizing abortions were the result of venereal disease, particularly syphilis.

Her conclusions have not gone unchallenged. Belsey (1976:324, 330) noted that her diagnoses were based on subjective clinical assessments and on serologic tests whose results could be confounded by crossreactions to yaws. He further noted that data from her 1973 studies in Upper Volta did not support a major role for syphilis in abortion and childlessness in two of the three villages studied. He and others (e.g., Gray 1977:21) felt that the observed association between syphilis and low fertility may merely reflect the presence of gonorrhea, because societies with high rates of syphilis also have high rates of gonorrhea.

Syphilis is, nevertheless, an undisputed and important cause of pregnancy loss and neonatal death on the individual level; in populations with high rates of infection, syphilis, though not a cause of childlessness or depopulation, can depress fertility rates somewhat via increased rates of pregnancy loss. The following discussion covers all aspects of syphilis and reproductive potential: coital inability, conceptive failure, and pregnancy loss. Special attention will be given to the effects of syphilis on pregnancy loss, particularly in terms of the variability of pregnancy outcome as to stage of syphilis, gestational age at time of infection, and the protective aspects of immunity.

Coital Inability

There is little evidence linking syphilis with significant levels of coital inability. Persons with neurosyphilis (about 8% of all persons with syphilis [U.S. Public Health Service 1968:76]), especially those with tabes dorsalis, frequently become impotent as the disease progresses. But because late syphilis usually occurs at the end of the reproductive period the impact on population fecundity is minimal.

Conceptive Failure

Syphilis is not an important cause of conceptive failure. Stokes (1935:222) noted that men with congenital syphilis have a tendency toward sterility because of syphilitic epididymitis. Syphilis may also cause male sterility via chronic orchitis. However, such cases are rare and syphilis can be considered only a very minor cause of conceptive failure (Barlovatz 1955:366).

Other Intermediate Variables

Although syphilis is not an important cause of either coital inability or conceptive failure, a few students of syphilis have reported that a large proportion of syphilitic couples are childless. Stix (1941:297) speculated that physicians "would doubtless have advised them to use contraceptive measures both for prophylaxis of the disease and to prevent pregnancy, and it is therefore probable that many of the childless syphilitic couples were childless because of their use of contraceptives."[3] Some of the older medical textbooks took this advice one step further and said intercourse should be avoided altogether for 2 years after infection. And one writer in the late nineteenth century questioned whether syphilitics should marry at all (see U.S. Public Health Service 1968:12). If this view seems a bit extreme, it should be remembered that

---

[3]This point is debatable. First, it is unlikely that the contraceptive methods used early in the century, no matter how carefully practiced, could have been so successful. Of course, abortion was used by some women if an unwanted pregnancy occurred. How many women used abortion can only be guesstimated, and how many of these women were aborting because they feared congenital syphilis is indeterminate. Second, it is not clear that physicians encouraged syphilitic patients to use contraception. A study in the early 1900s among a group of indigent urban women receiving therapeutic abortions showed that not one of these women, who had preexisting medical conditions that made pregnancy dangerous, had been instructed by a doctor in how to prevent conception.

between 1937 and 1946—that is, between the time states began to require a blood test before issuance of a marriage license and the time when a practical cure for syphilis was introduced—many syphilitics in the United States were effectively forbidden to marry. Interestingly, the U.S. birthrate began to rise after 1936, and it is possible that excluding syphilitics from marriage helped increase the birthrate. Probably then, syphilis had a greater effect on fertility levels via intermediate variables such as contraceptive use, coital frequency, and marital frequency than via coital inability or conceptive failure.

Pregnancy Loss

Even the very earliest accounts of syphilis noted that the disease occurred in newborns. At first, infection at the time of parturition or via infected milk was suspected. Paracelsus was the first, in 1530, to report that the child was infected in utero. But he and others were misled by the fact that so many mothers of syphilitic children appeared to be uninfected and thought the fathers were responsible, directly infecting the ovum at the time of conception. This misconception persisted until serologic tests were developed in the early twentieth century revealing that the mother was always infected.

Outcome of Pregnancy in Regard to Duration of Maternal Infection and Fetal Age at Time of Infection

The outcome of pregnancy in syphilitic women varies greatly. The pregnancy may terminate as a second- or third-trimester abortion, stillbirth, or live birth with a congenitally infected infant who may show signs of infection immediately after birth and die neonatally or who may appear normal at birth but develop signs and symptoms of congenital syphilis in the future. Or the pregnancy may terminate with the birth of a normal child. Two interdependent variables determine the outcome: (1) the stage of syphilis the mother is experiencing and (2) the stage of gestation at which the fetus is infected. The first variable, stage of maternal infection, influences whether or not the fetus will be infected and the severity of that infection. Generally, if the mother is experiencing primary or secondary syphilis spirochetemia is intense; the fetus has little chance of escaping infection and the fetal infection will be severe. The second variable, gestational stage at time of fetal infection, now comes into play. If the maternal infection occurs just prior to or early in pregnancy the fetus is likely to be infected early in gestation and fetal death is the most probable outcome. If the woman is infected later in pregnancy, the child will be born alive but will soon develop severe early congenital syphilis. If, on the other hand, the mother's infection is old and spirochetemia less intense, even children infected early in pregnancy may be born alive and suffer only mild congenital syphilis. And with even older infections spirochetemia may be very low or absent, so the child is spared altogether. Thus, the spectrum of possible outcomes in pregnant women with syphilis depends on the stage of the disease and how early the fetus is infected.

When Syphilis Is Transmissible to the Fetus as Reported in the Literature

Unfortunately, the literature does not present a unified front with regard to when syphilis may be transmitted to the fetus; this has created a great deal of confusion and some misconceptions about the impact of the disease on population subfecundity. Generally, early sources reported that syphilitic infection in a pregnant woman, duration unspecified, results in fetal infection, whereas more recent sources allotted risk according to the duration of the mother's infection, recent infections resulting in fetal involvement but infections of 2 or more years' duration posing little threat to the child. However, even some of the more recent sources have reported an extended period, often of unspecified duration, during which syphilis is infectious to the fetus. For example, Witters and Jones-Witters (1980:328) stated a woman can infect the fetus in the latent stage even when she is not infectious to anyone else. Cave *et al.* (1971:947) agreed, saying that women with latent syphilis frequently give birth to children with congenital syphilis. And a 1972 article in *Newsweek* (1972:48) stated: "But the mother, even in the latent stage, can infect her unborn child, causing death or severe deformities of the bones and teeth." Similarly, the U.S. Public Health Service (1968:74–75) reported that although syphilis is rarely communicable to others after the first few years, it can still be transmitted to the fetus. And Brown *et al.* (1970:26) reported that late syphilis is not infectious except to the fetus. A most extreme view is taken by Siegler (1944:427), who stated that even a woman with congenital syphilis can infect her child. Holder and Knox (1972:1152–1153) also said that third-generation syphilis exists, but added that it is extremely rare and suggested that some cases undoubtedly represent superinfection. However, most workers (e.g., Brown *et al.* 1970:26) believe that only women with acquired infections can transmit the infection to the fetus.

We agree that fetal infection may occur during latency, but it is regrettable that some of these authors did not specify that only early latency is a significant risk to the fetus, not latency of 5, 10 or 15 years' duration. One of these authors, Witters and Jones-Witters (1980:328), did go on to say that the more recent the infection, the more likely it was that the fetus would be infected. We do not believe that fetal infection during late syphilis or third-generation syphilis is possible; cases so recorded almost certainly represent superinfection. Finally, we believe that if spirochetemia is present, as it must be for fetal infection to occur, other body fluids may contain spirochetes and therefore contacts, as well as the fetus, are at risk.

Other authors agree with this position. In 1961 Blattner (1961:626) stated that ''pregnancy occurring in women with recent infection results almost invariably in miscarriage, stillbirth, or in congenital syphilis in the child. *Women who become pregnant some years after infection give birth to normal children as a rule''* [emphasis added]. Kissane (1975:58) further clarified the risk:

> Congenital syphilis is acquired by the fetus of an infected mother by passage of *Treponema pallidum* across the placenta. Since intrauterine infection requires spirochetemia (spirochetes circulating in the blood) in the mother, the maternal infection is usually recently acquired, almost always within two years. Pregnancies beyond this period usually produce normal infants even when the mother has received no treatment. (From John M. Kissane, 1975, *Pathology of infancy and childhood* [2nd edition]. St. Louis, MO: The C. V. Mosby Co.)

Probability of Fetal Infection as Reported in the Literature

Concomitant with the development of a refined definition of when syphilis is transmissible to the fetus came changes in assessments of the proportion of syphilitic pregnancies that have a negative outcome. Early in this century Stokes (1919:82) said that 75% of children born to syphilitic parents would be aborted, stillborn, or die of congenital syphilis before their first birthday. In the early 1930s McCord (cited in McKelvey and Turner 1934:506) found a 66% stillbirth rate in one series of syphilitic mothers and an 80% stillbirth rate in a second series. McKelvey and Turner (1934:506) found a significantly lower 46% stillbirth rate in their series. They reasoned that this lower rate was possibly due to (1) routine serologic testing in their clinic over a period of many years, which would add to the group of syphilitic mothers many women who would have otherwise passed unrecognized and (2) the use of a sensitive serologic test that identified women with long-standing infections who would be more likely to give birth to normal children. And Brown *et al.* (1970:26) felt that even McKelvey and Turner's estimates were too high because the study sample was a relatively small group of clinic patients among whom health standards were low and morbidity indices for all diseases high.

It seems likely then that many of the earlier assessments of risk were based on the outcome of pregnancy in women with visible signs of syphilis (lesions of primary or secondary syphilis) or with titers high enough to be detected by tests insensitive by today's standards (titers are highest during secondary and early latent syphilis). Also, in these women unfavorable pregnancy outcomes were probably attributed to syphilis even though in some cases a coexisting factor may have been the cause. Hence, to say a pregnant woman with syphilis, duration of disease unspecified, suffers the outcomes experienced by these women is to overstate the case grossly.

Nevertheless, many workers continue to cite the results of early studies. Farley (1970:222), using sources from the 1940s and early 1950s, stated that, if no care is given, 30–50% of pregnancies in syphilitic women will end in fetal deaths, and of those infants born alive up to 20% will die of congenital syphilis shortly after birth. He went on to quote Moore (1941, cited in Farley 1970:222), who said that "a syphilitic woman, untreated, has only one chance in six of bearing a healthy live infant as compared with a normal woman's three chances in four." Citing a 1941 article by Top, Bwibo (1971:188) also recounted that an untreated woman with syphilis has only one chance in six of having a healthy child. Similarly, a 1972 article by Holder and Knox (1972:1152), relying on Thomas's 1949 data stated that "normal children are born to only about 30 percent of women who have an untreated *late* syphilitic infection" [emphasis added].

The above assessments are more accurately applied to women with early syphilis, that is, with primary, secondary, or early latent syphilis. Barrett-Connor (1969:281) reported a 30% fetal death rate and a 70% congenital syphilis rate in live-born infants for women with untreated syphilis, but specified that this applies only to women with untreated early syphilis. Bai *et al.* (1972:174) reported similar figures, and they too specified that such outcomes apply only to early syphilis. And Gray (1977:21) reported that high rates of spontaneous abortion are associated only with early syphilis, the risk of fetal loss in late syphilis approaching normal levels. In many cases those who overstate the case know that risk decreases substantially with time but fail to be specific, and therefore their statements are misleading. Thomas Parran (1937:300), whose book *Shadow on the Land* did so much to awaken Americans to the syphilis problem, noted that the chances of bearing a diseased child decrease with time and previous treatment, but still made the blanket statement that five of six children born to untreated syphilitics will be dead or diseased.

Our view is that the fetus is at significant risk only when the mother's infection is of less than 2 years' duration. Even the most conservative estimates do not place the child at risk if the infection is of more than 4 years' duration. After this time an untreated woman has every reason to expect a healthy child. And even before this time chances are good an unaffected child will be born if the infection is of more than 1 year's duration. Syphilis, then, is not a cause of low fertility. Perhaps one child, even two, is lost early in reproductive life due to syphilis, but that is all. And although a sterilizing infection is possible following a spontaneous abortion, especially in developing countries, this probably does not occur with sufficient frequency to be important on the population level. Thus, fertility rates may be lowered somewhat if syphilis is very prevalent, but syphilis is not an important cause of low fertility and/or childlessness.

The Placental Barrier

The syphilis literature has been marred by still other erroneous fixed ideas. For example, vaccine research was stymied for decades because a misclassification of *T. pallidum* went unchallenged until the mid-1970s (see "Treatment" section). One of the most persistent myths in the syphilis literature is that of the placental barrier. For many years the placenta was believed to be a barrier that could permit oxygen and nutrients to pass to the fetus but would selectively exclude harmful substances and organisms. This was shown to be more wishful thinking than scientific fact after the tragic sequelae of congenital rubella were identified and the teratogenic potential of thalidomide revealed. It soon became apparent that pathogenic organisms, drugs, and chemicals of every sort could pass the placenta. Nevertheless, a certain element of the placental barrier theory persisted, namely, that the Langhans' layer of the chorion acts as a mechanical barrier to the spirochete of syphilis until after the sixteenth week of pregnancy. At this time the layer supposedly atrophies and fetal infection becomes possible.

The theory that the early placenta was impenetrable by *T. pallidum* was widely accepted and appeared in textbooks of obstetrics, pediatrics, and pathology. The theory was based on the observations of Dippel in 1944 and of a number of earlier workers that congenital syphilis did not occur until after the first trimester of pregnancy. But as early as 1962 Silverstein suggested that the reason for this was not due to a placental barrier but to the fact that not until the second trimester has the fetus developed an immune system capable of recognizing the antigen of syphilis as foreign and mounting an inflammatory response that culminates in fetal death and expulsion and is recognized by the physician as congenital syphilis. Before this time the immunoincompetent fetus lives in harmony with the spirochete and other pathogens, such as *Toxoplasma gondii*, the parasite that causes congenital toxoplasmosis. Modern electron microscopy supports Silverstein's theory, as electron micrographs show that the cells of the Langhans' layer do not disappear and there is no evidence that the placenta becomes more permeable as pregnancy progresses (Benirschke 1974:143).

Harter and Benirschke (1976:709–710) further debunked the placental barrier theory by finding spirochetes in 40% of the aborted fetuses of women with recent syphilitic infections. These fetuses were only of 9 to 10 weeks' gestation. The authors were not surprised that earlier studies did not detect signs of congenital syphilis as the spirochetes were scarce and were not associated with tissue destruction or an inflammatory response. In addition, earlier studies had very few early gestations (< 18 weeks) to investigate, and frequently specimens were not fresh. Because organisms were so rare in the early fetus, the authors concluded that there must be an initial barrier to their transmission. But they felt it is more likely a biochemical barrier, not a mechanical one.

Despite Silverstein's work in the early 1960s on the development of immunological competence in the fetus and the doubt this cast on the placental barrier theory, many workers continued to cite this theory. The section on congenital syphilis in the U.S. Public Health Service (1968:86) publication *Syphilis, A Synopsis* begins: ''After the 18th week of gestation, when the Langhan's cell layer of the early placenta has atrophied, the treponeme may cross the placenta to infect the fetus.'' Even as late as 1974 many textbooks in obstetrics still stated that congenital syphilis occurs only in the second half of pregnancy because of the placental barrier (see Benirschke 1974:143).

Congenital Syphilis

Congenital syphilis has a broad spectrum of manifestations. The child may be spontaneously aborted sometime after the fourth month, be stillborn, be born alive but soon die from a fulminating infection, or be born alive but not show signs of congenital syphilis for months, years, or even decades. And many congenital syphilitics remain asymptomatic their entire lives.

Congenital syphilis has been divided into two categories (U.S. Public Health Service 1968:86–89): early congenital syphilis, in which signs and symptoms appear before age 2, and late congenital syphilis, in which signs and symptoms have persisted or appear beyond 2 years of age. In early congenital syphilis, the earlier the onset of symptoms in the first few weeks of life the poorer the prognosis. Signs and symptoms of early congenital syphilis include bone changes, anemia, hepatosplenomegaly, and skin and mucous membrane lesions, which are essentially those of secondary syphilis. (There is no primary stage in congenital syphilis because the treponemes are introduced directly into the fetal circulation.) However, unlike the secondary lesions of acquired syphilis, these are frequently fluid- filled (vesicular) and are extremely infectious.

It was originally thought that if the child did not exhibit signs and symptoms of congenital syphilis by 6 months it was not infected. Of course this is not true. Often congenital syphilis is not apparent until the second or third decade of life. For example, interstitial keratitis,[4] a type of blindness caused by syphilis, usually appears during puberty. Deafness, a rare manifestation of congenital syphilis, also usually appears during puberty, but may be delayed until middle age. Paresis (syphilitic insanity) may also be delayed until adulthood. Fortunately, the signs and symptoms of congenital syphilis are often less debilitating than these examples. Frequently only bone or tooth development is altered. Unusually shaped teeth such as notched, barrel-shaped incisors (Hutchinson's teeth) or round molars (Moon's molars) may be seen. And thickening of the tibia causes a skeletal deformity called saber shins. And in 60% of persons with congenital syphilis the disease is latent and a reactive serologic test is the only indication that the individual is infected (U.S. Public Health Service 1968:86–91).

Concomitant with the post-1957 rise in the incidence of infectious syphilis there was an increase in congenital syphilis worldwide. Nevertheless, because of good prenatal care congenital syphilis remains a rarity in the developed countries. But in some developing countries congenital syphilis is a problem. Congenital syphilis is reported to be common in Ethiopia, Uganda, and Mexico (Willcox 1977:216) and in Nairobi, Kenya (Bwibo 1971:187). But just as the prevalence of acquired syphilis in the tropical world is difficult to measure because of difficulties

---

[4]Interstitial keratitis was an important cause of blindness. In 1940 it was responsible for an estimated 7.9% of all legal blindness in the U.S. By 1957 this figure was reduced to 3.8%. In children of school age syphilis was a cause of blindness in 5.2% of all cases in 1934, but in only 1.4% in 1955. Encouraging as these figures are, it should still be noted that in 1957 in the United States there were an estimated 12,800 cases of legal blindness caused by syphilis (Brown *et al.* 1970:131, 133).

in making a differential diagnosis, so too is the prevalence of congenital syphilis there made more difficult because of confusion with other common disorders. In the past, for example, cases of kwashiorkor and sickle-cell disease were probably misdiagnosed as congenital syphilis (Bwibo 1971:185).

A diagnosis of congenital syphilis rests on a positive serologic test together with any clinical signs and symptoms of disease. If congenital syphilis is suspected at birth, a serologic test should be done immediately. A positive test at this time does not necessarily mean congenital syphilis, however, because the child may have passively received antibodies from the mother. But if the child's serum is reactive at two tubes higher dilution than the mother's, this is evidence of fetal infection. A rising titer is also diagnostic, as is a test (the fluorescent treponemal antibody absorption test, immunoglobulin M; FTA-ABS IgM) that detects a class of antisyphilis antibodies of high molecular weight, which are almost always fetal in origin because they are too large to cross the placenta. If congenital syphilis is suspected but the serologic tests are negative, the tests should be repeated a few weeks later because the fetus may not be immediately seropositive if it was infected late in pregnancy (Holder and Knox 1972:1157–1158).

Diagnosis

Difficulties in Making a Diagnosis

Before the development in 1906 of the Wasserman test a diagnosis of syphilis was based on clinical observations. Given that syphilis is frequently asymptomatic in the early stages, that lesions may be confined to inapparent sites such as the cervix, and that when symptoms are apparent they resemble those of many other conditions, the physician's task of establishing a diagnosis was difficult indeed. (The signs and symptoms of the different stages of syphilis have already been discussed in the section ''Pathophysiology.'')

That job was and still is particularly difficult for physicians in the developing world where there exist many diseases that resemble syphilis clinically, and some (endemic syphilis, yaws, and pinta) that are clinically similar *and* give a positive reaction to all available serologic tests and dark-field microscopy. Scragg (1957:92), for example, found no syphilis in New Ireland in the 1950s and believed that earlier reports of syphilis were probably LGV or yaws. He also believed that the syphilis that was reported in New Hebrides was, in fact, yaws. And Bwibo (1971:185) reported that studies in the 1920s and 1930s that found congenital syphilis to be a major cause of infant death in Mulago Hospital in Kampala, Uganda, were probably cases of kwashiorkor or sickle-cell disease misdiagnosed as congenital syphilis. He speculated that positive serologic tests in the past were not due to syphilis but to yaws, which was common in Kampala then.

Making a differential diagnosis of syphilis is still difficult in the developing world. Willcox (1977:211) believed that in some developing countries the incidence of syphilis is overstated because chancroid, herpes, and other genital sores may be diagnosed as syphilis on clinical grounds and serologic results confused with past yaws. And Arya and Lawson (1977:54–55) noted that in yaws-endemic areas, where a differential diagnosis may be impossible, health workers—aware of the dangers of untreated syphilis—opt to diagnose all genital sores as syphilis and treat accordingly.

A positive diagnosis is more easily made in the United States and other developed countries where serologic testing is widely employed and there are no coexisting treponematoses. Routine serologic testing of young people at several important points in life (before marriage, during pregnancy, and upon entering the armed forces) has allowed many subclinical cases to be diagnosed and treated. However, some U.S. health officials have suggested that states abandon the required premarital exam for syphilis because it is not, in their view, cost-effective; $80 million is spent each year to test about 4 million people, fewer than 500 of whom are found to be infected (see Kotulak 1981:14H). These individuals have noted that in the United States syphilis is primarily a disease of homosexuals, who do not apply for marriage licenses, and have maintained that prenatal exams would effectively limit the risk of congenital syphilis. Other health workers have rigorously opposed any move to abolish the premarital exams that have been in effect since the late 1930s, noting that these exams have been so successful in containing the disease that it would be risky to discontinue them.

Laboratory Diagnosis

Because the signs and symptoms of syphilis resemble those of so many other diseases, laboratory tests are a necessary adjunct to the clinician's observational skills. Two types of laboratory tests are available for the diagnosis of syphilis, dark-field microscopy and serology.

Dark-field Microscopy

Although the results of serologic tests make a good case for or against a treponemal infection, dark-field microscopy is the only test that allows a diagnosis to be made with 100% confidence. In addition, it is the only test that can be used in the very earliest weeks of the infection before the serum has become reactive. Dark-field microscopy is, however, not available at all health facilities, as it requires a specially adapted microscope and, more importantly, an experienced observer.

The spirochete of syphilis must be observed in the living state to permit accurate identification. Usual microscopic techniques with the light entering from below are not adequate. But with the light source at the side, the spirochetes reflect the light and are easily visible against the dark background. In the living state the pathogenic treponemes of yaws, pinta, and syphilis demonstrate characteristic movements that, together with certain morphological features, enable an experienced observer to differentiate them from nonpathogenic treponemes that are common in healthy individuals.

Syphilis may be diagnosed by dark-field microscopy only during the primary and secondary stages, during infectious relapses, and in early congenital syphilis when there are accessible skin and mucous membrane lesions from which infected fluid can be drawn. Frequently, enlarged lymph nodes are associated with these lesions and these too usually yield large numbers of organisms. If the initial attempt reveals no spirochetes, additional attempts should be made on the next 2 days before a negative diagnosis is rendered. The patient should be questioned as to whether local antiseptics have been applied to the lesions or antibiotics taken, as the spirochetes will be immobilized under such conditions, giving negative test results. Dark-field microscopy will also be negative if the lesions are old and beginning to heal or if they are the lesions of late syphilis (gummas).

Serology

Since Wasserman's discovery of a serologic test for syphilis over 200 such tests have been devised, of which only a few are currently used. These tests fall into two categories, the nontreponemal tests and the treponemal tests. Wasserman's original test was a nontreponemal test in that it tested for a substance in the blood called reagin, which, although produced by the body in response to syphilis, is also produced in response to a number of other nontreponemal diseases. Thus, per-

sons with a positive Wasserman or other nontreponemal test,[5] such as
the Venereal Disease Research Laboratory test (VDRL), must be given
a second, more specific test, the treponemal test. The treponemal test
looks for antibodies that can immobilize *T. pallidum* or form antibody–
antigen complexes with extracts of treponemes. The treponemal tests
are positive only if the patient has at some time been infected with *T.
pallidum* or one of the other pathogenic treponemes.

The treponema immobilization test (TPI), the earliest of the treponemal tests, is rarely used because it is time-consuming, technically difficult, and costly. Nevertheless, its great specificity makes it the standard
by which all treponemal tests should be evaluated. The treponemal test
most widely used because it is as specific as the TPI is the FTA-ABS.
The virulent Nichol's strain of *T. pallidum* is used as the antigen, but
has been pretreated so that antigens common to nonpathogenic treponemes such as *Treponema microdentia* are absorbed from the sample.
Hence, only antibodies raised against a pathogenic treponeme such as
T. pallidum will give a positive result.

But *T. pertenue* and *T. carateum* will also give a positive result. Thus,
by serology and dark-field microscopy the pathogenic treponemes are
indistinguishable. Together with the similarity of their clinical symptoms, this accounts for the extreme difficulty in making a positive diagnosis when two or more of these diseases coexist.

False-Negative and False-Positive Results   Occasionally the serologic tests for syphilis give erroneous results. False-negative results are
obtained under certain circumstances. The best nontreponemal tests are
highly sensitive and give a positive reaction in the great majority of persons who have syphilis, but when titers are low, as in primary syphilis,
some cases may be missed. The VDRL test, for example, though completely accurate in detecting secondary syphilis, gives false-negative results in about 25% of cases of primary syphilis, even 4–6 weeks
postinfection (Hyde 1979:450). False-negative reactions are also seen
with the treponemal tests. The TPI test, for example, is not usually positive in the early weeks of infection, and does not become positive until
after the reagin tests are positive. (It appears, then, that the body produces reagin before it produces immobilizing antibody.) However, the
FTA-ABS test is positive at the beginning of the primary stage (Nicol
1971a:329), yet another reason why this test has superseded the TPI
test.

[5]The nontreponemal test most frequently used is the VDRL test. Other nontreponemal tests include the Kahn, Kline, Mazzini, Kolmer, and rapid plasma reagin tests.

The possibility of false-positive reactions must also be considered when interpreting the results of serologic tests. The treponemal tests are highly specific and only rarely give false-positive results. False-positive results are more frequent with the nontreponemal tests because the substance they test for, reagin, is produced in response to a number of other infections and conditions besides syphilis (see Table 11.5). Indeed, the primary purpose of treponemal tests is to check whether a positive nontreponemal test indicates syphilis or whether the person is giving a positive reaction for some other reason.

Table 11.5

Conditions Giving False–Positive Reactions to a Nontreponemal Test

Acute false-positive	*Chronic false-positive*
Atypical pneumonia	Addison's disease
Chancroid	Aging
Chicken pox	Alcoholic cirrhosis[a]
Glomerulonephritis	Congenital hemolytic anemia
Histoplasmosis	Convulsive disorders
Infectious hepatitis	Diabetes
Infectious mononucleosis	Gaucher's fever
Leptospirosis	Herpes simplex virus type 2 infection[a]
Lymphogranuloma venereum	Hodgkin's disease
Measles	Leprosy
Pneumococcal pneumonia	Liver disease
Pregnancy[a]	Lymphatic leukemia
Scarlet fever	Lymphosarcoma with autoimmune
Smallpox vaccination	hemolytic anemia[a]
Subacute bacterial endocarditis	Malaria
Upper respiratory tract infections	Metastatic carcinoma
Viral pneumonia	Multiple sclerosis
	Myocardial infarction
	Narcotics addiction
	Periarteritis nodosa
	Pernicious anemia
	Postencephalitic Parkinsonism
	Rheumatic fever
	Rheumatic heart disease
	Rheumatoid arthritis[a]
	Sarcoid
	Systemic lupus erythematosus
	Tuberculosis
	Viral hepatitis

[a]These conditions also give false-positive reactions to a treponemal test, the FTA-ABS test.

A person who has no history or clinical evidence of syphilis or other treponematosis and gives a positive reaction to a nontreponemal test but a negative reaction to the confirmatory treponemal test is classified as a biologic false positive (BFP). Normal, healthy individuals rarely (< .1%) give a false-positive reaction. However, a variety of infections and immunizations and narcotics addiction are frequently accompanied by an elevated reagin titer, which usually returns to normal in less than 6 months. These persons are classified as acute false-positive reactors. If the elevated reagin titer persists for more than 6 months the person is a chronic false-positive reactor, and further investigation often reveals a serious underlying disease (see Table 11.5). It should be noted that before the first treponemal test was available it was extremely difficult to distinguish between chronic false-positive reactors and persons with latent syphilis.

Although it is generally agreed that all the conditions listed in Table 11.5 may give a false-positive reaction, the frequency with which they do so was overstated in the early literature largely because the early nontreponemal tests were less specific than current tests. Sparling (1971:647) reported that the frequently cited 5% false-positive rate in persons with pneumococcal pneumonia, TB, subacute bacterial endocarditis, measles, chicken pox, and scarlet fever is too high when applied to current serologic tests. He also reported lower figures for smallpox vaccination, atypical pneumonia, and infectious mononucleosis. The false-positive rate for pregnant women has also been adjusted downward. Some studies (e.g., Salo *et al.* 1969:335) have continued to report very high (28%) false-positive rates for pregnant women, but more recent reports (e.g., Holder and Knox 1972:1154; Sparling 1971:647) have indicated that less than .05% of pregnant women give a false-positive reaction. Pregnancy is, however, one of only four or five conditions that can also give a false-positive reaction to the FTA-ABS test (Holder and Knox 1972:1154; Sparling 1971:644).

Whereas more specific nontreponemal tests have resulted in lower false- positive rates for many conditions, these tests have also confirmed that some conditions are indeed frequently associated with elevated reagin titers (cf. Sparling 1971:647). Leprosy, primarily lepromatous leprosy, carries a false-positive rate of 8 to 28%. And 10% of persons aged 70–80 years give a false-positive VDRL. Persons addicted to narcotics have a false-positive rate of 20 to 25%, and this elevated rate may persist for more than 1 year after drugs are stopped. Cushman and Sherman (1974:346) reported that in their study of 69 heroin addicts, 23% were biologic false-positives. After approximately 2 years of methadone this rate had dropped to 6%. They remarked that the cause of the elevated titers in heroin addicts is undetermined, but presumably is the result of exposure to an unknown antigen.

Serologic Changes The nontreponemal tests, particularly the VDRL, are easily performed, are quantifiable, and are inexpensive. Hence they are the standard tests for screening purposes and for following the serologic response to treatment. The titer and the patient's history and physical evidence help the physician to determine what stage of syphilis the patient is experiencing; changes in titer enable the physician to determine if the infection is recent and how the patient is responding to treatment.

Titers are low or nil during the first few weeks following infection but then begin to rise; the highest titers during the course of syphilitic infection occur during secondary syphilis. Thereafter, titers decline rapidly and are low by early latent syphilis. Low but detectable levels persist for many years afterwards. By late syphilis many cases are only weakly reactive and about one-third of cases are nonreactive. Occasionally, however, late syphilis, particularly late benign syphilis, is associated with some of the highest titers recorded.

Changes in titer accompany a variety of events. A rising titer may indicate recent infection. It may also indicate reinfection in an adequately treated patient or relapse in an inadequately treated patient. Hence, monitoring titers following treatment allows the physician to evaluate the adequacy of the treatment. Following treatment of primary syphilis, titers should become negative within 6 to 12 months. Following treatment of secondary syphilis the patient's serum should be nonreactive within 2 years. But treatment during latency or late syphilis has little or no effect on titers and should not be used to gauge the adequacy of treatment. Generally, the longer the duration of infection before treatment the greater the possibility of life-long seropositivity.

Treatment

At the time of the first syphilis epidemics in Europe in the late fifteenth century many treatments were tried. The most common was mercury, which the Arabs had used for centuries against scabies and yaws. In 1530 treatment with arsenic was suggested but abandoned when its fatal toxic effects became known. Thus, for 400 years mercury was essentially the only treatment for syphilis. In very limited amounts and in special situations, mercury therapy was of some slight value in treating syphilis. But frequently it was improperly administered, with disastrous results; severe ulceration of the gums and palate, loosening of the teeth, and gastrointestinal disorders were common complications. In an effort to avoid the toxicity of mercury a number of exotic concoctions of questionable efficacy were tried. Another heavy metal, bismuth, was introduced into syphilis therapy in 1884. Though more effective and less toxic than mercury, it did not supplant mercury as the most widely used antisyphilis agent until after World War I (Brown *et al.* 1970:11–14).

In 1907 Paul Ehrlich discovered an arsenic compound, variously called arsphenamine, Salvarsan, or 606, which was effective against syphilis, and this became the overwhelming treatment of choice until penicillin. Arsphenamine was unquestionably effective against early syphilis, but its ability to cure syphilis if used later was questioned. It was not, for example, effective in preventing cardiovascular syphilis in persons treated during latency (Kampmeier 1974:1351). And arsenotherapy could be very dangerous. There were many instances of poisoning from improperly supervised treatment or individual hypersensitivity. Aplastic anemia, encephalitis, and hemorrhaging are only some of the possible untoward effects.

Ten years after Ehrlich introduced arsphenamine, Wagner von Jauregg showed that syphilitic infection could be arrested by elevating body temperature. Exactly how this worked was unknown, but it was suggested that high temperatures destroyed the spirochete, interfered with its reproduction, or reduced its virulence. Fever therapy offered hope to patients suffering from some types of late syphilis, particularly neurosyphilis, as these were refractory to all forms of heavy metal therapy (mercury, bismuth, and arsenic). About 20–30% of these cases did respond to fever therapy (U.S. Public Health Service 1968:11–12), and the introduction of fever therapy in the United States in 1923 initiated a decline in the number of deaths from paresis. Some physicians still recommend fever therapy for an occasional case of neurosyphilis (Cave *et al.* 1971:948).

Fever therapy was not a new idea. The Sudanese had treated syphilis for centuries by burying patients in sand heated by the noonday sun (Adler 1980:208). But von Jauregg made the procedure more systematic, and in 1927 he received the Nobel Prize in medicine for his achievement. Two major types of fever therapy were used. One was the fever box, such as that designed by the Kettering Institute in Dayton, Ohio. Application of the Kettering Hypertherm, which was used for the treatment of syphilis and resistant and complicated gonorrhea, required that the patient stay in the box with only the head protruding for 8 hours at a temperature of 41° C (Adler 1980:208). The second type of fever therapy was no more attractive and involved raising body temperature by giving the patient malaria or typhoid fever, illnesses characterized by recurrent periods of high fever.

None of these therapies was wholly satisfactory. Fever therapy was considered "hazardous, unpredictable, and generally unsatisfactory" (Brown *et al.* 1970:16). All the heavy metals are extremely toxic and some are of questionable efficacy. And although arsenic was definitely effective against early syphilis, its usefulness at later stages was undetermined. Arsenotherapy also had the drawback that the patient had to come to the treatment center almost every week for 60 to 70 weeks. This treatment regimen did not change until the years immediately preceding World War II when a new intensive arsenotherapy schedule of 8 to 10 weeks was introduced and was fairly effective.

The long and painful nature of syphilis treatment in the prepenicillin era meant that few persons ever presented for treatment, and of those who did only 20–30% remained in treatment programs long enough that their infections were arrested. A survey by Edwards and Kinsie (1940:1) of the person on the street revealed that many persons felt that self-treatment or drugstore remedies were more successful in treating venereal disease than physician's care or clinic therapy. Many druggists, especially those in the poorer neighborhoods, profited from these feelings; they offered a diagnosis based on the customer's description of the symptoms and sold bottled remedies.

Many physicians also had reservations about existing treatments in the prepenicillin days and wondered whether it was not better to withhold treatment and allow the host's natural immunity to keep the spirochetes in check. They noted that few patients ever completed the course of arsenotherapy and that such spotty treatment just enhanced the hazards because it interfered with the development of immunity and thereby predisposed to infectious relapses (Kampmeier 1974:1350). In addition, the data regarding outcome of treated versus untreated syphilis were mixed; some studies showed a more favorable outcome following treatment, whereas some showed increased mortality rates following treatment (Kampmeier 1974:1351).

It was against this background that the Tuskegee Study was initiated in 1932 to study the outcome of untreated syphilis in black men of rural Alabama. The study has been severely criticized for withholding treatment, but supporters of the study have noted that no treatment at that time offered any real hope for these men because all were in late latency. In addition, said Moore (1933, cited in Kampmeier 1974:1351), "can any sensible person believe that any illiterate man would trudge miles weekly for these many months through heat and dust, cold, rain, and mud of rural Alabama in 1933, to welcome a nauseating intravenous dose of something or a painful injection into a buttock for no other reason than that some doctor or nurse said, 'So be it'."

All this changed by the middle of World War II. In 1943 the Lanham

Act established Rapid Treatment Centers throughout the United States that used arsenicals in a 5- to 10-day inpatient treatment regimen. That same year John Mahoney demonstrated that penicillin, which had been discovered 15 years earlier by Sir Alexander Fleming, was effective against syphilis. The first penicillin regimens required inpatient care, the patient receiving injections at 2 to 3 hour intervals around the clock. Later, outpatient care consisting of 1 shot per day for 7 to 10 days was available. And by 1953 one shot of penicillin was curative in early syphilis, although a number of visits were still required in later stages of the disease. It should be remembered that penicillin, although producing almost miraculous cures early in the disease, cannot reverse existing damage—late manifestations have been laid down by the end of the second decade following infection in almost all instances (Kampmeier 1974:1352)—and therefore is of limited value in some long-standing infections.

Although penicillin became available to persons with syphilis in 1944, it was not until 1947 that the infectious syphilis rate began to drop. Most workers (e.g., Lucas 1972:1082; U.S. Public Health Service 1968:15) have attributed this not to more syphilitics seeking treatment, but to the coincidental cure of many patients when they received penicillin for some other condition. But physicians gradually became aware that the nonspecific use of penicillin for nearly every condition was not good medicine. Some persons were severely allergic to the drug and, even more important, many organisms that were initially very sensitive to the drug were beginning to exhibit a degree of resistance. More discriminate use of penicillin coupled with less discriminate sexual activity resulted in a worldwide resurgence of syphilis in the 1960s.

With any infectious disease, one of the primary goals of medicine is to prevent infection by the immunization of susceptibles. Unfortunately, development of an antisyphilis vaccine has long been stymied by the inability to grow virulent *T. pallidum* in cell culture, a necessary first step in vaccine production. In 1973 Kiraly (1973:121) stated that "the greatest obstacle in anti-treponemal vaccine research is the *impossibility* of cultivating pathogenic treponemes *in vitro* [emphasis added]." Yet the following year Cox and Barber (1974:123) reported that they had reviewed the literature dealing with the growth requirements of *T. pallidum* and found evidence for its being classified as an anaerobe unsatisfying. Indeed, their own experiments showed that *T. pallidum* is in fact an aerobe, requiring oxygen for its growth and reproduction. Much valuable time had been lost in the search for a vaccine simply because old truths were accepted without question. It is hoped this new information will facilitate vaccine development.

CHAPTER 12

Genital Herpes

Introduction

The disease is incurable; once infected, individuals carry potentially infectious organisms in their bodies for the rest of their lives. Although in many persons the disease remains latent following the initial infection, some victims experience frequent recurrences of painful active infections. In women the disease is particularly worrisome because it is associated with a greatly increased risk of cervical carcinoma, and if transmitted to the fetus or newborn may result in death or serious permanent damage. The disease is genital herpes, and although it was rarely seen before 1965, some workers (e.g., Rapp 1978, cited in Gotwald and Golden 1981:261) believe it has become the major venereal disease in the United States and the world. In the United States, for example, an estimated 5–20 million persons were infected by the late 1970s, with .5 million new cases occurring each year.

Genital herpes is caused by herpes simplex virus type 2 (HSV–2)—a naturally occurring variant of herpes simplex virus type 1 (HSV–1), which is the virus that causes the painful blisters around the mouth commonly known as cold sores or fever blisters. Although the two viruses produce almost indistinguishable lesions, they are antigenically, biologically, and epidemiologically unique. For example, each virus has its own anatomical affinities, HSV–1 usually infecting oral tissue (lips, oral mucosa) and HSV–2 urogenital tissue (vulva, vagina, cervix, penis, testis, urethra, and bladder); HSV–2 is spread venereally and HSV–1 is spread by nonsexual contact; antibodies produced to one can be distinguished from those produced to the other; and whereas HSV–2 probably has oncogenic potential (the ability to produce cancer), no such capability has been described for HSV–1.

History

Genital herpetic infections were first described in France in the eighteenth century and by the nineteenth century were well recognized by European clinicians. It was not until the 1920s, however, that these infections were found to have a viral etiology. The 1960s saw not only the beginning of a tremendous increase in the prevalence of the disease but also the beginning of a tremendous increase in herpes research activities. Recognition of the possible oncogenic potential of HSV–2 gave a strong impetus to herpes research. But so too did the recognition that the disease is a cause of pregnancy loss and neonatal death; abortion, prematurity, and congenital and neonatal disease are all possible sequelae of herpes infection during pregnancy.

Prevalence

Developed World

By the late 1970s, 5–20 million persons in the United States alone were infected with genital herpes, with an additional 500,000 infections occurring each year (Brody 1980:C1; Raeburn 1981:E14; Subak-Sharpe 1978:155; *Time* 1980a:76). Although there are fewer new cases of genital herpes than of gonorrhea each year, the incurability of herpes means an ever-increasing pool of infected persons, a sizable proportion of whom experience one or more recurrences of active infection. Hence, if recurrent infections as well as initial infections are included, genital herpes may be the most common sexually transmitted disease (STD) (Bowie 1980:18).

Exactly how many persons are infected with genital herpes is, however, unknown, and the figures just given are only estimates. This is true for several reasons. There is still some confusion with classification of the virus; more important, by 1980 genital herpes was still not a reportable disease in the United States except in Massachusetts. Furthermore, many persons are asymptomatic, especially women because lesions are frequently confined to the cervix. In fact, a survey of mothers of children with neonatal herpes revealed that 70% were unaware they were infected (Brody 1980:C1).

National statistics on the numbers of persons infected with HSV–2 are, therefore, largely extrapolations from survey data, which use cytologic, virologic, or serologic techniques to detect persons carrying the virus. Serology detects all persons with a herpes infection, active or latent, whereas cytology and virology detect active infections only. Hence, only 2–4% of a random sampling of U.S. women were HSV–2-positive by cytology and virology (Monif 1974:53), but an estimated 15–30% of all sexually active adults in the United States are seropositive (Gotwald and Golden 1981:261; Holmes and Puziss 1980:640; *Time* 1980a:76).

In 1970 only 5% of sexually active adults in the United States were infected with HSV–2, but by 1980 this figure had risen three- to six-fold. With this increase genital herpes broadened its socioeconomic base; though still more frequent among members of the lower socioeconomic class, 20–60% of whom are infected, genital herpes is appearing with increasing frequency among the middle and upper classes, 10% of whom are infected (Benenson 1975:151; Pariser 1978, cited in Gotwald and Golden 1981:261). No matter which socioeconomic group one is investigating, the rates will always be highest among the most sexually promiscuous members of the group, that is, among adolescents and young adults. Among female prostitutes rates are extremely high; Pariser (1978, cited in Gotwald and Golden 1981:261) estimated that almost 100% of these women are infected with HSV–2.

The rate of increase in genital herpes may be slower in the future. Widespread publicity about herpes has undoubtedly sensitized the public to the dangers of the disease and encouraged, at least among some persons, greater discretion in sexual activities. More people can now recognize herpes sores and take proper precautions against spread. Some treatments have been offered that promise hastening of healing, thereby shortening the infectious period. But genital herpes will never be adequately controlled until the disease can be cured or prevented. Unfortunately, prevention via vaccination with killed or inactivated viruses does not seem possible because such viruses appear to be more capable of causing cancerous changes in cells than is the case with normal viruses (Barlow 1979:67). And finding a cure may be equally difficult, as no present drug is capable of eradicating the virus from the body.

Developing World

The prevalence of genital herpes in the developing world is unknown, but there are some indications that it may be almost as prevalent as in the developed world. Arya and Lawson (1977:54) reported that genital herpes is quite common in the tropics. A serologic survey in Ibadan, Nigeria (Montefiore *et al.* 1980:49–50), revealed the following seropositivity rates: blood donors, 20.6%; antenatal clinic patients, 27.9%; family planning clinic patients, 27.7%; venereal disease (VD) patients, 34.1%. The authors noted that these rates are comparable to those from the developed world, citing an 18% seropositivity rate among blood donors in Bristol, England, and a similar figure for asymptomatic pregnant women in the United States.

Primary Infection and Initial Infection

An individual's first experience with a herpes simplex virus usually occurs during childhood, at which time many persons are infected with HSV–1. Indeed, more than 60% of children aged 5 have antibodies against HSV–1, and by adult life 70–95% are HSV–1-positive (Barlow 1979:63; Benenson 1975:151). This initial HSV–1 infection, called the primary (herpes) infection because it is the first infection with any herpes simplex virus, is usually asymptomatic and therefore goes unnoticed. Recurrences are symptomatic, however, apparent as cold sores or fever blisters which appear on the lips.

Infection with HSV–2, which is transmitted almost exclusively through sexual contact, does not usually occur until puberty or thereafter. However, Montefiore *et al.* (1980:49, 52–53) reported that in Ibadan, Nigeria, children start to acquire HSV–2 antibodies much earlier, between ages 3 and 5, and that from ages 5 to 20 the seropositivity rate remains fairly constant at 12%. They noted that the rate of inactivation of the virus is known to vary considerably under different environmental conditions and suggest that in the tropics the virus can remain active long enough to allow nonvenereal transmission via shared towels and bed linens to occur.

If the individual has been previously infected with HSV–1, antibodies produced to this variant cross-react with HSV–2 and mollify the severity of the initial HSV–2 infection. Painful blisters in the genital area and local symptoms such as dysuria, itching, and dyspareunia are frequently the only symptoms. If, however, there has been no prior infection with HSV–1, the initial HSV–2 infection is usually much more severe. This infection, which in this instance is the individual's primary (herpes) infection, is frequently accompanied by viremia and resulting systemic symptoms such as fever, malaise, and muscle aches.

Fortunately, most persons have preexisting cross-reacting antibodies to type 1 at the time of their initial type 2 infection. Montefiore *et al.* (1980:53) estimated that by the time individuals in their study population in Nigeria began to develop HSV–2 antibodies over 50% had been exposed to HSV–1, and an even higher figure has been cited for the developed world (Barlow 1979:63; Benenson 1975:151). This is important to remember because viremia, which threatens the developing fetus, is normally associated only with primary infections (i.e., infections that occur in the absence of preexisting cross-reacting antibodies) (Monif 1974:55).

There is, unfortunately, no unanimity in the literature as to what constitutes a primary infection versus an initial infection. We have adopted the nomenclature of Josey *et al.* (1969:162) and Nahmias *et al.* (1975a:183–184), who defined a primary infection as that which occurs in an individual *with no preexisting antibodies to either type 1 or type 2 virus.* Monif (1974), on the other hand, applied the term *primary infection* to the *initial* infection with HSV–2 (or HSV–1) without regard to any prior infection with a herpes simplex virus. Indeed, he noted (1974:55) that "most persons with primary infection to *Herpesvirus hominis* type II have preexisting cross-reacting antibodies to *Herpesvirus hominis* type I." Such persons would not be considered to have a primary infection using the definition of Josey *et al.* (1969) or Nahmias *et al.* (1975a).

Knowing which type of infection is being referred to is essential in analyzing the literature because the probable effects on reproductive potential differ with each type. Primary infections—initial infections in which there are no preexisting cross-reacting antibodies—are the most severe. Viremia and resulting systemic reactions such as fever, malaise, and muscle aches are present. Lesions are more dispersed and more numerous, and swollen glands are more likely than with other types of infection. The viremia introduces the possibility of transplacental infection and fetal loss or congenital disease, the greater severity of the infection results in a more dramatic maternal reaction with an increased risk of fetal loss or premature birth, and the numerous florid lesions increase the chances of neonatal infection. An initial HSV–2 infection occurring in the presence of type 1 antibodies is not usually associated with viremia or systemic reactions, but is more severe than recurrent infections in that more lesions are present; there is also a greater risk of neonatal infection than during recurrent infections (Nahmias *et al.* 1975a:185). Thus, a recurrent infection presents the least risk to the child and a primary infection presents the greatest risk.

Course of the Disease

Primary and Initial Infections

In a susceptible person, sexual contact with an infectious case of genital herpes usually results in signs of infection within 1 week. If the individual has no preexisting antibodies to HSV–1 the infection is apt to be particularly severe. Viremia and systemic reactions such as fever and malaise are common. Lesions are larger, more numerous, more dispersed, and take longer to heal than in other types of attacks. In initial infections in which there are preexisting HSV–1 antibodies, viremia and constitutional symptoms are usually absent. Lesions are not as florid and there will be less tissue destruction than with a primary attack.

Herpetic lesions usually heal within 2 to 6 weeks without leaving a trace, although pregnancy slows resolution of the sores and a supervening secondary bacterial infection may not only slow healing but may result in scar formation as well. The healing of the sores signals that the virus has left the surface of the body and has moved along the nerve pathways to the sensory nerve ganglia near the lower spinal cord. Here the virus remains for the life of the host.

In about one-third of infected persons the virus remains sequestered in these nerves and they will never again experience an active infection. But in the remaining two-thirds the latent virus, for any of a number of reasons, is reactivated and creeps back along the nerves to the urogenital area, causing a recurrent infection.

Recurrent Infection

The recurrent infection is apt to be milder than the initial infection, especially if the initial infection was also the primary infection. The lesions are few, small, and localized. Frequently vaginal discharge, dysuria, and dyspareunia, which are common to all types of herpes infection, will be the only symptoms. It is not unusual for recurrent infections to be altogether asymptomatic. In women, for example, lesions in recurrent infections are frequently confined to the upper vagina and cervix, and because this area is relatively insensitive to pain such lesions are both painless and hidden. And often the lesions are atypical. Hence, Nahmias *et al.* (1975a:185) stated that laboratory methods are often necessary to diagnose a case of recurrent herpetic cervicitis. Men may also be asymptomatic, no lesions being obvious but herpesviruses being present in the urine (Amstey 1973:719), suggesting a herpetic urethritis.

Some persons experience only an occasional recurrence, but others experience serious painful outbreaks once a month or even more (Raeburn 1981:E14). Fortunately, most recurrences occur in the first year after infection; as time passes recurrences become less frequent and less severe. For example, a person who experiences 4–5 recurrences the first year after onset may experience only half that number the second year, and so on (Subak-Sharpe 1978:155).

It should be noted that the various disease manifestations discussed earlier as characteristic of primary infections, initial infections, and recurrent infections describe only the average cases and that some persons with primary infections have no symptoms whereas some persons with recurrent infections experience severe, painful outbreaks of disease (Nahmias *et al.* 1975a:184).

Factors Affecting Rates of Recurrent Infection

Scientists have been able to identify a number of factors—general health, physical trauma, emotional stress, and hormonal changes—that can trigger reactivation of the virus. Some of these can be avoided, thereby lowering recurrence rates, but some cannot. Persons with good general health will have few recurrences, whereas persons taking certain drugs and individuals with poor diets, infection, fever, immune deficiencies and cancer will experience more recurrences (Brody 1980:C6; Ely 1979:43; Young 1972:1176). Physical trauma to the urogenital area may also trigger an attack (Brody 1980:C6; Young 1972:1176). Indeed, in some persons intercourse is a precipitating factor. Emotional stress is a widely cited reactivation factor (Amstey 1974:134; Brody 1980:C6; Subak-Sharpe 1978:156), premenstrual tension being forwarded as being particularly important (Young 1972:1176). Frequently the relationship between stress and recurrences becomes a cyclical one, recurrences causing stress and stress causing more recurrences.

Hormonal changes, such as those associated with menstruation and pregnancy, are also believed to trigger the appearance of active disease (Brody 1980:C6; Ely 1979:43; Nahmias *et al.* 1975a:184; Subak-Sharpe 1978:156). Women in whom menstruation precipitates active infection may frequently be helped by oral contraceptives (Brody 1980:C6). De Lora *et al.* (1981:254) reported that women not taking the pill averaged one recurrence every 52 days whereas those taking the pill averaged only one recurrence every 82 days. Women using the pill were three times as likely to stay free of recurrences as nonusers. The severity and duration of recurrences were not, however, influenced by pill use.

Transmission

A person with active genital herpes may spread the disease to sexual contacts or, if pregnant, to the fetus or newborn. Given the possible gravity of herpes infection, infectious periods must be recognized and all available measures taken to avoid transmission. Unfortunately, this is not always possible. Many infections, especially recurrent infections, are completely asymptomatic. In the rare instance of a primary infection during pregnancy there is no way to prevent viremia and possible transplacental transmission because there are no effective, safe antiviral agents.

Sexual Contacts

It is believed that for all practical purposes genital herpes can be transmitted to sexual contacts only when sores are present. But not uncommonly these sores are hidden from view, particularly in women because the cervix is so frequently the site of infection. Inapparent infections are less common in men because the penis is most frequently involved. However, in some men only the urethra is involved and the infection therefore goes unnoticed. (Nahmias *et al.* [1975a:185] suggested that herpetic involvement of the urethra may be one of the causes of nongonococcal urethritis.) Even when lesions are apparent their clinical appearance is so diverse that the infection can easily be misdiagnosed or overlooked. Furthermore, when gonorrhea is also present, a not-infrequent occurrence, this bacterial infection may mask the herpes infection. In one study (Jeansson and Molin 1975:190) genital herpes infections were more than twice as likely to be asymptomatic if there was a concomitant gonorrhea infection.

Hence, one cannot with certainty avoid contracting genital herpes by avoiding sexual contact with persons with genital sores. One woman, assured by her physician that genital herpes was not contagious unless sores were present, slept with her boyfriend who was known to be infected but showed no signs of present active infection. Within a week she developed genital herpes (*Time* 1980a:76).

Fetus

Transplacental transmission of HSV–2 to the fetus is possible, in which case the pregnancy may terminate either as a spontaneous abortion or in the birth of a congenitally infected infant. Some workers (e.g., Nahmias *et al.* 1975b:66) have felt that transplacental transmission of HSV–2 is not proved and that the apparent increased abortion rate in women with active disease during early pregnancy may be related to a nonspecific maternal reaction to a severe infection and not to transplacental infection of the fetus. Amstey (1973:722), however, reported that HSV–2 had been isolated from an aborted fetus. And Florman *et al.* (1973:129) noted that five cases of intrauterine infection with HSV–2 appeared in the literature and reported that they found an infant infected in utero with HSV–1. These congenitally infected infants showed neurological and ocular damage similar to that seen in infants with neonatal herpes and in infants with other congenital diseases such as toxoplasmosis, rubella, and cytomegalovirus.

Amstey and Monif (1974:394) concluded that transplacental passage does occur but is exceedingly rare. Monif (1974:54–55) explained why transplacental infection is so exceptional, stating that transplacental infection requires viremia and viremia occurs only during a primary infection (i.e., in infections where there are no preexisting antibodies to either type 1 or type 2 virus, either type of antibody effectively aborting viremia). Because the vast majority of women of childbearing age have such antibodies, the chance that pregnancy and a primary infection would coincide is rather remote.

Newborns

A greater risk to the child comes from lesions in the genital tract. Such lesions may contaminate the child in two ways: (1) by an ascending infection following rupture of the membranes just before or during labor and (2) by the child coming into direct contact with lesions during its passage through the birth canal.

For women with active genital lesions in the immediate antepartum period delivery by cesarean section is recommended. Such women must be watched carefully and delivered within 4 hours of rupture of the membranes. After this it is probable that the child has already been contaminated by an ascending infection and vaginal delivery should be allowed because it presents no additional risk of infection and is safer than a cesarean.

Effects on Fecundity

From the preceding discussion it is clear that genital herpes can have a significant impact on fecundity and fertility. Coitus may for all practical purposes be impossible during severe attacks; pregnancy loss and neonatal death and disease are important sequelae of maternal herpes.

Coital Inability

Genital herpes, especially if there is a severe attack with many painful sores on the vulva or penis, can make intercourse so painful as to be impossible (cf. Monif 1974:53; Subak-Sharpe 1978:155). Although coital ability returns when the lesions heal and the overall effect is one of lower coital frequency, in some persons the emotional trauma associated with these episodes and their interference with normal sexual activity create a tension that carries over into periods of latency. This is particularly true for couples where one or both partners experience frequent recurrences; serious sexual problems occur in some of these couples (*British Medical Journal* 1980:1335; Gardner 1979:554). Such stress predisposes to more recurrences and the problem becomes a cyclical one whose resolution may require professional help.

Impotence has also been mentioned as a possible concomitant of herpes infection of the anus (herpetic proctitis) (Corsaro and Korzeniowsky 1980:55). In the large cities of the world—New York, London, and Paris—ano-rectal herpes of homosexual men has created a rather serious problem, as it is becoming more common and is very difficult to diagnose (Nahmias *et al.* 1975a:188).

Conceptive Failure

Conceptive ability is only rarely affected by genital herpes. Urethral strictures secondary to herpetic urethritis could possibly affect male fertility, but although herpetic urethritis is commonplace in both sexes complications are relatively rare (Nahmias *et al.* 1975a:185).

Pregnancy Loss

In 1969 Josey *et al.* (1969:163) reported that there was some evidence of an increased risk of spontaneous abortion if a woman had a genital herpes infection during the first trimester of pregnancy. In 1971 a study by Nahmias *et al.* (1971:832) quantitated this risk, noting that a woman with active genital herpes during the first 20 weeks of gestation has a risk of spontaneous abortion three times that for the general population. If the infection was the mother's first the risk was even higher, Edwards (1978, cited in Nass *et al.* 1981:496) placing it at five times that for the general population.

Workers have been unable to determine whether such pregnancy losses are the result of herpes infection of the fetus or if they are secondary to a maternal response to infection. Nahmias *et al.* (1971:832) looked at the placentas from such abortuses and found no clear evidence of viral invasion, although there was evidence of a lethal effect (unspecified) on the child before its expulsion. And although a number of cases of proved intrauterine infection with HSV–1 and HSV–2 have appeared in the literature, these are very few in number because, as noted earlier, most adults have circulating antibodies to HSV–1 or HSV–2 that effectively abort viremia. Hence, the three- to fivefold increase in the abortion rate in women with a genital herpes infection early in pregnancy probably reflects an as yet unspecified maternal reaction to the infection. Perhaps some toxic factor is released by the multiplying virus, or perhaps the fevers that accompany some severe infections are of sufficient height and duration to terminate the pregnancy.

Neonatal Infection

Although a child born to a woman with herpes usually possesses antibodies to the virus passively acquired via the placenta,[1] neonatal infection is possible because (1) the virus can multiply in the presence of significant antibody levels (which is clearly illustrated by the recurrent attacks that occur in adults) and (2) the newborn does not possess, at least in full measure, that other vital component of immunity necessary to combat infection: cellular immunity (Amstey 1974:134).

If maternal lesions are present at the time of parturition there is at least a 40% chance that the child will be infected unless it is delivered within 4 hours of rupture of the membranes (Edwards 1978, cited in Nass *et al.* 1981:488; Nahmias *et al.* 1971:833). It has been estimated (Amstey 1974:134; Monif 1974:54; *Time* 1980a:76) that 60–90% of these children will die from a fulminating infection; most of the survivors will suffer permanent neurological or ocular damage.

Even though a cesarean section can reduce fetal risk, each year in the United States several hundred children are born with neonatal herpes and more than half of these die (*Time* 1980a:76).

Prematurity

Nahmias *et al.* (1971:832–833) noted that whereas active herpes during the first half of pregnancy is associated with a greater risk of spontaneous abortion, active infection later in pregnancy is a cause of

[1]The one exception to this rule occurs in children born to mothers with a recently acquired primary infection.

premature delivery. Again, the risk is greater during the first HSV-2 infection. Edwards (1978, cited in Nass *et al.* 1981:496) estimated that a pregnant woman with active genital herpes runs a 20% greater risk of premature delivery than does the general population.

Again, the exact cause of the observed increase in premature deliveries in women with active genital herpes is unknown.

Cervical Carcinoma

A number of other disorders can be caused by HSV-2. One of these is herpes keratitis, a serious eye infection that is a leading cause of blindness in young adults. Care must therefore be exercised in cleaning the hands thoroughly after touching a herpes lesion to avoid contamination of the eye and other sites.

A more common and equally feared disease associated with genital herpes is cervical carcinoma. Cervical cancer strikes 16,000 U.S. women each year in its serious form and contributes to 7,400 deaths (*Time* 1980a:76). Whether HSV-2 actually *causes* cervical cancer is debated. Although HSV-2 has been isolated from human cervical tumor cells and it is possible that the virus caused the cells to become cancerous, it is also possible that these altered cells are simply more susceptible to infection with HSV-2 (Amstey 1973:722).

Although the experimental evidence is mixed the epidemiological evidence showing an association between cervical carcinoma and genital herpes is very strong, women with HSV-2 antibodies and/or a history of genital herpes having significantly higher rates of cervical cancer than control women (Nahmias *et al.* 1975a:185-186). The risk of developing cervical cancer is increased fivefold for women with HSV-2 antibodies (Nass *et al.* 1981:488). For women with cytologically detected infection the risk is even higher, such women showing an eightfold greater risk (Blough and Giuntoli 1979, cited in DeLora *et al.* 1981:254; *Time* 1973:55). Cervical dysplasia or carcinoma therefore occurs in about 1 in 10 women with a history of genital herpes.

Pap smears, recommended for all women of childbearing age and beyond, are extremely important for women with a history of genital herpes because periodic testing can detect cellular abnormalities in the precancerous stage, when a 100% cure rate is realizable. However, the surgery and radiation used to treat cervical cancer frequently leave the woman with greatly diminished fecundity. Radiation therapy of the cervix leaves a scarred structure capable neither of secreting cervical mucus nor of containing the fetus in the uterus. And surgical removal of the cervix may be necessary and thus absolute sterility is the result.

Hence, the increase in genital herpes is likely to result in an increase in cervical dysplasia and carcinoma. Although early detection of these pathological conditions will save many lives, many women will be rendered sterile by the treatment. Most affected women will be in their late 40s or 50s and for the most part past their childbearing years, but some younger women will undoubtedly be affected.

Summary

Genital herpes is, therefore, a significant factor in human procreative activity. During severe attacks coitus may be impossible. In persons with frequent recurrences the emotional trauma associated with periodic disruption of normal sexual activity may cause sexual difficulties even during symptom-free periods. Pregnant women with an active infection early in pregnancy, especially those with their first HSV–2 infection, are three to five times more likely to experience a spontaneous abortion. Later in pregnancy an active infection is associated with a slightly (20%) increased risk of premature delivery. Maternal infection at parturition is associated with a 40% risk of neonatal infection, due to infection of the child as it comes into contact with infectious material just before or during birth. More than half of these children will die and the survivors will be permanently damaged. The risk of neonatal infection can be minimized, however, by performing a cesarean section within 4 hours of rupture of the membranes. Finally, epidemiological studies have shown that women with a history of genital herpes have a five- to eightfold greater risk of cervical carcinoma, which, even if treated early enough to save the woman's life, usually leaves her incapable of bearing children.

These adverse sequelae loom even darker when it is realized that 5–20 million persons in the United States are already infected with this incurable disease, with .5 million new cases occurring each year. Estimates are that 20–60% of persons in the lower socioeconomic classes are seropositive and 10% of those in the upper socioeconomic classes have been infected.

Diagnosis

A diagnosis of genital herpes may be made on the basis of clinical observations and/or the results of a number of laboratory tests. A diagnosis based solely on clinical observations may miss the mark, however, because the vesicular lesions of genital herpes may be confused with a number of other diseases, particularly chancroid and syphilis, and in the pregnant patient may resemble cervical carcinoma (Josey *et al.* 1969:166; Nahmias *et al.* 1975a:186). Because HSV–2 often coexists with gonorrhea and other STDs such as trichomonas and condyloma acuminatum, a multiple diagnosis must not be missed (Nahmias *et al.* 1975a:186). As noted earlier, HSV–2 infection may be masked by concomitant gonorrhea.

For these reasons, many physicians are reluctant to make a diagnosis without the benefit of a number of laboratory tests that can confirm their suspicions. Microscopic examination of cells scraped from the surface of a lesion (exfoliative cytology) may reveal characteristic findings of giant multinucleated cells with intranuclear inclusions, although this is only presumptive evidence of genital herpes because other herpesviruses produce similar changes (Josey *et al.* 1969:163; Nahmias *et al.* 1975b:65). Conclusive proof therefore requires isolation and characterization of the virus through tissue culture and biochemical techniques. Immunological techniques such as the radioimmunoassay (RIA) or immunofluorescence (IMF) may also be used to establish a diagnosis (Nahmias *et al.* 1975b:65). By using these techniques scientists can also differentiate genital infections caused by HSV–2 (90% of cases) from those caused by HSV–1 (Nahmias *et al.* 1975a:184).

Treatment

The treatment of genital herpes is difficult because of an almost total lack of safe and effective antiviral agents. A large number of treatments have been used in the past—vitamin C therapy, injection with inactivated herpes, photoinactivation, ether, dietary supplements of zinc, antimetabolites such as idoxyuridine, repeated vaccinia vaccinations, etc.—most of them ineffective and some of them dangerous. Photoinactivation (painting the lesions with certain dyes and then exposing to fluorescent light) and idoxyuridine may themselves cause cancer (Brody 1980:C6). And experimental studies have shown that the oncogenic potential of inactivated herpesvirus is greater than that of the normal virus (Barlow 1979:67); hence, it cannot be used to treat sufferers or to immunize susceptibles.

In the late 1970s researchers at the University of Pennsylvania reported that a sugar, 2-deoxy-D-glucose, was effective in healing lesions in 90% of women treated, and there was hope that a cure had been found. Unfortunately, researchers are not so optimistic now about this compound. Another drug, acyclovir, shows promise of reducing the severity of initial episodes of genital herpes, but is worthless for persons battling recurring outbreaks of the disease (Haney 1982:1B). So until a safe and effective antiviral drug is available, herpes sufferers will simply have to wait out their attacks and treat the pain with aspirin and local anesthetics.

Those persons not yet infected with genital herpes may be spared this dangerous and painful disease if the work of a group of scientists with the New York State department of health proves successful. Using the new cut-and-paste method of manipulating genes, these scientists have inserted bits of herpes virus DNA into the DNA of the smallpox vaccine virus. This new vaccine, when injected into rabbits, produced large quantities of antibodies specific to herpes simplex. More importantly, mice immunized with the genetically engineered herpes vaccine remained healthy when exposed to herpes virus. Even with 10–20 times the lethal dose of virus, all of the mice survived. This vaccine is particularly exciting because there is no danger of getting the infection since the virus itself is not present in the formula (*Time* 1983:82).

CHAPTER 13

Genital Mycoplasmas

Introduction

In 1937 Dienes and Edsall isolated a mycoplasma, probably *Mycoplasma hominis*, from an abscess of Bartholin's gland. This was the first reported recovery of a mycoplasma from a human. Since then six species within the family Mycoplasmataceae have been found to infect humans. Two of these, *Mycoplasma hominis* and *Ureaplasma urealyticum*, are frequent inhabitants of the human genital mucosa; they are found in the urethra or vagina of 50% of sexually experienced adults (Taylor-Robinson and McCormack 1980b:1067).

The mycoplasmas are the smallest organisms that can grow on artificial media. About the size of the larger viruses, they form colonies clearly visible under the light microscope. *Ureaplasma urealyticum* forms very small colonies, hence its early name T[tiny]-mycoplasma. Both organisms may be acquired at birth upon delivery through an infected birth canal. The respiratory and/or genital mucosa is often colonized (more frequently with ureaplasmas), but such infections tend not to persist. In late childhood the genitals of most boys are mycoplasma-negative, whereas only 9–22% of girls are *U. urealyticum*-positive and only 8–9% are *M. hominis*-positive (Taylor-Robinson and McCormack 1980a:1004).

After puberty, genital colonization occurs primarily as a result of sexual contact; colonization rates are higher for persons with more sexual partners (Mardh *et al.* 1975:58; Taylor-Robinson and McCormack 1980a:1004). Hence, mycoplasmas are rarely found in nuns but are prevalent among persons in venereal disease (VD) clinics (Monif 1974:158).

Colonization rates also differ by socioeconomic status and are higher in persons of lower status, possibly due to an environmental factor or to differences in sexual activity (Taylor-Robinson and McCormack 1980a:1004). Recovery rates are higher in blacks even after controlling for differences in sexual experience (Taylor-Robinson and McCormack 1980a:1004). And recovery rates are elevated two- to threefold if there is an inflammation of the genital tract, as with trichomonas or gonorrhea (Monif 1974:156), supporting the notion (Taylor-Robinson and McCormack 1980a:1007) that the genital mycoplasmas may not be primary pathogens but simply opportunistic organisms that prefer to grow in damaged tissue.

Once it was established that the genital mycoplasmas were frequent inhabitants of the human genital tract, interest was stimulated in knowing if they played a role in genital tract disease. In women the organisms have, at one time or another, been implicated in the following disorders: lower genital tract infections, endometritis, pelvic inflammatory disease (PID), infertility, spontaneous abortion, stillbirth, neonatal death, prematurity, low birth weight, and maternal perinatal morbidity (Babson and Benson 1971:26; Eschenbach 1980:143S; Gnarpe and Friberg 1972:727; Harrison *et al.* 1975:607; Matthews *et al.* 1975:988; Monif 1974:156). In men, the genital mycoplasmas have been implicated in nongonococcal urethritis (NGU) and infertility (Gnarpe and Friberg 1972:727; Matthews *et al.* 1975:988).

Much evidence both for and against a role for *M. hominis* and *U. urealyticum* in these pathological conditions has been presented in the literature. This body of knowledge has been expertly reviewed by Taylor-Robinson and McCormack (1980a, 1980b) who concluded (1980b:1066): "We have been discouraged by our review of the recent literature. Many of the studies have been poorly designed and have predictably been uninterpretable, inconclusive, or both." They went on to say that if better studies are to be forthcoming, (1) the epidemiology of the organism must be understood and workers must be sensitive to the fact that the mycoplasmas coexist with many other organisms whose effects must be taken into account; (2) controls should be comparable in terms of sexual experience and other relevant variables; (3) researchers should, if possible, differentiate by serologic techniques colonization (low antibody titers) from infection (high or rising antibody titers); and (4) workers should use quantitative cultures whenever possible to determine the number of organisms and, therefore, the severity of the infection.

The role of *M. hominis* and *U. urealyticum* in human reproduction will now be considered. The review by Taylor-Robinson and McCormack (1980a, 1980b) is more detailed than this discussion and should

Table 13.1

Summary of the Association of Genital Mycoplasmas with Human Disease[a]

Condition	Evidence suggesting mycoplasma as a cause		Comments
	Mycoplasma hominis	Ureaplasma urealyticum	
Nongonococcal urethritis	None	Strong	Ureaplasmas cause some cases but the proportion is unknown
Prostatitis	Weak	None	An association with a few cases of chronic disease has been reported but a causal relation is unproved
Epididymitis	None	None	Mycoplasmas are not an important cause
Abscess of Bartholin's gland	Weak	None	*Mycoplasma hominis* may cause some disease, but is not an important cause
Vaginitis and cervicitis	None	None	*M. hominis* often associated with disease but a causal relation is unproved
Pelvic inflammatory disease	Strong	Weak	*M. hominis* causes some cases but the proportion is unknown
Postabortal fever	Strong	None	*M. hominis* is responsible for some cases but the proportion is unknown
Postpartum fever	Strong	None	Recent work indicates that *M. hominis* may be a major cause
Involuntary infertility	None	Weak	Ureaplasmas are associated with altered motility of sperm
Repeated spontaneous abortion and stillbirth	None	Weak	Maternal and fetal infections have been associated with spontaneous abortion but causal relation is unproved
Chorioamnionitis	None	Strong	An association exists but a causal relation is unproved
Low birth weight	None	Strong	An association exists but a causal relation is unproved

[a]Source: Taylor-Robinson and McCormack (1980b:1066). Reprinted by permission of the *New England Journal of Medicine*, 1980, **302**, 1063.

be read by anyone with a particular interest in the genital mycoplasmas. Information from this review summarizing the association of the genital mycoplasmas with conditions related to subfecundity is presented as Table 13.1.

Mycoplasma hominis

Effects on the Female Reproductive System

Because so many women of reproductive age are infected with *M. hominis,* determination of its role, if any, in reproductive disorders is imperative. The association between *M. hominis* infection and lower and upper genital tract infections, postabortal and postpartum fevers, and low birth weight infants has been extensively studied. Unfortunately, as noted by Taylor-Robinson and McCormack (1980b), many of these studies are flawed and therefore their conclusions must be viewed with some serious reservations.

Lower Genital Tract Infections

Mycoplasma hominis adheres to the surface epithelial cells of the vagina, and several researchers (e.g., Akerlund *et al.* 1975:172; Mardh *et al.* 1975:56) have felt the organism may play a role in lower genital tract infections. Although approximately 50% of women of childbearing age who are sexually active and have signs of a lower genital tract infection are *M. hominis*–positive, less than 5% of control women with no signs of inflammation harbor the organism (Mardh *et al.* 1975:56). Taylor-Robinson and McCormack (1980a:1007) noted, however, that *M. hominis* is frequently associated with other pathogens (it was noted in the ''Introduction'' section that recovery rates increase two- to threefold if other pathogens such as *Neisseria gonorrhoeae* are present), so it is hard to decide whether the mycoplasmas caused the disease or are simply opportunistic organisms that prefer to grow in damaged tissue. The authors noted that in some mixed infections with *Haemophilus vaginalis* eradication of that organism resulted in eradication of the disease but eradication of *M. hominis* did not. Yet Mardh *et al.* (1975:56) noted that in women with lower genital tract infections harboring *M. hominis* treatment with antibiotics to which the mycoplasma is susceptible usually produces cure. Evidence is therefore mixed, and the role of *M. hominis* in lower genital tract infections is still undetermined.

There is some question as to whether mycoplasmal infections of the lower genital tract are a hazard to the fetus. Colonization of the new-born's respiratory and/or genital mucosa is common following passage through an infected birth canal but represents only superficial contamination. Furthermore, significant infections are rare, suggesting that *M. hominis* is a pathogen of low virulence (Monif 1974:157). However, infection of the lungs following aspiration of infected amniotic fluid may adversely affect the fetus. Monif (1974:157) reported that *M. hominis* can be isolated from the lungs of 8 to 10% of spontaneously aborted fetuses, although available data do not allow a conclusion as to whether the organism was causally related to the abortion or was simply an opportunistic commensal. After reviewing the available studies, Taylor-Robinson and McCormack (1980b:1066) concluded there is no evidence linking *M. hominis* with pregnancy loss.

Pelvic Inflammatory Disease

Although Eschenbach and Holmes (1975:39) found no difference in the rate of isolation of *M. hominis* from the cervices of women in a VD clinic and those with acute salpingitis, they remarked that other studies have found an association between the organism and PID. In one study (Taylor-Robinson and McCormack 1980a:1008) *M. hominis* was isolated from the tubes in 4 of 50 women with acute salpingitis but in none of 50 controls. And in those women with *M. hominis* in the tubes there was a significant rise in antibody titer.

Further confirmatory evidence comes from infected organ cultures and from the experimental infection of grivet monkeys. If organ cultures of fallopian tubes are infected with *M. hominis,* the mycoplasmas multiply and cause swelling of the cilia observable under the electron microscope (Westrom and Mardh 1975:161). And when Moller *et al.* (1978:248ff) deposited *M. hominis* in the lumen of the fallopian tubes of grivet monkeys, although no signs of disease were clinically apparent antibody levels rose fourfold and the tubes showed redness and swelling. Histologically there was an inflammatory reaction in the muscle layer, but at all times the lumen of the tube remained normal. The infection was self-limiting, the tubes returning to normal 4–5 weeks post-infection. Such evidence has led researchers (e.g., Taylor-Robinson and McCormack 1980b:1066) to conclude that the evidence linking *M. hominis* and PID is strong but that the proportion of cases with this etiology is unknown. Because the lumen of the tube is not affected, salpingitis caused by *M. hominis* is not as likely to cause sterility as salpingitis caused by gonorrhea or chlamydia. Nevertheless, involvement of the muscular layer of the tube could disturb ovum transport and *M. hominis* could therefore be an important cause of ectopic pregnancy.

Postabortal and Postpartum Fever

Taylor-Robinson and McCormack noted that earlier suggestive evidence that *M. hominis* has a role in postabortal fever was supported by a prospective study by Harwick *et al.* (1970, cited in Taylor-Robinson and McCormack 1980a:1008) in which *M. hominis* was isolated from the blood of 7.8% of women with fever and abortion but not from women who remained afebrile after abortion nor from women with a normal term delivery. The serologic data also support a role for *M. hominis*, fourfold or greater rises in titer being noted in about half the febrile women and only 14% of the afebrile women. Thus, Taylor-Robinson and McCormack (1980a:1008) concluded that *M. hominis* causes some cases of fever after abortion. Because the site of the infection causing the fever has not been documented, it cannot be stated whether or not the infection could have residua that might affect fecundity.

It has been suggested (Bowie 1980:18; Mardh *et al.* 1975:59; Monif 1974:157) that *M. hominis* may cause some cases of postpartum fever. Taylor-Robinson and McCormack (1980a:1008–1009) noted that *M. hominis*, like other vaginal organisms, appears transiently in the bloodstream following a vaginal delivery. This invasion by *M. hominis*, which is associated with a serologic response (i.e., production of antibody), does not persist and is not associated with fever. However, in individual patients with postpartum fever *M. hominis* may be isolated from the blood a day or more after delivery (also accompanied by a serologic response), whereas *M. hominis* is seldom recovered at that time from postpartum women who are afebrile. They further noted that fever is much more common in women with low or absent antibody titers to *M. hominis* at delivery who then convert to antibody-positive status than it is in nonconverters. After reviewing available studies the authors concluded that *M. hominis* is a major cause of contemporary postpartum fever and that the fever is caused by an endometritis. Fecundity could be reduced in some of these women because a severe endometritis can be followed by intrauterine adhesions, which contribute to pregnancy loss. Pregnancy loss may also follow if there is a chronic subclinical endometritis. (See discussion of endometritis in the section ''*Ureaplasma urealyticum.*'')

Low Birth Weight

Although some authors (Taylor-Robinson and McCormack 1980b:1066) found no relationship between infant or maternal colonization with *M. hominis* and birth weight, others (e.g., Di Musto *et al.* 1973:36) have noted an association between maternal colonization and lower birth weight infants. The association, when noted, between *M.*

hominis and lower birth weight is not as striking as with the ureaplasmas, although the combined effect of both organisms is greater than that of the ureaplasmas alone (Taylor-Robinson and McCormack 1980b:1066). But, after considering all the available evidence, Taylor-Robinson and McCormack (1980b:1066) concluded there is no strong evidence linking *M. hominis* with lower birth weight.

Effects on the Male Reproductive System

The role of *M. hominis* in infections of the male genital tract appears to be very limited. There are no indications that it is a cause of either urethritis or epididymitis (Taylor-Robinson and McCormack 1980a:1005–1006). Mardh *et al.* (1975:57) reported finding *M. hominis* in 10% of 79 patients with chronic prostatitis but in none of 20 age-matched controls. However, Taylor-Robinson and McCormack (1980a:1006) felt that it is unclear if these results indicate a causal relationship between *M. hominis* and chronic prostatitis.

Ureaplasma urealyticum

Ureaplasma urealyticum is the second member of the family Mycoplasmataceae that is a frequent inhabitant of the human genital tract. Colonization of the genital and/or respiratory mucosa of newborns is frequent following passage through an infected birth canal. In fact, the genitals of 30% of all newborn females are colonized. By age 1 year this figure has dropped to less than 10% and then remains fairly constant until puberty. Incidence rises after puberty as the ureaplasmas, like *M. hominis,* are spread by sexual contact; there is a positive correlation between the number of consorts and the rate of colonization with these organisms. In general, about 50% of all sexually active men and women of childbearing age have ureaplasmas in the lower genital tract. The incidence decreases during reproductive life so only a small proportion of postmenopausal women are colonized (Mardh *et al.* 1975:58; Monif 1974:157).

Effects on the Female Reproductive System

Lower Genital Tract Infections

Although the presence of ureaplasmas in semen adversely affects sperm and therefore possibly conceptive ability (see the section ''Effects on the Male Reproductive System''), ureaplasmas in the female lower genital tract do not appear to affect sperm motility or viability or the physiologic characteristics of vaginal fluid or cervical mucus (Desai *et al.* 1980:470). Furthermore, epidemiological evidence does not even suggest a role for *U. urealyticum* in lower genital tract infections because the organisms are isolated as frequently from the lower genital tract of controls as from patients (Akerlund *et al.* 1975:172; Mardh *et al.* 1975:59; Taylor-Robinson and McCormack 1980a:1007). And Taylor-Robinson and McCormack (1980b:1064) felt that available evidence did not support an association between mycoplasmal colonization of the lower genital tract and fetal loss. Nevertheless, a study from Ethiopia has suggested that an ascending infection during pregnancy could be a cause of perinatal mortality. Tafari and associates (1976:108, 109) reported that in their study in Addis Ababa there was evidence that almost 8% of all perinatal deaths were caused by *U. urealyticum* ascending from the cervix to infect the fetal membranes.

Endometritis

Endometrial colonization with *U. urealyticum* has been associated with a subclinical endometrial inflammation, which could interfere with implantation and cause very early pregnancy loss that appears to be infertility. In one report (see Desai *et al.* 1980:470) endometrial colonization was noted in 50% of infertile women and only 7% of fertile women. Stray-Pedersen and her colleagues (1982) also reported recovering ureaplasmas more often from the endometrial aspirates of infertile (28%) than fertile (8%) women, although the isolation rate was about the same from women with unexplained infertility as from women for whom the cause of infertility was known. The association between ureaplasmas and female infertility appears to be further weakened by a study (Nagata *et al.* 1979, cited in Taylor-Robinson and McCormack 1980b:1064) showing that conception rates among a group of untreated ureaplasma-positive infertile women was the same after 1 year (28%) as it was for untreated infertile women not colonized by *U. urealyticum* (27%).

That ureaplasmal endometritis may play a role in recognizable pregnancy loss has also been proposed. Theoretically, the endometritis could cause a spontaneous abortion by spreading to the fetal membranes—ureaplasmas are more frequently isolated from the membranes of fetuses aborted spontaneously than from those aborted therapeutically (Taylor-Robinson and McCormack 1980b:1064)—or by producing intra-uterine adhesions that result in a loss of uterine elasticity with subsequent expulsion of the growing fetus. Stray-Pedersen (1978, cited in Taylor-Robinson and McCormack 1980b:1064) isolated ureaplasmas more often from the endometria of women with repeated spontaneous abortions (28%) than from the same site in a control group (7%). And Kudsin and colleagues (cited in Taylor-Robinson and McCormack 1980b:1065) have reported successful pregnancies after tetracycline treatment in women colonized by ureaplasmas who had frequent spontaneous abortions. However, Taylor-Robinson and McCormack (1980b:1065) were unwilling to draw the same conclusions from these data because other organisms that might cause endometritis, such as *Chlamydia trachomatis,* were not sought and because the antibiotic trials were not controlled. Thus, although *U. urealyticum* is more frequently isolated from the endometria of infertile women or women with repeated spontaneous abortions and is associated with a subclinical inflammation of the uterine lining, evidence for a causal association with reproductive failure, as provided by existing studies, is weak.

Pelvic Inflammatory Disease

Evidence that ureaplasmas play a role in PID is weak (Taylor-Robinson and McCormack 1980b:1066). Although these organisms have been isolated from the tubes and peritoneal exudates of a small percentage of women with acute PID and although antibody responses to *U. urealyticum* have been noted in PID patients (Taylor-Robinson and McCormack 1980a:1008), there is no proof of a causal relationship. Furthermore, organ cultures of fallopian tubes inoculated with *U. urealyticum* show no pathological changes, although experimental infections in animals would be more conclusive because they would allow for the interplay of the host's immunologic responses, which may play an important part in formation of disease (Taylor-Robinson and McCormack 1980a:1008).

Postabortal and Postpartum Fever

McCormack *et al.* (1975, cited in Taylor-Robinson and McCormack 1980a:1008) recovered *U. urealyticum* from the blood of 15 of 327 women a few minutes after delivery, but the bloodstream invasion did not persist nor was there an antibody response to the invasion. Thus, Taylor-Robinson and McCormack (1980a:1008–1009) concluded there is no evidence that *U. urealyticum* plays a role in postpartum or postabortal fever.

Low Birth Weight

Shepard (1970:1338) reported that more infants of low birth weight (<2500 gm) have nasal and pharyngeal colonization with ureaplasmas. And Taylor-Robinson and McCormack (1980b:1066) cited a number of studies showing that colonized infants have a statistically lower mean birth weight than noncolonized infants. In addition, a prospective study by Braun *et al.* (1971, cited in Taylor-Robinson and McCormack 1980b:1066) showed that women colonized with ureaplasmas gave birth to infants with a statistically lower birth weight. Taylor-Robinson and McCormack (1980b:1066) concluded that the evidence linking *U. urealyticum* and low birth weight is strong. Nevertheless, they did have some reservations, noting that women who have a predisposition to smaller babies may be selectively colonized. Lower socioeconomic class women, for example, are both more likely to have smaller babies (for many reasons) and to be colonized with genital mycoplasmas. Whether ureaplasmal colonization is a contributing factor in low birth weights in these women is yet undetermined.

Effects on the Male Reproductive System

Although many healthy men without apparent urethritis are colonized with ureaplasmas, recovery rates in NGU patients following administration of selective antimicrobial agents have established an association between *U. urealyticum* and NGU (Felman and Nikitas 1981:382–383). Meheus *et al.* (1980:239) believe *U. urealyticum* may be responsible for 20 to 30% of NGU cases. Taylor-Robinson and McCormack (1980a:1004–1006) have critically reviewed the literature and have concluded that evidence for an etiologic role is strong but that the proportion of NGU cases caused by *U. urealyticum* is still unknown. (See Chapter 10 for a more detailed discussion.)

There is little evidence for a role for *U. urealyticum* in prostatitis or epididymitis (Taylor-Robinson and McCormack 1980a:1006). This suggests that ureaplasmal urethritis is a self-limiting infection that does not spread posteriorly. Thus, although urethral strictures could follow infection of the male genital tract with ureaplasmas and could affect coital frequency if there is pain upon ejaculation, neither functional damage to the sperm due to prostatitis nor sterility due to epididymitis would follow such an infection.

It would then appear that ureaplasmal infection of the male genital tract has little effect on conceptive ability. But Gnarpe and Friberg (1972:730) noted that ureaplasmas seemed to be attached to spermatozoa, and Fowlkes and colleagues (cited in Taylor-Robinson and McCormack 1980b:1063) have found that sperm in semen samples containing ureaplasmas are fewer and have poorer motility and more aberrant forms than do sperm in samples without ureaplasmas. These workers subsequently showed that successful treatment of the infection was associated with considerable improvement in sperm motility and a decrease in certain abnormal morphological features.

Can these observations, however, be correlated with observable differences in conceptive ability? Neither Harrison *et al.* (1975:606) nor Matthews *et al.* (1975:989) found any difference in the frequency of ureaplasmas in fertile and infertile couples. And Harrison *et al.* (1975:605), in a well-controlled study, found that conception rates in infertile couples with genital mycoplasmas were the same whether they received antibiotic therapy or a placebo. But Gnarpe and Friberg (1972:727) reported that T-mycoplasmas were found significantly more frequently in infertile couples than fertile couples and later reported (Friberg and Gnarpe 1974:333) that pregnancy occurred in 25% of ureaplasma-positive couples shortly after eradication of the mycoplasmas. Toth and associates (1983:505) reported similar findings. In their study 161 men were ureaplasma-positive, and the antibiotic doxycycline was given to them and their partners. In those couples freed of the infection, 60% achieved pregnancy compared to only 5% of those who still had the infection. *U. urealyticum* is found so frequently in the genital tracts of both fertile and infertile couples, one research team (Cassell *et al.* 1983:502) suggested that the bacterium interferes with conception only when the couple has some other problem that has lowered their fertility.

Summary

Adadevoh (1974:18) noted in his study of the causes of subfertility and infertility in Africa that although there were indications that the ureaplasmas might be important in NGU and subsequent subfecundity, the neglect of the study of male infertility by researchers made assessment of its importance impossible. The report of a WHO Study Group on the Epidemiology of Infertility (World Health Organization 1975:18) noted that the role of the genital mycoplasmas in pregnancy loss had not yet been defined. In the years since, many studies of the genital mycoplasmas and their association with human reproduction have been published but, as noted by Taylor-Robinson and McCormack (1980b:1066), they have generally been of such poor quality that few conclusions can be drawn from them. Taylor-Robinson and McCormack have critically reviewed these studies and have concluded that there is strong evidence only for an association between *M. hominis* and PID and postabortal and postpartum fever and between *U. urealyticum* and NGU and low birth weight.

Mycoplasma hominis appears to be a cause of PID. Animal studies have suggested that the salpingitis caused by *M. hominis* spares the lumen, although the muscle layer is involved. Hence, sterility would not be a frequent sequela of such infections, although ectopic pregnancy resulting from damage to the tubal transport mechanism might be anticipated. *Mycoplasma hominis* also appears to be an important cause of postabortal and postpartum fever. Such postpartum fevers are secondary to an endometritis, which if persistent could diminish fecundity by causing pregnancy loss by interfering with implantation or, if intrauterine adhesion should form, by causing spontaneous abortion.

Studies suggest that *U. urealyticum* is an important cause of NGU. Although chlamydia probably causes 40–50% of cases, some authors believe that *U. urealyticum* may cause 20–30%. Other workers believe that the ureaplasmas are definitely a cause of NGU but that the proportion of NGU cases with this etiology is simply not known. *U. urealyticum* apparently does not spread posteriorly because involvement of the accessory glands or epididymis with these organisms has not been documented. However, urethral strictures may follow a urethritis and these may cause pain during ejaculation, which could in turn lower coital frequency. But even an uncomplicated infection may alter fertility, since the quantity and quality of sperm are lower in semen samples containing ureaplasmas than in uninfected samples. In women, *U. urealyticum* probably lowers infant birth weight and may therefore contribute to higher rates of perinatal mortality. And although one study has stated that the organism is a frequent cause of infertility (Toth *et al.* 1983), acceptance of this position must await confirmatory evidence. One research team suggested that *U. urealyticum* (a frequent inhabitant of the genital tracts of both fertile and infertile couples) may be an infertility promoter, interfering with conception only when the couple has some other problem that has lowered their fertility (Cassell *et al.* 1983).

CHAPTER 14

Genital Chlamydia

Introduction

Chlamydia trachomatis is an aerobic bacterium responsible for three important diseases in humans: lymphogranuloma venereum (LGV) (serotypes L_1, L_2, L_3), hyperendemic blinding trachoma (serotypes A, B, B_a, C), and ocular-genital infections (serotypes D–K). The latter is responsible for proctitis, urethritis, epididymitis, prostatitis, cervicitis, and salpingitis in adults, and inclusion conjunctivitis and pneumonia in newborn infants (Melo 1979:520). Trachoma is not of interest here because it does not affect fecundity, and although LGV may have some impact on fecundity we felt that it was not prevalent enough to merit discussion here. The focus of this discussion, therefore, will be ocular–genital chlamydia, which we shall simply call chlamydia. (Much information dealing with chlamydial infections has already been covered in Chapter 10, and the reader is referred to that chapter for additional information.

Uncomplicated chlamydial infections are associated with a urethritis in men and a cervicitis in women. When symptomatic, these infections mimic those of gonorrhea. But infection is usually asymptomatic in women and mild or asymptomatic in men. Frequently even examination of the cervix of an infected woman yields no evidence of abnormality (Paavonen *et al.* 1979:301). With a frequency equal to that seen in gonococcal infections, *C. trachomatis* ascends to produce a salpingitis (Bowie 1980:21). Complications in men are probably also common. In nongonococcal urethritis (NGU), 40–50% of which is chlamydial in origin, epididymitis occurs in 4% of cases and prostatitis even more frequently. Permanent sequelae are similar to those seen following a gonococcal infection. Tubal abnormalities causing sterility or ectopic pregnancy occur in women, and in men urethral strictures have been noted.

Prevalence

Developed World

In the developed world, genital chlamydial infections may be more common than gonorrhea. This is particularly true among those of higher socioeconomic status. In one group of women of high status chlamydia was isolated nine times more frequently than gonorrhea (Bowie 1980:24). The disease is particularly prevalent among young, sexually active, single, white males who belong to the middle or upper socioeconomic class (*Time* 1978a:73). Background infection rates for developed countries have been reported to be 1–2% for asymptomatic males and 5% for asymptomatic females (Muir and Belsey 1980:918). Alexander and associates (1977:151) found a 13% infection rate in an obstetric population, but others (see *Time* 1978a:73) found only 5% of pregnant women to be infected. Alexander *et al.* suggested at that time that their high figure was probably due to certain characteristics of their study population and to more sensitive diagnostic techniques. However, Alexander more recently stated (see *Philadelphia Inquirer* 1982:13D) that about 10% of all pregnant women are infected with *C. trachomatis,* basing this conclusion in part on a study he conducted in the late 1970s with Martin and others at the University of Washington (Martin *et al.* 1982). Indications are thus that chlamydial infections are increasing.

By collating the data from a number of studies in the developed world (Bowie 1980:24; Eschenbach 1980:143S; Felman and Nikitas 1981:385; Mardh *et al.* 1977:1377; Oriel 1977a:231), we arrived at the following isolation rates: 0% for women with no genital tract infection, 6% for women with a lower genital tract infection, 10–20% for women in sexually transmitted disease (STD) clinics, 20–36% for women with acute salpingitis, 30–60% for women with gonorrhea, and 60–80% for women whose male partner has a chlamydial infection. (The rates for women with acute salpingitis may be lower than expected because, according to Mardh *et al.* [1981:128], the rising antibody titers associated with an acute infection may result in lower isolation rates from the cervix.) In men *C. trachomatis* can be isolated in 0 to 7% of men with no genital tract infection, 20 to 30% of men with gonorrhea, and 30 to 50% of men with NGU (Meheus *et al.* 1980:239).

Developing World

In the developing world the importance of *C. trachomatis* is unmeasured. Although most cases of cervicitis and salpingitis and of urethritis and epididymitis in the developing world are believed due to *Neisseria gonorrhoeae*, there are indications that among persons of higher socioeconomic status gonorrhea is less important, allowing a greater role for *C. trachomatis*. Thus, although more than 80% of urethritis cases in Rwanda, Kenya, Malaysia, and Swaziland are gonorrheal, among higher-status men in Ibadan, Nigeria, only 33% of cases are due to gonorrhea (Meheus *et al.* 1980:243–244). And although *C. trachomatis* is found in 1% of males with gonorrhea in Swaziland, this figure is 25% for white males in Johannesburg (Meheus *et al.* 1980:244).

Mafiamba (unpublished, cited in Muir and Belsey 1980:918) did a serologic survey in Cameroon to determine how widespread chlamydial infections were. Antibodies to chlamydia were detected in 50% of the population, and in 16% of the population were high enough that recent infection was suspected. However, only 63 blood samples were assayed, so the findings are very preliminary. Whether antigen specific to serotypes D–K was used was not stated, but this is important to know because LGV and trachoma are also endemic in the developing world, and ocular–genital chlamydia can be differentiated from them only by using type-specific antigen.

Evidence for a Role
in Genital Infections

The higher isolation rates of *C. trachomatis* in men and women with infections of the lower or upper genital tract is one of the strongest bits of evidence supporting the role of the organism as a primary pathogen. Other significant correlates are (1) seroconversion during the first clinical attack, (2) rising antibody titers associated with active infection, (3) eradication of genital tract infection in chlamydia-positive but not chlamydia-negative cases after treatment with drugs effective against chlamydia, and (4) the appearance of salpingitis in monkeys experimentally inoculated with *C. trachomatis* (see Eschenbach 1980:143S; Holmes and Hobson 1977:4; Mardh *et al.* 1977:1379). In the experiments of Moller and Mardh (1980:117ff), *C. trachomatis* inoculated onto the cervix or into the uterus of grivet monkeys moved along the mucosal surface, just as *N. gonorrhoeae* does, to produce an endosalpingitis. At sacrifice several weeks postinoculation there were persistent changes in the tubes—thickening, adhesions, degenerative changes in the epithelial cells—that could impair fecundity.

Effects on Fecundity

Coital Inability

Although chlamydial infection in women does not cause sequelae that could interfere with coital ability, such sequelae are possible in men. Urethral strictures have been noted in men following chlamydial infection, and Masters and Johnson (1970:293) noted that urethral strictures may cause severe pain during ejaculation. Prostatitis is seen during chlamydial infections; Masters and Johnson noted that infections of the prostate and other accessory glands may cause an intense burning sensation during and immediately after ejaculation. In such cases coital frequency would probably be reduced, and in severe cases coital inability would be a possibility. Although any negative effects on coital ability caused by an acute prostatitis subside as the infection subsides, strictures are permanent features whose correction requires dilation or sometimes surgery.

Conceptive Failure

Many authors (e.g., Felman and Nikitas 1981:383; World Health Organization 1975:15) have suggested that because chlamydia can cause epididymitis and pelvic inflammatory disease (PID) it may also be involved in male and female infertility. Punnonen et al. (1979, cited in Muir and Belsey 1980:918) found antibodies to C. trachomatis in 57% of infertile women and only 29% of fertile women, a difference that is statistically significant. Paavonen et al. (1979:301) found such antibodies in 19.6% of infertile women and 9% of fertile women, which, though suggestive, is not a statistically significant difference.

Sequelae in men have not been as extensively studied, although urethral strictures have been reported and occlusion of the genital ducts and functional damage to sperm are possible because both chlamydial epididymitis and prostatitis have been reported. (The reader is referred to Chapter 10 for a more detailed discussion of chlamydia and infertility.)

Pregnancy Loss

In chlamydial infections of the fallopian tube, as in gonorrheal infections, tubal occlusion and sterility is only one possible negative outcome. Often the tubes are only partly occluded and/or the ciliated epithelial cells are so damaged that conception is possible but the fertilized ovum cannot reach the uterus and implants ectopically. Pregnancy loss is the almost inevitable result in an ectopic pregnancy, and frequently the tube is surgically removed along with the pregnancy because of irreparable damage. Hence, an ectopic pregnancy is not only a cause of pregnancy loss but lowers conceptive ability as well.

In the discussion of *N. gonorroheae* (Chapter 10), it was mentioned that in the first trimester gonorrhea is a cause of spontaneous abortion; late in pregnancy it is a cause of premature rupture of the membranes and prematurity, which could compromise fetal well-being, and of postpartum fever, which could threaten future conceptive ability. Whether chlamydia can cause similar effects is unknown but seems probable. One bit of confirmatory evidence on one of these points comes from Rees *et al.* (1977:146), who noted that postpartum pelvic infections, presumably chlamydial, were frequent in mothers whose infants had a neonatal chlamydial infection. Also, *C. trachomatis* has been implicated in habitual abortion in domestic animals, and some workers have suspected a similar effect in humans (Greenberg 1979:319). Indeed, a study by Martin *et al.* (1982) showed that in a sample of 256 pregnant women, those with chlamydial infections were *10 times* more likely to experience spontaneous abortion or to lose their babies during the first month of life. Although the sample was too small to permit definite conclusions and the magnitude of the association greater than what could reasonably be expected, the study was the first to show a cause-and-effect relationship between chlamydia and pregnancy loss.

Other Effects

Since 1975 *C. trachomatis* has been linked to 20 medical conditions of previously unknown origin. It has been recognized that this organism is the commonest cause of infant conjunctivitis and perhaps of infant pneumonia as well (Holmes and Puziss 1980:640). Although Rees *et al.* (1977:146) suggest that the baby may be infected in utero, *C. trachomatis* ascending from the cervix, most workers (e.g., Evans 1979:441; Felman and Nikitas 1981:383) have felt the infant is infected as it passes through the birth canal. An estimated 40–50% of infants born to mothers with a cervical infection will develop conjunctivitis (Alexander *et al.* 1977:151; Galton 1980:16; *Time* 1978a:73). Because about 5% of all newborns are exposed (*Time* 1978a:73), such eye infections occur in 2 to 2.5% of newborns. The risk of an exposed infant developing pneumonia is only 5–10% (Galton 1980:16). Nevertheless, chlamydia accounts for 30% of pneumonia cases in infants under 6 months of age (Felman and Nikitas 1981:383).

Summary

Chlamydia trachomatis is capable of causing genital infections in men and women that, if extending beyond the anterior urethra or cervix, may cause male coital inability, male and female conceptive failure, and pregnancy loss. An infant born to a mother with a cervical infection has a 40–50% chance of contracting an eye infection and a 5–10% chance of developing pneumonia. The statement by Berger and associates (1978:304) is thus very apt: "The morbidity caused by *C. trachomatis* now parallels and rivals that caused by *N. gonorrhoeae.*"

Diagnosis

The clinical picture of a chlamydial infection is very similar to that of gonorrhea, but in most cases is milder. Women with a chlamydial cervicitis are overwhelmingly asymptomatic. Fewer men are asymptomatic, but their symptoms are generally mild and frequently overlooked or ignored. Whereas gonorrhea in the male frequently presents as an acute urethritis with copious amounts of a purulent discharge, chlamydial urethritis is mild with a scant, mucoid discharge that frequently requires penile stripping to be expressed. But differentiating a chlamydial infection from a mild gonorrheal infection may be difficult if physical criteria alone are used. Thus, whenever possible the physician should use serologic and tissue culture techniques to confirm the clinical diagnosis.

Tissue culture techniques for chlamydia have been vastly improved during the 1970s. Before then infections caused by *C. trachomatis* were generally missed because routine bacteriologic culture methods were inadequate for isolation of this organism, which is unique among bacteria in that it requires living cells for its growth. Now McCoy cells are used to isolate *C. trachomatis* and present methods fail to diagnose only a very few acutely infected cases. But techniques for culturing chlamydia are not available at all medical facilities, and physicians must frequently base their diagnoses on symptoms and a history of contact with persons with a nongonococcal infection (Bowie 1980:27).

Serologic techniques for detecting active and past infections with chlamydia have also been developed. Conversion from a seronegative to a seropositive status occurs during the first infection. Low titers reflect past infection and high or rising titers indicate present infection. High antibody titers, however, may obscure a bacteriologic diagnosis; Mardh *et al.* (1981:128) noted that *C. trachomatis* is isolated more often in women with no or low antibodies and suggested that high antibody levels destroy chlamydial organisms, resulting in negative cervical cultures.

Treatment

A chlamydial cervicitis or urethritis will subside after several months even without treatment, although treatment will shorten this period and substantially lower the risk of complications. As with gonorrhea, effective immunity is not produced and reinfection is possible (Wang *et al.* 1975:40). Because chlamydia is not susceptible to penicillin, amoxicillin, ampicillin, or spectinomycin, a misdiagnosis of the infection as gonorrhea means a persistence of the infection (Oriel 1977a:231). Tetracycline and erythromycin will, however, effectively eradicate the disease. In the past complications frequently developed because the infection was misdiagnosed, poorly treated, or left untreated because it was regarded as trivial.

Complications of chlamydial infections—PID, epididymitis, prostatitis—are handled the same way as complications of gonococcal infections, except that tetracycline or erythromycin is substituted for penicillin. Secondary invaders are even more frequent than in gonococcal infections and, if present, may require the use of additional antibiotics. It should always be kept in mind that tetracycline given to a pregnant woman will darken the primary teeth of the offspring and interfere with growth of the long bones. Therefore, erythromycin is the drug of choice for pregnant women.

IV

Events Predisposing to Pelvic Inflammatory Disease and Other Reproductive Problems

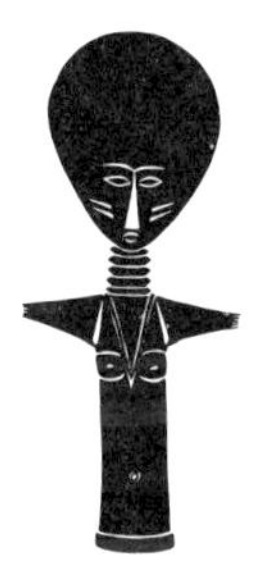

Induced Abortion

Introduction

Infection of the upper female genital tract always involves some risk to future fecundity. Intrauterine adhesions, kinking and partial or complete occlusion of the fallopian tubes, and tubo–ovarian abscesses are just some of the sequelae of pelvic infection that can compromise reproductive ability. Infections of the lower genital tract are the most important source of pelvic infections. *Neisseria gonorrhoeae* is the most frequent cause of such infections, but other sexually transmitted pathogens such as *Chlamydia trachomatis* or *Mycoplasma hominis* may also be important. In addition, members of the normal vaginal flora such as the anaerobic streptococci can ascend to the uterus and tubes, either as secondary invaders following a gonococcal or chlamydial salpingitis or by themselves. Other types of female pelvic infections are the consequence of infections that have their primary focus elsewhere and only secondarily infect the genitals. Among these are genital tuberculosis and genital schistosomiasis.

Important as these types of pelvic infection are, they may be responsible for fewer cases of pelvic infection in some parts of the world than septic complications following genital tract interference. The most important of these so-called iatrogenic causes of pelvic inflammatory disease (PID) are abortion and childbirth. Pelvic infections have also increasingly been linked to use of intrauterine devices (IUDs), and attention has been drawn to the fact that female genital mutilation (circumcision) may be a cause of pelvic infection and subsequent sterility in some parts of the world. Starting with this chapter on induced abortion, each of these four causes of pelvic infection will be discussed and evidence for the purported effects on female reproductive ability will be reviewed. In addition, noninfectious processes that are associated with induced abortion, childbirth, the IUD, and female circumcision and that may affect reproductive potential will also be discussed.

History

Abortion (interruption of a pregnancy before the period of viability, approximately 28 weeks [Potts 1970:65]) as a means of fertility control is as old as history. Chinese writings 5000 years old refer to mercury as an effective abortifacient. The Greeks favored abortion on social and economic grounds. Plato even recommended obligatory abortions for women over 40. And in Roman civilization it was fashionable for a woman to obtain an abortion early in pregnancy to maintain a youthful figure. But widespread acceptance of abortion in Western civilization waned with the growth of Judaism and especially Christianity (M. Guttmacher 1967:175–176). Criticisms of abortion, which appear in the Old Testament, became stronger during the Christian era (*Population Reports* 1980a:107), Judeo–Christian ethics proclaiming the sanctity of human life and labeling abortion a pagan practice. Religious proscriptions were followed by legal ones and abortion, except under conditions of medical necessity, was considered a serious crime throughout the Middle Ages and into modern times (M. Guttmacher 1967:176–177). However, under the principle of common law, induced abortion before quickening (the feeling of fetal movement, which occurs at approximately 16 weeks) was not an offense. Thus, in mid-nineteenth century America, for example, the fetus did not exist in the eyes of the law or in the collective opinion of the majority of people until it had quickened (Mohr 1978:73–74). The nineteenth-century woman seeking an abortion did not, therefore, have to face the same moral agonies as her twentieth-century counterpart. And women who may have had moral reservations about abortion even before quickening were protected by the contemporary medical opinion that a diagnosis of pregnancy was equivocal until quickening occurred. A woman could therefore be treated early on for ''obstructed menses,'' the treatment being the same as that used to induce abortion (Mohr 1978:15–16). In practice, then, abortion was common, particularly in nineteenth-century Europe and the United States (*Population Reports* 1980a:107–108); in fact, abortion is believed to be one of the primary factors underlying the remarkable decline in fertility in these areas that spanned much of the nineteenth and early twentieth centuries (see, e.g., Potts and Selman 1979:172).

Prevalence

Developed World

Soviet Union

The first modern nation to make abortion legal was the Soviet Union, which issued a decree in November 1920 making hospital-based abortions available on demand and at no expense. Within 4 years the demand for abortion was so great that a charge based on family income was exacted, the proceeds to be used in the building of new abortion facilities. However, by 1935 the original decree was greatly modified to disallow first pregnancies, pregnancies of more than 3 months' gestation, and performance of a second abortion less than 6 months after a prior termination. And in mid-1936 a very restrictive law went into effect, allowing abortion only if the life or health of the woman was threatened or if a serious disease of the parents could be inherited (M. Guttmacher 1967:177–178). The reasons for this startling reversal are unclear. It is probable that an increasing need for workers was a major factor. A second reason may have been that although abortion-related maternal mortality rates were low, morbidity rates may have been high, especially in women with repeated operations. Sterility was reported in a high proportion of such cases, and subsequent pregnancies in these women were reportedly often ectopic or associated with high complication rates and increased perinatal mortality. Thus, fears of "racial deterioration" may have prompted the government to restrict access to abortion (Taussig 1944:41). However, the morbidity data from the Soviet Union are considered controversial, as they do not reflect the experience of other countries at that time (M. Guttmacher 1967:178).

The Soviet Union has since relaxed its abortion laws, and abortion as a means of birth control is widely used because contraceptives are unpopular and hard to find (*Time* 1981a:27). In the late 1970s an estimated 2500–4000 abortions occurred for every 1000 live births (Davis and Feshbach 1980:13). The abortion rate per 1000 women of reproductive age is the highest in the world—twice that of Rumania, which has the second highest rate, and six times that of the United States. Incredibly, the average woman in the Soviet Union has six abortions in her lifetime

(*Time* 1981a:27). The infant mortality rate (IMR) in the Soviet Union is also quite high, especially for a developed nation; it rose phenomenally from 22.9 per 1000 live births in 1971 to 31.1 per 1000 live births in 1976 (Davis and Feshbach 1980:12). By comparison, the U.S. rate was only half this in 1976 and has declined since (*Philadelphia Bulletin* 1980a:A3). One reason forwarded for the increase in the IMR is the frequent use of abortion; reports indicate that women with a history of multiple induced abortions are more likely to give birth to premature infants, who have an IMR many times that of full-term infants (Davis and Feshbach 1980:13). It would not be unexpected then for the Soviet Union to reinstate more restrictive laws governing abortion and/or make contraceptives more available.

United States

From colonial times until the latter part of the nineteenth century there were few statutes regarding abortion in the United States, and the practice, if not approved of, was at least tolerated (Mohr 1978:145–146). During the mid-nineteenth century abortion became more common in the United States than ever before. Whereas the majority of American women who sought abortions during the eighteenth and early nineteenth centuries were poor, unwed, and socially desparate, women seeking abortions after 1840 were more likely to be older, married, and desiring to limit family size (Mohr 1978:240–241). A demographic profile of these women described them as primarily married, Protestant women, frequently of high social standing, usually native-born, and from all parts of the country (Mohr 1978:100). Their numbers must have been quite large because estimates by physicians of the day of the proportion of pregnancies terminated by abortion range from a high of 1 in 3 to a low of 1 in 10 (Mohr 1978:82). Generally it is thought that although 1 in 25 to 1 in 30 pregnancies ended as an induced abortion during the first 3 decades of the nineteenth century, by the 1850s and 1860s this figure had jumped to 1 in 5 or 1 in 6 (Mohr 1978:50; Potts and Selman 1979:201).

But between 1860 and 1880 the situation changed dramatically, largely as a result of the pressure exerted by physicians on legislators and on public opinion. Physicians had traditionally been opposed to abortion, both because it violated the Hippocratic oath and because some felt it was morally wrong. But many physicians opposed the procedure for more self-serving reasons. University-trained physicians, or regulars as they were called, were losing patients to untrained practitioners or irregulars who made their living largely by performing abortions. Restricting abortion would put the irregulars out of business, thereby allowing the regulars to regain their sagging prestige and restore their economic base (Mohr 1978:34–35).[1] Although some states had enacted anti-abortion legislation prior to 1860 and the physicians' crusade, such laws usually included the quickening doctrine and did not recognize the criminal liability of women. Anti-advertising laws prior to 1860 were uncommon, and existing laws were weak and did little to stop the widespread advertisement of abortion in the popular press. But under pressure from physicians and because of the shift in popular opinion that the physicians worked to bring about, legislators dropped traditional quickening rules, revoked common-law immunities against criminal prosecution for women, and passed effective anti-advertising and anti-obscenity laws (Mohr 1978:224–225).

It was the anti-advertising and anti-obscenity laws that did the most to limit the number of abortions effectively, driving the abortionists underground or out of business. A highly visible casuality of the new laws was Madame Restell, one of the most successful abortion specialists of the mid-nineteenth century. Madame Restell (née Ann Lohman) was an Englishwoman who migrated to New York City and began performing abortions on a commercial scale in the 1830s. By the mid-1840s she had branch offices in Boston and Philadelphia. Her salesmen peddled pills on the road, instructing women that if the pills failed to produce the desired result they should go to one of the main clinics for more extensive treatment. In 1871 Madam Restell's empire was so large that an estimated $60,000 was spent each year on advertising alone. But Madame Restell was arrested under the new anti-obscenity laws, and one day before her trial was to begin, in April 1878, she committed suicide (Mohr 1978:48, 52, 199).

Despite restrictive laws, abortion continued to be a factor in fertility regulation after 1880. Reportedly, a greater proportion of women seeking abortions after 1880 were young and unmarried, much like those who sought abortions in the early part of the century. And although it is likely that some older, married women still sought abortions, a greater reliance on contraception helped limit the number of unwanted pregnancies (Mohr 1978:241–243). Data on the frequency of abortion in the United States between 1900 and 1920 are nonexistent and estimates are based on tangential information. One such estimate by Taussig (1936, cited in Mohr 1978:254) placed the number of abortions early in the century at more than 500,000 per year. Another study about this time

---

[1]There is evidence that a fair number of regulars succumbed to patients' offers of large fees to perform abortions; complaints about the involvement of regular physicians in the abortion trade were extremely common in the medical press of the period (Mohr 1978:95, 285).

(Whelpton 1944:22) estimated that 350,000 abortions were performed each year, meaning that almost 13% of all pregnancies terminated as an abortion. Urban rates were believed to be much higher than rural ones, there being an estimated 1 abortion for every 6 confinements among urban women and 1 for every 9 confinements among rural women (Dunn 1944:5). A survey by Kinsey in the 1950s revealed that 90% of premarital pregnancies in the women he surveyed ended as abortions, and that 22% of married women had an abortion while married (see Mohr 1978:254). Indeed, Kleegman (1967:255) reported that 90% of all abortions at this time were among married women with three or more children. By the late 1960s anywhere from 0.2 to 1.2 million abortions were being performed annually in the United States (Mohr 1978:254). Maternal deaths reached 500–1000 per year (Nathanson 1979:193), a remarkably low number considering that an Institute for Sex Research survey showed that many abortions were being done by incompetent physicians, quacks, alcoholics, and drug addicts (Horton and Leslie 1974:212). One reason why women continued to resort to abortion was that some did not know proper contraceptive techniques. It was not until the late 1930s that the American Medical Association recommended the teaching of contraceptive methods in medical schools (Kleegman 1967:261), and this information was not made widely available to the public. Indeed, one study showed that even women with medical conditions that contraindicated pregnancy were not taught by their physicians how to avoid conception (see Kleegman 1967:254).

It should be noted that there is an almost total lack of information about abortion among U.S. blacks prior to the twentieth century (Mohr 1978:287). And for the first half of the twentieth century information on abortion among blacks is equally as sketchy as it is for whites. However, there is no compelling reason, given the readiness with which blacks used legal abortion in the 1970s, to assume that behavior in this regard was markedly different from that of whites. However, because prior to legalization therapeutic abortions were more easily obtained by private patients (Kleegman 1967:256), it is likely that a disproportionate amount of maternal mobidity and mortality occurred among black women who had to rely more often on self-induced or back-alley abortions.

When individual states began to liberalize their abortion statues during the 1960s and New York State adopted its ''abortion on demand'' statute in 1970, women in unanticipated numbers filled the abortion clinics. The floodgates were really opened in 1973 when the Supreme Court decision in *Roe* v. *Wade* forbade any state to limit abortion during the first 3 months of pregnancy and placed only moderate restrictions on abortions between 3 and 6 months' gestation, primarily to protect the mother's health. Only during the last trimester did the interests of the unborn child override those of the mother and abortion at this time was allowed only to preserve the life or health of the mother (Mohr 1978:248–249). Under this liberal law the number of legal abortions performed each year in the United States grew from 22,000 in 1969 to 1.5 million in 1980 (Leary 1982:4A).

Data collected between 1973 and 1977 show that U.S. women obtaining abortions were overwhelmingly young (one-third were teenagers), white, and unmarried. Abortion rates were highest among women 18–19 years of age, nonwhites (three times the white rate), the unmarried (four times the married rate), and the very poor (Forrest *et al.* 1978:274–275). Between 1973 and 1977, 4 million U.S. women obtained 5 million abortions, and by 1977 there were 385 abortions for every 1000 live births (Forrest *et al.* 1978:271–272). But even in 1977 30% of women who wanted an abortion were unable to obtain one, largely because abortion services were unavailable in their communities or nearby (Forrest *et al.* 1978:271). Many of these women were probably from rural areas where abortion is much less frequent; in 1976 and 1977, 95% of all abortions were performed in metropolitan areas (Forrest *et al.* 1978:272). Since the Supreme Court decision there has been a steady trend toward the performance of abortions earlier in pregnancy when they are safer. In 1976, 50% of abortions were performed at 8 weeks' or less gestation, whereas 90% were performed at 12 weeks or less (Forrest *et al.* 1978:274). Earlier-term abortions are one important factor responsible for the substantial decrease between 1970 and 1979 in the maternal mortality rate (from 6.2 per 100,000 to 1.5 per 100,000) (Leary 1982:4A).

Developing World

General

Although abortion is legal in China, Japan, and India, it is illegal in most of the other countries of Asia. It is also illegal in most of Africa, Latin America, and the Middle East. Nevertheless, abortion is common throughout the developing world, but is more common in Asia and Latin America than in the Middle East and Africa. Indeed, it is as common in some countries where it is illegal, especially in Southeast Asia, as it is in some countries where it is legal. And rates of illegal abortion are increasing in some developing countries. The type of woman seeking an abortion tends to differ according to region. In Asia, Latin America, and the Middle East the average woman seeking an abortion is older, married, of high parity, and wishes to limit births; her counterpart in Africa is more often a young, unmarried student without children who wishes to postpone childbearing and often fears expulsion from school if the pregnancy is detected. Young women in Latin America are also turning to abortion in larger numbers (*Population Reports* 1980a:106, 135).

Illegal abortion is a major cause of maternal mortality in the developing world, accounting for 4 to 70% of maternal deaths in hospitals and an unknown number of additional deaths outside of hospitals (*Population Reports* 1980a:105). Very high rates of abortion-related mortality have been recorded in particular locales. In Kinshasa, Zaire, for example, an autopsy series revealed that 95% of all maternal deaths were due to septic or hemorrhagic complications of illegal induced abortion (Smith *et al.* 1976:640).

Maternal morbidity secondary to induced abortion is also very high in the developing world. Postabortal hemorrhage and infection are more threatening to women in developing countries (1) because these women are frequently undernourished and are therefore more susceptible to infection, and (2) because many have chronic anemia, which both limits their ability to withstand an acute blood loss and further increases the risk of infection. In addition, menstrual irregularities caused by poor nutrition may postpone recognition of pregnancy, resulting in later abortions with greater risks (Cates *et al.* 1980:131). Thus, postabortal sepsis is common in the tropics and, according to Grech *et al.* (1973:126), "many countries both within and without Africa would rate septic abortion before either gonorrhea or puerperal sepsis in aetiological importance" to pelvic infection.

Africa

Restrictive abortion laws, primarily a legacy of the region's colonial past, are the rule in most of Africa. In Zambia abortion is allowed if continuation of the pregnancy would be a threat to the woman's physical or mental health, if there is a potential fetal deformity, or if an additional child would threaten the physical or mental health of existing children. Elsewhere abortion is forbidden entirely or allowed only if the mother's life or health is threatened (*Population Reports* 1980a:141). Illegal abortion has therefore become an increasing problem in Africa, especially in urban areas where socioeconomic pressures to space and limit births—crowding, high unemployment, and increased educational opportunities for women—are greatest. In urban areas traditional methods of birth control such as postpartum abstinence have been abandoned, yet there is almost a complete absence of commercially available contraceptives or extensive family planning programs. As a result the number of abortions is increasing, and many are performed in the second trimester with associated high risks of complications (*Population Reports* 1980a:143). In Kenya, for example, between 1971 and 1975 the number of septic abortions doubled (*Population Reports* 1980a:142).

The magnitude of the problem is difficult to assess because a considerable degree of underreporting occurs in African survey research (*Population Reports* 1980a:142). African gynecologists agree, however, that complications from spontaneous or illegal abortion are one of the most frequent causes of hospitalization (*Population Reports* 1980a:141). In fact, septic complications following abortion may be the most important cause of pelvic infections in some parts of the developing world (Grech *et al.* 1973:126). Kinshasa may be one of these areas. An extensive autopsy series there revealed that 95% of all maternal deaths were hemorrhagic or septic complications of induced abortion, which in almost all cases was illegal. In the same study 20% of all women autopsied had active or healed pelvic infections (Smith *et al.* 1976:640, 642). It is likely, therefore, that a substantial proportion of these infections were the result of postabortal sepsis. Charlewood (1956:55) has also noted increasing rates of criminal abortion among the urbanized Bantu with resulting sterility and complaints of dyspareunia (painful coitus). Because African women turn to abortion early in reproductive life—the majority are less than 25 years old (*Population Reports* 1980a:142)—the effect on population fecundity and fertility, especially in urban areas, could be great.

Latin America

The laws regarding abortion are very restrictive in Latin America. Nevertheless, in many countries illegal abortion is a lucrative business (*Time* 1981a:27). Prosecutions are few and the incidence of illegal procedures is believed to be very high. In some Central American countries, for example, there may be 1 abortion for every 2 live births (Hellman *et al.* 1971:519). The International Planned Parenthood Federation in 1974 estimated that 5 million abortions occur annually in Latin America (*Population Reports* 1980a:144).

The typical woman in Central or South America seeking an abortion is older, married, and has several living children and desires no more. However, this profile may be changing. Abortion among unmarried women is not rare and may be increasing. And growing numbers of women may be seeking abortions to space or postpone births. In addition, in the past most women receiving abortions were from the middle socioeconomic stratum of society and abortion was less frequent among richer and poorer women; however, women from all social strata have more frequently been seeking abortion (*Population Reports* 1980a:144, 148–149.

Asia

In Asia abortion rates are very high regardess of legal status. Japan, where abortion is legal, has one of the highest abortion rates in the world. So too do many countries in Southeast Asia where abortion is illegal. Indeed, abortion rates in many of these countries are higher than in the United States and other countries where abortion is legal and are exceeded only by rates in Eastern European nations. And in India, where abortion is legal, bureaucratic red tape translates to limited access to legal procedures and illegal abortion therefore remains a major health problem (*Population Reports* 1980a:135–136). For example, during the 3 years following passage of the reformed abortion law in 1972 there were only 250,000 legal operations performed, but an estimated 4 million back-alley abortions took place each year (Potts and Selman 1979:318). A similar situation exists in Hong Kong where abortion is legal and cheap but subject to much government red tape and long waits. Consequently, well-to-do women go to Japan or Singapore to get abortions but the poor wait, go to back-alley abortionists, or cross the border and get abortions in the Chinese cities of Shumchun or Guangzhou (Canton). Although abortion is cheap in China, the facilities are often inadequate and sanitation poor (*Intercom* 1978a:5).

Middle East

In Tunisia abortion is available on request. Elsewhere in the Middle East laws are very restrictive as a result of nineteenth-century colonial tradition and the influence of Islamic law. Only a threat to the mother's life or health is an acceptable reason for termination. However, the laws are rarely enforced and physicians perform illegal abortions openly in private clinics and hospitals (*Population Reports* 1980a:139).

Summary

Starting in the late nineteenth century anti-abortion sentiment grew. Restrictive laws were passed forbidding abortion unless the life or health of the mother was threatened. Indeed, the restrictive laws seen in many developing countries date from nineteenth-century colonial rule (*Population Reports* 1980a:108). However, in the developed world, starting with the Soviet Union in 1920 and followed in midcentury by other developed nations (by Japan in 1948 and progressively since 1955 by countries in Eastern Europe [Kerslake and Casey 1967:35]), the trend toward less-restrictive legislation began. In some instances the impetus for change came at the governmental level and was primarily motivated by socio-economic considerations. In other cases it was public opinion that shifted and called for more relaxed laws. For example, the thalidomide scandal called attention to the fact that grave medical hazards often confront the fetus rather than the mother. The tragedy of congenital rubella drew additional support for elective abortion on grounds of ''protecting'' the offspring from a life of grave physical and mental disability (Horton and Leslie 1974:213; Mohr 1978:252–253). Studies in midcentury allayed fears about the safety of abortion because they showed that first-trimester abortions performed by a competent physician in an appropriate facility were safer than full-term deliveries (Mohr 1978:254).

Between 1965 and 1980, 17 countries liberalized their abortion laws and 7 countries toughened their laws (*Time* 1981a:27). Several of the latter countries were among the first to enact liberal laws, but sagging birthrates prompted the governments to limit access to abortion. In 1981, 9% of the world's people lived in countries that totally forbade abortion and 38% lived in nations where abortion is available on request. The rest lived in countries where abortion was allowed under conditions that range from saving the mother's life to economic hardship (*Time* 1981a:27). It is estimated that 40–55 million abortions occur each year; half of these occur in the developing world and about half are illegal (*Intercom* 1976:9; *Population Reports* 1980a:105, 108).

It is probably true that ''abortion is an inescapable part of fertility control'' (Potts and Selman 1979:204). It was practiced by the ancients and is frequent in modern societies. It is found in the villages and cities of the developing world and the rural and urban areas of the developed world. Whether it is legal or illegal, women of all ages who wish to limit, space, or postpone births will often resort to abortion. In Colombia and Egypt, which have two of the world's strictest abortion laws, denying the operation even if the mother's life is threatened, half the beds and budgets of maternity hospitals in the large cities are devoted to women suffering the complications of criminal abortion (*Intercom* 1976:9). In Mexico City, where abortion is illegal except in cases of incest or a threat to the mother's life (*Population Reports* 1980a:144), herbal abortifacients are readily available and 80% of the beds in the Women's Hospital are filled by women suffering complications of illegal abortion (*Time* 1981a:27).

The reasons for seeking an abortion are diverse. In nonindustrial societies two major reasons have been noted (Potts and Selman 1979:165) that may, in a broader sense, be important in all societies. The first reason is that life is hard and there is a constant struggle for survival, which will only be intensified by increased numbers. This reason frequently motivated abortion among Australian aborigines and Eskimos. In other more economically secure societies abortions are performed so "status" goods can be conserved and the standard of living maintained. Thus, the Tikopia (of Tikopia in the Solomon Islands) limit births to ensure there will be no shortage of ceremonial food such as coconut cream.

Variables Affecting the Outcome of
Induced Abortion

Introduction

It is evident then that abortion is found in all societies among women of all ages and parities. The abortions these women receive may be performed by an experienced physician or, as is more often the case in the developing countries, by a traditional midwife. Or the abortion may be performed by a back-alley abortionist or be self-induced. The physician may perform the abortion using modern equipment such as a vacuum aspirator, the midwife may massage the abdomen until vaginal bleeding is initiated, the illegal abortionist may use a catheter (a piece of flexible tubing), or the women may try to abort the fetus herself by inserting the rib of an umbrella or a crochet hook into the uterus. All these procedures, even those performed by a physician in a hospital setting with modern equipment, carry some risk to the woman's general health and, as many studies have suggested, to her reproductive health in particular. The risk is increased considerably when the provider is untrained, the setting unsanitary, the equipment crude, and postoperative care nonexistent, a scenario common to criminal abortion (*Population Reports* 1980a:116).

The most common early complications of abortion are infection, hemorrhage, and shock. Late complications include chronic pelvic infections and reproductive problems such as sterility, ectopic pregnancy, spontaneous abortion, or dyspareunia. It has long been recognized that pelvic infection resulting from a septic abortion can compromise later fecundity. What has only relatively recently been recognized is that fecundity may be compromised even in the absence of any early indications of trouble. A cervix too forcibly dilated may be rendered incompetent in future pregnancies, a hysterotomy (removal of the fetus through an incision in the uterus) may result in endometriosis, and a curettage that cuts too deep may leave intrauterine adhesions in its wake. Thus, the problem of subfecundity following abortion may be far greater than the number of postabortal infections would indicate. And, indeed, it is being recognized that adverse sequelae—pelvic infections, damaged cervices, etc.—are not limited to the criminal abortions, but are also seen following hospital- or clinic-based procedures. The following discussion of the various abortion methods and their inherent dangers will show that any technique, even in the most experienced hands, involves some measure of risk.

Abortion Techniques

Abortion techniques fall into two major categories, mechanical and chemical, although often more than one method in either or both categories may be used. In Thailand, for example, some women combine oral abortifacients (chemical) with uterine massage (mechanical) to induce abortion (Narkavonnakit and Bennett 1981:60), and in the developed nations curettage (mechanical) often follows saline injection (chemical) to ensure complete removal of the products of conception.

Mechanical Techniques

Mechanical means are the most frequently employed of all abortion methods and include everything from the dilatation and vacuum aspiration performed by a physician, to the catheter inserted by a quack, to the uterine massage done by the village midwife, to the crochet hook used by the woman herself. In each case the objective is to damage the fetus, disrupt the feto–placental organization, or excite the uterus. The fetus is thereupon spontaneously expelled or, to speed the process, is removed by the operator.

External Procedures External methods of disrupting the uterine contents, such as uterine massage, are found in many traditional societies. Uterine massage is usually performed by the village midwife, who massages the lower abdomen to relax the stomach muscles and raise the uterus and then presses hard on the fetus until vaginal bleeding signals the onset of the abortion. If bleeding is not produced within a reasonable amount of time, the client may have to return for one or more repeat treatments (Narkavonnakit and Bennett 1981:60–61). In other cases, the midwife may escalate the procedure and begin pounding on the abdomen with her heel and elbow (Potts and Selman 1979:201–202). Severe complications such as uterine rupture might be anticipated following such violence to the pregnant uterus, and this would have implications for future fecundity. But the more moderate massage techniques seem to be associated with lower complication rates than several other means of illegal abortion. In rural Thailand, for example, where uterine massage is the most commonly used method of abortion (other popular methods are uterine injections and oral abortifacients), it is also the least debilitating (Narkavonnakit and Bennett 1981:60–61, 64).

Internal Nonmedical Procedures Mechanical methods that cause abortion by introducing an object into the uterus are the most frequently used of all abortion techniques. In self-induced abortions the object inserted into the uterus is usually a familiar item found around the house such as a knitting needle, crochet hook, or umbrella rib. The Eskimos use a thinly carved rib from a walrus for this purpose (Gordon 1977:37). In many societies a stick or twig is used. On the Indian subcontinent the pregnant woman squats over a stick held upright by a number of stones. Friends then push on her shoulders to drive the stick into the uterus (Potts and Selman 1979:200). When available, more professional equipment, such as a catheter, is used (Gordon 1977:38). Although the flexibility of the catheter seemingly has the advantage of lowering the risk of lacerating the cervix or perforating the uterus or vagina, it is one of the methods most likely to lead to hospitalization, perhaps because it is the most common method of illegal abortion worldwide (*Population Reports* 1980a:114). A study in Italy showed that about 50% of cases of catheter insertions by persons not medically trained were admitted to the hospital (World Health Organization 1978b:17). The most usual complications following insertion of a twig, catheter, or similar object are cervical laceration, uterine and intestinal perforation, and peritonitis. Hemorrhage, localized infection, and shock are also seen (*Population Reports* 1980a:106, 105, 113).

Internal Medical Procedures Although morbidity (and mortality) rates are higher for illegal than legal abortions, this is to a great extent a consequence of the procedure. An illegal abortion performed by a physician is apt to be no more hazardous than a legal one, largely because the physician is able to use a safer procedure (*Population Reports* 1980a:114). There are approximately six basic procedures used by contemporary physicians, and which procedure is used often depends on the duration of the pregnancy. If it has been 2 weeks or less since the missed menstrual period, a procedure called menstrual regulation is used. Other first-trimester pregnancies are usually terminated by a D & C (dilatation and curettage, sharp curettage) or vacuum aspiration (dilatation and suction). Second-trimester abortions may be performed using a modification of the D & C called a D & E (dilatation and evacuation) or by chemical means (discussed in the next section). Infrequently a hysterotomy (removal of the fetus through an incision in the uterus) or hysterectomy (removal of the uterus itself) is performed late in pregnancy.

Menstrual regulation is the removal of the endometrium when pregnancy is suspected but unproven. This is accomplished by a hand-operated syringe and cannula (tube) within 14 days of a missed menstrual period (*Population Reports* 1974:49). Where moral or legal restraints against abortion are operative, the ambiguous nature of the procedure makes it attractive. But from a medical point of view the procedure has several drawbacks. First, the woman may not be pregnant, in which case she has undergone an unnecessary procedure. Second, the products of conception are so small that they may be missed, making a second procedure necessary (Potts and Selman 1979:136). Minor uterine infections may also be troublesome (*Population Reports* 1974:64). However, menstrual regulation has the distinct advantage of not requiring cervical dilatation because a very fine cannula can remove the products of conception at this stage of development (*Population Reports* 1974:52; Potts and Selman 1979:136).

Once a pregnancy has progressed beyond 4 or 5 weeks' gestation the products of conception have reached a size when dilatation of the cervix is necessary for their removal. If the pregnancy is within the first trimester, a D & C or vacuum aspiration is usually performed. The sharp curettage associated with a D & C has been shown to cause injury to the muscular wall of the uterus (smooth muscle tissue has been noted during histological analyses of scrapings) three times as frequently as vacuum aspiration; such injury carries a serious risk of intrauterine adhesions (Edstrom 1975:126). Thus, reproductive potential may be jeopardized more by a D & C than by vacuum aspiration.

Once the pregnancy has entered the second trimester chemical means such as saline or glucose instillation have routinely been used. In the late 1970s the D & E (dilatation and evacuation) was introduced, in which the cervix is dilated and the fetus removed after dismemberment by a sharp instrument. Complications are believed to be less frequent and less severe following a D & E than following instillation procedures, primarily because there is less chance of retaining products of conception, which carries an increased risk of hemorrhage and infection (Cates *et al.* 1980:130–131).

One possible complication of all procedures involving dilatation of the cervix—the D & C, vacuum aspiration, and D & E—is trauma to the cervix. Many cervical injuries are associated with excessive force applied in use of dilating instruments (Edstrom 1975:131; *Population Reports* 1977:85), although tears may also be caused by the tenaculum, an instrument used to stabilize the cervix during dilatation (*Population Reports* 1977:85). The greater the duration of pregnancy, the wider the cervical diameter must be to remove the uterine contents effectively;[2] if the cervix is not adequately dilated there is the chance of incomplete evacuation, postabortal bleeding, and infection (*Population Reports* 1977:86). If the cervix is dilated 10 mm or less, full recovery to normal size will occur in 6 weeks. A midtrimester abortion requires at least 12 mm, and if dilatation should exceed 12–14 mm there could be risks for future reproductive performance, primarily cervical incompetence with possibly increased rates of spontaneous abortion (Cates *et al.* 1980:131; *Population Reports* 1977:85), stillbirths and premature births (*Population Reports* 1977:85), or low-birth-weight infants (World Health Organization 1978b:23–24).

One study showed cervical trauma in less than 1% of cases if the pregnancy was less than 9 weeks' gestation, but noted trauma in 2.5% of cases where gestation length was 9–12 weeks (Edstrom 1975:131). Although the risk of cervical injury is likely to increase as the pregnancy advances, the evidence is not clear-cut because in some instances the cervix softens in the later stages of pregnancy, making dilatation easier. On the other hand, a softened cervix may be more likely to suffer tenaculum damage (*Population Reports* 1977:86). It is certain, however, that the risk of cervical injury is greater in nulliparous than in parous women, because more force is necessary to dilate the cervix of a woman who has never borne a child vaginally (World Health Organization 1978b:27).

A survey of abortion studies found the reported incidence of cervical injury to be anywhere from 0 to 5% (*Population Reports* 1977:86). It is felt that studies vary widely on the reported incidence of cervical trauma because of differences in the method and degree of dilatation and because of differences in the type or severity of injury; an injury that one physician regards as important enough to report may be viewed as insignificant by another physician. It is also likely that reported incidences are underestimates because some cervical injuries may be difficult to detect and some physicians may be reluctant to report cervical injuries because they feel it reflects badly on their skill.

Safer, more "physiologic," methods do exist for dilating the cervix than the widely used metal expansion devices. One of these methods is the laminaria tent, a centuries-old method. These tents are simply

---

[2]Cervical dilatation of 4 man is necessary to remove a pregnancy of 1–4 weeks' gestation, 8 mm for 5–8 weeks', 10 mm for 9–10 weeks', 12 mm for 11–12 weeks', and 14 mm for 13–14 weeks' gestation (*Population Reports* 1977:86).

pieces of seaweed—*Laminaria digitata* or *L. japonica*—that are cut into shape and placed in the cervix. Intensely hygroscopic, the substance slowly absorbs body fluids and the swelling of the tent causes a slow, progressive dilatation and softening of the cervix (*Population Reports* 1977:92). Unfortunately, this method is unacceptable in most clinic situations because it takes so long (Cates *et al.* 1980:128). A vibro-dilator has been developed that proponents claim to be less traumatic than conventional methods. However, results with this device fall far short of those obtained with laminaria tents; in one study (see Edstrom 1975:131) serious lacerations of the cervix were noted in 12 of 165 women using the vibro-dilator and in only 1 of 500 women using the laminaria tents. In sum, most evidence points to the fact that the method of cervical dilatation may be more important than the method of uterine evacuation in preventing abortion morbidity which compromises reproductive potential (*Population Reports* 1977:85).

Two other mechanical methods of terminating a pregnancy are hysterotomy and hysterectomy. Both are rarely used for a number of reasons. First, they usually cause the fetus to be born alive, struggling briefly before dying. Second, major complication rates are very high; they have been reported at 2.5, 9.4, and 38.0% for hysterotomies and at 17.1 and 51.2% for hysterectomies (see Edstrom 1975:127). Future childbearing is obviously impossible following a hysterectomy, but reproductive potential may also be compromised following a hysterotomy because endometriosis has been noted following this operation (Edstrom 1975:127; Tietze and Lewit 1977:25). Infertility has been estimated to be present in 40 to 50% of women with endometriosis (Spangler *et al.* 1971:850). Endometriosis can interfere with conceptive ability if the errant tissue blocks the fallopian tubes (*Newsweek* 1976:62) or if implants on the tubal serosa irritate and scar the tube (Clark 1978:71). In many cases infertility is noted even though the tubes remain patent (Israel 1967:348). Thus, in many cases the exact relationship of endometriosis to infertility remains unclear (Spangler *et al.* 1971:850). If there is extensive growth of the endometrial tissue in the pelvic area, dyspareunia may result as well (Israel 1967:347; Masters and Johnson 1970:285–286).

Chemical Techniques

Oral Procedures   Using chemical means to induce abortion is also widely practiced. Abortifacient substances may be taken orally or may be introduced directly into the genital tract. Oral abortifacients might well be the oldest of all methods of abortion; the earliest reference to abortion, a Chinese text 5000 years old, mentions mercury as an effective

abortifacient (M. Guttmacher 1967:175). Oral abortifacients have continued to be popular means of initiating abortion despite their often
wrenching effect on the woman's body. Some oral abortifacients—such
as the emmenagogues, which cause uterine bleeding—affect the uterus
directly. Other oral abortifacients affect the uterus only indirectly by severely irritating the digestive system or causing convulsions, which in
turn causes uterine contractions and expulsion of the fetus (Devereux
1976:37–39).

The effectiveness of any oral abortifacient varies directly with its
toxicity. Some folk recipes have known and appropriate effects whereas
others are semimagical. Although paste of mashed ants, foam from a
camel's mouth, and tail hairs of the blacktail deer dissolved in bear fat
would seem to be in the semimagical category, they may have some
abortifacient chemical properties. Formic acid is presumably found in
the powdered bodies of certain ants, camel's sputum does have irritant
properties, and the concoction of deer hairs and bear fat causes gastric
irritation and hence possibly also uterine contractions (Devereux
1976:37–38). Herbal medicines for abortion are commonly used, and although some produce a strong and unpleasant effect on the woman's
system they do not always succeed in producing an abortion (*Intercom*
1978a:5).

Nevertheless, oral abortifacients must be effective in a fair proportion of cases, as they reportedly accounted for 7 to 14% of successful
abortions in the 1970s (Gordon 1977:36). However, they are from all
indications rather dangerous. Intense vomiting leading to dehydration
and death is a real possibility (*Population Reports* 1980a:106). In Mexico
City, where herbal abortifacients are openly sold in the marketplace despite the fact that abortion is illegal, four out of five beds in the Women's
Hospital are filled by women suffering complications of illegal abortion
(*Time* 1981a:27). A study in rural Thailand (Narkavonnakit and Bennett
1981:60–61, 64) found that emmenagogues, which were used by about
10% of women who had an illegal induced abortion, were the most dangerous method—more dangerous than uterine massage, which was used
by 59% of women, and uterine injection, which was used by 23%. A far
greater proportion of women using emmenagogues were hospitalized,
many because of heavy uterine bleeding. Heavy bleeding predisposes
to infection; if blood volume drops to the point where adequate tissue
perfusion cannot be maintained, bacteria can grow virtually unchallenged because cellular defenders carried in the blood reach the infection site in insufficient numbers (McFee 1973:157–158). Therefore, oral
abortifacients that act in this manner can jeopardize future fecundity.

Other oral abortifacients, which irritate or poison the body or digestive system thereby causing uterine excitation and expulsion of the fetus, although a serious threat to a woman's general health, would probably have a smaller residual effect on fecundity.

Intragenital Procedures   Chemicals that are introduced directly into the genital tract include everything from folk recipes placed in the vagina to salt solutions instilled into the amniotic sac. The Yoruba of Nigeria insert a variety of substances—a mixture of potash and lime juice, washing blue and gin, or local herbs—into the vagina to abort unwanted pregnancies, such as those occurring during lactation, which are believed to be a threat to the unweaned child. Such caustic compounds are reported to cause secondary sterility by severely damaging the vagina (Olusanya 1974:50–51). Other substances inserted into the genital tract include tar, pepper, potassium soap, and utus paste (Edstrom 1975:127; Gordon 1977:38). These methods are most commonly used in countries with poor health statistics, so complication rates are difficult to estimate (Edstrom 1975:127).

Introducing chemicals into the genital tract, albeit in a more sophisticated way, is a common method of inducing second-trimester abortions in the developed world. A portion of the amniotic fluid is withdrawn and replaced with a hypertonic solution—usually saline, less commonly dextrose. Although the mechanism of action is unknown, after a variable amount of time uterine contractions begin and the fetus, usually dead, is expelled. In the past dextrose, a sugar, was used in lieu of saline to bypass the problem of excessive sodium levels in the blood, a particular problem in women with kidney problems. However, dextrose is now infrequently used because of a greater risk of infection (Edstrom 1975:127; World Health Organization 1978b:31).

Some early studies (see Fullerton 1971:130) indicated high rates (22%) of infection following saline abortion as well, but most data show that although infections are not common after saline abortions, they are more common than after first-trimester abortions (see Edstrom 1975:127). This is probably the result of incomplete expulsion of the uterine contents, the immunoincompetent fetal tissue being an excellent sustainer of bacterial growth. Retention of tissue following saline abortion has been reported at extremely varying rates (Edstrom 1975:127). The World Health Organization (WHO) (1978b:33) estimated that 30% of second-trimester abortions are incomplete, the proportion decreasing with advancing gestation. As a result many centers routinely perform a curettage after expulsion of the fetus (Cates *et al.* 1980:132; Edstrom 1975:127;

World Health Organization 1978b:33). This introduces some risk of intrauterine adhesions should the curet cut too deep and damage the myometrium.

An additional risk associated with saline abortion is that if the cervix should fail to dilate properly despite powerful uterine contractions, the fetus could be expelled through an abnormal cervical tear opening directly into the vagina instead of through the cervical canal. Such an occurrence is difficult to detect and may go untreated, developing into a permanent cervicovaginal fistula that could adversely affect the woman's subsequent reproductive performance (*Population Reports* 1977:87).

Skill of the Provider

The technique used in inducing an abortion, although extremely important, is only one of several factors that determine the frequency of early and late complications. Naturally the skill of the provider and the conditions under which he or she works are vitally important. But it would be misleading to assume that accepted procedures performed by a physician in a clinic are safe and reflect minimal rates of risk. For example, two investigative reporters revealed appalling conditions in four of six Chicago abortion clinics. Unsanitary conditions, inexperienced or unqualified personnel, and haphazard procedures were all noted. Abortions were often performed in 3 minutes; a safe abortion takes approximately 15 minutes. One doctor went from patient to patient without washing his hands or putting on gloves. Some patients were not even pregnant. It is not surprising then that cases of uterine or vaginal perforation were reported, as were severe infections and a case of internal damage that later required a hysterectomy (*Time* 1978b:52). The long-term consequences for reproductive ability in some of these cases could be substantial. In addition, abortions performed in such haste must have involved even more forceful cervical dilatation than normal, and cervical incompetence may be an important problem for these women.

Maternal Factors and Abortion-Related Factors

Certainly the type of procedure and how well it is performed are important determinants of complication rates and may explain why various studies have come to different conclusions regarding the risk to subsequent reproduction of induced abortion (Daling and Emanuel 1975:172). But many maternal factors such as age, parity, race, socioeconomic status and health status, and factors related to abortion itself, such as length of gestation at time of abortion and the number of prior abortions, can also affect complication rates. The way in which these factors relate to an unfavorable outcome will be discussed, with emphasis on the interactive relationships among many of these factors.

Age is reported to affect abortion-related morbidity and mortality, rates being higher among the very young and older women (Edstrom 1975:130; World Health Organization 1978b:15). Parity is also believed to affect morbidity rates (World Health Organization 1978b:15), a relationship that has been supported by some studies but refuted by others (see Edstrom 1975:130). Some surveys (see *Population Reports* 1980a:115) see the relationship as being important only when comparing parous to nulliparous women. This is probably particularly true with regard to complications involving the cervix because the nulliparous cervix is much harder to dilate, increasing the risk of trauma and subsequent reproductive problems.

The length of gestation is a most important risk factor, complication rates invariably increasing with fetal age in weeks (Edstrom 1975:131; *Population Reports* 1980a:113; World Health Organization 1978b:15). Abortion at advanced stages of pregnancy is more common among very young women (Tietze and Lewit 1977:23), who, out of ignorance, fear, or other factors, deny the symptoms of pregnancy until they become unmistakable. Thus, very young women are at multiple risk of suffering complications following abortions: They are at risk because of their age, they are more likely to be nulliparous and require more forceful cervical dilatation, and they are more likely to seek an abortion when the pregnancy has advanced to the point where all complications—hemorrhage, infection, cervical trauma, etc.—are more frequent and more severe.

The same multiple-risk pattern exists for nonwhites, in large part because of their lower socioeconomic status. For example, black women in the United States have more late abortions than white women, a phenomenon that studies have shown to be related to their lower socioeconomic status (Tietze and Lewit 1977:23; World Health Organization 1978b:27). But more factors must be involved because abortion-related mortality (and, presumably, morbidity) in the United States for nonwhite women is more than twice that for white women even after controlling for stage of gestation (World Health Organization 1978b:28). Other important risk factors such as a history of repeat abortions and poor health status are probably more frequently seen in nonwhites, again largely as a consequence of poorer economic circumstances. Black women do have a higher abortion rate than white women (Forrest *et al.* 1978:274), and thus more black women suffer the accumulated risk associated with multiple procedures. In addition, the health of black women is poorer on the average than that of white women, and this also influences complication rates. Edstrom (1975:130) noted that among women with a preexisting condition, 23.3% of abortions had complications of some sort and 3.5% had major complications; for healthy women these figures were 11.1% and 1%, respectively. Yet these two risk factors—the number of repeated abortions and health status—may not be entirely independent if the results of a study by Carlsson and Hamilton (1970, cited in Jacobsson *et al.* 1976:75) are verified. This study found that women who applied for one or more repeat abortions were in a poorer state of physical and mental health than other abortion applicants.

Additional risk factors associated with both abortion behavior and possible complications of abortion, especially poor future reproductive performance, are being identified. Smoking, for example, may be more frequent in European women who have had an abortion, according to the World Health Organization's Task Force on Abortion Sequelae (see Logrillo *et al.* 1980:18). Because smoking is associated with adverse pregnancy outcome, especially low-birth-weight infants, differential smoking habits between aborters and nonaborters could be a confounding variable. Differential use of drugs and intake of alcohol between aborters and nonaborters should also be considered (Logrillo *et al.* 1980:18).

Effects on Fecundity

The risk of early and late complications following abortion depends, as just noted, on a large number of factors including the type of procedure, the skill of the provider, certain characteristics of the woman such as age and parity, and abortion-related factors such as the number of repeated abortions and the length of gestation. (Length of gestation and type of procedure are linked factors, pregnancies of greater duration requiring procedures that are innately more hazardous.) For legal procedures complication rates are very low and cervical trauma, much of which is unrecognized or unreported, is probably the most frequent complication and one which may have important repercussions on fecundity. Pelvic infections are rare, although the conditions reported in the Chicago clinics (*Time* 1978b:52) illustrate that not all legal procedures are equally safe and that serious complications such as pelvic infection and uterine perforation may occur with greater than expected frequency after legal abortion. Also, in developing nations such as China, where abortion is legal but resources are limited, the procedure is undoubtedly more hazardous. In countries such as India where most abortions are performed by back-alley abortionists because access to legal procedures is limited by an inefficient bureaucracy, complication rates are higher also. There the situation is much as it is in the many developing nations of Latin America, Africa, and Asia where abortion is still illegal. In these countries pelvic infection and severe hemorrhage following criminal abortion contribute to rates of maternal morbidity and mortality that are often incredibly high. Here ectopic pregnancy rates are inflated by post-abortal infections that have left the tubes damaged but not occluded. And here sterility rates are elevated because of tubal occlusion, tubo–ovarian abscesses, and other sequelae of septic abortion.

Coital Inability

The unfavorable late sequelae of septic abortion include not only effects on conceptive ability and rates of pregnancy loss, but effects on coitus as well. Dyspareunia is a common sequel to septic abortion, and although coitus may not be impossible it may be so painful that coital frequency is greatly diminished. The causes of dyspareunia are many-fold. Acute and chronic infections of the uterus or the broad ligaments supporting it and generalized pelvic infections that result in adhesions between loops of bowel, the omentum, and pelvic tissue can all cause the pelvic organs to become rigid and fixed and make coitus extremely painful (Masters and Johnson 1970:285; Rankin 1970:771; Rendle-Short and Stewart 1967:398). Even nonseptic abortions can result in scars in the vagina or tears in the broad ligaments, which can cause dyspareunia (Masters and Johnson 1970:268, 280). Although most cases of dyspareunia are associated with criminal abortions, this problem can arise following legal procedures, and is especially frequent in women with repeated abortions (Jacobsson *et al.* 1976:85).

Conceptive Failure

When comparing legal and illegal abortion perhaps the most re-markable difference is in the incidence of pelvic infection. Though rare following a legal procedure, pelvic sepsis is not uncommon following criminal abortion, especially if the provider is unskilled. In fact, posta-bortal sepsis has been forwarded as an important cause of pelvic infec-tion and sterility in some parts of the world. However, although some workers feel that postabortal sepsis is an important cause of reproductive failure, others maintain that it is not. The difference of opinion seems to hinge upon whether postabortal sepsis causes an endosalpingitis, which has grave consequences for fecundity, or a perisalpingitis, which is less serious. It has even been theorized (World Health Organization 1975:15) that although in the developed countries the tube is most often infected from without with a perisalpingitis, this is not the case in the developing countries where most women suffer from a number of endemic diseases and deficiencies so that the mucosa is more likely to be involved (endosalpingitis) with resulting sterility. However, reasons for such a change in the natural history of postabortal sepsis are not forwarded. Are there two alternate routes of tubal infection? Are different organisms involved that exhibit their own preferential routes of attack? Does maternal health status affect which route the organism will take? These and many other questions should be addressed before any statements can be made regarding the impact of postabortal sepsis on fecundity.

Pelvic infections may be caused by a wide variety of viral, bacterial, parasitic, and fungal agents. The organism may be normally pathogenic to humans, as in the case of *Mycobacterium bacillus* or *N. gonorrhoeae*, or it may be only potentially pathogenic as are some members of the normal vaginal flora, such as *Bacteroides fragilis*, which causes trouble only when found in the upper genital tract. The infectious agent may reach the pelvis secondary to an infection elsewhere, as in the case of an infected appendix where the organisms reach the genital tract by contiguous spread. More commonly the lower genital tract is the primary infectious focus for the organism, pelvic infection being initiated when the organism ascends. One of the most frequent instances of an ascending infection is that of gonorrhea, where *N. gonorrhoeae* moves from the cervix to the upper genital tract aided by the reflux of menstrual blood (Eschenbach and Holmes 1975:40). Organisms may also ascend when the cervix is breached, as in childbirth, spontaneous abortion, and induced abortion, as well as during surgical procedures such as D & C, insertion of an IUD, and hysterosalpingography. In most of these cases the opportunity is also present for the introduction of exogenous organisms on nonsterile instruments (Hajj 1978:289; Jacobson and Westrom 1969:1094; Thompson and Hager 1977:105; Westrom and Mardh 1975:157).

Once the infectious organism has reached the upper genital tract the pathological process begins, varying somewhat depending on the organism involved. Tuberculous infections of the fallopian tubes, unless detected and treated early, are usually associated with complete and irreversible sterility. Even if the tube remains patent, free passage of gametes is hindered by a labyrinth maze resulting from intratubal adhesions and by damage to the ciliated epithelium and the muscularis, which together comprise the tubal transport mechanism. Gonorrheal infections of the tubes are also devastating, but often repeated infections are necessary before sterility becomes inevitable (Westrom and Mardh 1975:162). However, even one attack can leave a woman sterile or with damage to the tubal mucosa, which substantially increases her chances of having an ectopic pregnancy. Nongonococcal salpingitis, and infection of the tubes in which the gonococcus cannot be isolated from the endocervix (and which in most series refers to spontaneous infections, not ones preceded by abortion, childbirth, or other predisposing events where the cervix is breached), is believed by most researchers to be an even more serious threat to fecundity than gonococcal salpingitis, subsequent tubal occlusion being two or three times more common. Belsey (1976:329), for example, reported tubal occlusion in 16.6% of cases of nongonococcal salpingitis and only 5.5% of cases of gonococcal salpingitis. One reason for this may be that the organisms seen in such infections are not as sensitive to the commonly used antibiotics as is *N. gonorrhoeae* (Belsey 1976:329; Eschenbach and Holmes 1975:48).

In gonococcal salpingitis and some types of nongonococcal salpingitis, spread from the vagina to the tubes is via the mucosa and the result is destruction of the mucosal folds and ciliated epithelium with partial or complete occlusion of the tubal lumen unless early and vigorous treatment is initiated (Thompson and Hager 1977:108). But many workers believe that if the pelvic infection has been preceded by abortion or childbirth, any spread of organisms[3] to the uterus and the adnexa— tubes and ovaries—will have been via the lymphatics, venous sinuses, or loose cellular tissue, not via the mucosa (Curtis and Huffman 1950:205, 565). The resulting tubal infection is therefore stated to be not an endosalpingitis, but a perisalpingitis. A perisalpingitis carries a much more favorable prognosis for future childbearing because the tubal mucosa is spared even though the tube may be kinked and the ovum transport mechanism disturbed due to peritubal adhesions and damage to the muscularis (Curtis and Huffman 1950:209; Rankin 1970:771). Although tubal pregnancy is a real possibility if such damage is present (Hellman *et al.* 1971:536–537), the prognosis for a successful pregnancy following therapy is far better than following an endosalpingitis of equal

---

[3]These include enterococci, *Bacteroides* species, streptococci (especially *Peptostreptococcus*), staphylococci, *Clostridium welchii*, and *Clostridium tetani*, the latter two being extremely serious (Curtis and Huffman 1950:213; Czernobilsky 1968:25; Hellman *et al.* 1971:520–521; *Population Reports* 1980a:122; Santamarina and Klein 1970:779; Westrom and Mardh 1975:160).

severity (Curtis and Huffman 1950:565) and Hellman *et al.* (1971:991), in referring to postpartum sepsis, which is agreed to have essentially the same pathogenesis as postabortal sepsis (Curtis and Huffman 1950:214), stated that "most often tubal patency is maintained, and subsequent fertility is not impaired." In addition, some workers (e.g., Fisher 1967:9) have not even mentioned salpingitis as a sequel to septic abortion, citing septicemia and peritonitis as the usual sequelae of infected abortion. And Hellman *et al.* (1971:521) claimed that infections following abortion are most commonly confined to the uterus.

However, the position of some of those who maintain that a perisalpingitis predominates in cases of septic abortion (e.g., Curtis and Huffman 1950:565) is shaken when they say that "sterility subsequent to abortion occurs very frequently" (1950:565) and that "the number of families deprived of offspring because of visits to abortionists during early marriage is beyond the comprehension of physicians and undreamed of by the laity" (1950:562). The issue has been confused even further by the statement (World Health Organization 1975:15) that although postabortal sepsis appears most often as a perisalpingitis in developed countries, in the developing world, among women suffering from a variety of endemic diseases and deficiencies that make them more susceptible to infections and their sequelae, the natural history of postabortal infections may be altered so that endosalpingitis and sterility are more frequently encountered.

The association of endosalpingitis with postabortal infections in the developing world is supported by Rendle-Short and Stewart (1967:407) who said that "both gonococcal and post-abortal infections tend to produce an endosalpingitis first." Further, Edstrom (1978:31) listed postabortal and postpartum infection as one of the causes of tubal occlusion in Africa. But data from developed countries (Westrom 1975:711) also suggest that endosalpingitis frequently follows postabortal infections, because tubal occlusion occurs even more frequently (27% of cases) than following gonococcal (6%) or nongonococcal (17%) salpingitis. Indeed Westrom and Mardh (1975:162) stated that "infections preceded by, e.g., parturition, curettage, or abortion, generally ran a *more severe* course than most 'sexually transmitted' cases of salpingitis" [emphasis added]. This is probably because of associated conditions, such as tissue trauma or hemorrhage, and because in almost all cases the organism is not the gonococcus (Westrom 1975:711) and, therefore, sensitivity to usual antibiotics is not as great (Thompson and Hager 1977:107; Westrom 1975:712).

The most reasonable assumption then is that a postabortal infection can result in either an endosalpingitis or a perisalpingitis. Indeed, Czernobilsky (1968:30) and Westrom and Mardh (1975:158) noted that an unchecked postabortal infection can move to the tubes via the mucosa to produce an endosalpingitis as well as via the lymphatics, venous sinuses, and interstitial tissues to produce a perisalpingitis.

What then determines which route the organism will follow? The two most important determinants are (1) whether or not there has been serious trauma to the genital tract and (2) the type of organism involved. If the genital tract has been substantially traumatized (i.e., if the cervix has been lacerated or the vagina or uterus perforated), organisms are offered direct access to the subepithelial lymphatics and vessels or to the pelvic cavity itself (Czernobilsky 1968:31; Rankin 1970:766; Rendle-Short and Stewart 1967:401). The result is likely to be a pelvic cellulitis, an infection of the pelvic cellular tissues. This may be a generalized infection or it may be localized in the broad ligaments as a parametritis or in the fallopian tubes as a perisalpingitis. The condition tends to be unilateral, the affected side being the site of entry (Rankin 1970:766); bilateral involvement is seen in only 25% of cases (Czernobilsky 1968:31). Indeed, the better fertility prognosis seen in such cases is probably due in large part to the fact that one tube and ovary are frequently normal.

The second determinant of whether an endosalpingitis or perisalpingitis will occur is the type of organism involved, because organisms differ in how they traverse a structure. Monif (1974:103) clearly illustrated this difference in his description of the two distinct routes of infection of *N. gonorrhoeae* and the Group A beta-hemolytic streptococcus, an organism frequently associated with postabortal and postpartum infections (Eschenbach *et al.* 1975:170).[4] *Neisseria gonorrhoeae* takes the path of least resistance, spreading transmucosally. There is a sequential infection due to contiguous bacterial replication and dissemination along the mucosal surface, resulting ultimately in an endosalpingitis. The Group A beta-hemolytic streptococcus, on the other hand, pursues a transorgan route. Once the epithelium of the uterus is penetrated, the following structures are sequentially involved: the endometrium, myometrium, and then adjacent soft tissues or peritoneal serosa. Thus, this organism would produce a perisalpingitis.

From such observations a gonococcal–nongonococcal, transmucosa–transorgan dichotomy sprang up (Moller *et al.* 1978:254–255), which lent support to the notion that postabortal and postpartum infections, which are usually nongonococcal, are associated primarily with perisalpingitis. However, this gonococcal-nongonococcal, transmucosa-

---

[4]Organisms frequently associated with infected abortions are the Group A and Group B beta-hemolytic streptococci and Group D streptococci (Eschenbach *et al.* 1975:170).

transorgan dichotomy has been proven wrong by the experiments of Moller and Mardh (1980:107ff), which showed that a nongonococcal organism, *C. trachomatis*, spreads from the cervix to the tubes via the mucosa and produces an endosalpingitis. Studies have also shown that other nongonococcal organisms, specifically the endogenous bowel organisms that are frequently found in the vagina, can ascend and cause an endosalpingitis. However, they are unlikely to do so unless there is some structural or functional alteration in the cervico-uteral junction, which normally provides an effective barrier to their ascent, or in the fallopian tubes themselves. Hence, tubal infection with bowel organisms, so-called endogenous nonvenereal PID, is usually seen in older women (structural changes in the cervico–uteral junction subsequent to child-bearing may facilitate spread) and in women with a prior episode of PID (fibrosis subsequent to healing of the inflamed tube renders the part more susceptible to infection).

It is probable that an induced abortion also dramatically alters the integrity of the cervico–uteral junction and predisposes to ascending infection with the potentially pathogenic bacteria of the vaginal flora. Tubal infection is even more likely in those women undergoing abortion whose tubes have been damaged by a prior episode of salpingitis. And Muir and Belsey (1980:920) suggested that tubal infection is probably also more common in women with genital schistosomiasis or genital filariasis, because both of these disorders can irritate and weaken the tubes and render them more susceptible to infection. Genital filariasis, for example, is associated with impaired lymph drainage of the genital tract. The ability of the tubes to resist infection subsequently drops, and organisms that before were transient visitors from the lower genital tract now become initiators of pelvic infection.

In sum, a perisalpingitis is more likely following induced abortion if there has been laceration or perforation of the genital tract, regardless of the organism involved. Indeed, even *N. gonorrhoeae* may cause a perisalpingitis if conditions are right (Monif 1974:103). In the absence of genital tract trauma a perisalpingitis or endosalpingitis may occur, depending on the organism involved. A perisalpingitis is more likely if an organism such as the Group A beta-hemolytic streptococcus, which spreads by a transorgan route, is involved. (This highly pathogenic bacterium is not an inhabitant of the female genital tract, and is introduced by nonsterile instruments.) On the other hand, if infection is due to one of the potentially pathogenic bacteria that normally inhabit the lower genital tract, an endosalpingitis is more likely. But because the innate virulence of these organisms is low, it is likely that they will initiate an infection only if the host tissue has been compromised by a prior salpingitis or by other infections of the genital tract such as schistosomiasis or filariasis. It may be for this very reason, as suggested by a WHO Study Group on Infertility (World Health Organization 1975:15), that postabortal infection in women in developing countries is likely to be an endosalpingitis. But even in the developed world endosalpingitis is frequent (Westrom and Mardh 1975:162). Perhaps the lower risk of genital tract trauma associated with better abortion methods and widespread legal abortion, coupled with an increased number of women with prior tubal infections, has produced a situation that results in fewer cases of perisalpingitis and more cases of endosalpingitis than in the past.

Finally, it should be noted that although consideration of the effects of septic abortion on conceptive ability has focused almost exclusively on tubal factors, some subsequent reproductive problems are doubtless due to ovarian involvement. Certainly there is ample opportunity for involvement of the ovary in the infectious process. And if there is substantial fibrosis upon healing, the eggs may not be able to escape (Decker and Loebl 1978:96; Sweeney 1968:251–252).

Pregnancy Loss

Ectopic Pregnancy

Septic abortion, whether associated with a perisalpingitis or an endosalpingitis, can result in tubal changes that predispose to ectopic implantation and subsequent pregnancy loss. In both perisalpingitis and endosalpingitis the muscularis is frequently affected and there may be permanent damage to the tubal transport mechanism. Both conditions may also result in peritubal adhesions so that the tubes are kinked and distorted. In either case, the risk of ectopic implantation is increased considerably. An endosalpingitis may further increase the risk, because although the tube may remain patent, the lumen is frequently narrowed or the ciliated mucosal cells damaged and thus normal transport of the fertilized ovum is affected. By one account (Westrom 1975:710) a prior episode of salpingitis—gonorrheal, postpartum, postabortal, etc.—increases a woman's chances of an ectopic implantation sixfold from 1 in 147 to 1 in 24. Hence, in tropical countries where ruptured tubal pregnancy is the commonest surgical emergency among women, the high rates of ectopic pregnancy are believed due to widespread pelvic infection, with septic abortion the most important factor in some areas, especially urban ones (Grech et al. 1973:126). Muir and Belsey (1980:923) cited two studies showing that of women in Kampala, Uganda, and Benin, Nigeria, with ectopic pregnancies, 17.5% and 26.5%, respectively, previously had abortions.

In the developed world pelvic infection following abortion is much less frequent. Only about .5% of the 1.5 million abortions performed each year in the United States end in sepsis, for example. Nevertheless, ectopic pregnancy rates in the developed world are increasing, paralleling the increase in all types of pelvic infections, most of which are associated with sexually transmitted diseases or the IUD. However, a not insignificant number of ectopic pregnancies are associated with abortion. Muir and Belsey (1980:923) reported that even in Sweden, where abortions are legal and skillfully performed, a prior abortion increases a woman's chances of having an ectopic pregnancy by 50%; women with a prior live birth have 1 chance in 68 of having an ectopic implantation, and women with a prior abortion have 1 chance in 46. It is likely that in some cases there is no history of pelvic infection, the postabortal infection being mild or completely asymptomatic.

Endometritis

We have concentrated on how septic abortion affects the fallopian tubes, as this organ is the most vulnerable to disorganization capable of profoundly affecting fecundity. But certainly the other genital organs and pelvic tissues may be infected with a subsequent negative impact on reproductive potential. The uterus, for example, is frequently infected in septic abortion, the organisms involved having been introduced by a dirty instrument or having ascended from the vagina (Rendle-Short and Stewart 1967:401). Uterine infection (endometritis) is most likely to occur when the abortion is incomplete because the products of conception are immunoincompetent and cannot resist infection. If strong chemicals have been introduced into the uterus, the resulting necrotic tissue also offers an excellent culture medium for bacterial growth (Rendle-Short and Stewart 1967:412). Such infections may leave in their wake intrauterine adhesions, which are associated with higher rates of pregnancy loss because the uterus can no longer expand to accommodate the growing fetus.

Spontaneous Abortion and Reproductive Failure

We have so far discussed septic abortion as it relates to induced abortion. But is it not possible for an infection to follow a spontaneous abortion? Many workers have felt that it is, especially where medical treatment is inaccessible (*Population Reports* 1980a:121) and where people are debilitated and live in poor surroundings (Rendle-Short and Stewart 1967:401). In the latter case, spontaneous abortions are likely to be more numerous as well, due to adverse health factors that increase the risk of premature termination of pregnancy. Women in developing countries, for example, have higher rates of malaria and syphilis, which are abortifacient. Indeed, Retel-Lauretin (1974:73) has stated that venereal disease, especially syphilis, is associated with a high risk of abortion and subsequent sterilizing pelvic infections and, consequently, with low fertility. However, others (e.g., Romaniuk 1967, cited in Belsey 1979:258; Scragg 1957) have felt that spontaneous abortion is not a cause of low fertility. And Trichopoulos *et al.* (1976:647) made the point that although the association between spontaneous abortion and subsequent infertility is "statistically highly significant and very strong," this may be due to the fact that those endocrine or local factors that cause spontaneous abortion also eventually cause infertility.

Frequency of Reproductive Problems Following Induced Abortion

Illegal Abortion

Illegal induced abortion is undoubtedly associated with a significant threat to health and fecundity (*Population Reports* 1980a:115),but quantitating this risk is extremely difficult because data on the frequency of illegal abortion and its complications are "limited" and "fragmentary" (World Health Organization 1978b:17). Two possible data sources for information about the frequency of illegal abortion and its complications are hospital records of septic and hemorrhagic complications of abortion and statistics on postabortal maternal mortality.

Muir and Belsey (1980:917) presented data from hospital records from 12 countries showing the proportion of gynecologic admissions for septic abortion. Particularly noteworthy were the Philippines and Thailand where 10–30% of ward admissions were for infected abortions. Similarly, a study in Benin City, Nigeria (Okojie 1976:517–519) showed 25% of beds in the gynecologic ward were occupied by women with botched abortions. And in Latin America 20–48% of women required hospitalization after their last spontaneous or induced abortion (*Population Reports* 1980a:113). Of course, these data probably underestimate the frequency of complications following illegal abortion, as it is likely that only the most desperately ill women make their way to medical facilities.

Maternal mortality rates following abortion are yet another barometer of the frequency of illegal abortion from which approximations of the frequency of fecundity impairment can be derived. But mortality rates are also problematic because they often lump together deaths from spontaneous and induced abortions (*Population Reports* 1980a:110). Nevertheless, where deaths from abortion are extremely high it is reasonable to assume that illegal abortion and its complications are high also. In Kinshasa, for example, where 95% of all maternal deaths are the result of hemorrhagic or septic complications of induced abortion (Smith *et al.* 1976:640), illegal abortion is undoubtedly very common and very dangerous and fecundity impairment is probably substantial. In the Kinshasa study 20% of all women over age 10 had evidence of active or healed pelvic infection, a very high rate and one undoubtedly linked to the high rate of postabortal sepsis. Although certainly not all areas where abortion is illegal report such high rates of morbidity and mortality, wherever abortion is *self-induced or performed by unskilled persons*, as is the case in Kinshasa, the death rate will be much higher than elsewhere. Thus, whereas 50–100 deaths can normally be expected for every 100,000 illegal procedures, the death rate will be 1,000 deaths per 100,000 procedures when the abortionist is unskilled or is the woman herself (*Population Reports* 1980a:110).

Although maternal morbidity and mortality rates are a reflection of the number of abortions being performed and the level of skill of the abortionist, they can only suggest the level of abortion-related damage to the reproductive system. And even if it were possible to record the number of complications—the numbers of injured cervices, damaged endometria, etc.—the proportion of these that could result in reproductive problems would still be unknown. It is even difficult to determine whether a pelvic infection has caused infertility. Although certain diagnostic procedures such as tubal insufflation, laparoscopy, and hysterosalpingography are useful in detecting tubal abnormalities, these procedures give variable numbers of false-positive and false-negative results. And even if the tubes appear patent by one or more of these procedures, there is no assurance that tubal function is unaltered. Thus, only a full-term uterine pregnancy is unequivocal proof that reproductive ability is intact. Hence, difficult and time-consuming as it may be, accurate evaluation of abortion sequelae must rely on studies of reproductive performance.

Developed World

Some reports on illegal abortion in the developed world have suggested very high rates of fecundity impairment. Pantelakis and associates (1973:799) reported that in Greece approximately one-third of women subject to an induced abortion subsequently become sterile and concluded that induced abortion is a "very important cause" of the population decrease in that country. Similarly, a study by Trichopoulos *et al.* (1976) reported that women with a prior induced abortion had a 3.4 times normal risk of secondary sterility. However, such estimates seem inordinately high, especially because most abortions, though illegal, are performed by physicians under the guise of correcting a menstrual irregularity (Valaoras *et al.* 1969:14). Indeed, a re-analysis by Hogue (1978, cited in Daling *et al.* 1981:61) of the Trichopoulos *et al.* (1976) study showed no association between prior abortion and infertility. And the additional data of Pantelakis *et al.* (1973:802), which showed an increased risk of premature birth in women who had an abortion, is of little value because no separate analysis of induced versus spontaneous abortions could be done. Nevertheless, because abortion is probably the most widely used form of birth control in Greece (Pantelakis *et al.* 1973:802), used by 35% of women in one cross-sectional study (Valaoras *et al.* 1969:14), additional more strictly controlled studies should be done.

Developing World

Data on the late sequelae of illegal abortion in the developing world are extremely scarce. A study (Okojie 1976:517ff) in Benin City, Nigeria, found that 25% of beds in the gynecologic wards were occupied by women with postabortal complications. Uterine perforation, cervical laceration, and anemia were commonly recorded. The effect on population fecundity of these illegal abortions is potentially great because the women involved were usually young and nulliparous, with one or two prior abortions and no knowledge of contraception. The low fertility rate in this area, which is a major problem, is believed due in large part to tubal occlusion and to repeated spontaneous abortions arising from cervical incompetence, both possible sequelae of induced abortion.

Another African study (Smith *et al.* 1976:640), in Kinshasa, also revealed high rates of pelvic infection concomitant with extremely high rates of abortion-related morbidity and mortality. In the Kinshasa study 20% of all women over age 10 had evidence upon autopsy of active or healed PID. Because illegal induced abortion is very common in Kinshasa and very crudely performed, septic and hemorrhagic complications accounting for 95% of all maternal deaths, there can be little doubt that septic abortion is a major etiological factor in sterility and other reproductive problems in the city.

These studies can only suggest that late complications are very frequent after illegal induced abortion; they are unable to quantify the effect. Thus, conclusions regarding the frequency of late complications must be guarded. However, in the developing world where most abortions are performed by unskilled persons, where many women are suffering from a number of endemic diseases and nutritional deficiencies which can increase the risk of infection, and where health services are scarce (decreasing the likelihood of early and adequate treatment of complications), illegal induced abortion poses a greater hazard and substantially higher rates of subsequent reproductive problems would be anticipated.

Legal Abortion

Some studies have suggested that even legal induced abortion is not without risk. Although that risk seems to be minimal for the major early complications such as hemorrhage and infection, there has been increasing interest in the possibility that late complications that reduce reproductive potential are not uncommon.

The first experience with widespread legal induced abortion and its sequelae was in the Soviet Union in the first half of this century. In 1920 free hospital-based abortions were made available on request. Although the demand for abortions was great, by 1936 the government had re-enacted restrictive abortion laws. This move was believed by some (e.g., Taussig [1944:41]), to have been motivated by fears that the reportedly high rates of reproductive failure seen in women with repeated abortions would ultimately lead to "racial deterioration." Relying heavily on the Soviet Union data, Taussig cited rates of sterility following abortion of 5.4, 10, 14, 19, and 27% noting, however, that some of these data will not stand up to critical analysis. He also noted an increase in spontaneous abortion rates, strikingly higher rates of ectopic pregnancy, increased rates of complications of labor and delivery, more menstrual disturbances, and higher rates of psychosexual problems (Taussig 1944:41–45). Taussig observed that late complications—sterility, complications in subsequent labors, menstrual and endocrine disturbances—were even more frequent following legal abortion (27.9%) than following spontaneous (11.6%) or criminal (12.3%) abortion, and he attributed this to damage secondary to curettage (Taussig 1944:39–40). Whether the surgical techniques used in the Soviet Union were improper or whether the data on pregnancy outcome are incorrect is not known, but no other experience with widespread legal abortion has ever recorded such high rates of unfavorable outcome (A. Guttmacher 1967:12).

There is a considerable body of literature concerning the impact of legal abortion, as currently practiced, on subsequent reproductive performance. Some of these studies have indicated that whereas pelvic infection and subsequent sterility are rare following induced legal abortion—only an estimated .5% of abortions in the United States are followed by a tubal infection (*Family Planning Perspectives* 1980b:206)—rates of spontaneous abortion, prematurity, and low-birth-weight infants are substantially increased. Three variables seem to be associated with an increased risk of adverse outcome: (1) the number of abortions, (2) the method used, and (3) the length of time between an induced abortion and conception.

Many studies have indicated that if any risk to future fecundity exists it is limited to women with two or more abortions. A study in Boston (Levin *et al.* 1980, cited in *Family Planning Perspectives* 1981b:238) reported no greater risk of spontaneous abortion for women with one prior induced abortion, but women with two or more abortions were significantly more likely to experience pregnancy loss (2.3 times as likely to have a first-trimester abortion; 3.3 times as likely to have a second-trimester abortion). Losses early in pregnancy were attributed to the possibility that multiple induced abortions may somehow alter the viability of the developing pregnancy or impair implantation or placentation; losses later in pregnancy were attributed to abortion procedures that damage the body of the uterus or cervix, promoting cervical incompetence.

A multinational WHO study indicated that women with a history of repeated abortions are also significantly (2.5 times) more likely to have premature (<37 weeks) and low-birth-weight (≤2500 gm) infants (*Family Planning Perspectives* 1979:39–40; *Population Reports* 1980a:115). However, a study in Taiwan (Daling and Emanuel 1975:170–172) noted no such adverse effects unless the number of abortions exceeded four, and even then there was only a suggestion of reduced birth weight. This study reported that age, parity, prior fetal death, and socioeconomic status, which are significant indicators of pregnancy outcome, also showed a statistically significant relationship to abortion status. It concluded that if study and control groups are not matched for these factors, abortion appears to increase prematurity rates by 52% and low birth weight by 21%, whereas if the two groups are matched abortion shows no effect on pregnancy outcome.

A study in Hawaii by Smith *et al.* (1980, cited in *Family Planning Perspectives* 1981b:238–239) suggested that the interval between induced abortion and subsequent conception is a very important determinant of pregnancy outcome and may have confounded the results of some studies. In the Hawaii study there was no increased risk of spontaneous abortion with one prior induced abortion, and only a slight increase with two prior induced abortions. But if the index pregnancy occurred within 1 year of an induced abortion it was much more likely to end as a spontaneous abortion; 33% of conceptions occurring within 6 months of an induced abortion ended as a spontaneous abortion, whereas <8% of those occurring more than 1 year following an induced abortion ended so. The authors noted that a short interval between birth and subsequent pregnancy is also believed to lead to a greater risk of spontaneous abortion, and they therefore concluded that the spontaneous abortions are not necessarily related to induced abortion per se. The further noted that other studies may have found an increased risk associated with induced abortion because they were limited to 1 year in length and therefore to pregnancies closely following an induced abortion.

There is, therefore, little unanimity about the effects of induced abortion on future reproductive potential. In 1975 Edstrom (1975:129–130) charged that the literature was a "study of biases and their effect upon research" and made a plea for additional studies, more carefully controlled, in a large number of women. But selecting the variables to be controlled is no easy matter, as illustrated by the problems encountered by a prospective study conducted among a large group of women in New York State. The interim report of this study (Summary of Progress 1978)—which matched more than 20,000 women who had ended their first pregnancy as an induced abortion between July 1, 1970, and June 30, 1971 (study group), and an equal number of women matched by race, age, education, gravidity, and residence who had a live birth during the same period (control group)—showed that subsequent pregnancies in the study group had much less favorable outcomes than did subsequent pregnancies in the control group. Increased rates of spontaneous abortion (almost double), low-birth-weight infants, premature births, and complications of labor and delivery were noted. However, the final study report (Logrillo et al. 1980:23–24, 26–28) showed that these differences were attributable primarily to the fact that the study group was experiencing its first live birth, which is itself associated with poorer outcome. When the study group's pregnancies were compared to the first pregnancies of the control group, no statistically significant differences in outcome were noted, with the exception of complications of labor (premature separation of the placenta, placenta previa, prolapse of the cord, etc.). These complications were particularly evident when the abortion was a D & C or suction abortion; the risk following saline abortions was only half that of these procedures.

Diagnosis and Treatment

Septic abortion is usually not difficult to diagnose, although it may be confused at first with gonococcal or nongonococcal salpingitis because fever, vaginal discharge, and lower abdominal pain are common features of all three conditions. Septic abortion may also present a clinical picture similar to an incomplete spontaneous abortion because a dilated cervical os, hemorrhage, and retained products of conception are seen in both instances. However, when the hemorrhage is significant a diagnosis of illegal induced abortion is almost always correct (*Population Reports* 1980a:121). This can further be confirmed by looking for any trauma to the genital tract that may have been caused by instrumental interference.

The treatment of septic abortion is a three-pronged attack involving antibiotic therapy, monitoring and correcting blood volume, and early removal of any retained products of conception. Antibiotics are given in large doses to arrest the infection; fluid therapy is initiated to correct blood volume, which may have dropped significantly following extensive hemorrhage; and the uterus is evacuated as soon as possible, as risk of a fatal infection is greater if this is delayed (*Population Reports* 1980a:122, 124, 125–126).

The prognosis is best if the infection is confined to the uterus and its contents, and worst if the infection spreads not only to adjacent pelvic structures but beyond as well (*Population Reports* 1980a:122). The vast majority of cases of septic abortion can be controlled by immediate, aggressive therapy, but in a small number of treated cases and in many untreated cases the disease becomes chronic. Tubo–ovarian or other pelvic abscesses may form. These are often difficult, if not impossible, to eradicate and are a cause of chronic pain and ill health and, almost certainly, of sterility. And if the abscess should rupture a life-threatening condition such as peritonitis is possible. Unfortunately, in many patients drugs are being used inappropriately and cases of chronic pelvic infection are on the increase (Rendle-Short and Stewart 1967:398).

The most serious complication of septic abortion is septic shock, which is caused by a toxic substance (endotoxin) produced by certain bacteria. Blood circulation is reduced, there is inadequate tissue perfusion, cells become oxygen starved, and metabolic acidosis develops. The percent of septic abortions complicated by septic shock was 1.8–3.8% in the United States before legalization, 15.6% in Egypt in 1973, and 10.25% in India in 1970. Mortality rates are high in developing countries, sometimes close to 50%, and septic shock accounts for the majority of abortion-related deaths (*Population Reports* 1980a:122, 124).

Summary

In 1944 Siegler (1944:416) stated that "induced abortion . . . must be considered as the etiology of the frequent involuntary sterility following voluntary termination of pregnancy." And in a 1950 review Caine and Wilson (1950, cited in Wilson 1967:195, 197) estimated that of women having an abortion—self-induced, criminal, or therapeutic—about 20% would never have children because of abortion-related infections or a "change in attitude" toward the husband. In the late 1950s Halbrecht (1956, cited in Israel 1967:463) stated that "ascending post-abortal and post-puerperal infection of the endosalpinx is doubtless the most frequent cause of tubal occlusion in secondary sterility." Ryder (1959:417) suggested that "abortion procedures may play an important role in reducing the fecundity of most, if not all, populations."

Such dire assessments predate widespread experience with legal abortion, except in the Soviet Union, and were therefore probably based on impressions that complication rates were high following criminal abortions. Although the data for illegal procedures still remain sketchy, better data now exist on the frequency of complications following legal abortion.

Legal Abortion

It does appear that legal abortion can be followed by pelvic infection, tubal damage, and sterility, although this occurs in only a small percentage of cases (see Hacker 1976:D15; *Newsweek* 1976:62). It has been estimated that .5% of legal abortions are followed by tubal infections (*Family Planning Perspectives* 1980b:206) and that about 15–20% or more of these will end in sterility despite antibiotic therapy (*Family Planning Perspectives* 1980b:206; Westrom 1975:711; Westrom and Mardh 1975:157, 1978:21). Thus, about 5000 of the 1–1.5 million abortions performed in the United States each year will be followed by a tubal infection, leaving about 1000 women sterile. Sterility is therefore a rare sequela to legal induced abortion and is no more frequent than after delivery in comparable circumstances (World Health Organization 1978b:23).

But some other types of reproductive problems occur with much greater frequency. Many studies have suggested that spontaneous abortion rates may be higher in women whose abortions involved cervical dilatation. And for women who have had two or more abortions, spontaneous abortion rates may be elevated two- or threefold. Prematurity and low birth weight are also reported to be more common in women with repeated abortions. But because many studies that have shown higher rates of spontaneous abortion, prematurity, and low birth weight have been criticized as being flawed, confirmation of these findings must await further investigations. Regardless, when there is a deviation from normal operating standards, as was observed in the Chicago clinics, high complication rates would be anticipated.

Illegal Abortion

Illegal induced abortion is associated with substantial risks to health and fecundity. About 3% of abortions in the United States prior to legalization were associated with severe side effects (Potts 1970:68). Higher rates would be anticipated in the developing world, and these would vary with the type of abortion, skill of the provider, etc. In Latin America, for example, 20–48% of women required hospitalization following their last spontaneous or induced abortion (*Population Reports* 1980a:113). Other areas have recorded substantially lower rates, however. In a study in rural Thailand by Narkavonnakit and Bennett (1981:63, 60), 24% of illegal abortions were followed by some sort of early complication, but only one-tenth of these were serious enough to require hospitalization, yielding a figure (2.4%) not very different from the U.S. figure for serious side effects. In this study the risk of early complications was not evenly distributed by method, however, the risk being highest for oral abortifacients and lowest for uterine massage. Indeed, the complication rate for uterine massage was surprisingly low. It may be that such traditional methods, which are performed by midwives, carry less risk than the instrumental abortions performed by the unskilled abortionist. Thus, it is probably in the urban areas of the developing world—where socioeconomic forces increase the demand for abortion and where the unskilled abortionist uses primitive, dirty instruments—that complications, especially those that affect fecundity, are most often seen.

Septic abortion is one of the most commonly treated conditions in the obstetric and gynecologic services in developing countries (*Population Reports* 1980a:121). (See Muir and Belsey [1980:917] for a table showing the proportion of gynecologic admissions due to septic abortion for nine developing countries.) In many areas it is a more important cause of pelvic infection than either gonorrhea or postpartum sepsis (Grech *et al.* 1973:126). At the same time, tubal occlusion, a possible sequela of septic abortion, is believed to be the most important cause of infertility in Africa south of the Sahara and other areas where a high prevalence of infertility exists (World Health Organization 1975:15), accounting for three-fourths of the cases of infertility in the developing world (Guest 1978:27). As a result, septic abortion has been suggested as one cause of the high rates of secondary sterility seen in parts of Africa (see, e.g., *New York Times* 1978:8; Prothero 1972:106). However, such conclusions have been criticized because they have relied, albeit of necessity, on anecdotal evidence (*Population Reports* 1980a:115).

It is true that no hard evidence exists on the sequelae of illegal abortion. Even for legal procedures reliable data are scarce. But certainly indications are that infection following criminal abortion is an important cause of sterility, and perhaps ectopic pregnancy, in the developing world. These indications include (1) the fact that most abortions are practiced by unskilled practitioners, especially in urban areas where abortion is more frequent; (2) the high rates of maternal death due to septic complications of abortion; (3) the poor health status of women, which decreases their resistance to infection; (4) the high incidence of prior pelvic infections, especially gonorrheal salpingitis, and of genital schistosomiasis and genital filariasis, all of which make it more likely that a sterilizing endosalpingitis will follow an induced abortion; (5) the tendency for women to seek abortions late in pregnancy when complication rates are much higher; and (6) the limited access to and use of health services. And reproductive problems resulting from cervical laceration or endometrial damage are admitted to be more frequent in areas where unskilled abortion is frequent. However, it has been concluded (World Health Organization 1975:17) that they do not contribute significantly to pregnancy wastage in sub-Saharan Africa. We feel that this conclusion is premature. Indeed, Okojie (1976:521) noted that in Benin City, Nigeria, where unskilled abortion is rampant, women frequently suffer repeated spontaneous abortions because of cervical incompetence.

There is much to be learned about the effects of induced abortion—legal and illegal—on reproductive ability. But certainly present data, though not irrefutable, strongly suggest that legal abortion is followed, if not by sterility then by increased rates of misadventures during pregnancy—spontaneous abortion, prematurity and low-birth-weight infants. For illegal abortion such repercussions are probably more frequent. But because methods of legal and illegal abortion are so different, assigning the same sequelae to each its risky. However, if sequelae such as prematurity and low birth weight are seen following illegal abortion, their impact in the developing world is undoubtedly great because a further reduction in birth weight or a shortening of the gestational period may prove fatal to the newborn in areas where health services are poor. Finally, although pelvic infection and sterility are rare following legal abortion, illegal induced abortion is associated with a substantial threat of a sterilizing postabortal infection.

CHAPTER 16

Childbirth

Introduction

Like abortion, childbirth may be associated with pelvic infection and sterility. Indeed, postpartum infections were frequent prior to the introduction of aseptic obstetrical practices and were probably an important cause of secondary sterility in historical populations in Europe and elsewhere (Gray 1979:242). Postpartum sepsis is not infrequent now in the developing world and has been cited as a cause of secondary sterility there (Hull and Tukiran 1976:21). The pathogenesis of the infection is the same as for a postabortal infection. Many of the same microorganisms are involved and the lesions are essentially the same, although they may be even more serious if the birth is traumatic and there is extensive tearing of tissue (Curtis and Huffman 1950:214). And again the same difference of opinion exists over whether postpartum infections affect the inside (endosalpingitis) or the outside (perisalpingitis) of the fallopian tubes. Curtis and Huffman (1950:214) stated that a perisalpingitis occurs. Hellman and associates (1971:991) agreed, saying that ''most often tubal patency is maintained, and subsequent fertility is not impaired by the puerperal infection.'' But the Scientific Group on the Epidemiology of Infertility of the World Health Organization (World Health Organization 1975:15) proposed that although a perisalpingitis may follow an infected delivery in the developed world, the natural history of the infection may differ in women in developing countries and more serious sequelae (i.e., an endosalpingitis and sterility) may be encountered. As with abortion, we again assume an intermediate position and maintain that either a perisalpingitis or an endosalpingitis is possible; the latter is more likely if the tube has suffered prior damage and a perisalpingitis is more likely if there has been tearing of the genital tissue so that organisms have direct access to the abdominal cavity.

Causes of Postpartum Infection

Whenever there is a breach of the cervix—due to childbirth, abortion, dilatation and curettage (D & C), hysterosalpingography, or other causes—an infection of the pelvic organs becomes more probable for three reasons: (1) The cervix and its mucus plug, normally effective barriers to ascending infection, have been disturbed, allowing endogenous organisms from the lower genital tract to ascend; (2) there is the possibility of the introduction into the uterus of exogenous pathogens, such as the beta-hemolytic streptococcus, on nonsterile instruments; and (3) there is the likelihood that there has been some tissue trauma that thereby enhances the chances of infection; perforation of the vagina and laceration of the cervix are frequent sequelae of criminal abortion, difficult childbirth may be associated with extensive tearing of the tissues or uterine rupture, and even a D & C may cut too deep and injure the muscle layer of the uterus.

Developed World

In the developed world, the widespread hospitalization of births, aseptic conditions in the labor room, and the presence of birth attendants who are medically trained professionals translate into few postpartum infections. And if fever should signal trouble in the postpartum period, powerful antibiotics are readily available. Therefore, postpartum infections and adverse sequelae are rare.

What infections do occur appear to be due largely to two sexually transmitted pathogens, *Mycoplasma hominis* and *Neisseria gonorrhoeae*, which are frequently encountered in the lower genital tract of sexually active women. Taylor-Robinson and McCormack (1980a:1009) reported that *M. hominis* is believed to be a major cause of contemporary postpartum fever. Although it causes no inflammatory reaction in the lower genital tract, it may ascend during a vaginal delivery to cause an endometritis. Such infections are self-limiting and the patient recovers quickly even without treatment.

Neisseria gonorrhoeae may also be an important cause of postpartum infection in the developed world, as postpartum fever has been noted in about 30% of women with gonorrhea at parturition (Charles *et al.*

1970:598). Some studies (e.g., Handsfield *et al.* 1973:697; Sarrel and Pruett (1968:670) have indicated that gonorrhea may cause premature rupture of the membranes, which in turn is a cause of postpartum infection (*Population Reports* 1980a:121).

Developing World

In the developing world sexually transmitted pathogens, especially *N. gonorrhoeae,* are also an important cause of postpartum sepsis. Nasah and Eyang (in press, cited in Muir and Belsey 1980:916) found that in Cameroon *N. gonorrhoeae* could be isolated twice as frequently from women with postpartum sepsis as from postpartum women with no signs of infection. But in the developing world—particularly in rural areas where most births take place at home, where septic conditions during labor and delivery are the rule, and where the only birth attendant is usually the village midwife—not only are postpartum infections much more frequent, but a greater proportion are probably due to exogenous organisms introduced by the midwife. According to Olusanya (1974:49–50),

> The woman in labour usually lies on a dirty mat or sometimes on the bare floor and the traditional midwife uses his or her bare hands, often unwashed. Almost invariably, unsterilized instruments such as a blade or a piece of broken bottle are used for cutting the umbilical cord. Under such conditions there is a fifty-fifty chance of the mother's organs being contaminated, quite apart from the high incidence of peri-natal mortality that may result. *The number of children the woman ultimately has thus depends on her luck in escaping contamination on each confinement* [emphasis added].

Even attempts by midwives to prevent infections often cause reproductive problems. The Hausa pour nearly boiling water into the genital tract following delivery to decrease the risk of some infections, which in turn increases the risk of burns and scar formation that could alter reproductive potential (Belsey 1977:13). And in Uganda midwives use native medicines with oxytocic properties to shorten labor, but if the labor is obstructed these medicines can cause rupture of the uterus with maternal infection and death (Trussell *et al.* 1968:147). Hence, the traditional methods and medicines used by midwives undoubtedly contribute to higher rates of complications and subsequent subfecundity. It is felt, however, that improving midwifery services will eventually reduce the incidence of postpartum infection and its sequelae in developing countries (Grech *et al.* 1973:126). So too will the trend toward more hospitalizations of births. Indeed, Romaniuk (1980b:304) has noted that the increase in the number of births taking place in hospitals in Zaire has been paralleled by a rise in fertility.

Obstructed Labor and Postpartum Infection

Some workers (e.g., Stewart 1967a:243) have believed that serious infections are rare after normal labor and spontaneous delivery even under the most unsanitary conditions, provided there has been no interference or vaginal examination. But instrumental interference and vaginal examination are probably frequent in areas such as Africa because of the high incidence of obstetric difficulties. In fact, obstetric difficulties are believed to be a possible major cause of pregnancy wastage and secondary sterility in Africa (World Health Organization 1975:12).

The most frequent obstetric difficulty in obstructed labor. Obstructed labor caused by extensive scarring of the external genitals following circumcision is important in some parts of Africa and the Middle East (see Chapter 18). But obstructed labor most frequently arises when the pelvic outlet is too small to allow the fetal head to pass freely (cephalo–pelvic disproportion) (Lawson 1967e:172). Labor may be prolonged and/or require a high forceps delivery. In very severe cases the uterus may rupture (Trussell *et al.* 1968:147). In any case there is ample opportunity for the introduction of exogenous pathogens or the ascension of organisms from the lower genital tract.

In addition, the devitalized tissues of the genital tract offer an excellent growth medium for bacteria; the mother—exhausted, dehydrated, and suffering from acute blood loss—can offer little resistance to their spread (Stewart 1967a:243). Acute blood loss is particularly important in regard to postpartum sepsis, as it predisposes to infection because of inadequate tissue perfusion. This means that less oxygen, fewer phagocytes, fewer antibodies, etc. arrive at the site of bacterial entry and the infection is allowed to proceed virtually unchecked (McFee 1973:158). Anemia, though often stated to be a cause of more frequent and more severe postpartum infections due to diminished resistance to infection (see, e.g., Lawson 1967a:86–87; Masawe *et al.* 1974:314; Stewart 1967a:243), does not, according to McFee (1973:157–158), have this effect except in patients with very severe anemia (hemoglobin less than 8 gm percent).[1] If, however, anemia is the result of acute blood loss, as

---

[1]Hemoglobin levels are usually lower during pregnancy because the increase in red cell volume of 20–30% does not keep pace with the increase in total blood volume of about 50%. A hemoglobin level of 12 gm percent (36% hematocrit) for nonpregnant women and 11 gm percent (33% hematocrit) for pregnant women is considered a low normal value. A pregnant woman is considered mildly anemic if her hemoglobin level is 10–11 gm percent and more severely anemic if the level is below 10 gm percent. A value of 8 gm percent constitutes a very severe anemia (see McFee 1973:153–154).

just discussed, or is associated with severe malnutrition or protein deficiency (these are associated with reduced antibody formation and diminished phagocytic activity), then infections will be more frequent and more severe (McFee 1973:157–158).

Obstructed labor is also associated with higher rates of perinatal mortality, primarily intrapartum death from asphyxia due to prolonged labor and birth trauma due to mechanical difficulties (Platt 1971:335; World Health Organization 1975:17).

The frequency of obstructed labor in Africa due to cephalo–pelvic disproportion should not be underestimated. In fact, when malaria was found to cause intrauterine growth retardation and was subsequently identified as one of the major causes of the low-birth-weight tropical neonate, some concern was expressed at to the wisdom of eradicating the disease and thereby raising birth weights and possibly increasing the problem of cephalo–pelvic disproportion (E. Jelliffe 1967:34).

Age

There are several reasons why cephalo–pelvic disproportion is so frequent in Africa. One is early age at marriage, which often means the bearing of the first child before adult stature is attained. Such pregnancies, noted Adadevoh (1974:16), often result in stillbirths. Ibeziako (1974:92–93) noted that in some areas of Nigeria where marriages are contracted at very young ages and pregnancies consequently occur between ages 14 and 16, obstructed labor due to cephalo–pelvic disproportion occurs more frequently. If medical services are inadequate, as is the case in much of Africa, this phenomenon assumes far greater significance, as there is no antenatal care and obstructed labor develops at home. Ibeziako (1974:93) described such a labor and its sequelae: ''The duration of labour may be up to three or four days and during this period interference by traditional birth attendants is common. Thus, in addition to prolonged and obstructed labour severe pelvic sepsis invariably sets in.''

Infertility in these women may be secondary to tubal infection, or it may be the result of an amenorrhea, which is probably the result of failure of the uterus to respond to hormonal stimulation because of extensive tissue devitalization. Tissue devitalization also frequently occurs in the bladder and rectum due to prolonged pressure on these organs during labor. The necrotic tissue sloughs off after delivery and the woman is left with a vesicovaginal fistula and perhaps a rectovaginal fistula as well. Often such women are rejected by their husbands because of the associated unpleasant odor and are deprived of demonstrating their reproductive potential (Ibeziako 1974:93). Some women with fistulas may, however, be sterile due to genital blockage, which can remain even after surgical repair (Adadevoh 1974:10).

Nutritional Deficiencies

The negative reproductive sequelae of young age at marriage are probably greatest in Africa and other areas where there exists the additional factor of growth impairment due to environmental causes such as malnutrition (see Adadevoh 1974:10). Thus, a second major cause of cephalo–pelvic disproportion is skeletal deformity secondary to nutritional deficiencies. Such deformities may be in the form of rickets, osteomalacia, or contracted pelvis.

Rickets

Rickets is normally a disease of young children and is the result of a deficiency of vitamin D, which is necessary for the absorption of calcium from the gut. In the absence of sufficient calcium, normal bone development cannot occur and the bones are soft and easily distorted.

Even if the diet is deficient in vitamin D the body can, if exposed to sunlight, synthesize sufficient amounts in the skin. Thus, rickets is rare in the tropics except in dark, crowded slums, and is found mainly in temperate and relatively sunless areas of the world (Cruickshank 1967:20). But, not surprisingly, rickets is often seen in Muslim countries (Davidson *et al.* 1975:318) where, despite abundant sunlight, skin synthesis of vitamin D is minimal due to the wearing of clothing that covers most of the body. If diet improves or exposure to the sun increases after the second or third year of life, deformities in the bond tend to heal spontaneously. Otherwise, permanent deformity is likely.

Osteomalacia

Osteomalacia is a second, but rarer, form of skeletal deformity. Whereas rickets develops in childhood while bones are developing, osteomalacia develops in adults as a result of decalcification of fully formed bones (Mukherjee 1967:29). Osteomalacia is caused by a disequilibrium in the supply and demand of calcium or vitamin D. Calcium deficiencies may be due to inadequate intake or to an increased demand for the mineral, as during pregnancy and lactation. Or, through calcium may be present in sufficient amounts, vitamin D, which is necessary for its absorption, may be lacking due to inadequate dietary intake or insufficient exposure to sunlight (Cruickshank 1967:21; Mukherjee 1967:29).

Osteomalacia is most frequently seen in women because of the nutritional demands of pregnancy and lactation. It is stated to be found most frequently in tropical areas and is endemic in the northern and central zones of India, the northern part of China, and certain areas of Japan. In the 1920s, 10% of the women of childbearing age in China and 3% in India had osteomalacia. But by the 1960s the latter figure had dropped to just under 1% in endemic areas (Mukherjee 1967:31). Osteomalacia has also been reported (Grossman and editors 1971:318) to be common among women in Muslim countries who spend much of the day indoors and are completely shrouded against the sunlight when they do go outside.

The typical woman with osteomalacia is 26 years old with frequent gestations (Mukherjee 1967:30). Osteomalacia is seldom seen in the first pregnancy (unless rickets in childhood has been followed after puberty by persistent nutritional deficiency), but becomes worse with each subsequent pregnancy as the bones are progressively demineralized and become increasingly softer (Mukherjee 1967:37–38). The most characteristic change is in the pelvis, where the shape of the outlet becomes increasingly triradiate (Mukherjee 1967:32). Thus, each pregnancy is met with a progressively more difficult labor until a destructive operation must be performed to overcome major obstruction. Premature rupture of the membranes is common and uterine rupture is a grave risk. Studies show that women with osteomalacia have a twofold greater risk of perinatal loss and a greatly increased risk of dying following childbirth as a result of shock and infection. The pelvic abnormalities are not only a threat to fecundity because of higher rates of pregnancy wastage and secondary sterility due to postpartum infection, but are a threat to coital ability as well. Dyspareunia was reported in 20% of women with osteomalacia in one series, and in the past was severe enough in some cases to render coitus impossible (Mukherjee 1967:37–38, 40–41).

General Pelvic Contraction

Although rickets and, to a lesser extent, osteomalacia may currently be important causes of cephalo–pelvic disproportion in selected areas, the commonest cause is general pelvic contraction. No specific nutritional deficiency has been defined as the cause of contracted pelvis; rather, the condition seems to be related to impairment of growth by general ill health and malnutrition in childhood and adolescence (Lawson 1967e:172). Contracted pelvis is not only widespread in the developing world but was also important in historical populations. Therapeutic abortion, which was no longer allowed when Judeo–Christian ethics became predominant, was reintroduced in the eighteenth century for cases of grossly contracted pelvis that made vaginal delivery of a living infant impossible. During the last quarter of the nineteenth century abdominal delivery became safer, although mortality rates still approached 20% (Williams and Sun 1926:745), and contracted pelvis was no longer an indication for therapeutic abortion (A. Guttmacher 1967:13).

Summary

Thus, obstructed labor due to cephalo–pelvic disproportion caused by contracted pelvis, osteomalacia, or rickets is associated with higher rates of pregnancy wastage and postpartum infection. Childlessness, one-child sterility, or low fertility are all possible outcomes, depending on how many live births precede a sterilizing infection. Subsequent ectopic pregnancies are also a possibility, as they are for postabortal infections. In addition, some pelvic deformities such as osteomalacia can cause dyspareunia. And even if the skeletal deformity does not cause dyspareunia, this may develop following delivery. Unrelieved obstructed labor, for example, can cuase very severe damage to the lower genital tract, and severe dyspareunia or even apareunia may develop because the vagina may become occluded by fibrous tissue and be difficult to repair (Lawson 1967f:210–211). A difficult forceps delivery may also cause dyspareunia if the broad ligaments supporting the uterus are damaged (Masters and Johnson 1970:280).

Other obstetric complications that may affect fecundity are precipitate delivery (dyspareunia may result if the broad ligaments are damaged [Masters and Johnson 1970:280]) and major bleeding (already discussed as an important predisposing factor in postpartum infection [see McFee 1973:158]). Delivery of twins is associated with increased hazards, and the high frequency of twinning in certain groups may make them more susceptible to future reproductive problems. In the Yoruba of western Nigeria, for example, a high rate of twinning (1 in 22 deliveries) has been noted (D. Jelliffe 1967:255).

In certain populations complications of childbirth may assume particular significance. Henin (1969:191–192) noted that the incidence of sterility and pregnancy loss among the nomadic populations of the Sudan was high as compared to the settled populations, and he attributed this in part to the many adverse health conditions associated with childbearing among the former. A survey among the nomads revealed that during a journey only 4% of deliveries were assisted by a midwife. And if bleeding or some other serious complication developed there were no health services available and all the woman could do was visit the religious man or drink certain potions believed to have healing properties. Although Henin conceded that the evidence was not conclusive, he felt that the poor health of the nomads, the lack of antenatal and postnatal care, and unsanitary midwifery or no obstetrical assistance at all might well have contributed significantly to the relatively high incidence of sterility and pregnancy loss.

Postpartum Infections and Population Subfecundity

The contribution to population subfecundity of postpartum infections and other adverse sequelae of childbirth has not been systematically studied. Gray (1979:242) has proposed that postpartum infections were frequent in historical populations in Europe and elsewhere and were probably an important cause of secondary sterility. The World Health Organization Scientific Group on the Epidemiology of Infertility (World Health Organization 1975:12, 15) listed postpartum infections as a potentially major cause of infertility in sub-Saharan Africa, but hesitated to draw final conclusions as to their importance because sufficient data were not yet available on the frequency of postpartum infections there and on the risk of subsequent infertility.

Some scattered reports may, however, be found in the literature, and these indicate at least the importance of postpartum infections relative to other causes of pelvic inflammatory disease (PID). A study in Uganda by Grech and associates (1973:123) showed that 10.4% of cases of PID were due to postpartum infections. Shah *et al.* (1978, cited in Muir and Belsey 1980:918) reported that 15.3% of pelvic infections diagnosed during 7 years in an Indian hospital were due to postpartum sepsis, and Lithgow and Rubin (1972, cited in Muir and Belsey 1980:918) reported an identical figure for a South African hospital. Muir and Belsey (1980:917), in an excellent review of the causes and consequences of PID in the developing world, reported that in the Philippines, Zambia, and Thailand postpartum infection accounted for a minority of the cases of PID—19%, 17%, and 23%, respectively; postabortal sepsis and acute salpingitis were more important. In Egypt and Pakistan, however, postpartum sepsis accounted for the majority of PID cases, 57% and 72%, respectively. This is consistent with their being Muslim countries, Islamic law forbidding abortion and highly valuing chastity in the unmarried woman and fidelity in the married woman. It would be interesting to know what role rachitic pelvis, osteomalacia, and genital mutilation played in these cases of postpartum infection, because these conditions are more prevalent in Muslim countries.

The proportion of these women who subsequently become sterile following postpartum infection or have other reproductive problems is not known. Westrom (1975:711) reported that for Swedish women with pelvic infection following childbirth, abortion, curettage, etc., tubal occulsion occurred in 27% of cases. Because these women were given optimal care, we would expect rates of tubal occlusion and sterility to be higher yet in the developing countries. Thus, given the high frequency of obstetric difficulties in Africa and other parts of the developing world, the scarcity of skilled medical assistance, and the unsanitary conditions that accompany most deliveries, postpartum infections are a significant contributor to population subfecundity through secondary sterility and through pregnancy loss due to ectopic pregnancy.

Postpartum Infections and U.S. Black Fertility: 1880–1936

Between 1880 and 1936 the U.S. black population experienced a precipitous decline in its birthrate. Negative health conditions among blacks during this period are often cited as contributing factors. Venereal diseases such as syphilis and gonorrhea and nutritional diseases such as pellagra have been mentioned as causes of the black fertility decline (Farley 1970:215–226). Indeed, we have proposed in Chapters 3 and 19 that genital tuberculosis was probably not uncommon among blacks and may have been one cause of the extraordinarily high rates of childlessness observed during the period. And an article by Cutright and Shorter (1979) proposed that changes in the prevalence of pelvic deformities and subsequent postpartum infections and secondary sterility in black women were largely responsible for the decline and later recovery of black fertility between 1880 and 1936 (see Figure 19.1). We shall now explore the merits of this hypothesis.

Diets were extremely poor among blacks following Emancipation, and specific deficiency diseases such as rickets were seen in a large number of blacks. Indeed, a 1917 survey of black infants in a poor section of New York City noted rickets in 90% of cases (Hesa and Unger 1917, cited in Cutright and Shorter 1979:197). Rickets would be expected to be more prevalent in the North because of reduced sunlight and to be especially prevalent in northern cities where smog further blocked ultraviolet rays. And blacks would be particularly liable to suffer since their dark pigmentation reduces the amount of ultraviolet radiation that can penetrate the skin. (Adequate synthesis of vitamin D in the skin of blacks, as compared to whites, requires even greater exposure to sunlight.)

Because rickets had been crucial in the etiology of pelvic deformity in Europe, Cutright and Shorter (1979:197) felt that it was probably just as important in the rise in pelvic deformities noted among American black women. Data on the frequency of pelvic deformities in black women are limited, but do indicate a substantial rise in frequency over time—from 0.5 cases per 1000 mothers in Washington, D.C., in 1875, to 330 per 1000 in Baltimore at the turn of the century, to 390 per 1000 in Baltimore in the 1920s; rates for white women in the Baltimore series were 75% lower. There are six types of contracted pelvis listed by Williams and Sun (1926), authors of the Baltimore study, and whereas typical general contracted pelvis contributed substantially to the total amount of pelvic abnormality in both populations (white, 35%; black, 39%), rachitic pelvis played a negligible role in the genesis of abnormal pelvises in white women (6%) but a major role in black women (36%). In fact, the increase in the incidence of contracted pelvis between 1900 and 1920 for blacks was almost exclusively the result of the increase in rachitic pelvis (Williams and Sun 1926:737–738).

These data are consistent with the notion that women born and raised in slavery had diets sufficient to allow normal skeleton growth, whereas those born after Emancipation had much poorer diets and a substantial proportion developed general contracted pelvis and particularly rachitic pelvis. Thus, according to the Cutright and Shorter (1979) hypothesis, during the immediate post–Civil War period black women had high birthrates, but as the reproductive cohorts became increasingly filled by women with pelvic abnormalities more women experienced difficult labors and an increased risk of postpartum infection and secondary sterility; consequently, birth rates began to fall. Indeed, Williams and Sun (1926:745, 746, 747) noted that black women were more liable to infection and experienced "considerably higher" rates of postpartum fever following even a normal labor. It is likely that this greater disposition to infection was the result of dietary deficiencies, especially of protein (Cutright and Shorter 1979:196; Farley 1970:219; White *et al.* 1964:956), which increases susceptibility to infection (McFee 1973:157–158).

Although Cutright and Shorter did not discuss childlessness as a consequence of contracted pelvis, we believe that childlessness may occur if the sterilizing infection follows the first pregnancy and the child dies from asphyxia or birth trauma because of the difficult birth. Fetal mortality rates are definitely increased if there is pelvic contraction. Even in a hospital setting, where emergency surgery such as cesarean section is available to save the baby, fetal mortality rates are quite high. In the Baltimore series 11.71% of children born to women with contracted pelvis died even though cesarean sections were performed when necessary. However, less than half of these deaths could be attributed directly to the difficult labor (Williams and Sun 1926:747). Because prior to the 1940s the overwhelming majority of black births were not hospitalized, the fetal mortality rate for the entire population was probably much higher.

In the late 1930s, with the rising standard of living, diets for most blacks began to improve (Farley 1970:227, 235–236). Concomitantly there was a dramatic increase in the number of hospitalized births; in 1935 only 17% of black births were hospitalized, but in 1940 this figure was 27% and by 1945 had jumped to 40% (Farley 1970:229). These two developments would have the effect of steadily decreasing the number of women with contracted pelvis in the reproductive cohort and reducing rates of perinatal mortality and postpartum infection in women with obstetric difficulties. The role of powerful antibiotics in controlling infection in the post–World War II years must also be considered. These changes would be reflected in lower rates of maternal mortality, perinatal mortality, postpartum infections, and primary and secondary sterility. Thus, the trends in the prevalence of contracted pelvis and those in childlessness and low parity women are in phase, and it is reasonable to assert, as did Cutright and Shorter (1979), that postpartum infection did play some role in the U.S. black fertility decline.

CHAPTER 17

The Intrauterine Device and Fecundity

Introduction

Many centuries ago Arabs and Turks inserted pebbles into the wombs of their camels to prevent them from becoming pregnant during long journeys across the desert. By the eleventh century devices were also being inserted into the genital tract of the human female as a means of birth control. These early devices were not strictly intrauterine devices (IUDs), as they remained in the vagina, and it was not until the late nineteenth century that devices that protruded into the uterus were introduced. The first entirely intrauterine appliance was a circular device of silkworm gut designed in 1909 by a German physician, Richard Richter. In the late 1920s a similar circular device of gut and silver developed by Ernst Gräfenberg became the first widely used IUD. By the 1930s gold and gold-plated silver rings were available in Japan that were claimed by their developer, Tenrei Ota, to be even more effective than Gräfenberg's devices.

Initial enthusiasm for these IUDs was soon met, however, with skepticism and charges that they were not only ineffective but dangerous. The Japanese government outlawed Ota's rings and German physicians were reluctant to use Gräfenberg's device because of fears of uncontrollable pelvic infection. The IUD seemed dead. However, two major technological advances prompted a reappraisal of the IUD in the late 1950s: (1) advances in antibiotic therapy that dispelled fears of infection and (2) the introduction of polyethylene, a biologically inert plastic that could be molded into any shape, straightened in a narrow tube for insertion into the uterus (making cervical dilatation unnecessary), and then extruded, whereupon its original shape was restored (*Population Reports* 1979b:51–52). These advances made the IUD an acceptable means of birth control for many women. The IUD gained further popularity in the early 1970s when reports surfaced about the harmful side effects of oral contraceptives (the pill). Thousands of women abandoned the pill at that time and turned to the IUD because they believed it was a safer means of birth control (*Time* 1980b:60).

Prevalence of Use

By the late 1970s 50–60 million women were using IUDs. Of these, 40 million live in China where 50% or more of rural contraceptors may use IUDs. Another developing country where IUD use is high is Taiwan, where 32% of married women of reproductive age are users. In the Republic of Korea and Colombia this figure is 8%, in Thailand 6%, in Fiji, Sri Lanka, and Costa Rica 5%, and in Egypt, Tunisia, Indonesia, Ecuador, Jamaica, Mexico, and Paraguay 5% or less. Among the developed nations Finland and Sweden report the highest rates of IUD use, 20% among married women of reproductive age. In France, Japan, and Denmark this figure is 7–9% and in the United States, England, and Wales it is 6% percent (*Population Reports* 1979b:52–53).

Problems Associated with Use

In most developing countries the proportion of IUD acceptors has been falling even though the total number of acceptors has, in some cases, increased. This is probably because in these areas oral contraceptives and sterilization have increased even more rapidly than IUD use (*Population Reports* 1979b:56). The relative unpopularity of the IUD is due largely to personal dissatisfaction with the method because of associated pain and/or excessive bleeding, but it is also due in part to adverse publicity concerning serious complications such as uterine perforation or septic abortion. The rarity of these complications is, however, seldom appreciated; many women in developing countries say they do not want an IUD because it "wanders round your insides" (Savane 1979:8), and in the United States the proportion of married women of reproductive age using IUDs fell from 6.7% in 1973 to 6.1% in 1976 following widespread publicity of a score of IUD-related deaths caused by septic abortion (*Population Reports* 1979b:52).

The device most often associated with the fatal cases of septic abortion was the Dalkon Shield, and all uninserted devices were recalled in 1974. In 1980 the H. R. Robins Company, manufacturer of the Dalkon Shield, suggested that all these devices should be removed because of an association in long-term IUD users (all Dalkon Shield users had the device inserted prior to 1975, so all are in the long-term use category) with an often-serious pelvic infection, actinomycosis. In addition, the National Medical Committee of the Planned Parenthood Federation of America recommended removal of any IUD and concomitant antibiotic therapy if the user's Pap smear is positive for the bacterium *Actinomyces* (*Family Planning Perspectives* 1980a:306). Indeed, many reports have indicated that not only actinomycosis but other pelvic infections as well may be more frequent in IUD users, and the risk may be greatest for young, nulliparous women. Because of such reports the U.S. Food and Drug Administration issued an advisory bulletin to physicians suggesting that women requesting an IUD be advised of the possibility of their becoming sterile because of the device (see Dreifus 1980:D9).

Still other problems associated with IUD use have detracted from its popularity. Some women are reluctant to use the IUD because of reports that it increases their chances of having an ectopic pregnancy (see *Population Reports* 1979b:70–72). And some women who choose an IUD subsequently request removal because of increased menstrual bleeding and pain (Eschenbach and Holmes 1975:36). The popularity of the IUD has further been diminished by reports that the action of the device is not to prevent conception but to prevent implantation of a fertilized ovum (Tatum 1977:194–195; *Time* 1980b:60), although more recent evidence suggests that an equally or more important action is destruction of sperm entering the uterus (*Popline* 1981:4). Nevertheless, couples opposed to abortion might find this means of birth control unacceptable.

Have the shortcomings of the IUD been overstated, or is the device actually linked to significant amounts of septic abortion, pelvic infection, ectopic pregnancy, and sterility? As yet, not all the necessary studies with all the necessary controls have been done that would allow definitive answers on all these points. However, enough data do exist to reach conclusions with an acceptable level of confidence.

Mechanism of Action

The pathological conditions associated with IUD use can be better understood through a knowledge of the mechanisms by which the device prevents births, although admittedly even the experts are not absolutely certain about what mechanisms are involved. There are two basic types of IUDs, nonmedicated and medicated, and each type prevents births in a somewhat different way. The nonmedicated IUDs are made of an inert plastic and most probably work by stimulating an inflammatory or foreign body reaction in the uterus (and, as research has shown, in the tubes as well [*Population Reports* 1979b:67]), mobilizing leucocytes, plasma cells, macrophages and other host defender cells that can engulf (phagocytize) spermatozoa or the fertilized ovum (*Population Reports* 1979b:59). It is also possible that this inflammatory reaction produces changes in the endometrium that create an environment inhospitable to implantation (*Population Reports* 1979b:59; Tatum 1977:194).

The medicated IUDs also stimulate a local inflammatory reaction and phagocytic activity. In addition, the metal, hormone, or antibleeding agent that has been added to the plastic device heightens its effectiveness and/or reduces adverse side effects. Metallic copper not only increases the inflammatory response but also interferes with the enzyme systems of the spermatozoa, with the cellular DNA content of the endometrium, and with estrogen uptake by the uterine mucosa (*Population Reports* 1979b:59). There are also reports that copper can affect sperm penetration and ascent through the cervical mucus and may even cause a very rapid disintegration of the human ovum while it is suspended in the fallopian tube fluid (see Tatum 1977:195). The progesterone-carrying IUDs maintain high progesterone and low estrogen levels and thereby keep the endometrium in the decidual or progestational stage in which implantation is unlikely (*Population Reports* 1979b:59). Other pharmacologic agents added to IUDs include fibrinolytic inhibitors, which reduce heavy menstrual bleeding (*Population Reports* 1979b:82). But of all the modes of action of the various IUDs, it is probably the inflammatory response in the uterus and tubes that is responsible for most of the unfavorable sequelae associated with IUD use.

Sequelae

Cervical Injury

Injury to the cervix is always a possibility whenever this barrier to the uterus must be breached, whether it is to remove the products of conception, perform a curettage, or insert an IUD. The amount of cervical dilatation necessary to perform the procedure, the physical state of the cervix, and the skill of the physician all determine outcome. Whether or not the cervix must be dilated in order to insert an IUD depends on a number of factors including the type of device and the timing within the menstrual cycle. The Lippes Loop, for example, the most widely used plastic IUD, can usually be inserted without cervical dilatation. This is generally true of plastic devices, which can be placed into a long, narrow tube, passed through the cervix, and then extruded into the uterus where they resume their original shape (*Population Reports* 1979b:52). Also, insertions done during or immediately after menstruation not only assure that the woman is not pregnant but further reduce the necessity for mechanical dilatation as the cervical os is already slightly dilated (*Population Reports* 1979b:59). Thus, problems with cervical laceration and uterine perforation should be much fewer with IUD insertions than with abortion procedures, where greater dilatation is necessary to effect removal of the products of conception. Nevertheless, the greater force necessary to dilate the nulliparous cervix makes the nulliparous group of women particularly susceptible to cervical injury even when only a small opening is needed. In addition, tears may also be caused by the tenaculum, an instrument used to stabilize the cervix during insertions. Therefore, the risk of cervical damage and subsequent reproductive problems cannot be dismissed entirely in regard to IUD insertion, especially in nulliparous women. Also to be considered is the skill with which the insertion is performed, as this determines not only the frequency of cervical damage, but also rates of expulsion, uterine perforation, infection, bleeding, etc. (*Population Reports* 1979b:59).

Pelvic Infection

It is becoming increasingly clear that IUD users run a higher risk of pelvic infection—not only immediately after insertion, as was previously thought (Tatum 1977:197), although the risk is particularly high then, but for as long as the device remains in place (*Family Planning Perspectives* 1981c:182–183; *Population Reports* 1979b:67). Indeed, a study (Burkman and the Women's Health Study 1981, cited in *Family Planning Perspectives* 1981c:182–183) has shown that the increased risk persists for approximately 12 months after removal. The infection may be caused by *Neisseria gonorrhoeae*, by *Escherichia coli*, by a staphylococcus or one or more of the other members of the vaginal flora, or by *Actinomyces israelii*, a highly pathogenic bacterium (*Family Planning Perspectives* 1980a:306; *Population Reports* 1979b:67, 69). Although IUD users with a positive cervical smear for gonorrhea have a significantly greater chance of developing a pelvic infection than gonorrhea-positive nonusers (Curran 1979:179; Thompson and Hager 1977:105), IUD use increases the risk of nongonococcal infection even more than a gonococcal infection (Eschenbach 1980:146S; *Population Reports* 1979b:67).

The pelvic infection may take the form of an endometritis, an endosalpingitis, or a pelvic actinomycosis. Tubo–ovarian abscesses have been observed (Eschenbach and Holmes 1975:36; Hacker 1976:D14–D15; *Population Reports* 1979b:67; Thompson and Hager 1977:105) and, indeed, pelvic abscesses may be more frequent in IUD users (Curran 1979:179). The excavation of the mucosal surface of the uterus by the IUD exposes the submucosal lymphatics and thus a perisalpingitis or even a generalized pelvic cellulitis may follow. Despite such possible sequelae the infection is often mild or asymptomatic and may heal without treatment (*Population Reports* 1979b:67), as is true for pelvic infections of most any etiology. Indeed, examination of the tubes removed from 1500 apparently healthy, previously fertile Thai women seeking sterilization revealed evidence of past pelvic infection in 12.3% of IUD users, three times the rate seen in nonusers (*Population Reports* 1979b:67). Nevertheless, there is always the danger of a sudden flare-up complicating a spontaneous abortion or of a progressive tubal infection leading to scarring with subsequent sterility (*Newsweek* 1976:62; *Time* 1980b:60; *Population Reports* 1979b:67). Hysterectomy may sometimes follow a far-advanced case that does not respond to therapy (*Time* 1980b:60).

Factors Affecting the Risk of Developing Pelvic Inflammatory Disease

Of women seeking treatment for pelvic infections, more use IUDs than any other type of contraception (Eschenbach and Holmes 1975:36; Thompson and Hager 1977:105). In general, IUD users stand a two to nine times greater risk of developing pelvic infections than nonusers (Eschenbach and Holmes 1975:36; *Family Planning Perspectives* 1980b:207; Thompson and Hager 1977:105), a risk that varies with age, race, socioeconomic status, sexual activity, and other factors that influence risk of pelvic infection (*Family Planning Perspectives* 1980b:207) and with whether the control group uses no contraception or uses the pill or one of the barrier methods, as these appear to protect against pelvic inflammatory disease (PID). These variables must therefore be controlled for in studies attempting to define strictly *IUD-related risk factors*. Several such factors have already been defined; these include nulligravidity, duration of use, and type of IUD.

Parity and Gravidity   Eschenbach *et al.* (1977:838) noted a substantially greater risk of infection for young, nulliparous IUD users, and Westrom (1980, cited in *Family Planning Perspectives* 1980b:207) further distilled this to an increased risk among never-pregnant women (3.4 infections/100 woman-years of use for ever-pregnant women versus 11.8 infections/100 woman-years of use for never-pregnant women), an increased risk that was not seen with any other contraceptive method. The reason for this differential risk is not known, but Westrom and Mardh (1978:14) suggested it could be due to differences in muscular activity between the never-pregnant and ever-pregnant uterus.

Duration of Use Duration of use may be another important risk factor, although some studies (e.g., Burkman and the Women's Health Study 1981 and Vessey *et al.* 1981, both cited in *Family Planning Perspectives* 1981c:182–183) have not reported that the incidence of PID increases with duration of use.[1] Preliminary studies by Kaufman *et al.* (1980, cited in *Family Planning Perspectives* 1980b:207) have suggested a doubling of infection risk if the device has been in place for more than 5 years. This increased risk with duration of use is particularly strong in the etiology of pelvic actinomycosis (*Family Planning Perspectives* 1980a:306), an infection that was once quite rare but has been reported in a number of IUD users including women with severe pelvic infections and those in whom evidence of disease was found only at the time the IUD was removed (*Population Reports* 1979b:69). The cause of the increased risk of infection with duration of use has not been defined, but is probably associated with progressive damage to the endometrium and endosalpinx caused by chronic inflammation.

Type of Intrauterine Device Differential risk of infection has also been reported according to the type of IUD used although, again, not all studies have reached this conclusion (*Family Planning Perspectives* 1981a:151). In general, the copper devices have been associated with the least risk of infection, perhaps because of a mildly antiseptic property of copper (*Family Planning Perspectives* 1980a:307) or, perhaps even more likely, because there are fewer long-term users as these devices are relatively new (Kaufman *et al.* 1980, cited in *Family Planning Perspectives* 1980b:207). The Dalkon Shield, on the other hand, has frequently been associated with pelvic infection. Although infections now associated with the device, especially pelvic actinomycosis, may simply be a result of long-term use, it is true that a Dalkon Shield left in place during preg-

---

[1]The British study by Vessey *et al.* (1981, cited in *Family Planning Perspectives* 1981c:182–183) found that the incidence of acute PID was highest in IUD users in the first 12 months of use. The incidence declined thereafter but rose after 6 years or more of use. The U.S. study (Burkman and the Women's Health Study 1981, cited in *Family Planning Perspectives* 1981c:182–183) found that recent insertion or reinsertion was associated with an increased risk of PID, but otherwise duration of use was not associated with infection.

nancy is three times more likely than other IUDs to result in a septic abortion (*Population Reports* 1979b:69). The multifilamented tail of the Dalkon Shield was found to have wicking properties that could contribute to the transmission of bacteria from the vagina or cervix to the uterus (Tatum 1977:194). However, two sizes of the Dalkon Shield with the same tail were marketed, and only the larger model was associated with increased maternal morbidity and mortality (*Population Reports* 1979b:69). Perhaps then it was improper placement that contributed to problems associated with the Dalkon Shield;[2] because the larger device was more likely to be improperly inserted it was associated with more problems.

Causes of the Increased Risk of Pelvic Inflammatory Disease

As yet the question of whether tails, multifilamented (as in the Dalkon Shield) or single-threaded, increase the risk of infection has not been resolved (*Population Reports* 1979b:69), although Sparks *et al.* (1977, cited in Eschenbach 1980:146S) have shown that whereas the endometria of all 50 non-IUD users and 2 tailless-IUD users in the study were sterile, bacteria were present in the endometrial cavity of all 11 women with tailed IUDs 1 wcck to 9 years after insertion. Indeed, why IUDs cause higher rates of pelvic infection is not well established.

That the chronic inflammation seen in the uterus and tubes of users—one study showed a sterile salpingitis in 47% of IUD users and in only 0.7% of nonusers (Smith and Soderstrom 1976:161)—decreased host resistance to bacterial infection is the most reasonable schema and may also explain some symptoms commonly associated with IUD use such as heavy, noninfectious leukorrhea and chronic pelvic discomfort (*Population Reports* 1979b:67). This is a case where the initial inflammatory response of the uterus (mobilization of macrophages, etc.), which is necessary for the effectiveness of the IUD (phagocytosis of spermatozoa and fertilized ova), goes too far and results in a more serious and widespread inflammation in which host immunological responsiveness is diminished, making the uterus and tubes more receptive sites for bacterial infection. At this point the mechanism of action vis-à-vis birth con-

---

[2]Some workers (e.g., Cates *et al.* 1976:1158) have suggested that the increased problem of septic abortion associated with the Dalkon Shield, as compared to other devices, may have arisen in part because many doctors, unfamiliar with this new device, did not place it adequately in the uterine cavity but inserted it only as far as the internal os of the cervix. The full contraceptive effectiveness of the Shield was, therefore, not realized and more than the expected number of pregnancies occurred, a proportion of which were septic; hence the observation that more Dalkon Shield users than users of other IUDs experienced septic abortion. It seems possible that this improper placement within the cervical os may have also damaged the cervix.

trol might also change from one of strictly phagocytosis of germ cells or fertilized ova to one of this *and* an inhospitable environment for uterine implantation and an altered tubal environment. This hypothesis correlates with other observations about long-term IUD use, including (1) increasing effectiveness against uterine pregnancy (*Population Reports* 1979b:71) (2) possibly greater proportions of ectopic pregnancies if used more than 4 years (*Family Planning Perspectives* 1980c:157), and (3) greater risk of infection (Kaufman *et al.* 1980, cited in *Family Planning Perspectives* 1980b:207).

We propose yet another mechanism whereby IUDs may increase the risk of pelvic infection. It has been observed that pelvic infections often occur at the time of the menses—the loss of the cervical mucus plug, the greater patency of the cervix at this time, and the reflux of menstrual blood aiding the ascent of bacteria from the endocervix to the upper genital tract. The IUD increases not only the volume of menstrual flow (by 50 to 100%) but also its duration (by 1.5 days on the average) (these aspects are discussed in the section "Bleeding and Anemia"); perhaps it thus increases the probability of an ascending infection. This hypothesis in reverse has already been proposed by Osser and associates (1980, cited in *Family Planning Perspectives* 1980b:207) regarding the protective action of oral contraceptives on the risk of pelvic infection (see subsequent discussion in this section), because the volume and duration of menstrual bleeding are diminished by the pill (*Family Planning Perspectives* 1980b:207). Indeed, those devices associated with the least blood loss (e.g., the Copper 7) are associated with the lowest rates of infection and those with the greatest blood loss (e.g., the Dalkon Shield) are associated with the highest rates of infection (*Family Planning Perspectives* 1980b:207). In general, the larger the device, the greater the bleeding (*Population Reports* 1979b:65; Tatum 1977:196).

Interestingly, whereas the IUD appears to enhance the chances of developing a pelvic infection, oral contraceptives appear to have the opposite effect, reducing the relative risk of infection by two-thirds (*Family Planning Perspectives* 1980b:207). Thus, assignment of risk based on comparisons between IUD users and users of other types of contraceptives (oral contraceptives, barrier methods, etc.) overstate the case. Indeed, whereas IUD users have a fivefold-greater risk of developing a pelvic infection compared to oral contraceptive users and a fourfold greater risk compared to women using barrier methods, the risk is only one-and-a-half times greater when the proper control group—sexually active, noncontracepting women—is used (Westrom 1980, cited in *Family Planning Perspectives* 1980b:207).

Exactly why oral contraceptives protect against pelvic infection is now known, although Osser *et al.* (1980, cited in *Family Planning Per-*

spectives 1980b:207) have hypothesized that the protection may be due to hormone-induced thickening of the cervical mucus and shortening of the period of menstrual bleeding. Whatever the reason, oral contraceptives may have an added value in areas of the world, such as developing countries, where sterility subsequent to pelvic infection is a problem (*Family Planning Perspectives* 1980b:208).

Sequelae of Pelvic Infection

When a pelvic infection develops in a woman with an IUD, the possible reproductive sequelae are the same as those seen following other types of pelvic infection: sterility and ectopic pregnancy. Sterility follows in an estimated 20% of cases (Dreifus 1980:D8), a figure comparable to that given for pelvic infections of other etiologies (see *Family Planning Perspectives* 1980b:206). According to one estimate (*Family Planning Perspectives* 1980b:207) there are 100,000 cases each year of IUD-related salpingitis in the United States; thus, if 20% become sterile, 20,000 women each year become sterile because of IUD use. Given that 2 million U.S. women use an IUD, an IUD user stands 1 chance in 20 (5%) of developing PID and 1 chance in 100 (1%) of becoming sterile each year she wears the device. And if the woman should retain the ability to conceive, the chance that the conceptus will implant ectopically is increased sixfold because of tubal damage. Even in the absence of a history of pelvic infection, a woman with an IUD in place is at greater risk of an ectopic implantation is she should become pregnant.

Ectopic Pregnancy

Pregnancy in a woman using an IUD is a cause for concern because such pregnancies are ectopic in 1 to 5% of cases (*Population Reports* 1979b:72); and even if the pregnancy is within the uterus, spontaneous abortion frequently occurs (see the section ''Abortion and Septic Abortion''). Because 1–6% of all IUD users become pregnant each year (*Population Reports* 1979b:49) these complications are of considerable importance.

The chances that a pregnancy will be ectopic are roughly 7–10 times greater for a woman with an IUD than for a nonuser. And a number of studies (e.g., Tatum and Schmidt 1977:413; Vessey *et al.* 1979:548) have concluded that the longer an IUD has been in place, the greater the risk will be. This has been confirmed by a study (Ory and the Women's Health Study 1981, cited in *Family Planning Perspectives* 1981a:151) that showed that long-term users (>24 months) have a threefold greater risk of ectopic pregnancy than short-term users (1–24 months). Even after removal the elevated risk persists for approximately 1 year, suggesting a residual alteration of tubal function that is not reversed until about a year after removal. The nature of the chance in the fallopian tubes has not been determined with certainty, although it may well be the chronic noninfectious inflammation that Smith and Soderstrom (1976:161) noted in 47% of women with an IUD but in less than 1% of women without an IUD.

It has also been suggested that the increased risk of an ectopic pregnancy in IUD users—1 of 30 such pregnancies is ectopic versus 1 of 250 in the general population (*Population Reports* 1979b:70)—is the result of an increased incidence of subclinical pelvic infection. (It is known that pelvic infections are much more frequent in women using an IUD and it is likely that a certain proportion of these infections are mild or completely asymptomatic.) Weeks and Hutchins (1976:105), for example, could not elicit a history of PID from either of two IUD users in their study who had a ectopic pregnancy, despite histological evidence of a prior pelvic infection. However, because the risk of ectopic implantation returns to normal about 1 year following removal of an IUD, pelvic infection residua cannot be responsible for the majority of cases.

Despite the increased risk of an ectopic implantation in a pregnant woman with an IUD, the relative rarity of pregnancy in such women means that the overall risk of an ectopic pregnancy is less for women who use an IUD than for women who use no contraceptive at all (*Time* 1980b:60). However, if an ectopic pregnancy does occur, it is a medical emergency that may seriously jeopardize not only a woman's immediate health if a rupture should occur but her future reproductive health as well, because extensive tubal damage may occur and removal of the tube may be required in some cases. Even in developed countries such as the United States and Great Britain, 10% of maternal deaths are due to ectopic pregnancies (*Population Reports* 1979b:70). Ectopic pregnancies are especially dangerous in developing countries where emergency surgical care is seldom available and medical personnel need to be alerted to the fact that the symptoms of ectopic pregnancy (i.e., pain and bleeding) are similar to and must be distinguished from those commonly associated with IUD use (*Population Reports* 1979b:50).

Abortion and Septic Abortion

If an accidental pregnancy occurs in an IUD user there is a 40–50% chance of a spontaneous abortion if the device remains in place, a rate three to eight times above normal (*Family Planning Perspectives* 1980c:156; *Population Reports* 1979b:69; Tatum 1977:199). This figure is almost halved if the device is expelled or is removed (*Population Reports* 1979b:69; Tatum 1977:199). For pregnancies proceeding with the IUD in place there is also evidence of substantially increased rates of premature delivery and of some increase in the number of stillbirths and low-birth-weight infants (*Family Planning Perspectives* 1980c:156–157; *Population Reports* 1979b:69; Tatum 1977:199). Studies have indicated that there is probably little variation in the outcome of pregnancy resulting from the type of device (*Family Planning Perspectives* 1980c:157).

A particularly grave threat to pregnant women with an IUD in place is septic abortion. IUD users are twice as likely as nonusers to develop signs of infection (e.g., fever) at the time of a spontaneous abortion (*Population Reports* 1979b:69). However, severe cases of septic abortion that are life-threatening are rare; there have been only 15 deaths per 100,000 pregnancies where the IUD remained in place. Although septic abortion can occur with any IUD it was first linked to the Dalkon Shield, which was subsequently removed from the market. Further studies showed that compared to other IUDs the Dalkon Shield was associated with only a threefold greater risk, less than first suspected (*Population Reports* 1979b:69) (see footnote 2).

The increased risk of abortion in IUD users is probably due to uterine irritation caused by the device, and the increased risk of septic abortion probably represents a flare-up following the abortion of a low-grade, previously asymptomatic infection (*Population Reports* 1979b:67). Because removal of the device as soon as pregnancy is detected reduces the risk of abortion by half and of septic abortion to almost nil, recommendations by the U.S. Food and Drug Administration and the manufacturer of the Dalkon Shield that IUDs be removed as soon as a pregnancy is detected resulted in no septic abortion deaths in the 17 months following the request (*Population Reports* 1979b:70). However, in developing countries such ready medical care once a pregnancy is detected (or even early detection of pregnancy) is improbable, and thus the risk of spontaneous abortion and of postabortal infection is substantial there. Indeed, infection may be a much more frequent sequela of IUD-associated abortion in developing countries, as it has been noted that spontaneous abortion is more likely to be followed by pelvic infection in debilitated women suffering from a number of endemic diseases and nutritional deficiencies.

Congenital Malformations

As with many of the other types of contraceptives, particularly oral contraceptives, there was some fear expressed about the effects of IUD use on the offspring of future pregnancies. Fears were particularly strong in regard to the toxic effects of any residual copper in women using those medicated devices. But studies have shown (1) that copper levels in the muscular layer of the uterus, which are elevated when the device is in place, fall to normal levels upon removal (*Population Reports* 1973:17), (2) that in laboratory animals metallic copper does not result in any demonstrable congenital defect (Tatum 1977:199), and (3) that there is no increase in the rate of malformed infants after discontinuing use of the IUD (or pill) (*Family Planning Perspectives* 1980c:156). The number of accidental pregnancies is too small (more than 50,000 births would be necessary) to allow confident conclusions about congenital malformation rates with the IUD in place. However, that malformation rates are normal after removal should be somewhat reassuring (*Family Planning Perspectives* 1980c:157).

Bleeding and Anemia

Most IUDs are associated with an increased volume and duration of menstrual bleeding (*Population Reports* 1979b:64–66). The nonmedicated devices are associated with the greatest blood loss, which is twice the 35-ml average loss experienced before insertion; the copper devices are associated with only a 50% greater-than-normal loss, this lower figure being related to their smaller size and not the addition of copper. The progesterone-carrying devices actually reduce blood flow, the 40–50% reduction being comparable to the flow associated with the steroidal oral contraceptives.

Prolongation of the menstrual flow is noted with all the devices, being approximately 1–1.5 days longer for the nonmedicated and copper devices and up to 3–4 days longer for Progestasert, the progesterone-releasing device. However, in the latter case blood flow during these 3–4 days is minimal, described as spotting. Intermenstrual or midcycle bleeding has also been noted with all the IUDs and may be somewhat more frequent with progesterone-releasing devices. Among IUD users in a Canadian study, 40% reported midcycle bleeding but stated that blood loss was small (< 10 ml) and declined with time elapsed after insertion.

The cause of midcycle bleeding, at least with the nonmedicated and copper devices, is damage to the endometrium. The prolongation of menstrual bleeding is believed due to hormonal asynchronization. And the increased volume of flow is believed due to enzymes that concentrate in the endometrium adjacent to the device and destroy fibrin, which is essential to the formation of blood clots.

Many women request IUD removal because of this heavy and prolonged bleeding (Eschenbach and Holmes 1975:36). For women in developed countries this is usually because of associated inconvenience. But for women in certain developing countries, where menstruating women are not allowed to carry on usual household tasks, perform religous rites, or engage in sexual intercourse, prolonged and midcycle bleeding mean substantial family disruptions and may even prompt a husband or mother to force the woman to have the device removed (*Population Reports* 1979b:66). The increased blood loss is also problematic as more than 50–80% of women of reproductive age in developing countries are anemic, and heavy bleeding increases the dangers of anemia (Masawe *et al.* 1974:314; *Population Reports* 1979b:66). Work is proceeding on devices that reduce blood loss, and the addition of antifibrinolytic agents to plastic IUDs is in the experimental stage. Of the available devices copper IUDs, which cause less bleeding, are recommended for women in developing countries who have bleeding problems with the Lippes Loop (*Population Reports* 1979b:80). Although the progesterone-releasing devices reduce the volume of blood loss even below normal levels, they have several drawbacks including prolonged bleeding, a possible association with more ectopic pregnancies, and an effective life of only 1 year (*Population Reports* 1979b:50).

Fecundability after Removal of an Intrauterine Device

Thus, intrauterine devices may be associated with a number of undesirable side effects such as cervical injury, pelvic infection, ectopic pregnancy, abortion, septic abortion, and anemia. Indeed, some of these adverse reactions may not be remediable by improving these devices; they may be unavoidable because they are a consequence of the contraceptive action of the devices. It seems probable, for example, that the sterile inflammation of the uterus (and tubes) seen in IUD users is responsible for preventing births *and* for an increased risk of pelvic infection and ectopic implantation.

Unfortunately, studies have shown that removal of an IUD is not immediately followed by a return to preinsertion conditions. As mentioned earlier, the risk of pelvic infection and ectopic implantation, which is increased in women with an IUD, does not return to normal levels until 1 year after removal. Studies have suggested that fecundability also does not return to normal levels until many months following removal.

Although one study (Tatum 1977:198) of short-term users (1–3 years) did show that when an IUD was removed because pregnancy was desired normal fertility returned within the normally expected time, a study of several thousand Taiwanese women who had a Lippes Loop removed showed increasing rates of sterility and decreasing fecundability with increased duration of use. Among the older women in this study the failure to conceive within 36 months of discontinuation was three times higher in users than nonusers (Jain and Moots 1977:146). However, a study by Vessey *et al.* (1978:265) on a smaller group suggested that although women using an IUD are slower to recover their fertility than women abandoning the diaphragm or other traditional contraceptive methods—after 1 year 48.5% of prior IUD users had not become pregnant compared to 29.4% of the control group—virtually all do so eventually.

Although it is significant that in the Vessey *et al.* (1978) study fertility returned after 3.5 years in almost all IUD users, suggesting a reversibility of any tubal damage, the difference between users and nonusers in the length of time necessary for the return of fertility is probably greater than the data indicate because the control group, which was abandoning traditional methods of contraception, is biased toward lower-fertility women; the more fertile women who chose these methods have dropped out of this group due to accidental pregnancies associated with their lower effectiveness. In the first year of use, for example, there were 13.1 pregnancies per 100 women associated with diaphragm use and only 4.2 pregnancies per 100 women associated with IUD use. Hence, we believe that present studies do not allow firm conclusions to be drawn about the return of full fecundability following removal of an IUD.

Summary

The IUD, like every other available effective method of birth control, is not perfect. In some women the IUD may even be an unacceptable method of birth control; this is especially true for never-pregnant women because the risk of pelvic infection which is about 5% for all IUD users, is greatest in this group. In addition about 4% of IUD users become pregnant each year, and of these pregnancies 40–50% will end as spontaneous abortions if the device remains in place. And even if the device is removed as soon as pregnancy is detected, only one-half of these pregnancies can be saved. A further drawback is that approximately 5% of all pregnancies in users implant ectopically. Therefore, pregnancy in an IUD user always calls for prompt medical assistance, either to remove the IUD (thereby halving the chances of a spontaneous abortion and eliminating the possibility of a potentially fatal septic abortion) or to remove an ectopic pregnancy surgically.

Studies that have examined the tubes of apparently healthy IUD users have indicated chronic sterile inflammation in about 50% of cases and actual tubal adhesions indicative of pelvic infection in about 12% of cases. Thus, fears that IUD use may have lingering effects on reproductive potential are justified. A number of studies have already been conducted on resumption of fecundity following discontinuation of use, but the results have been mixed and more studies are necessary before any firm conclusions can be drawn.

Population planners often favor the IUD over other forms of birth control for use in developing countries because the effectiveness of the device, though intrinsically lower than that of the pill, is user-independent and therefore may be associated with fewer accidental pregnancies than methods requiring daily or precoital action by the user. However, the drawbacks of the IUD—pelvic infection, spontaneous abortion, septic abortion, ectopic pregnancy, increased bleeding—though of concern to every woman using an IUD are of particular importance to women in developing countries, where there is less accessibility to prompt, high-quality medical care. Because pelvic infections are more likely to occur in IUD users, this means of birth control is not recommended for areas—and this includes many developing nations—where gonococcal and nongonococcal salpingitis are already a major problem; oral contraceptives, which seem to protect against pelvic infection, are a better choice for such areas. Women with a history of pelvic infection should not be provided with IUDs, yet this not infrequently happens in developing countries for a variety of reasons. In a family planning clinic in Nairobi, 9 of 100 women who had a Dalkon Shield inserted were subsequently treated for pelvic infections, and all of these were judged to be exacerbations by the IUD of a chronic pelvic infection (Hopcraft *et al.* 1973:585). The increased bleeding associated with most IUDs is also problematic because it is a danger to those many women of reproductive age in developing countries who are anemic. Oral contraceptives are the superior method in this respect, too, as they reduce menstrual blood loss. Thus, when deciding which types of birth control to introduce in a particular area, population planners should consider not only the effectiveness with which each method will be used, but also coexisting health problems in the area that could detract from the attractiveness of each method. But because death rates from childbearing reach 600–700 per 100,000 women in the poorest countries of Africa and Asia (*Popline* 1981:2), the relative risk posed by the IUD in these areas is quite low.

CHAPTER 18

Female Circumcision

Introduction

Any surgical interference in or near the female genital tract carries with it some risk of unfavorable reproductive sequelae. Cauterization of the cervix, if too deep or too extensive, can permanently damage the glands that secrete mucus favorable to sperm survival (Harrison 1977:97), thereby lowering conceptive ability. Hysterosalpingography, where a radiopaque substance is injected into the uterus and tubes to visualize via X rays any abnormality, may be associated with pelvic infection and subsequent sterility (Jacobson and Westrom 1969:1094). Neither of these procedures could have any impact on population fecundity because the number of women involved is so small. However, a rarely discussed yet widely performed procedure, female genital mutilation, may have a considerable impact on the fecundity of some populations. In black Africa alone about 20 million women are affected by genital multilation (*People* [UK] 1979:24), which has been cited as a cause of coital pain, coital inability, pelvic infection leading to sterility, and difficulties in childbirth resulting in considerable maternal morbidity and perinatal morbidity and mortality.

Female genital mutilation involves removal of part (circumcision) or all (excision) of the clitoris, often coupled with removal of the labia minora and sometimes the labia majora as well. In infibulation, the most radical procedure, the clitoris is excised, the labia cut away, and the scraped tissue sewn together. The term *circumcision* is not synonymous with genital mutilation but is customarily used so, and to prevent confusion will also be used here to refer to any of the various types of genital mutilation.

Reasons for the Procedure

Contrary to popular belief, female circumcision did not originate in Islamic tradition. It is practiced by both Christians and Muslims and there is evidence that the practice existed long before Christianity or Islam (Assaad 1980:4–5), dating from at least ancient Egypt (Verzin 1975:169). However, the strength of this practice in many parts of the world lies in Islamic tradition where it is seen as a means of preserving female modesty and chastity, which are highly valued (Assaad 1980:5). Removing the seat of female sexual pleasure is seen as a way of preserving the virginity of the young girl and the fidelity of the married woman, and thus has become one of Africa's most valued traditions (Ogunmodede 1979:30; *Population Reports* 1980b:446).

Female circumcision has also been justified as a hygienic measure (Assaad 1980:7; Verzin 1975:169); it is believed that a woman with a clitoris is dirty, that she smells bad, and that only such women have a white discharge (Epelboin and Epelboin 1979:28). Frequently it is seen as a rite of passage to true femininity or as an embellishment to secure a husband (*Population Reports* 1980b:446). Some women even believe that if the clitoris is retained the girl will develop masculine characteristics, thereby jeopardizing her chances for marriage (Assaad 1980:9). The Bambara group of Mali believe that a man, upon entering an uncircumcised woman, could be killed by poison secreted by the clitoris; thus failure to circumcise a girl would certainly jeopardize her chances for marriage (Epelboin and Epelboin 1979:28). Female circumcision is also believed to ensure fecundity. According to some groups in Mali an evil power, Wanzo, resides in the clitoris and will prevent fecundity if not removed. The presence of the clitoris is also felt to be dangerous during childbirth, contact between the head of the fetus and the clitoris causing death. The excised clitoris of young women is believed able to heal those who are sterile (Epelboin and Epelboin 1979:28).

But it is tradition that most assures the continuing practice of female circumcision, just as it does for male circumcision in the developed world, a procedure with no medical justification but possible complications such as hemorrhage and infection (*Time* 1981c:57). Although female circumcision is forbidden in Egypt, Ivory Coast, Somalia, and Sudan, it persists in these and in most countries where it has been banned (Assaad 1980:5; *People* [UK] 1979:40; Verzin 1975:163). Despite the pain that most women have endured because of circumcision and despite the often-recounted death of a friend or sister, many women do not question the value of the procedure and cannot believe there are ''real'' women who have not been circumcised. And even if a mother should decide she does not want her daughter circumcised, a grand-mother or aunt will often make sure the daughter is made acceptable by "cutting" her by surprise (Epelboin and Epelboin 1979:28–29).

Thus, arguments that female circumcision is disfiguring, an infringement of human rights, a threat to physical, obstetrical, and psychological health, and a cause of disharmony in marital relationships (Assaad 1980:7) usually fall on deaf ears and must be funneled to the people through trusted social institutions if any significant change of attitude is to occur (*People* [UK] 1979:2). Raising the general level of education of the populace will also help to stop the practice of female circumcision, as better-educated women and those of higher socioeconomic status are less likely to be circumcised and fewer have intentions of circumcising their daughters. Thus, although at least 75% of Egyptian women are circumcised, the modernized and privileged upper class has been spared (Assaad 1980:4, 6, 7).

Variations in Procedures

Most female circumcisions are performed by traditional midwives. These *dayas* account for about 50% of all operations performed in Egypt, and gypsies, barbers, aunts, female neighbors, and, increasingly, doctors and nurses do the remainder. In sub-Saharan Africa the situation is similar with the circumcision usually performed by a midwife but also by other villagers of certain castes (*Population Reports* 1980b:446) and occasionally by medical personnel. In Somalia, for example, the operation is done in special hospital units to prevent the unnecessary tragedies that occur when native surgeons using dirty instruments do the job (Ogunmodede 1979:30).

The age at which a girl is to be circumcised varies by region. In Ethiopia and Arabia it is done during the first days or weeks of life; among the Masai of Kenya it is done shortly after marriage, and among some Swahili-speaking tribes it is performed after bearing children. But these are exceptional cases, and most female circumcisions are performed on prepubescent girls (Verzin 1975:163). Hanry (1965, cited in Belsey 1976:335) noted, for example, that 84% of Muslim girls in a Guinean school had had a clitoral excision between ages 8 and 11.

The type of procedure also varies considerably from region to region. The two commonest procedures are the sunna and pharaonic circumcisions. The sunna, which is widely practiced in Egypt, is the more conservative procedure, as recommended by Islam, and involves removal of only the labia minora and part of the clitoris. In Sudan the pharaonic form of circumcision predominates and is a radical operation involving removal of all the labia minora, labia majora, and clitoris (Assaad 1980:4). In this case infibulation is often performed, which entails joining together the two sides of scraped vulva with catgut, metal wire, or the thorns of the acacia tree. The raw areas are left to heal around a small sliver of wood, which ensures an opening through which urine and menstrual blood can pass (Ogunmodede 1979:31; *Population Reports* 1980b:446; Verzin 1975:163). The vulva has now been replaced by almost a solid wall of flesh that joins the thighs from the pubis nearly to the anus, with the exception of a small orifice approximately the size of a pencil (Pieters and Lowenfels 1977:730).

Prevalence

Female circumcision is practiced on every continent (Verzin 1975:163), but is most prevalent in Africa and the Middle East. The most radical procedure, pharaonic circumcision, often with infibulation, is seen primarily in Sudan, Ethiopia, and Somalia but is also reported in Kenya, Mali, and Nigeria (Epelboin and Epelboin 1979:25; Verzin 1975:163). The more conservative sunna procedure or simple excision may be found in at least some areas of the following countries: Mauritania, Senegal, Gambia, Guinea-Bissau, Sierra Leone, Liberia, Ivory Coast, Mali, Upper Volta, Ghana, Togo, Benin, Niger, Nigeria, Cameroon, Central African Republic, Chad, Sudan, Zaire, Botswana, Lesotho, Mozambique, Malawi, Tanzania, Kenya, Uganda, Ethiopia, and Somalia. Some cases of female circumcision have also been reported in Algeria, Libya, Jordan, Syria, Saudia Arabia, and Yemen (*People* [UK] 1979:25).

The exact prevalence of female circumcision is unknown and some African observers (see *People* [UK] 1979c:2) have objected that certain reports (e.g., Epelboin and Epelboin 1979; Ogunmodede 1979) have exaggerated the problem of female circumcision. Nevertheless, solid data do exist that at least in Egypt and Sudan the proportion of women circumcised is extremely high—a reported 70–85% (Assaad 1980:6–7; *Population Reports* 1980b:446). A 1977 survey in Cairo of primarily middle-class women revealed that 82% were circumcised, and a study in Alexandria the same year showed that 70% of middle-class women were circumcised. Surprisingly, the majority (59%) of these circumcisions were the pharaonic type, not the more conservative sunna type that is believed to predominate in Egypt (Assaad 1980:6–7).

Effects on Fecundity

Female circumcisions are often performed by untrained persons. Anesthetics are not normally used and the girl struggles out of pain and fear, increasing the chances of a misplaced or too-generous cut. The instruments used—a knife, razor, piece of glass, or even a fingernail—are frequently dirty, and the traditional dressings often contain bits of soil and are applied without antiseptic precautions (Epelboin and Epelboin 1979:26). It is not surprising then that female circumcision produces short- and long-term complications (*Population Reports* 1980b:446), many of which are inimical to reproduction.

Early Sequelae

Hemorrhage and infection are the two major early sequelae of female circumcision, although the frequency with which they occur is debated. Belsey (1977:14) said there is a very high immediate risk of hemorrhage and infection in infibulation, whereas Pieters and Lowenfels (1977:730) believed these complications are rare. The incidence of severe hemorrhage may be less than expected, however, because the genitalia are not as well vascularized as in the adult (Verzin 1975:164). Nevertheless, fatal hemorrhage has been noted (Epelboin and Epelboin 1979:27; Ogunmodede 1979:31). Severe, potentially fatal infections such as septicemia and tetanus have also been recorded (Epelboin and Epelboin 1979:26). Much more common, however, are the less-severe and apparently localized infections of the external genitals. Whether such infections can spread to the uterus and tubes and thereby cause sterility is uncertain; and pros and cons of this hypothesis are treated in the section ''Conceptive Failure.''

Late Sequelae

While the early sequelae of female circumcision threaten a young girl's life, the late sequelae threaten her general health and, most especially, her future reproductive health. Threats to her general health include kidney and other urinary tract infections secondary to retention of urine which follows damage to, or partial obstruction of, the urethral opening (Epelboin and Epelboin 1979:27; Ogunmodede 1979:31; Pieters and Lowenfels 1977:731; Verzin 1975:167), and bladder and bowel incontinence and other disorders resulting from damage to the urethra or anus (Epelboin and Epelboin 1979:27; Ogunmodede 1979:31; Verzin

1975:165). The effects of female circumcision on reproductive health are many and can cause coital inability, conceptive failure, or pregnancy loss.

Coital Inability

Adverse effects on coitus are one of the most obvious outcomes of female circumcision and are largely the result of extensive scar tissue formation. Coital inability is rare, although Aziz (1980:562) reported that a "tight" circumcision that prevented penetration caused 60% of cases of infertility in a large group of women with pharaonic circumcisions. And in some cases of infibulation the vaginal opening may be so narrow that surgery is necessary before coitus is possible (Verzin 1975:166).

A lower-than-normal coital frequency must, however, be anticipated in those many circumcised women who receive little sexual pleasure because the clitoris has been removed (Verzin 1975:167) or who experience considerable discomfort because the scar tissue that replaces the labia makes penile penetration and thrusting painful (Belsey 1977:14; Epelboin and Epelboin 1979:27; Verzin 1975:166). In some instances anal intercourse may replace vaginal intercourse (Verzin 1975:167). The degree of narrowing of the vaginal opening and of any resulting dyspareunia vary, of course, with the operation, and are greatest for infibulation. But even if the scraped labia are not sewn together, extensive scarring and narrowing of the vaginal opening with dyspareunia can result. Even when only the clitoris is removed a neuroma (tumor composed of nervous tissue) may form due to severing of the clitoral nerves, and this also causes dyspareunia (Epelboin and Epelboin 1979:27). Interestingly, it has been proposed (*People* [UK] 1979:31) that the effect of dyspareunia on fertility may be opposite to that which would be expected, because a circumcised woman is highly motivated to become pregnant as often as possible so she can avoid regular intercourse during pregnancy and the postpartum period.

Conceptive Failure

It has been stated that female circumcision causes sterility (Belsey 1977:14; Epelboin and Epelboin 1979:27; Ogunmodede 1979:31; Verzin 1975:167), although admittedly the frequency and exact causes are not really understood (Epelboin and Epelboin 1979:27). It has been proposed (Epelboin and Epelboin 1979:27) that stasis of vaginal secretions and the menstrual flow caused by a greatly narrowed vaginal opening predispose to infection of the upper genital tract with resulting intrauterine adhesions and tubal obstruction. This seems a reasonable hypothesis because it is known that even a normal menstrual flow aids the ascent of bacteria to the upper genital tract. However, most workers (e.g., Belsey 1977:13; Verzin 1975:167) have felt that pelvic infections secondary to female circumcision represent an infection that has ascended from an initial focus in the external genitals following a non-sterile procedure. Verzin (1975:164) stated that the tendency for such an infection to spread to the tubes is enhanced by the presence in prepubescent girls of a thin and unprotected vaginal epithelium and non-menstruating endometrium that makes for particular susceptibility to upward spread of infection. To the countrary Kraus (1972:1118) felt that the absence of menstruation is a factor in the low prevalence of pelvic infection in prepubescent girls, because menstruation aids in the ascent of organisms to the upper genital tract.

If pelvic infections secondary to *infected* circumcisions are important in the etiology of the infertility in certain areas, two facts should be observable: (1) The number of pelvic infections among prepubescent girls, which ordinarily is quite low (Eschenbach and Holmes 1975:39), should be considerably higher than expected and (2) primary sterility should be an important contributor to the infertility in the area. However, if pelvic infections are the result of *stasis* of the menstrual flow, older, menstruating young women would be the most frequent victims. Here too the youth of the persons involved makes primary sterility the expected outcome.

Chronic pelvic infection is common among the Sudanese (who practice the radical pharaonic circumcision) and it is tempting, according to one worker (Verzin 1975:167), to conclude that this is due in part to acute ascending infections following circumcision. Indeed, Mustafa (1966, cited in Belsey 1977:14) claimed that 20–25% of cases of infertility in Sudan are due to infibulation. All this is just speculation, however. Other workers have speculated on different roles for female circumcision in sterility. Meuwissen (1967a:225) examined 398 infertile women in Ghana and found that 10.3% had vaginal changes, primarily fibrous narrowing, resulting from circumcision and native treatments. However, the proportion of fertile women with these changes is not given and the contribution of the narrowing to infertility is questionable. Additional more systematic research is therefore necessary before the importance of female circumcision in infertility can be determined.

One possibility that deserves investigation is whether endometriosis is more common in circumcised women, particularly those who have undergone infibulation, because it has been noted that obstruction of the menses can cause endometriosis (Schifrin *et al.* 1973:973). Obstructed menses is a consequence of the scar tissue that appears following female circumcision and completely or partially closes the vulva (Epelboin and Epelboin 1979:27). It may be so serious that, according to Ogunmodede (1979:31), a girl may writhe in pain because she cannot have a normal menstrual flow due to the restricted opening of the vagina. Endometriosis, which is a serious threat to fecundity because infertility is present in about 40 to 50% of cases (Spangler *et al.* 1971:850), is then a real possibility in such cases and should be explored.

Pregnancy Loss

The excision of the labia, especially when followed by infibulation, may result in a vaginal opening that is too small to allow normal delivery, even after reopening upon marriage, either by the husband's penetration or with a small knife (Epelboin and Epelboin 1979:26; Pieters and Lowenfels 1977:730). Prolonged labor due to obstruction will then occur (Belsey 1977:14; Epelboin and Epelboin 1979:27; Ogunmodede 1979:31; World Health Organization 1975:17). A radical upward episiotomy is often necessary to avoid injury to the mother, such as a rectovaginal or vesicovaginal fistula (see discussion of fistulas in Chapter 16) (Epelboin and Epelboin 1979:27; Pieters and Lowenfels 1977:731; Verzin 1975:169). It may also be necessary in order to avoid the otherwise high rates of perinatal morbidity (Ogunmodede 1979:31) and mortality (Belsey 1977:14). It is surprising then that the effect of female circumcision on pregnancy wastage has not been evaluated (World Health Organization 1975:17). Neglected too has been its role in secondary sterility, which may be substantial because obstructed labor is often associated with nonsterile instrumental interference and with tissue trauma, both of which increase the chances of postpartum infection (see Chapter 16).

Summary

Much about female circumcision remains shrouded in mystery. Although the practice is believed to be very prevalent in some areas of the world such as Africa, no firm statistics on its prevalence exist. The degree of mutilation, the skill of the operator, and the cleanliness of the cutting instrument, the dressing, and the general environment vary to an unknown extent. However, these variables are extremely important in determining the frequency of possible late sequelae—coital difficulties, conceptive failure, obstructed labor—that affect fecundity.

Coital difficulties are a frequent sequela to female circumcision, especially infibulation. And although we believe that local infection is possible after any type of circumcision, there is no solid evidence that this infection does ascend and cause pelvic infection. There simply are no reports of pelvic infection being widespread among young girls in affected areas. The observation that endometriosis, which causes infertility in 40 to 50% of cases, can follow obstructed menses is potentially very important, however, and infertile women in areas where circumcision is common should be investigated for this possibility. This aside, existing evidence suggests that if female circumcision is to have a marked effect on population fecundity, it is likely to be through pregnancy loss and postpartum infection leading to secondary sterility, and then only in women having undergone infibulation. This entire area is an important one for further research.

V

Overview

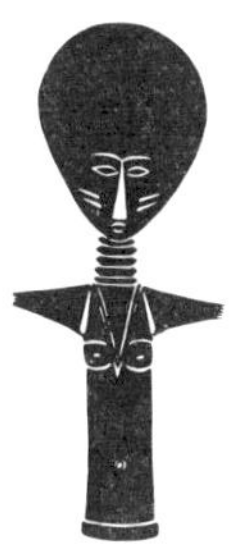

The Effects of Venereal Disease and Genital Tuberculosis on U.S. Black Fertility: 1880–1960

Introduction

The object of this volume is to familiarize the reader with the available facts about the pathophysiology of those diseases that are potentially important subfecundity factors. In this way the reader can assess the importance of these diseases to the observed fertility of particular populations. To provide an example of the utility of this type of information, this chapter assesses the role several diseases played in the 1880–1960 fertility swing in the U.S. black population.

In the latter part of the nineteenth century the U.S. black fertility rate began a sharp decline that continued until the mid-1930s, at which time it rebounded and continued to rise until 1960 (see Figure 19.1). The trend in childlessness was the reverse, rising during the first period and falling during the latter. Population students have long suspected that these trends were due almost entirely to changing health conditions. This health hypothesis holds that subfecundity-producing health conditions increased among blacks from 1880 to 1936, leading to widespread involuntary childlessness and subfecundity and a consequent fall in fertility. The subsequent rise in black fertility and decline in childlessness is attributed to a decrease in the prevalence of these conditions. Farley (1970) was the first to develop this idea systematically.

Other writers (Masnick and McFalls 1976, 1978; McFalls and Mas-

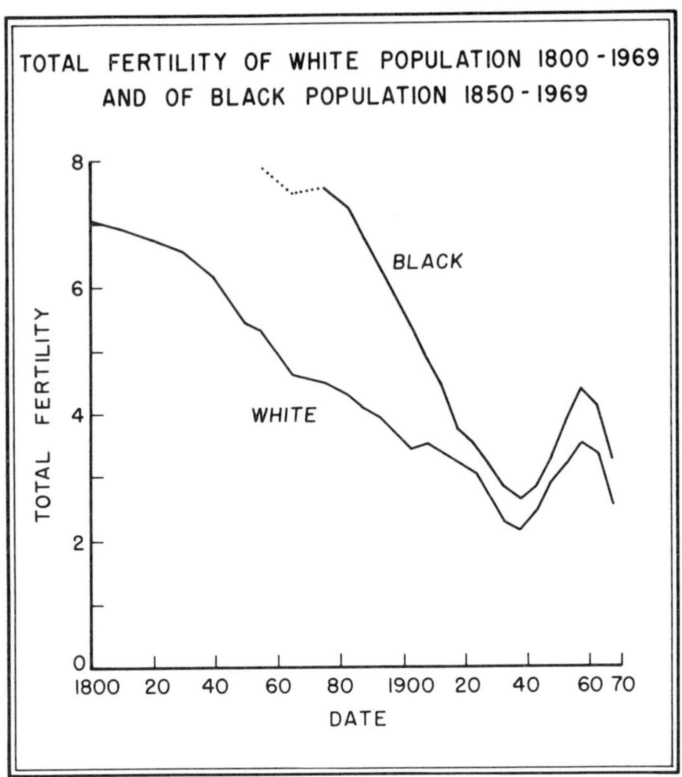

Figure 19.1 Total fertility of white population 1800–1969 and of black population 1850–1969. Source: Coale and Rives (1973, cover figure).

nick 1981; McFalls and Tolnay, forthcoming) have also concluded that subfecundity was a significant factor in the U.S. black fertility trend (certainly more so than in its white counterpart). However, they have also recognized two other factors as important determinants: (1) changes in the prevalence and effectiveness of various birth control practices and (2) changes in mate exposure variables such as the proportion of time spent in stable sexual unions. Despite disagreement on just how influential subfecundity was, there is a clear consensus that it was one of the important causes of the fall in black fertility from 1880 to the mid-1930s.

The causes of this subfecundity and their relative importance are still not clear. Early formulations of the health hypothesis focused mainly on the venereal diseases syphilis and gonorrhea. However, a subsequent critique (McFalls 1973) showed that their impact on black fertility and childlessness rates was exaggerated. Syphilis was demoted to a factor of only secondary importance. Gonorrhea was judged to be a primary cause of black subfecundity, but one given undue credit in the past for subfecundity produced by other causes. These underrated causes probably included genital tuberculosis (TB) and postpartum and postabortal infection, general undernutrition and specific deficiency diseases, and psychopathological disorders such as alcoholism and psychic stress.

This chapter combines findings from the aforementioned critique (McFalls 1973), new material, and information from Chapters 10 and 11 to yield more refined estimates of the impact of syphilis and gonorrhea on U.S. black fertility between 1880 and 1960. It also explores the role genital TB played in this fertility swing, using the information developed in Chapter 3 together with other previously unpublished work.

Syphilis

Central to any determination of the impact of venereal disease (VD) on the black fertility decline is how much VD prevalence increased between 1880, the year marking the beginning of the decline, and 1936, the year that black fertility reached its lowest point before turning upward. The prevalence of VD among slaves is unknown. Savitt (1978:76–80) felt that VD may have been common among slaves, perhaps even more common than among whites "because of the promiscuity engendered by the slave system." There are reports of prostitution and casual sexual liasons among slaves, suggesting there was ample opportunity for the spread of VD (Savitt 1978:78). Emancipation with its attendant social upheaval must have offered even greater opportunity for the spread of VD. But the actual prevalence of VD in 1880, at the beginning of the black fertility decline, is simply unknown. Had 3% been infected with VD? Had 6%? No one knows.

And although no one knows exactly how prevalent VD was at the end of the fertility decline in 1936 either, there are ancillary data on which a fairly reliable estimate may be made. Selective Service data for the first 2 million men recruited during World War II show that 35% of black recruits aged 31–35 were infected with syphilis (Vonderlehr and Usilton 1942). (There are no Selective Service data on the frequency of gonorrhea.) However, this figure probably overstates prevalence for all black men in this 1905–1909 birth cohort (which, incidentally, was the black cohort with the lowest fertility) because men tested by the Selective Service were not a representative cross-section of the black population. They were more often typical of the black military population—they were less educated, relatively fewer were married, had children or deferrable jobs, etc; in short, they were persons who would tend to have more syphilis. (This would be especially true of older men, those aged 31–35 at the time of testing.) Therefore, the actual rate for the entire 1905–1909 black male cohort was probably closer to 25 than to 35%. But to be on the safe side we use a 30% prevalence estimate in the model of syphilis' impact on black fertility.

The prevalence of syphilis in black women in the 1905–1909 cohort may be extrapolated from the male data using the sex differential in syphilis prevalence reported in the 1962 National Health Examination Survey. This study provides the best data available on this differential because it is based on a random sample and is not plagued by sex-related differences in (1) the frequency of symptomatic disease and (2) the likelihood of seeking medical attention once a problem is noted. It found that the ratio of male to female syphilis infections was approximately 1.4:1 (Brown *et al.* 1970:77). Because there is no reason to suspect that transmission patterns or susceptibility changed radically between 1940 and 1960 among blacks, about 21.4% of black females in the 1905–1909 cohort probably had syphilis, given the 30% male prevalence estimate.

All the data necessary to calculate the increase in syphilis prevalence have now been assembled: first, a "guesstimate" that by 1880 3–6% of the black population had experienced some venereal infection, which translates into a 2–4% syphilis rate. (Because gonorrhea is a more communicable disease than syphilis—shorter incubation period, greater likelihood of infection upon exposure, more frequent asymptomatic nature, etc.—there are usually more persons in a population who have been infected with gonorrhea than with syphilis. Hence, if 3–6% of a population has at some time been infected with VD [gonorrhea and/or syphilis], chances are that almost all 3–6% have experienced at least one gonorrhea infection, whereas only about 2–4% have been infected with syphilis.) And, second, a fairly reliable estimate that by 1940 30% of black men and 21.4% of black women in the low-fertility 1905–1909 cohort had syphilis. Given the most likely case of a 2% syphilis rate in 1880, the increase in the percentage ever-infected with syphilis would be 28 percentage points for black males and 19.4 percentage points for black females.[1]

What impact would such increases have on black fecundity? There would be no impact in men, in whom syphilis is rarely a subfecundity

[1]Although more men than women were probably infected in 1880 also, it is not necessary to account for this because the effect on the *difference* in prevalence would be negligible.

factor (McFalls 1973:13). But in women the increase would have an impact because syphilis can depress fecundity by increasing the probability that a pregnancy will end as a spontaneous abortion or stillbirth. However, as noted in Chapter 11, it is only during early syphilis that spirochetemia is present and fetal infection is possible. A woman is therefore at risk of pregnancy loss secondary to an intrauterine infection only during the first 2 years following infection. Because one infection, if untreated, confers long-lasting immunity against a second infection, an infected woman is temporarily subfecund for only 24 months during her entire reproductive life. Most women, then and now, were infected during their 20s (Brown *et al.* 1970:79; Frazier and Hung-Chuing 1948:32), and assuming that the average birth interval of a noncontracepting population during this decade of life is 30 months, an infected woman averts 4/5 of a birth. Because this 4/5 of a birth was averted by an additional 19.4% of black women in 1940 as compared to 1880, an average additional .16 of a birth was averted. The average family size of blacks shrank from 7 to 3 children between 1880 and 1940, and thus syphilis could account for only 3.9% of the 4-child decline using this model.

It is worth noting that this model substantially overestimates the impact of syphilis for the following reasons:

1. It assumes no birth control use at all during the 1880–1936 period, which is known to be untrue.
2. It assumes an average birth interval of 30 months, which may be too long for the early intervals of a noncontracepting population averaging 7 children.
3. It assumes *all* conceptions terminate as miscarriages during the infectious 2-year period, when not all do.
4. It assumes the infectious period (to the fetus) is 2 years for all women. But this too is a very generous figure because more than 75% of women are infectious for 1 year or less. These women never have a relapse to secondary syphilis during the second year. The real infectious period is therefore less than 1.25 years (.75[1] + .25[2] = 1.25 years). Just by using 1.25 instead of 2 years, the impact of syphilis on fecundity is almost cut in half.
5. It assumes that syphilis prevalence was conservatively low (2%) at the beginning of the 1880–1936 period and conservatively high (21.4% [which was based on a generous 30% male rate]) at the end, thus maximizing the increase over the period.

If none of these assumptions were made, syphilis could account for as little as .5% of the 4-child decline. This .5% figure will be used later in the calculation of the low estimate of the impact of VD (syphilis and gonorrhea) on black fertility. A figure of 1% will be used in the realistic estimate.

Gonorrhea

Because syphilis can account for only 0.5% to 4% of the black fertility decline, the VD hypothesis is in real jeopardy unless gonorrhea is able to account for the rest of the decline. How great was the increase in gonorrhea prevalence over the period, and for how much of the fertility decline could such an increase account?

Prevalence in 1880 and 1936

As with syphilis, the prevalence of gonorrhea among slaves is unknown. It certainly was present in the slave quarters and the social disorganization following Emancipation afforded opportunity for rapid spread. The percentage of blacks ever-infected with gonorrhea in 1880, at the beginning of the fertility decline, is unknown but a guess of 3 to 6% (i.e., virtually all those estimated to have had VD) is probably not far from the mark. It is important to emphasize that this figure represents the proportion of the population that ever had at least one infection. A fair number of persons had two or more infections because multiple infections with gonorrhea are common. Indeed, data on gonorrhea epidemiology indicate that there is a core of frequently infected, highly active transmitters (Yorke *et al.* 1978:56) who account for a disproportionate number of gonorrhea infections. In one study only .06% of the population were responsible for 22% of the gonorrhea cases recorded in 1 year (Brooks *et al.* 1978:163).

The percentage of blacks ever-infected with gonorrhea in 1936, at the end of the decline, is unknown but can be estimated by using the previously mentioned syphilis prevalence data. By relying on these data some workers have overestimated the number of persons ever-infected with gonorrhea because they have misinterpreted reports that in the preantibiotic era gonorrhea *infections* outnumbered syphilis *infections* by 3 or 4: 1 (Brown *et al.* 1970: 69, 84; Parran 1937:6). From such data they concluded that if 25% of the population had syphilis, then 100% must have had gonorrhea. This is not true for two reasons. First, in the preantibiotic era it was possible to be infected only once with syphilis because an untreated infection confers long-lasting immunity against subsequent infection. (Treatment with arsenicals became available in 1907 but few persons availed themselves of it, and of those who did few ever completed the lengthy regimen necessary to effect a cure.) But gonorrhea, which is significantly more communicable than syphilis, offers no such immunity and multiple infections have always been common. Hence, whereas gonorrhea infections may have outnumbered syphilis infections by 4:1, the ratio of the number of persons ever-infected with gonorrhea to the number ever-infected with syphilis must have been significantly smaller than 4:1, perhaps 2:1 or less, to allow for multiple gonorrhea infections in the same person, a very common occurrence. Second, in any population there is an upper limit on the proportion of the population at risk of developing any venereal disease. Hence, it is likely that although 50% of the black population was at such risk, the other 50% was not because they were in stable monogamous unions, sexually inactive, celibate, and so forth (McFalls and Tolnay, forthcoming). The 100% gonorrhea rate noted earlier in the paragraph would therefore be impossible. A model is thus proposed (see Figure 19.2) that allows that in intensely exposed groups VD rates will increase, but only to a certain upper limit (here 50%). In addition, the ratio of the percentage of persons ever-infected with gonorrhea to the percentage ever-infected with syphilis will steadily decline as the percentage ever-infected with syphilis increases. (In Figure 19.2 this ratio declines from 4:1 at age 16 to 1.2:1 by age 33.) To do otherwise would mean involving persons who simply are not at risk of acquiring any venereal disease. Because there is the same upper limit (here 50%) on the syphilis rate and the gonorrhea rate, the excess of persons ever-infected with gonorrhea over those ever-infected with syphilis approaches zero as this limit is approached.

According to this model, when relatively few members of a population acquire VD, as was the case for blacks in 1880, the greater communicability of gonorrhea results in a substantially greater chance of ever acquiring gonorrhea than syphilis. Hence the estimate earlier of a 50% higher ever-infected gonorrhea rate (3–6%) than ever-infected syphilis rate (2–4%) in 1880. It is not likely, however, that the same 50% differential holds when VD rates are very high. In 1940, for example, when syphilis rates were 30% for black men and 21.4% for black women, such a differential would mean that 45% of black men and 32.1% of black women had had gonorrhea at least once, figures that are unrealistically high. There were simply too many blacks, perhaps 50%, who were not at risk of acquiring a venereal disease. And of the 50% who were at risk, certainly not all acquired the disease. For example, a man runs only a 20–30% risk of a gonorrhea infection after one or two acts of coitus with

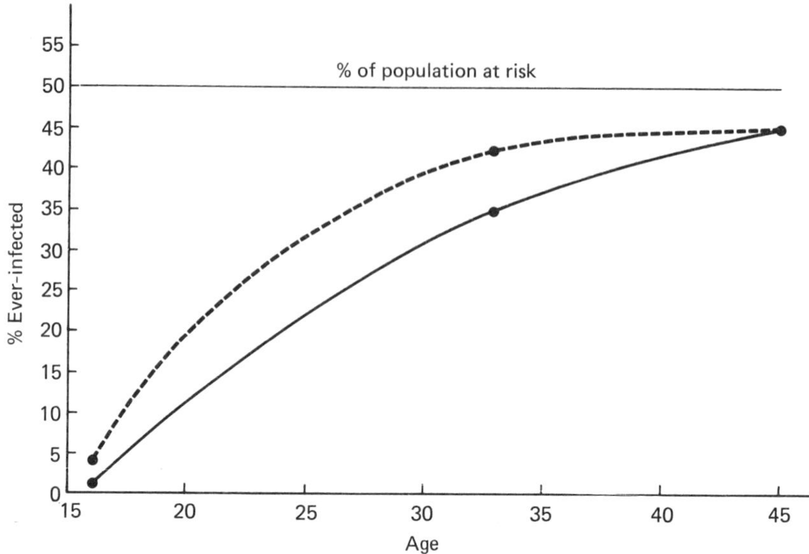

Figure 19.2 The cumulative frequency of those ever-infected with gonorrhea
(----) and syphilis (———) over time, in a hypothetical society in which 50% of the population is at risk of infection and 90% of those at risk become infected with both diseases.

an infected partner, although the risk for women is substantially higher,
50–70% (Pariser 1972:1127; Wigfield 1972:672). (Exposure to an infectious case of syphilis is even less likely to result in infection. Only 10%
[Benenson 1975:316] to 50% [von Werssowetz 1948, cited in Cannefax
1965:261] of persons acquire the disease following exposure.) Numerous
acts of intercourse with a *currently* infectious partner are therefore necessary to ensure infection. Thus not everyone at risk becomes infected.
Probably no more than 90% do. Hence, the effective upper limit of the
proportion of the population ever-infected with gonorrhea (or syphilis)
is probably about 45% (50% × 90%). (See Figure 19.2.)

Hence, more realistic estimates of the percent of blacks ever-infected with gonorrhea are 36% for males and 25.7% for females. These
estimates assume that about 20% more blacks in the 1905–1909 cohort
had had gonorrhea than syphilis. These estimates are used in the realistic models to be presented. However, high- and low-impact models
are also constructed. The upper-limit or high model assumes a 50% differential, which yields ever-infected estimates of 45% for males and
32.1% for females. The low model assumes a 0% differential, which leads
to ever-infected estimates of 30% for males and 21.4% for females. Now

that estimates have been made of gonorrhea prevalence in 1880 and 1936, the increase in prevalence can be calculated.

Other Factors in the Models

Aside from the increase in gonorrhea prevalence over the period, several more facts must be ascertained before an estimate can be made of the impact of this disease on black fertility. These include (1) the percentage distribution of the additional persons ever having gonorrhea in the 1905–1909 cohort compared to the cohorts reproducing around 1880 by number of lifetime infections, (2) the percentage of those infected who developed complications capable of causing subfecundity, (3) the percentage of those with complications who actually became sterile, and (4) the average number of children before sterility. These facts will first be determined for women and then models will be developed to estimate the contribution of female gonorrhea to the fertility decline. The same will then be done for men.

The distribution of the additional women ever-infected with gonorrhea in the 1905–1909 cohort compared to the earlier high-fertility cohorts by number of lifetime infections is not known, but can be calculated if two assumptions are made:

1. Gonorrhea infections occurred with four times the frequency of syphilis infections, which is what data from the preantibiotic era suggest (Brown *et al.* 1970:69, 84).
2. No one had more than 10 infections (data from the preantibiotic era actually suggest that it was rare for an individual to have more than five infections [Grimble 1972:614]).

The frequency distribution generated by adhering to these two assumptions and to the realistic assumption of a 3% ever-infected gonorrhea rate for black women in 1880 and a 25.7% rate in 1936 is shown for black women in Table 19.1. In this realistic model the *increase* over the period in the proportion ever-infected with gonorrhea is 22.7% (25.7–3%). Because gonorrhea infections occurred four times as frequently as syphilis infections, this same fourfold factor applied to the increase in syphilis infections over the period means that the increase in the total number of gonorrhea infections was 77.6 per 100 women (4 × [21.4% − 2%]). (It is the *increase* over the period that is important because it allows a determination of the proportion of the four-child decline attributable to an increase in VD prevalence.)

Table 19.1
Estimated Percentage Distribution of the Additional 22.7% of Black Women
Ever Having Gonorrhea in the 1905–1909 Cohort Compared to the Cohorts
Reproducing around 1880, by Number of Lifetime Infections

Number of lifetime infections	% of black women	Total infections[a]
1	6.4	6.4
2	4.6	9.2
3	3.3	9.9
4	2.4	9.6
5	1.7	8.5
6	1.2	7.2
7	.9	6.3
8	.6	4.8
9	.4	3.6
10 or more	1.2	12.0
	22.7	77.6

[a] The sum of the percentages does not equal the total because of rounding.

The next critical problem is to determine how many infected women went on to develop salpingitis. Although a frequently cited study of the preantibiotic era placed this figure at 14% (Rees and Annels 1969:206), that figure is suspect because it is lower than the contemporary rate of 20% (see, e.g., Eschenbach 1980:142S; Westrom 1975:707; Wiesner and Holmes 1975:19). The 20% salpingitis rate will therefore be used.

But how many women with gonococcal salpingitis actually became sterile? In the preantibiotic era a 60–70% sterility rate was recorded (Holtz 1930, cited in Thompson and Hager 1977:108; Westrom and Mardh 1975:162). This is an average figure because, as is still the case, second- and higher-order episodes of salpingitis are associated with a greater likelihood of sterility because the tube has been compromised by earlier infection (Thompson and Hager 1977:108). A 70% sterility rate is likely and will be used here.

The final question to be decided is how many live children on average do women who become sterile from gonorrhea have before childbearing ceases. An average of two children seems realistic for two reasons. First, the average age at first intercourse for the U.S. black population around 1936 was probably around 18 (McFalls and Tolnay, forthcoming). The mean age of initial syphilis infection for black females around 1936 was about 22.3 (Frazier and Hung-Chuing 1948), and because the distribution of gonorrhea cases by age is almost identical to that of early syphilis cases (Brown *et al.* 1970:85) the same 22.3 figure may be used for gonorrhea. Thus there is a 4–5-year interval between the average age of first intercourse and the average age of first infection. True, some individuals get gonorrhea in the first year, but some do not get it for 15 years—it is the average that is important. Second, an individual does not necessarily develop salpingitis or sterility with the first case of gonorrhea. The probability that these occur increases with the number of infections a person has. What this means in terms of the model is that the average length of time between first coitus and sterility is *longer* than the interval between first coitus and first infection. On average, the former is probably several years longer than the latter. But to be conservative only 1 year will be added to the first coitus to first infection interval. Thus, the average interval between the first coitus and sterility (when it occurs) is 5–6 years, or approximately 66 months. Assuming a reproductive life of 27 years (age 18–45) and recognizing that the early birth intervals are much shorter than the average birth intervals in high-fertility populations such as the black population in 1880, the average woman could easily have had 2–3 children during a 66-month interval.

The 2-child allowance is also sensible in the light of the research noted in Chapter 10 that gonorrhea is found with surprising frequency among high-parity women and among pregnant women.

Models for Women

Now that all the pieces are in place it is possible to construct a model of the impact on black fertility of an increase in gonorrhea based on realistic (i.e., moderate) assumptions. Table 19.2 shows how the calculations go. In line 1, an additional 6.4% of the black women in the cohort have *only* one infection. Because 20% get salpingitis and 70% of those become sterile, .90% become sterile (6.4 × .2 × .7 = .90). In line 2, an additional 4.6% of women have two infections, .64% become sterile with the first infection (4.6 × .2 × .7 = .64), and .55% become sterile with the second infection ([4.6 − .64 who are already sterile] × .2 × .7 = .55%). Adding .64 and .55, it is found that 1.19% are sterile. The other lines follow this same step progression. The bottom line is that 8.23% more women in this cohort than in the cohorts reproducing around 1880 are sterile due to gonorrhea.

To estimate the impact of this on the fertility decline—a 4-child average drop from 1880 to 1936—it is necessary first to calculate how much it would reduce the 1880 7-child average. This can be found by the following equation: (8.23% × 2 children before sterility) × (91.77% × 7

Table 19.2

Realistic Model of Impact of Increase in Gonorrhea on Fertility of Black Women

Number of lifetime infections	% of black women	% with gonorrhea who did not become sterile	% with gonorrhea who became sterile from infection number:										
			1	2	3	4	5	6	7	8	9	10	Total
1	6.4	5.50	.90										.90
2	4.6	3.41	.64	.55									1.19
3	3.3	2.10	.46	.40	.34								1.20
4	2.4	1.31	.34	.29	.25	.21							1.09
5	1.7	.80	.24	.20	.18	.15	.13						.90
6	1.2	.49	.17	.14	.12	.11	.09	.08					.71
7	.9	.31	.13	.11	.09	.08	.07	.06	.05				.59
8	.6	.19	.08	.07	.06	.05	.05	.04	.03	.03			.41
9	.4	.09	.06	.05	.04	.04	.03	.03	.02	.02	.02		.31
10 or more	1.2	.27	.17	.14	.12	.11	.09	.08	.07	.06	.05	.04	.93
	22.7	14.47											8.23

children) = 6.589 children. Subtracting from seven children, the impact is .411 children, which represents 10.3% of the 4-child decline. Thus, adhering to realistic assumptions, gonorrhea in women can be found to account for only 10.3% of the black fertility decline.

But what if this "realistic" model is too conservative; that is, it underestimates the increase in prevalence over the period and overestimates the average number of children before sterility? Perhaps the number of persons ever-infected with gonorrhea exceeded the number of persons with syphilis by 50% instead of 20%. This would mean that male gonorrhea prevalence increased by 42 percentage points ([1.5 × 30%] − 3% = 42%) and female rates by 29.1 percentage points ([1.5 × 21.4%] − 3% = 29.1%). And perhaps only an average of 1.5 children were born to infected women before the onset of sterility. The following discussion reveals what the impact on the fertility of black women would be under these conditions.

To calculate this impact, the percentage distribution of the additional 29.1% of black women ever having gonorrhea in the 1905–1909 cohort compared to the cohorts reproducing around 1880 must first be determined, as in Table 19.1. These values must then be substituted for those in column 2 of Table 19.2. Then, by simply employing the notion that 20% of women with gonorrhea get salpingitis and 70% of these become sterile, the rest of the values in this new table may be derived. Totaling all the new values in column 4 will show that in this "high" model 8.85% more women in the 1905–1909 cohort than those in the cohorts reproducing around 1880 are sterile due to gonorrhea. It is at first surprising that a substantial increase in the number of women with gonorrhea (29.1% in the high model versus 22.7% in the realistic model) results in only a small increase in the final number of women rendered sterile (8.85% versus 8.23%). But because both models adhere to the idea that gonorrhea cases outnumbered syphilis cases by a 4:1 margin, the number of gonorrhea infections is the same in both cases, necessitating that the same number of infections must be distributed among a larger group of women in the second model. This means that the average number of infections per woman is lower. Hence, in the second, high model, for example, only 63% of women with one gonorrhea infection go on to a second infection, whereas 72% do so in the first, realistic model.

The high model also assumes that a woman had only 1.5 children before sterility. The following computations reveal how much this would reduce the 1880 7-child average: (8.85% × 1.5 children before sterility) + (91.15% × 7 children) = 6.513 children. Subtracting from 7 children the impact is .487 children, which represents 12.2% of the 4-child decline. Hence, even when very generous assumptions are made, gonorrhea in women can account for only 12.2% of the black fertility decline.

But what if many of the assumptions, even those in the realistic model, are too generous? Perhaps the following assumptions prevail:

1. Gonorrhea was more prevalent in 1880, at a level of possibly 6%, and thus the increase over the period was overestimated in the two models.
2. Cases of gonorrhea outnumbered those of syphilis by only 2.5:1.
3. Gonorrhea affected the same number of persons as did syphilis (30% of black men and 21.4% of black women).
4. Couples averaged 2.5 children before sterility.

In this model, as in the earlier ones, complication rates and sterility rates remain at 20% and 70%, respectively, because these values are based on very reliable medical estimates. Again, by doing the calculations illustrated in Tables 19.1 and 19.2, it is found that 5.25% more women in the 1905–1909 cohort than in the 1880 cohort were sterile due to gonorrhea.

Given the 5.25% female sterility rate in this "low" model and a 2.5-child average before sterility, how much of the 4-child decline can be accounted for? Calculations will be made as before: (5.25% × 2.5 children before sterility) + (94.75% × 7 children) = 6.764 children. Subtracting from the 1880 7-child average equals .236 children, which is 5.9% of the 4-child decline. Hence, using modest assumptions, female sterility due to gonorrhea can be found to account for only 5.9% of the black fertility decline.

Models for Men

But what of male sterility due to gonorrhea? The same three models, high, realistic, and low, will be generated to determine the impact of additional male sterility due to gonorrhea on the black fertility decline. In all three models, as was the case in the female models, complication rates and sterility rates will be the same; it is estimated that before antibiotics 20% of men with gonorrhea developed epididymitis (the only complication proven to cause sterility) and 33% of these became sterile (see Pelouze 1939:240). In the high model the same assumptions will be made as were made in the high female model:

1. There was a 3% gonorrhea prevalence rate in 1880.
2. There was a 4:1 ratio of gonorrhea infections to syphilis infections.

3. There were a 50% greater number of persons ever-infected with gonorrhea than syphilis.
4. Couples had an average of 1.5 children before sterility.

In the realistic model assumptions 1 and 2 remain the same, but assumption 3 is reduced to a 20% greater rate and assumption 4 is increased to two children. In the low model assumption 1 is increased to a 6% gonorrhea prevalence rate in 1880, assumption 2 is dropped to a 2.5:1 ratio of gonorrhea cases to syphilis cases, assumption 3 assumes that the same proportion of persons got gonorrhea as got syphilis, and assumption 4 raises the average number of children before sterility to 2.5.

By performing the same calculations as before, one can use the high, realistic, and low models to account for 9.2%, 8.1% and 4.6% of the black fertility decline, respectively.

Combined Effect of Gonorrhea and Syphilis

The corresponding values for the three female gonorrhea models are 12.2%, 10.3%, and 5.9% (see Table 19.3). For syphilis, which is a

Table 19.3
Three Models of the Impact of Gonorrhea on the 4-Child Black
Fertility Decline, 1880–1940

	High model		Realistic model		Low model	
	Male	Female	Male	Female	Male	Female
Increase in the percentage ever-infected with gonorrhea, 1880–1940	42.0	29.1	33.0	22.7	24.0	15.4
Ratio of total gonorrhea cases to total syphilis cases	4:1	4:1	4:1	4:1	2.5:1	2.5:1
Percentage of infected persons who develop epididymitis or salpingitis	20.0	20.0	20.0	20.0	20.0	20.0
Percentage with epididymitis or salpingitis who become sterile	33.0	70.0	33.0	70.0	33.0	70.0
Average number of children before sterility	1.5	1.5	2.0	2.0	2.5	2.5
Percentage of the decline accounted for	9.2	12.2	8.1	10.3	4.6	5.9

subfecundity factor only for women, the figures are 3.9%, 1.0% and 0.5%. Given these figures, the impact of VD on the fertility decline can be estimated. Simply totalling the syphilis, female gonorrhea, and male gonorrhea figures will overestimate the impact of any series of models— high, realistic, or low—because persons with VD tend to have mates or spouses with VD. Because sterility in one member of a couple is sufficient to avoid childbearing, a more appropriate measure would be $p(M) + p(F) - p(MF)$, where $p(M)$ and $p(F)$ are the proportions of males and of females that are sterile, respectively, and $p(MF)$ is the proportion of males who are sterile and whose partners are also sterile. Taking such double counting into account, the three high models indicate that certainly no more than about 22% of the black fertility decline can be attributed to VD. The low models suggest that the impact could be as low as 9%. And the realistic models suggest a figure in the vicinity of 16%. Thus, based on the most realistic assumptions we conclude that VD accounted for about 16% of the black fertility decline between 1880 and 1936.

Once it is realized that VD can account for only 9% to 22% of the decline, it is no longer necessary to prove that the trends in VD and fertility were mirror images of each other from 1880 to 1936 (which is a requirement for the VD hypothesis). Indeed, the lack of symmetry between the two trends has always been problematic for proponents of the VD hypothesis; simply the wrong people had the low fertility and the high childlessness. Individuals with the lowest VD rates (the more educated, for example) had the lowest fertility and highest childlessness. And geographic areas, such as the North, that had the lowest VD rates again had the lowest fertility and highest childlessness. It is therefore necessary to forward other factors to help explain the decline. These determinants include other subfecundity factors, such as genital TB, as well as low mate exposure, contraception, and induced abortion. The possible contribution of genital TB to the black fertility decline will be explored next.

Genital Tuberculosis

It is possible that TB had a substantial impact on the natality history of the U.S. black population over the past 100 years. Following Emancipation, TB grew at an alarming rate among blacks. One factor that probably facilitated increased infection rates was increased exposure to tuberculous whites. This was particularly true for blacks who moved into urban areas where TB rates were higher. Another factor was the crowded, unsanitary conditions that were the norm for urban blacks. Development of tuberculous disease, which is more serious in blacks than whites,[2] was facilitated by poor nutrition and high disease rates and the stress associated with social disorganization (Lowell *et al.* 1969:84)—all of which blacks endured throughout this period in varying degrees. It was not until the late 1930s that health conditions for blacks greatly improved and a precipitous fall in the number of cases of TB was recorded. Intriguing then is the possibility that changes in the prevalence of TB, and consequently genital TB, were partly responsible for the dramatic changes in the fertility (see Figure 19.1) and childlessness rates of the black population between 1880 and 1960, a pattern that is still largely unexplained. That is, perhaps the steep decline in black fertility and the concomitant rise in childlessness between 1880 and 1936 are attributable partly to the tremendous increase in TB among blacks during this period. Similarly, perhaps the 1936–1960 increase in fertility and decrease in childlessness were due partly to the declining prevalence of TB.

It is not possible to study the relationship between genital TB and black fertility directly because data on genital TB are unavailable for blacks during this period. However, this relationship can be evaluated indirectly be exploring the extent to which trends and differentials in fertility are consistent with trends and differentials in the prevalence of extragenital TB, for which data do exist. As with the discussion of the impact of VD on U.S. black fertility, the following investigation will show how a detailed understanding of the pathophysiology of a disease can provide population students with important clues regarding the influence of the disease on fertility, even in the absence of reliable epidemiological data.

In checking the consistency of trends and differentials in fertility with those in TB, the essential question is how well the trends and differentials in TB are synchronized in the expected direction with those in fertility and childlessness. In other words, are the trends in phase?

---

[2]TB occurs with greater frequency and severity in blacks (Medlar *et al.* 1949:1080; Long 1971:300). It is believed that resistant stocks have not yet developed in blacks as in whites with whom natural selection against the disease has been operating for centuries (McKusick 1964:120–121). Other researchers (e.g., Payne 1949:335, 338) believe that the disease is more serious in blacks because they are the more intensely exposed group. That is, because of their living and working conditions blacks are less likely to encounter the small doses of bacilli that lead to development of acquired immunity. Rather, they are more likely to receive massive doses, which lead rapidly to serious disease in the non-immune.

The answer is yes, there is remarkable synchronization between changes in black fertility and childlessness and changes in TB prevalence. The exact relationship between the two will be discussed in some detail, but first it is important to reemphasize that any discussion of the relationship between TB and fertility must take into account two facts: (1) Genital TB is far more often a cause of primary than of secondary sterility, and thus childlessness, rather than simply reduced fertility, is the most frequent outcome;[3] and (2) development of tuberculous disease is a two-stage process dependent on both infection with the tubercle bacillus and subsequent reactivation of initial lesions to form active disease.

Tuberculosis and Sterility

As discussed earlier, TB of the genitals is a cause of conceptive failure because the nodules formed in the fallopian tubes or epididymis interfere with the normal passage of gametes. Majority opinion favors the view that primary sterility is the most frequent outcome of genital TB. This is compatible with two important facts discussed in Chapter 3: (1) In order for seeding of the genitals to occur, primary infection must occur approximately at the time of greatest vascular activity in the reproductive organs, usually adolescence, and (2) development of tuberculous disease usually occurs early in life, between ages 12 to 24, before childbearing normally begins. Thus, the effects of genital TB on fertility are best reflected in the amount of childlessness experienced. Increasing childlessness was, of course, a major factor in the decline of black fertility over the period 1880–1936, but whether that portion attributable to infecundity was due to conceptive failure or to pregnancy loss is unknown.[4] The results of one study (McFalls and Tolnay, forthcoming) of urban black women born 1916–1921 does suggest, however, that pregnancy wastage was not an important cause of childlessness among blacks. Almost 36% of the surveyed women were childless, but less than one-third of these women reported ever being pregnant. Thus, 71% of childless women and 26% of all women in this cohort never conceived. Such a high proportion of women never conceiving bolsters the position of genital TB as a possible determinant of trends in childlessness and fertility for the period.

---

[3]Pregnancy loss is also a possible outcome but a rare one, because only a small minority of women with genital TB can conceive.

[4]It should be emphasized again that infecundity was not responsible for all of the childlessness experienced by this cohort. Some of these women were voluntarily childless, achieving this status by minimizing the time spent in conjugal unions and/or by using birth control (McFalls and Tolnay, forthcoming).

The Risk of Developing Tuberculosis

It is important when determining the impact of TB on fertility to separate those factors that influence the chances of becoming infected from those that influence the chances of developing disease. Comstock (1975:371) described those factors that influence the chances of becoming infected as being primarily extrinsic ones. Crowding is one factor related to the probability of infection, but most important is the severity of disease in the source case. And whether or not disease will develop in an infected person depends, according to Comstock (1975:377–378), on certain intrinsic factors—age, sex, race, and body build. The first three factors are clearly not responsive to change. The tendency for quiescent lesions to be reactivated and for tuberculous disease to develop will always be higher in infected persons who are young (a study in Puerto Rico [Comstock *et al.* 1974, cited in Comstock 1975:374] showed case rates peaking between the ages of 12 and 24, while a study of Eskimo rates [Comstock *et al.* 1967, cited in Comstock 1975:374] showed a more prolonged peak to age 30), female (this excess is limited to the young adult years), and black (this excess is also limited to the young adult years and is accounted for by the high rates for black women during that period) (Comstock 1975:374–375). Body build may, however, be viewed not solely as an intrinsic factor, but as one sensitive to dietary inputs. Indeed, malnutrition is a widely cited factor in the reactivation of tuberculous lesions and the development of disease (Comstock 1975:377–378; McKeown 1976:134–136; Rich 1951:623) because it is a cause of immunodeficiency. Indeed, McKeown (1976:141) stated that increased resistance because of better nutrition was the single most important reason for the decline in TB. Although Comstock did not mention them, other conditions such as malaria and early syphilis are also causes of immunodeficiency and are associated with a reduced ability to curb tuberculous infection. In short, then, the probability of developing TB depends on the chances of becoming infected *and* the chances of experiencing a stressful event such as malnutrition, which lowers the body's defense mechanisms and allows the reactivation of quiescent lesions.

Infection Rates among U.S. Blacks

Those persons who give a positive reaction to the tuberculin test represent the pool of infected individuals who are at risk of developing TB. It is commonly thought that in the early years of the twentieth century in most U.S. cities virtually all adults reacted to the tuberculin test (Lowell *et al.* (1969:18). But Comstock (1975:366) revealed that the tuberculin tests administered at this time were inaccurate, biasing upward the number of positive reactors. More restrictive criteria (only reactions to smaller inocula of tuberculin and more intense reactions were scored as positive evidence of infection) reveal that, contrary to dogma, a child in the 1930s had a very good chance of reaching adulthood uninfected by the tubercle bacillus. This was especially true for whites. But the new criteria did not alter so drastically the acknowledged infection rates for blacks, because a large proportion of blacks reacted to the smaller doses of tuberculin and their reactions were substantially more intense than those of whites (Aronson 1931:380).

Because most tuberculin tests conducted early in the century were inaccurate, infection rates for the U.S. black (or white) population prior to 1940 are largely unknown. However, the trend in TB mortality for U.S. blacks[5] (see Figure 19.3) should suggest the trend in infection rates because infection rates are high when the death rate is high (Sartwell 1965:216). This is because it is those serious cases of pulmonary TB with active ulcerative lesions (i.e., those cases in which death is relatively near) that spew bacilli into the environment, infecting others. Indeed, the severity of disease in the source case is the most important factor influencing others' chances of becoming infected (Comstock 1975:371). The consistent decline in black TB mortality after 1910 should then have been accompanied by a decline in infection rates for U.S. blacks. Data to support this hypothesis have come from studies (Lowell *et al.* 1969:172; Comstock 1975:372) of infection rates in black persons of all ages living in several Southern communities. Data from these studies (see Figure 19.3) show that TB infection rates did begin a rapid decline for women born after 1912. Unfortunately, similarly reliable infection rates for persons born prior to 1890 are unavailable. Although it is generally held that TB was relatively unknown in slaves, newer data (see Kiple and King 1981; Savitt 1978) contradict this view and persuasively argue that TB was no stranger to the slave quarters. But even these data allow that TB mortality among slaves was only a fraction of what it was to become after Emancipation. It is reasonable to assume, then, that infection rates were moderate in the antebellum period but increased after Emancipation and did not decline until the early 1900s in response to declining mortality (i.e., serious cases).

---

[5]Because there was no nationwide vital statistics system until 1933 these rates are based on data from many studies, some of it conflicting. For example, although TB mortality rates almost certainly dropped during the 1920s in urban areas, the trend in rural areas is believed somewhat in question (Farley 1970:72–73).

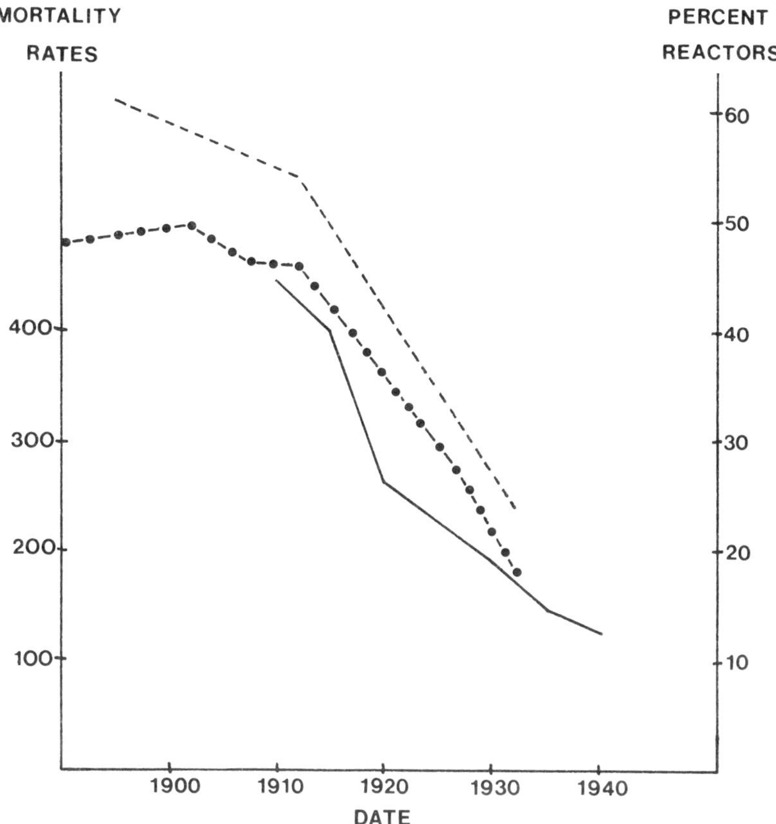

Figure 19.3 Nonwhite tuberculosis mortality rates by year and percentage of black women reacting to tuberculin, by year of birth. ———, Mortality; source: United States Bureau of the Census (1944b:29). ----, Reactors; source: Lowell *et al.* (1969:172). —•—•—, Reactors; source: Comstock (1975:372).

Diets among U.S. Blacks

The probability that tuberculous disease would develop in infected blacks was greatly enhanced by the widespread malnutrition that plagued the race. Prior to Emancipation the self-interest of slaveholders determined that the diets of slaves, though monotonous, provided sufficient nutrients and calories to ensure vigor (Farley 1970:36–37; Fogel and Engerman 1974:109–115).[6] But after Emancipation the diets of blacks

[6]Some workers (e.g., Kiple and King 1981:139–140) have contended that slave diets were deficient in certain nutrients essential to good health and the body's ability to fight infection. They have claimed that vitamin C was chronically absent from slave diets, vi-

became progressively worse, and the majority of the black population was suffering from severe malnutrition in the earlier part of this century (Myrdal [1944] 1972:375). Nutritional levels were characterized as ''very poor'' (Myrdal [1944] 1972:1289) and ''unhealthy'' (Farley 1970:72) for Southern blacks, and were perhaps only marginally better for their Northern counterparts (Myrdal [1944] 1972:375). Protein, the nutrient that plays probably the most decisive role in the development of TB (Payne 1949:337), was undoubtedly seriously lacking in the diets of U.S. blacks. It is certainly true that at least the diets of Southern blacks were protein-deficient; the high pellagra rate[7] among this group attests to that.[8] And Fogel and Engerman (1974:261) noted that the black share-croppers in the mid-1890s were both protein- and vitamin-starved. It was not until the late 1930s when the standard of living for the nation's blacks began to rise that diets improved (Farley 1970:227, 235–236).

Trends in Extragenital Tuberculosis

Many antebellum physicians stated that TB was uncommon among slaves, and this judgment is accepted by most modern authorities. Several medical historians cited by Farley (1970:59) stated, for example, that TB was almost unknown among slaves. But other medical historians, notably Savitt (1978) and Kiple and King (1981), have argued that TB was an important cause of death among slaves. Savitt (1978:143–145) presented data showing TB as the second leading cause of death for Virginia slaves from 1850 to 1860. He argued that had scrofula been included the TB mortality rate of blacks would have equaled or exceeded that of Southern whites. (Scrofula is an unusual manifestation of TB involving massive enlargement of the lymph nodes and was frequently not recognized as TB because physicians were more accustomed to seeing pulmonary disease.) Kiple and King (1981:139–146) also argued that many slave deaths from TB masqueraded as scrofula, dropsy, and even typhoid fever, largely because nineteenth-century U.S. blacks represented a ''virgin'' population in regard to tuberculous infection and

---

tamin A was available only seasonally, and essential amino acids were lacking or seriously out of balance. Fogel and Engerman (1974:114–115) disagreed and showed that slave diets exceeded modern recommended daily levels of these and other nutrients.

[7]In the early 1900s, 2–25% of the rural population of the South suffered from pellagra (Farley 1970:219). The disease was particularly serious in women, mortality rates being twice those for men (United States Bureau of the Census 1944a:236).

[8]Pellagra, though usually described as solely the result of a deficiency of one of the B vitamins, probably represents a deficiency of dietary protein as well (White *et al.* 1964:956).

the first two or three exposed generations suffer atypical extrapulmon-ary disease. They also argued that the impression that slaves did not suffer as much as whites from TB stems from the fact that they were rural dwellers and enjoyed the lower TB rates of this geographical area. In 1850, for example, the TB death rate for seven Southern states was 80 per 100,000 for whites and 60 per 100,000 for blacks, whereas the rate for Massachusetts was 344 per 100,000 (Kiple and King 1981:140).

Nevertheless, after the Civil War any prophylactic circumstances of slavery disappeared and the "flashpoint was reached for the disease to explode in epidemic form" (Kiple and King 1981:146). As Fogel and En-german (1974:261) noted, after Emancipation the diet of blacks, which was quite adequate under slavery, deteriorated badly and thus black sharecroppers in the mid-1890s were protein- and vitamin-starved. Eco-nomically blacks languished. They were squeezed out of crafts they had occupied during slavery. They were paid less for the same job as whites, and this salary gap continued to widen until World War II. The black population became increasingly urbanized as blacks migrated to the cit-ies in search of jobs. Not surprisingly, health deteriorated and disease rates in 1890 were 20% higher than what they had been on slave plan-tations. Thus U.S. blacks found themselves malnourished, socially dis-organized, economically destitute, increasingly urbanized, and in a state of poor health. All these factors were important determinants in the en-suing increase in black TB rates. Whereas black TB mortality was re-corded at 60 per 100,000 in the seven Southern states in the 1850s (Kiple and King 1981:40), by the early part of the twentieth century rates were 400 per 100,000 (Lowell *et al.* 1969:69). Calling TB "the scourge of the race," Scott and Winston (1976:706) went on to say:

> The health prospects of black Americans were so gloomy in the two gener-ations after Emancipation that in 1896 Frederick L. Hoffman, statistician of the Pru-dential Life Insurance Company, predicted that epidemic tuberculosis and social disorganization made inevitable the total extinction of the Negro population of the United States. [*American Journal of Diseases of Children*, 1976, **130**, 704. © 1976, Amer-ican Medical Association.]

TB mortality rates for blacks dropped dramatically between 1900 and 1920 (see Figure 19.3), at least in urban areas (Farley 1970:72), probably as a result of improved treatment methods. In response, infection rates began a rapid decline. But disease rates would not fall as precipitously until improvements in nutritional levels as well as lower infection rates were registered, as there remained a large core of persons infected in the past (and a smaller number of more recently infected persons) who remained at risk of developing TB. Indeed, the poor diet of blacks in the 1930s has been cited as responsible for their continued high rate of tuberculous disease during that period (Farley 1970:74). But in the late 1930s improved economic conditions for the nation's blacks meant better diets. The risk of infected persons developing TB therefore fell, and by 1940 the incidence of all forms of tuberculous disease had begun a precipitous decline (Lowell *et al.* 1969:171).[9]

If tuberculous disease of the genitals followed the same trajectory as the more visible extragenital TB, a portion of the drop in black fertility following 1880 and part of the subsequent recovery after 1936 could be explained. Indeed, genital TB is a particularly attractive explanatory variable for the black fertility trend because (1) most of the increase in TB occurred during the period (1880–1918) of greatest decline (80%) in black fertility (McFalls 1973:5) and (2) genital TB is usually a cause of childlessness, and high childlessness rates were a notable feature of the fertility decline.

Trends in Genital Tuberculosis

When analyzing how changes in childlessness are affected by the two risk factors associated with development of genital TB (infection rates and diet), it is instructive to work with birth cohorts. In this way the importance of these two risk factors during the critical years of early reproductive life can be evaluated and any effects on childlessness assessed. Figure 19.4 shows childlessness rates for selected cohorts of black women born between 1835 and 1944. It also shows TB infection rates for these same cohorts in the Southern communities studied in Figure 19.3.

The most striking feature is a general decline in childlessness as TB infection rates fall. However, there does appear to be a lag between the drop in infection rates and the drop in the childlessness rates. For example, childlessness rates for women born 1900–1910 continued to climb despite a drop in their infection rates. And whereas the 1915–1919 and the 1920–1924 cohorts experienced about the same percentage point drop in infection rates, the latter showed a much greater drop in the childlessness rate. Thus, substantial gains in reducing the childlessness rate did not come until the 1920–1924 cohort, that is, with those women who began childbearing in the period 1940–1944. (Urban black women of the period had their first child about age 22 [McFalls and Tolnay, forthcom-

[9]In the past, TB morbidity data (disease rates) were either not available or there was some doubt about their validity. Hence, mortality rates served as crude but useful indicators of the impact of the disease on a population. But once effective chemotherapy was available (post–World War II) death rates became useless for this purpose, as there could be significant levels of TB and few reported TB deaths (Lowell *et al.* 1969:74).

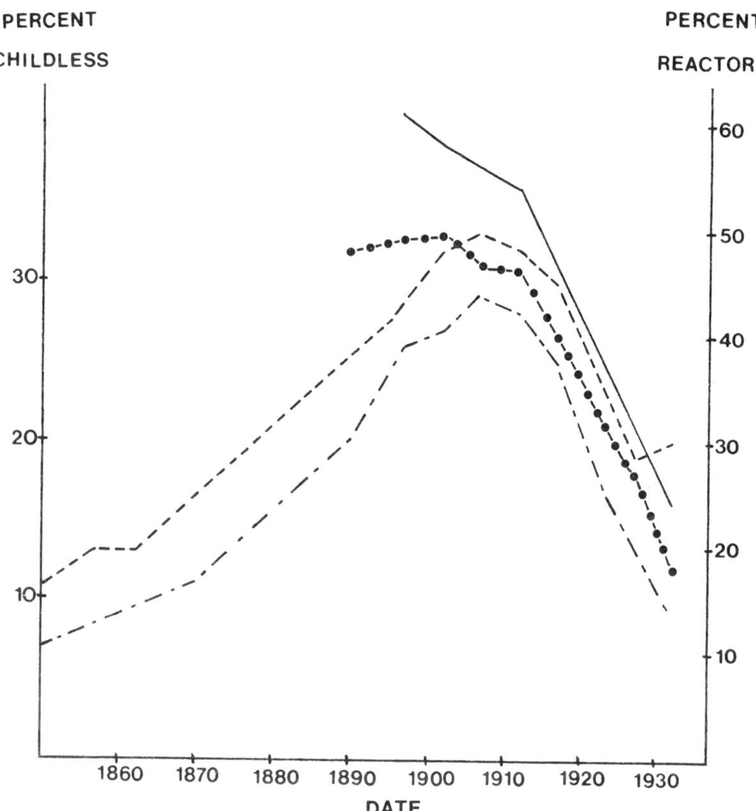

Figure 19.4 Percentage of total and ever-married black women childless, by year of birth; and percentage of black women reacting to tuberculin, by year of birth. — — — —, Total women childless; source: Farley (1970:95). — — —, Ever-married women childless; source: Farley (1970:95). ————, Reactors; source: Lowell *et al.* (1969:172). — •—•—, Reactors; source: Comstock (1975:372).

ing], so these dates approximate the onset of childbearing for this cohort.)

What experience distinguished this 1920–1924 cohort from the previous ones to explain the more precipitous decline in the rate of childlessness? Perhaps it was that substantially fewer of the infected women in this cohort ever developed genital TB because they were the first cohort of black women in 50 years to enter the childbearing years at a time—the late 1930s—when black diets were improving and the risk of developing tuberculous disease was falling. Thus, although declining infection rates meant that progressively fewer women were in the pool of infected persons who could ultimately develop genital TB and be rendered childless, the impact on the rates of childlessness would be relatively small as long as the chance of developing disease remained high. But when diets improved and the risk of developing tuberculous disease dropped dramatically for every infected person, a more significant change in the levels of genital TB and childlessness could be recorded.

Similarly, it is possible that the fairly constant infection rates for cohorts born around the turn of the century were accompanied by an increase in the rates of childlessness because TB disease rates were increasing. In fact, the highest rates of childlessness were reported for those women who would enter reproductive life in the 1920s, when economic conditions and diets were at a critical low point for the nation's blacks and the risk of developing tuberculous disease was very high.

Urban–Rural Differentials

Urban–rural differences in the prevalence of TB are also in phase with regard to differences in urban and rural childlessness rates. Usually TB is an urban disease; infection rates tend to rise as crowding heightens the chances of coming into prolonged close contact with an infectious case. An inspection of black childlessness in the period shows that urban areas had much higher rates (see Table 19.4). In 1910, 31% of ever-married urban black women were childless, whereas only 16% of rural women were; in 1940, 37% of urban black women were childless, whereas the childlessness rate for rural women was only 23%.

A closer inspection of urban and rural childlessness rates by region shows that the increases in childlessness between 1910 and 1940 were

Table 19.4
Percentage of Ever-Married Nonwhite Women
Childless, by Urban or Rural Residence:
1910 and 1940[a]

	Percentage childless	
	1910	*1940*
Total United States	21	32
Total urban	31	37
North and West	38	37
South	28	38
Total rural	16	23
Nonfarm	18	28
Farm	15	21

[a] Source: United States Bureau of the Census (1940: Tables 1, 2, 15, 16), cited in Farley (1970:110).

due entirely to large increases in the Southern rates. Because most rural blacks lived in the South, the increase of 7 percentage points in rural childlessness represents almost entirely an increase in childlessness in the rural South. And the increase in urban childlessness over the period was exclusively a reflection of an increase in the urban South. Here childlessness rose by 10 percentage points over the period, whereas in the urban North the rate remained unchanged.

Was genital TB increasing in the South over this period contributing to the rise in childlessness? An increase in the Southern cities would not be surprising, because the standard of living there experienced a decline between 1900 and the beginning of World War I, resulting in poorer diets (Farley 1970:219). And pellagra, a Southern disease that is more common in rural areas, increased greatly between 1900 and 1930, indicating that diets were worsening in Southern rural areas as well (Farley 1970:219). Rural rates of genital TB might also have risen because TB infection rates were rising as the interface with urban areas increased. In fact, the infection rates observed by Aronson (1931:392) in the rural South in 1930, being higher than usually assumed, led him to suggest that recent improvements in roads and better means of transportation had resulted in fewer isolated communities and greater chance for the spread of tuberculosis. (In this regard it is important to note that in Table 19.4 childlessness increased more dramatically in the more populous rural nonfarm areas [towns, villages] than in isolated rural farm areas.) It has also been suggested that mortality rates for rural blacks may have increased during the 1920s (Farley 1970:73), and a rise in TB mortality would translate into higher infection rates. It is possible then to conclude that by the turn of the century TB (as well as genital TB and any subsequent childlessness) had reached saturation level in the urban North, but that rates in the South (urban and rural) were increasing prior to 1930 because (1) Southern diets were worsening and (2) infection rates were possibly increasing.[10]

Occupational Differentials

Investigation of black childlessness rates in the early part of the century by husband's occupation (see Farley 1970:118) reveals that the usual differentials hold—wives of white-collar workers have high rates of childlessness and wives of farmers have low childlessness rates. Wives

---

[10]It should be noted that the data in Figure 19.4 for several Southern communities do not suggest that infection rates in the South were rising prior to 1930. It may be that this phenomenon did not occur in these selected communities or that infection rates did not increase in the South as suggested here and elsewhere.

of blue-collar workers occupy an intermediate position, with one notable exception—service workers. In 1910 childlessness rates were substantially higher for wives of service workers than for any other category. By 1940 all categories showed increased rates. Wives of service workers were still at the top of the list, but shared this position with wives of white-collar workers. The high rates of childlessness among wives of service workers is considered a mystery.[11] Yet this could be partly explained by the high rates of TB among service workers. Indeed, one reason given for the high rates of TB among blacks is their traditional employment in personal service capacities, which results in heavy extradomiciliary exposure to the bacillus (Payne 1949:335).

It is not likely that this childlessness is the result of genital TB in wives who have been exposed to tuberculous husbands because the average age at first union for these women falls several years after the critical age for developing genital TB. But the effect on male reproductive potential may be important, especially because employment in service occupations often occurred simultaneously with puberty. (Although the sequence of events of puberty currently spans ages 9–18 in boys [Tanner 1973:22], the average age of puberty probably occurred closer to the end of this interval in black males during the late nineteenth and early twentieth centuries than it does currently. It is believed that a century ago the average age of puberty was delayed by 3 to 4 years [Parkes 1976:7, 15; Tanner 1973:25]). DuBois's study of Philadelphia blacks in the late 1890s showed that many boys were leaving school at age 15 and finding work in service occupations and as laborers and porters. By age 20, almost 40% of black males were in service occupations (DuBois [1899] 1967:105). It is probable then that some service workers developed pulmonary and other forms of extragenital TB and that some also developed genital TB. The high rate of childlessness in women whose husbands were service workers could partially be the result of sterility in the husbands caused by genital TB.

The effect of service occupations on the fecundity of women so employed should not be overlooked. DuBois ([1899] 1967:104) noted that by age 18, 40% of black females in Philadelphia were employed as domestic servants, which was virtually the only occupation open to black women. These women, like their male counterparts, may also have had high rates of genital TB. It is also possible that persons employed in service occupations met and married persons engaged in the same oc-

---

[11]Frequently service workers, especially those engaged as house servants, are separated from their spouses for extended periods. However, this would be expected to result in low fertility, not childlessness.

cupation. In this case the high rates of childlessness recorded for couples where the husband is employed as a service worker could be, in part, the result of sterility subsequent to genital TB in the wife or husband or both.

Reduced Fertility in Parous Women

The discussion up to this point has focused on childlessness because genital TB is far more often a cause of infecundity prior to childbearing than after childbearing has occurred. But any discussion of the effects of genital TB on black fertility would be incomplete without consideration of genital TB as a cause of reduced fertility among parous black women. Genital TB can reduce the fertility of parous women through pregnancy loss, but this is a rare occurrence because only a small minority of women with genital TB can conceive. The effect almost always occurs through secondary sterility.

Genital TB and subsequent sterility in a parous woman may happen in any one of a number of ways. The individual may have been infected early in life, but reactivation of lesions and development of disease come after one or more children have been born. But because development of tuberculous disease is most likely to occur before the mid-20s, development of genital TB in this way (reactivation) is significantly more frequent in nulliparous than in parous women. Secondary sterility due to genital TB may also occur if pregnancy coincides with a woman's primary infection, because this predisposes her to developing progressive genital TB (Snaith and Barns 1962:715). This may not be so uncommon because a significant minority of women who will eventually become infected are not yet infected by their late teens and early 20s when childbearing commences. Yet another way to develop genital TB is by infection from an active pulmonary lesion. The frequency with which this occurs has been disputed. One reliable source (National Tuberculosis and Respiratory Disease Association 1969:11) stated that, because of acquired resistance, bacilli in a chronic infection are localized at the infection site and dissemination is infrequent. But perhaps blacks, because of their lower ability to acquire and maintain resistance (Rich 1951:145), are more likely than whites to develop genital disease secondary to pulmonary disease. Because pulmonary TB is a chronic disease, often of many years' duration, the initiation of a localized infection of the reproductive organs can probably occur at any time during the illness. Men and women so affected would be rendered sterile, and this sterility would be classified as secondary if a previous pregnancy has occurred.

The possible importance of secondary sterility in unions where at least one partner has tuberculosis is underscored by Downes's (1939) study of fertility in white couples who were so afflicted. Cumulative birth rates for two groups of tuberculous couples[12] were substantially lower than for matched nontuberculous couples in the rural North in the late nineteenth and early twentieth centuries. Perhaps intermediate variables such as contraception or low coital frequency were the cause of the lower birth rates. Or perhaps these couples were subfecund. Because childlessness has been controlled for,[13] secondary sterility would be important here.

Impact on the Black Fertility Decline

In sum, TB is an attractive explanatory variable for the black fertility trend. Among U.S. blacks, TB rates were rising as fertility rates were falling. It was only after black TB disease rates improved substantially that their fertility turned upward. Genital TB is usually a cause of primary sterility, and increasing childlessness was a notable feature of the black fertility decline. Where TB rates were the highest, namely in the urban centers, childlessness rates were highest. Where TB was less prevalent, as in the rural areas, childlessness rates were lower. In the early 1900s Southern cities and rural areas experienced a substantial increase in childlessness. It was during this period that the greater interaction of rural and urban areas could have increased rural infection rates. And it was during this period that deteriorating economic conditions in both areas meant poorer diets and a greater chance for development of tuberculous disease. One occupational differential in childlessness, the ''mysteriously'' high rates among service workers, is partly explicable by the fact that many service workers, who have a very high job-related

[12]One group consisted of tuberculous couples who built families between 1850 and 1890. In these couples one or both spouses died of TB before age 50 (Downes 1939:278). The second group consisted of tuberculous couples who built families between 1900 and 1929, identified by a case of pulmonary TB in one spouse (Downes 1939:280).

[13]No childless couples were included in the earlier (1850–1890) study sample. Childless couples were included in the later sample, but the rate of childlessness was the same (14%) in tuberculous and nontuberculous couples. That there is no difference in the childlessness rate between tuberculous and nontuberculous couples is not problematic for this analysis. Because primary sterility is proposed as the chief cause of childlessness during this period for white (see Kiser 1939:62) as well as black women and because cases of genital TB that result in primary sterility usually occur as a silent, isolated focus of the disease without any symptoms of pulmonary or any other extragenital tuberculosis, childlessness should be fairly evenly distributed between the two types of couples—those with and those without *manifest* tuberculosis.

risk of developing TB, were entering these jobs during their teens when the risk of developing genital TB subsequent to an initial infection was the highest. Last, the role of secondary sterility due to genital TB, though not so significant as the role of primary sterility, could be one explanatory variable for the observed differences in fertility rates between tuberculous and nontuberculous couples. Thus, genital TB had the power not only to cause childlessness but to reduce the fertility of black women at all parities.

What impact then did genital TB have on the black fertility decline? Muir and Belsey (1980:918) stated that female genital TB once accounted for a significant amount of pelvic inflammatory disease cases throughout the world, and still does in those countries where TB remains a major health problem. And Paulsen (1977:464) believed that male genital TB is responsible for a sizeable portion of male infertility where TB is a prevalent disease. Hallo (1971:138) went so far as to say that genital TB may be the *most* common cause of sterility where TB is a common disease. Indeed, many studies have reported high rates of genital TB among sterile patients. Bonafos *et al.* (1967:308) found genital TB in 25% of all cases of sterility in Algeria. In one study in India, where TB is common, 10% of unselected women subjected to endometrial biopsy had genital TB and this figure rose to 17% in women selected for sterility (Gupta 1957:184, 196). And in Israel an incredible 40% of patients with primary sterility and partial or total tubal occlusion were shown to have genital TB (Halbrecht 1956:369).

However, it would be improper to generalize from these studies and say that 10%, 20%, or even 40% of the black fertility decline was due to genital TB. First, some of the childlessness and low fertility during the period were probably the result of low mate exposure, contraception, and induced abortion. And, second, what sterility did exist was probably the result of many fecundity-reducing diseases, including gonorrhea, syphilis, postpartum and postabortal sepsis, as well as genital TB.

The only data from which any reliable estimate of the impact of genital TB on the black fertility decline can be extracted come from an autopsy study conducted by Medlar *et al.* (1949) at Bellevue Hospital in New York City between 1935 and 1944, just when black fertility had reached its lowest point and was beginning to rebound. They found that 3.1% of all males autopsied had urogenital TB, the rate being approximately 1.5 times higher, or 4.7%, if just black males were considered (Medlar *et al.* 1949:1087, 1080). Unfortunately, there are several problems with this study that make it unsuitable for our purposes of model building. First, it describes urogenital TB (i.e., TB of the kidneys and/or genital tract), and it is difficult to extract from these data just how many men had genital TB. Furthermore, Medlar and associates felt that their data indicated that genital involvement is almost always secondary to infection of the kidneys. Others (e.g., Monif 1974:225; National Tuberculosis and Respiratory Disease Association 1969:14) have stated, however, that genital TB usually has its initial infectious focus in the epididymis. This has been borne out by one clinical study (Pieterse 1973:2418) that showed renal involvement in less than 10% of cases of tuberculous epididymitis. It is also likely that the frequency of urogenital TB reported by Medlar *et al.* seriously underestimated the frequency of the disease because of problems associated with diagnosis. Indeed, Botella-Llusia (1967:514) reported that during successive reviews of the same endometrial biopsy material in a Madrid clinic, each review employing greater precision in examining the slides, the percent of specimens classified as tuberculous rose from 8.1% in 1944 to 10.6% in 1974, an increase of 30%. The frequency of urogenital TB in the black men in the Medlar *et al.* series could therefore be as high as 6.1%.

Because of these problems, it would be inappropriate to use the prevalence data of Medlar *et al.* to generate a model of the impact of genital TB on the black fertility decline. However, the study certainly does offer a feeling for what were reasonable rates of genital TB in the black population in 1940. High, realistic, and low estimates of genital TB in blacks can therefore be made, and the resulting impact on the four-child decline calculated. A 5% genital TB rate for black men in 1940 seems realistic, with a slightly (20%) higher rate of 6% for black women, because genital TB is believed to strike women with greater frequency (Fritjofsson and Kollberg 1973:292; Gupta 1957:182). A low estimate would be 3% for men and 3.5% for women. A high estimate would be 7% for men and 8.5% for women. The prevalence of genital TB in 1880 must also be estimated, because the model will measure what proportion of the four-child decline can be accounted for by the *increase* in genital TB over the period. The genital TB rate in 1880 is unknown, but a rate one-fifth of that in 1940 seems reasonable. (The TB mortality rate, an imperfect proxy for the TB morbidity rate but the only one available, suggests the disease increased fivefold over the period.[14] See earlier discussion in the section "Trends in Extragenital Tuberculosis.") Hence, for the high model 1880 rates would be 1.4% for black men and 1.7% for black women. The same rates for the realistic model would be 1.0% and 1.2%, and for the low model 0.6% and 0.7%. The increases in the

---

[14]Although TB mortality rates began to decline after the first two decades of the twentieth century, morbidity rates, for which there are no good data, are believed to have shown less improvement and in some areas may have actually increased during the Depression years.

percentage with genital TB would therefore be: high model, 5.6% for men and 6.8% for women; realistic model, 4% for men and 4.8% for women; low model, 2.4% for men and 2.8% for women (see Table 19.5).

The model needs only one more value to be complete—the average number of children before sterility. Because the average age of onset of genital TB is about age 20 (Rajan *et al.* 1974:12), cases of primary sterility frequently outnumber those of secondary sterility by 4 or 5:1 (see Bonafos *et al.* 1967:308; Rozin 1968:214), and even those with secondary sterility probably have only 1 child before childbearing ceases. Hence, an average of .2 children will be assigned to each individual with genital TB. All the values necessary for the model are now in hand. The following equation, which was used in the gonorrhea models, will now be applied to genital TB. For black men in the high model: (5.6% × .2) + (94.4% × 7) = 6.62. Subtracting from the 7-child average of 1880, it is seen that .38 fewer children would be born, which is 9.5% of the 4-child decline. In Table 19.5 the impact on the 4-child decline for men and women is shown for all three models.

In the gonorrhea models the values for men and women were not additive because persons with VD are more likely to have mates with VD. However, with genital TB random mating may be roughly assumed because the age at which tuberculous infection is most likely to result

Table 19.5

Three Models of the Impact of Genital TB on the 4-Child Black Fertility Decline, Varying by the Increase between 1880 and 1940 in the Percentage of the Black Population with Genital TB

	High model		Realistic model		Low model	
	Male	Female	Male	Female	Male	Female
Increase in percentage with genital TB, 1880–1940 (%)	5.6	6.8	4.0	4.8	2.4	2.8
Average number of children before sterility	.2	.2	.2	.2	.2	.2
Percentage of the decline accounted for by each sex	9.5	11.6	6.8	8.2	4.1	4.8
Percentage of the decline accounted for by both sexes combined	21.1		15.0		8.9	

in genital involvement precedes both sexual and marital activity. Hence, anywhere from 8.9 to 21.1% of the black fertility decline could be accounted for by genital TB, depending on which assumptions about its prevalence are used.

Conclusions

What these TB models show is that during the period genital TB could have been a negative force on black fertility equal to that of gonorrhea. Indeed, genital TB may have been even more important than gonorrhea because the trends and differentials with respect to TB and black fertility, especially childlessness, are in very much better alignment than those with respect to VD and black fertility (see McFalls 1973). Of particular importance is the finding that, unlike that for VD, most of the increase in extragenital TB, and undoubtedly in genital TB, occurred prior to World War I when 80% of the 1880 to 1936 decline in black fertility also occurred.

Discussion

Genital TB is not forwarded here as the dominant factor shaping the black fertility pattern from 1880 to 1960, but only as one of a number of important factors. Indeed, it has been argued elsewhere (Masnick and McFalls 1976, 1978; McFalls and Masnick 1981; McFalls and Tolnay, forthcoming) that these fertility patterns are the outcome of changes not only in the level of fecundity, but also in the use of birth control[15] and in the proportion of time spent in stable conjugal unions. And the fact that VD or TB could have accounted for a certain percentage of the fertility decline does not mean that that portion of the decline would not have occurred at least in part without them. These maladies were undoubtedly present in many couples who would have had fewer than seven children anyway either through birth control or low mate exposure. Thus, any accurate interpretation of the determinants of black fertility between 1880 and 1960 must be a balanced one, taking into account not only all three variables but the fact that two or more were present and interacting in many couples.

---

[15]One of the more interesting findings from these studies is that, contrary to popular belief, many black women were effective users of contraception and other forms of birth control prior to 1936.

CHAPTER 20

Conclusions and Research Pitfalls

The Disease–Subfecundity
Relationship

The idea of studying in detail the various diseases that might affect
fecundity was prompted by a reading of Reynolds Farley's health hypothesis as outlined in his important book *Growth of the Black Population*
(1970). This hypothesis, which focuses primarily on changes in venereal
disease (VD) prevalence, was forwarded to explain the decline and subsequent rise in U.S. black fertility during the first half of the twentieth
century. Although it was argued in an earlier paper (McFalls 1973) that
VD was not the principal cause of the secular decline in black fertility,
it did not exclude the possibility that VD and other health factors were
involved to some degree. Indeed, Farley did suggest that diseases such
as pellagra as well as VD might have influenced black fertility. But he
was unable to pursue in depth exactly *how* these diseases might affect
fecundity. Thus, this book was designed to examine closely all aspects—
medical, pathological, and epidemological—of those diseases that might
alter human reproductive potential, primarily as an aid to researchers
in estimating the impact of these diseases on the fecundity of populations they are studying.

The examination of the pathophysiology of the diseases contained
in this volume reveals the many ways in which diseases can affect fecundity. In contrast with the fixation of some researchers on tubal occlusion as the sole cause of disease-related subfecundity, this book has
shown that fevers, anemia, intrauterine adhesions, cervical injury, local
heat, inflammation of the accessory sexual glands, inflammation of other

reproductive organs, and so forth can all affect fecundity. The following sections examine these varied ways in which diseases can cause coital inability, conceptive failure, and pregnancy loss. Examples are given under each heading to illustrate how specific diseases can cause pathophysiological changes inimical to reproduction. This is not, however, an exhaustive compilation of the conclusions of this book, but rather an overview with some selected examples. The individual chapters should be consulted for more complete and detailed information.

Coital Inability

Absolute coital inability is an infrequent sequela of most of the diseases studied. Nonetheless, a few diseases are accompanied by impotence, complete or partial obstruction of the vaginal opening, or genital deformities that make coitus impossible. More frequently, coital inability subsequent to disease is the result of dyspareunia. In some cases the dyspareunia is temporary, but in others it is permanent. In some cases it is mild and coital activity continues, albeit at a lower frequency; in others it is so severe that coitus is abandoned altogether.

Diseases that can cause absolute coital inability include African sleeping sickness, filariasis, and schistosomiasis. In advanced-stage African sleeping sickness, especially the more prolonged Gambian type, neuroendocrinological changes occur that frequently cause impotence in affected males. Elephantiasis of the external genitals of males or females subsequent to infection with Bancroftian filariasis may, if severe, make coitus impossible. And severe schistosomiasis of the external female genitals may be associated with pseudotumors so large that coitus is not possible.

Many of the diseases covered in this book cause dyspareunia. In women a difficult labor with a forcible forceps delivery may injure the broad ligaments supporting the uterus, resulting in dyspareunia. And in some cases of pelvic inflammatory disease (PID) the infection is followed by the formation of fibrous adhesions that link the internal genital organs to other pelvic structures; the internal organs are then rigidly fixed and pain is common with penile thrusting and similar movements. Dyspareunia is also a common complaint among women who have a much narrowed vaginal introitus because they have undergone infibulation. (In some cases the vaginal opening is so small that penetration is impossible, and the woman must be ''cut'' on her wedding night.)

These are the more important causes of dyspareunia because they are permanent conditions. Many diseases, however, are associated with one or more temporary episodes of dyspareunia, which collectively may be of some importance.[1] In some men and women bouts of active genital herpes may be associated with lesions so numerous and so painful that coitus, if not impossible, is at least unwelcome. And inflammation of the male accessory glands during genital infection may be associated with pain during ejaculation. Finally, coitus is also painful during the acute stages of several diseases when there is inflammation of the genital organs and/or the adjacent lymph ducts and glands. An important example of this is the funiculo–epididymo–orchitis that occurs in the early stages of filariasis.

Conceptive Failure

Male Conceptive Failure

Conception is a very complicated event requiring the proper functioning and coordination of many processes in both the male and female. Hence, there are many opportunities for error. In the male the ducts that carry sperm, specifically the tiny epididymis, may be occluded by the fibrosis that follows genital infection or inflammation. Tuberculous and gonococcal epididymitis are two of the major causes of permanent occlusion of the male genital ducts. And even if the ducts are not occluded, concomitant infection of the accessory glands is frequent and associated with temporary, and in some cases permanent, changes in their secretory activity; this may impact on the fertilizing capacity of sperm. Other infections, such as filariasis, though not directly causing tubal damage may set the stage for future damage. Episodes of filarial funiculo–epididymo–orchitis, for example, may damage the lymphatics that drain the genitals, rendering the genital organs more susceptible to infection.

Recurrent high fevers, which are a common feature of several very prevalent diseases such as malaria and filariasis, are important causes of subfecundity. In men such fevers are associated with azoospermia followed by a 1–2 month period of oligospermia. Two episodes of fever each year is the norm even for "immune" men living in areas of hyperendemic malaria. Bouts of filarial fever are even more frequent, occurring 2–6 times a year early in the course of the disease. Because oligospermia is believed to be the most important cause of male infer-

---

[1]Dyspareunia can lead to inhibition in sexual drive and may also result in psychogenic impotence and vaginismus (McFalls 1979b:52–54). Thus even one bout with dyspareunia can bring about coital inability for long periods and even life.

tility in Africa, these two diseases are probably very important subfecundity factors.

Female Conceptive Failure

There are many reasons why a woman may fail to conceive. There
may be an endocrine problem, an immunological problem, or damage
to the ovaries or tubes. Or the woman may have endometriosis, a frequently asymptomatic condition often associated with the inability to
conceive. Diseases may produce all these pathological changes, and
more.

Advanced-stage African sleeping sickness is associated with damage to the hypothalamus. The hypothalamic–pituitary–gonadal axis is
therefore disturbed, and the resulting endocrine imbalance is frequently
associated with sterility and menstrual disorders.

Some women have difficulty conceiving for immunological reasons;
they produce antibodies to their husband's sperm. It has been suggested that antispermal antibodies may be produced by women with
genital schistosomiasis, which lowers their conceptive ability.

Damage to the ovaries and/or tubes is a common sequela of PID
(tuberculous, gonococcal, nongonococcal, postabortal, or postpartum)
and may occur following diseases such as schistosomiasis and filariasis
and following the use of an intrauterine device (IUD). In PID, purulent material dripping out of the fimbriated end of the tube may infect
the ovary and leave it so scarred that an egg cannot break through the
thick fibrous tissue encapsulating the ovary. A heavy schistosomal infection of the ovary may also leave the ovary scarred and the woman
sterile.

Damage to the fallopian tubes following PID is the most frequently
cited cause of sterility and certainly deserves this attention, as it is undoubtedly the most importance cause of conceptive failure worldwide.
And some disorders, though not a direct cause of tubal infection, contribute to salpingitis rates because they devitalize the tubal tissue,
thereby increasing susceptibility to infection. Some workers have suggested that genital schistosomiasis and genital filariasis work this way.
Schistosome eggs are believed to irritate and weaken the tubes. And
obstruction of the lymph drainage of the tubes by filariasis prevents removal of normal cellular breakdown products, the accumulation of
which damages the genital tissue and increases susceptibility to infection. The chronic sterile tubal inflammation seen in a large proportion
of IUD users also undermines tissue immunity and contributes to the
high rates of PID in IUD users.

Endometriosis is yet another condition that may result in conceptive failure. The causes of endometriosis are not well defined, but some workers have felt that stasis of the menstrual flow is one possibility. Because stasis of the menses is common in circumcised women, particularly those who have undergone infibulation, conceptive failure secondary to endometriosis may occur with greater-than-average frequency in these women.

Pregnancy Loss

Pregnancy loss sometimes occurs so early following conception that the woman is not even aware she is pregnant. On the other hand, she may complete 9 months of pregnancy and go through labor only to be delivered of a stillborn child. Pregnancy loss at any time from conception to birth may be caused by disease. The loss may be the result of problems in the tubes (kinking, partial occlusion, damage to the cells involved in tubal motility), uterus (intrauterine adhesions, failure to respond to hormonal stimuli, endometritis, uterine irritation), vagina (infibulation), or pelvic bones (pelvic contraction). Or the loss may be secondary to an endocrine problem, anemia, fever, transplacental transmission of infectious organisms, or placental parasitization.

Various diseases may damage the tubes (partial occlusion, kinking) so that the fertilized ovum is trapped and implants ectopically. The usual causes of PID (tuberculous, gonococcal, nongonococcal, postpartum, or postabortal infection) may be involved, but so too may a noninfectious inflammation of the tubes, such as that seen in women with an IUD. In either case, not only is the pregnancy lost—surgical removal of the pregnancy (and frequently the tube as well) is required because the tube cannot contain the growing fetus and will eventually rupture—but often the tube is so badly damaged that tubal occlusion or an even greater disposition to ectopic implantation results.

The fertilized ovum, upon reaching the uterus after a 5-day journey through the tube, may still be in jeopardy. It is believed that an endometrium affected by tuberculosis or one devitalized by a prolonged, obstructed labor is in some cases unable to respond to hormonal stimuli, thereby increasing the risk of pregnancy loss. If there are intrauterine adhesions—such as occur following serious injury to the endometrium, as following a postpartum or postabortal infection or a curettage that cuts too deep—the uterus will not be able to expand with the growing fetus and a spontaneous abortion will occur. A pregnancy that continues with an IUD in place frequently terminates as a spontaneous abortion, theoretically because of uterine irritation associated with the device. And in some cases (e.g., genital herpes) premature rupture of the fetal membranes allows dangerous organisms from the lower genital tract to reach and infect the child and can result in perinatal dealth.

Disorders of a more general nature—endocrine dysfunction, anemia, fever—are also capable of causing pregnancy loss. The endocrine dysfunction seen in advanced-stage African sleeping sickness is a cause of spontaneous abortion. Anemia is a frequent problem in pregnant women, especially in developing countries, and if severe may cause fetal death and stillbirth. Women with malaria are frequently anemic because of the destruction of parasitized red blood cells. And both early and advanced-stage African sleeping sickness are associated with a significant anemia.

Fevers, if sufficiently high (1.5–$2.5°$ C above normal), are a very important cause of pregnancy loss. The fevers associated with early-stage African sleeping sickness (Rhodesian), filariasis, and malaria (in poorly immune women) are sufficiently high to damage the fetus.[2] Two possible outcomes of elevated maternal temperature are (1) spontaneous abortion due to increased uterine activity, fetal hypoxia, placental necrosis, or embryonic damage incompatible with life and (2) birth of an infant with congenital anomalies. The particular outcome depends on (1) the stage of gestation—early pregnancy is more sensitive to temperature variations, (2) the height of the fever—lower fevers are more likely to result in a deformed offspring and high fevers in abortion, and (3) the duration of fever—prolonged temperature elevations for 1 or 2 days are generally believed to be necessary to cause damage, although adverse effects have been noted following spikes of temperature caused by certain infections or by sauna bathing and hot tubs (Arora *et al.* 1979; Morishima *et al.* 1975; Pleet *et al.* 1981). One researcher (Edwards, personal communication, 1981) believed that embryonic or fetal death, followed by resorption or abortion, is probably more common than congenital malformation under natural conditions where temperature height and duration are not tightly controlled. Because loss may occur very early in pregnancy with embryonic resorption, some cases of pregnancy loss due to high fever undoubtedly go unnoticed. Studies of birthrates in populations stricken by epidemics of febrile diseases such as smallpox, influenza, and dysentery support the notion that fevers are a cause of pregnancy loss early in pregnancy, because in these studies

---

[2]Smallpox, influenza, penumonia, and chicken pox are other diseases that are associated with high fevers and pregnancy wastage. The incidence of pregnancy loss (and maternal mortality) in women with severe influenza during the 1918 epidemic was very high (Bland 1919).

(Hotelling and Hotelling 1931; Leridon 1973b) fluctuations in birth rates did not occur until 7–9 months after the epidemic.

In many diseases the placenta becomes the site of transmission of infectious organisms from the mother to the developing fetus, frequently with disastrous results. Congenital syphilis is perhaps the best known of the transplacentally transmitted diseases; spontaneous abortion after 16 weeks' gestation, stillbirth, or birth of a child with congenital syphilis may occur. Chagas' disease may also be transmitted to the fetus in this manner, resulting in a similar spectrum of clinical responses. Genital herpes too may cross the placenta, but herpes viremia is rare in adults and, therefore, so is the incidence of congenital herpes.

Finally, placental parasitization with *Plasmodium falciparum* is very frequent in women living in hyperendemic areas. If severe, a spontaneous abortion may occur; more frequently, however, the result is intrauterine growth retardation.

Disease and the Other Davis–Blake Intermediate Variables

Disease may lower fertility rates by Davis–Blake intermediate variables other than subfecundity, particularly via the time spent in unions, coital frequency, and contraceptive use (see Table 1.8). The time spent in unions is frequently affected by disease. Women in societies where children are highly valued who suffer from diseases that leave them relatively subfecund (syphilis, for example, leaves a woman subfecund for 2 years following infection) may be deserted or divorced by a mate anxious to have children. Also, women who develop a vesico–vaginal fistula following a difficult birth may, because of the unpleasant odor associated with this condition, be rejected by the husband. Persons with greatly feared diseases such as syphilis and tuberculosis (TB) are less frequently chosen as mates. And in some areas there are even legal proscriptions against such persons marrying. In the United States, for example, states began to pass laws in 1937 forbidding the issuance of a marriage license to those persons with a positive serologic test for syphilis.

Coital frequency is, as noted earlier, frequently affected by disease. Some diseases such as genital herpes cause genital lesions so painful that coitus is virtually impossible during active disease. Coital frequency is probably also low with some of the debilitating diseases such as TB, malaria, and African sleeping sickness. And with some diseases coitus may be avoided for fear of infecting the partner. Genital herpes, syphilis, and gonorrhea are important examples. Indeed, some physicians in the early part of the twentieth century, unable to cure their syphilitic patients, recommended prolonged periods of abstinence to avoid transmission of the disease to the partner and to preclude the possibility of a syphilitic pregnancy.

Contraceptive use is also affected by disease. Women with debilitating diseases such as TB might wish to avoid the rigors of pregnancy and so use contraception. Often barrier contraceptives are used to prevent the spread of an infection that can be contracted via intercourse. Syphilis, gonorrhea, and genital herpes are important examples of such infections.

Hence, diseases may and do affect fertility rates in many ways. They may cause subfecundity—coital inability, conceptive failure, and/or pregnancy loss. Identifying and describing the ways in which diseases cause subfecundity has been the focus of this book. But diseases may affect fertility in yet other ways, including the time spent in unions, coital frequency, and contraceptive use.

Importance of Selected Diseases in Historical, Developing, and Developed Societies

Historical Societies

Many of the diseases discussed have been in existence for thousands of years and therefore have been impacting on human fecundity for many centuries. Gonorrhea, which has been known since classical times, is said to have depressed the fertility of historical European populations. Also implicated in the fertility of some historical societies is postpartum infection, whose risks were appreciated as early as 1000 B.C.; an Indian text of that time advised careful trimming of midwive's nails and postpartum vaginal fumigation (Sandison and Wells 1967:502). Infection after abortion was also important. For example, induced abortion was legalized in the Soviet Union in 1921 in order to combat the ''evil'' of growing ''underground abortion . . . [in which] 50 percent of women are infected . . . and up to 4 percent of them die'' (Decree on the Legislation of Abortion of 18 November 1920, cited in Potts *et al.* 1977:377).

Malaria, which is an important subfecundity factor, has been present at least since the fourth century B.C. Malaria was common in ancient Greece and, indeed, the decline in the brilliance of Greek civilization has been attributed to an increased prevalence of malaria (Jones 1967:175). Schistosomiasis is also a disease of great antiquity, existing for at least 3000 years. The papyruses of ancient Egypt mention hematuria (Sandison 1967:178) and eggs of *Schistosoma haematobium* have been found in Egyptian mummies (Ruffer 1967:177). Filariasis is also an ancient disease. As early as 1500 B.C. elephantiasis was graphically described by the Egyptians and in A.D. 1 Greco–Roman authors accurately described this and other sequelae of filarial infection (Schacher and Sahyoun 1967:234). African sleeping sickness, which probably originated in the large grazing animals of Africa, infected humans and their domestic animals during their prehistoric invasion of the continent (Jones 1967:52, 55). But perhaps the most ancient of all the diseases is TB. It cannot be said with certainty that TB has been with man throughout his evolution, but clearly some form of TB has existed since Neolithic times (Morse 1967:268).

Some of the subfecundity-producing diseases are relative newcomers. Syphilis made its first recognized appearance in the late fifteenth century in Europe, hence the notion that Columbus's sailors had brought the disease to Europe from the New World. In all probability this is not so. Probably a mutation occurred in a preexisting organism and manifested itself as venereal syphilis (Hackett 1967:162). How long Chagas' disease has been around is hard to say. Because of the great variation in the clinical picture of late Chagas' disease—megacolon, deformities of the esophogus, heart failure—it went unrecognized until 1909 when some sophisticated sleuthing by Carlos Chagas revealed the common origin of these abnormalities.

At least one important subfecundity-producing disease, smallpox—a most significant disease in human history and one that has definitely been in existence since the beginning of the Christian Era—has now been eradicated. Because it is no longer important, it was not discussed in the body of this text. Nevertheless, smallpox is a cause of obstructive azoospermia and one researcher (Razzell 1977) felt that it was important in reducing the fecundity and fertility of historical populations. (See Appendix C for further discussion.) Sudden declines in the incidence of subfecundity-producing diseases such as smallpox and TB are often accompanied by a rise in fertility, as happened in Europe during the nineteenth century and more recently in parts of the developing world. Although only indirect evidence of a cause-and-effect relationship, such associations do merit close attention. Indeed, in Chapter 19 we have discussed at length the evidence supporting an association between changes in the prevalence of TB among U.S. blacks between 1880 and 1936 and changes in their childlessness rate.

Developing Societies

Although the developing world is usually characterized as possessing high fertility, there are large areas where fertility levels are low and childlessness approaches 50%. Because many of the diseases that cause subfecundity are prevalent in these areas, it is likely that disease is a major reason for the low birthrates. And even in disease-affected areas where birthrates are not low, it is likely that they would be even higher in the absence of these diseases.

Although diseases such as African sleeping sickness probably affect fewer than 100,000 persons each year, others such as malaria, filariasis, schistosomiasis, and TB each count hundreds of millions of victims. Even the little-known Chagas' disease affects 25 million persons in Central and South America. The number of cases of PID resulting from sexually transmitted diseases such as gonorrhea or from postpartum or postabortal infections is probably staggering. And one conservative estimate suggested that female circumcision currently affects 20 million women in sub–Saharan Africa alone (*People* 1979b:24).

In many cases development has, in the short term at least, worsened rather than improved the health situation with respect to certain diseases. The Aswan High Dam and other irrigation projects have provided new breeding grounds for the snails that transmit schistosomiasis. Malaria is also resurging, in part because the *Anopheles* mosquito is finding new breeding pools in waters dammed for irrigation or hydroelectric projects and in the pools and streams of areas deforested for agricultural projects. And one of the reasons filiarsis is on the increase is that one of its vectors, the *Culex* mosquito, is thriving in the septic tanks and pit latrines that were built to control intestinal parasites.

Gonorrhea and the other sexually transmitted diseases are also on the increase because development has increased the contact between cities and the villages. In the cities of the developing world, rapid social change has resulted in a tremendous increase in pelvic infections due to self-induced or back-alley abortions. One study in Kinshasa, Zaire (Smith *et al.* 1976) attributed 95% of all obstetric fatalities to hemorrhagic or septic complications following illegal induced abortion. With development has also come the introduction of modern contraceptive methods—one of which, the IUD, has been associated with an increased risk of pelvic infection.

Several of the subfecundity-producing diseases, specifically PID following gonorrhea, childbirth, abortion, and IUD use, although seen in the developed world, are much more common in developing countries. For example, because diagnostic and treatment facilities are poor in many developing areas, more women with gonorrhea will go on to develop gonococcal PID. Postpartum infections are also more frequent, for two reasons: (1) Difficult births are more common in developing countries because of infibulation or cephalo–pelvic disproportion resulting from young age at marriage and/or actual pelvic deformity due to rickets or general malnutrition and (2) nonsterile interference by untrained attendants is more likely. Abortion in the developing world, especially in the cities, is extremely hazardous because most such abortions are self-induced or done by inexperienced back alley abortionists. In such cases complications such as infection are higher than following illegal procedures performed by experienced persons, and much higher than following legal procedures. Use of the IUD is also more hazardous in developing areas. The heavier bleeding associated with the inert IUDs often aggravates an existing anemia, leaving the woman even more vulnerable to many types of infections. Pregnancy in a woman with an IUD is a serious matter requiring expert medical attention at the earliest possible moment, in order to avoid a spontaneous abortion (sometimes septic) and to determine if there has been an ectopic implantation. But in the developing world delays are common because medical facilities may not be readily available and because pregnancy frequently goes unrecognized for longer periods due to menstrual irregularities associated with poor nutrition. Finally, medical personnel are not as well trained and may mistake the symptoms of ectopic pregnancy for those associated simply with IUD use, thereby subjecting the woman to the grave risk of a tubal rupture.

Developed Societies

Many of the infectious diseases that are so important in the developing world—malaria, schistosomiasis, filariasis, tuberculosis, African sleeping sickness, and Chagas' disease—are not often found in the developed world, either because they have been successfully controlled or eliminated or because the vectors, climatic conditions, etc. necessary for their survival never existed in these areas. Nevertheless, for some diseases such as TB there are scattered pockets of high prevalence. In the United States, for example, pockets of TB are seen in the Southwest among Mexican immigrants.

More important as subfecundity factors in the developed world are the sexually transmitted diseases. Disadvantaged minorities have the highest rates of venereal disease, but with the relaxation in sexual mores and abandonment of the condom (which helps prevent transmission of venereal disease) in favor of other contraceptive methods, venereal disease is on the increase in all segments of society. In the United States alone, 3 million cases of gonorrhea are reported every year, and a frightening number of young women, 50,000–100,000, are becoming sterile each year as a result. Nongonococcal urethritis and cervicitis (NGU/C) is increasing even faster than gonorrhea. And whereas gonorrhea is still predominantly a disease of the poor, NGU/C is seen mostly in sexually active singles from the middle and upper classes. Unfamiliar with NGU/C, many physicians misdiagnose and treat this disease as if it were gonorrhea. This can have serious repercussions because the organisms that are usually responsible for the infection, primarily *Chlamydia trachomatis*, are insensitive to penicillin and if they should ascend to the fallopian tubes the chances of tubal blockage are even greater than with gonorrhea.

Genital herpes is also an increasing public health problem in the developed world. In the United States anywhere from 5 to 20 million persons are already infected, with a half-million new cases occurring each year. Because genital herpes is incurable, the effect on fecundity is potentially great. Recurrent attacks, which may occur three or four times a year, may be accompanied by painful blisters that make coitus virtually impossible. And the spontaneous abortion rate among pregnant women with genital herpes during the first trimester is three to five times that of the general population.

The spread of genital herpes may, however, soon be contained if the work of scientists at the New York State Department of Health (see *Time* 1983:82) fulfills its promise. Using the new cut-and-paste methods of manipulating genes, these scientists have inserted bits of the genetic material of the herpesvirus into the virus (vaccinia) used to immunize against smallpox. This new virus proved capable of eliciting large quantities of antibody against herpesvirus when injected into experimental animals and protected immunized animals against doses of herpesvirus 10–20 times the lethal dose.

As exciting as the prospect of preventing genital herpes may be, it is dwarfed by the other potentialities of this technique. Scientists believe that this method will work for virtually any infectious disease—viral, bacterial, or parasitic. In addition, vaccinia is such a large virus that there is enough room to insert 12–15 foreign genes, creating a polyvaccine which would render a person immune to many diseases with just one inoculation. Such a vaccine would be cheap (about 30 cents), easy to use, and would not require refrigeration—all tremendous advantages in developing countries where infectious diseases are rampant. And because the vaccine does not contain the infectious organisms themselves, there is no danger of anyone actually contracting the diseases.

The impact of such a vaccine on the demographics of developing countries would be staggering. Mortality from the great killers such as malaria would drop precipitously. And fertility would undoubtedly rise as the many diseases which impact on fecundity were simultaneously eradicated. Without proper safeguards and planning, however, the resulting population increases could lead to adverse social and economic circumstances so severe that the net effect of the vaccine would be negative for some time.

Pitfalls in Population Subfecundity Research

During the course of this research many difficulties were encountered, difficulties undoubtedly encountered by countless researchers in the past and still awaiting future researchers. Although these difficulties were mentioned in those chapters where they specifically applied, it was felt that it would be helpful to discuss these pitfalls of subfecundity research in one place. The pitfalls can be divided into five general categories: (1) limitations of existing data on the prevalence of disease and/or subfecundity, (2) effects of the social setting on disease and subfecundity prevalence, (3) persistent myths about certain diseases, (4) the unreliability of indirect evidence, and (5) the variability of response to a disease by population.

Problems Associated with Existing Prevalence Data on Disease and Subfecundity

Underreporting and Misreporting

National statistics on the prevalence of disease and subfecundity are woefully inadequate for many countries, especially the less developed ones. Underreporting is the rule. And the accuracy of reported cases must often be questioned because of the difficulties in making an accurate diagnosis where monies for lab tests and sophisticated diagnostic equipment are limited—80% of the population of tropical areas are served by peripheral medical units having no lab facilities—and where many diseases with similar clinical presentations exist side by side. Even in advanced societies many diseases are frequently mistaken for one another. Nongonococcal urethritis and cervicitis are often mistaken for gonorrhea, for instance, thus boosting the apparent prevalence of gonorrhea.

Most information on the prevalence of disease and subfecundity in less-developed countries comes from surveys. But these too must be viewed with skepticism. Again there are the difficulties in making an accurate diagnosis where funds are limited and where many diseases that are clinically similar coexist. For example, tubal insufflation is the cheapest and easiest way to diagnose tubal occlusion and is therefore frequently used in areas where limited resources preclude hysterosalpingography or laparoscopy. But Carty and Chatfield (1972) have shown that tubal insufflation is an extremely inaccurate way to diagnose tubal blockage. It incorrectly diagnosed blocked tubes in 50% of women in their study, and in 10% gas was thought to pass freely in women who later showed bilateral blockage by another method. Because of the large number of erroneous results, especially false positives, studies using this method must be evaluated accordingly. Simple pelvic examinations are also notoriously inaccurate in establishing pelvic pathology. Jacobson and Westrom (1969:1096) reported that 25% of women thought to have pelvic swelling or masses were normal by laparoscopy. When blocked tubes or a pelvic mass is found, determining the cause is very difficult; all too frequently there is a tendency to attribute cases of pelvic pathology to the familiar gonococcal PID, excluding consideration of other possible etiologies, particularly genital TB.

Coverage of Both Sexes

Surveys often underestimate the prevalence of disease and subfecundity by focusing entirely on women. One study that clearly pointed up the need to extend studies to husbands and male sexual partners is that of Arya and Taber (1975) in Uganda. They found gonorrhea in 25% of the husbands of sterile gonococcal-negative women compared with only 7% of the husbands of fertile gonococcal-negative women. If they had not studied the husbands, they would have underestimated the role gonorrhea played in that society's subfecundity.

Self-assessments

Often in fecundity research the investigator is interested in past medical conditions that, in many cases, cannot be presently detected. He or she may wish to know if the patient had gonorrhea or some other venereal disease. Individuals are frequently asked if they have ever experienced symptoms suggestive of VD. Such self-assessments invariably over- or underestimate disease prevalence, depending on the population. Some studies (e.g., Henin 1969:188) have found that overestimates are a problem because minor diseases are frequently interpreted by some persons as being a serious venereal disease. On the other hand, Arya *et al.* (1973:592) noted that more than 50% of Teso men of Uganda with gonorrhea were not aware of a urethral discharge or any other symptom. And the asymptomatic nature of gonorrhea in the female is well appreciated. Scragg (1957:79, 90) and Hopcraft *et al.* (1973:581) further noted that a discharge and even a substantial degree of discomfort, such as that associated with salpingitis, is often ignored by native men and women, and only when debility occurs or an ulcer appears does the individual seek medical attention. Thus, self-assessments do not accurately reflect the importance of a particular disease.

Assessments by Local Physicians

Researchers must also be warned not to rely too heavily on assessments of the prevalence of disease or subfecundity as reported by local physicians. At times a physician will treat symptoms without knowing the origin of the disorder. Sudanese physicians who often treated patients for hydrocele and other sequelae of filariasis told a research team that filariasis was not found in their area. However, the research team's investigation revealed a 25% infection rate (Satti and Abdel Nur 1974:314–315).

Pregnancy History Recall

Fertility researchers are also interested in a woman's pregnancy history—the number of pregnancies, abortions, stillbirths, and live births. Frequently there is no documentation of these events and again the investigator must rely on patient recall. Inaccuracies are common both because of faulty memory and a desire to withhold some types of information. In some societies miscarriage is considered a shameful event or the consequence of a sexual taboo breach and is kept secret (Nag 1968:138). And in many parts of Africa there is a reluctance to mention children who have died, meaning that the investigator must check birth registrations (if available) to determine the number of children born. But in cases of neonatal death it is likely that neither the birth nor the death was registered (Romaniuk 1968:315, 317). To circumvent these problems some investigators have installed checks in their studies. Scragg (1957), for example, noting that spontaneous abortion was rarely reported among women in New Ireland, confirmed the absence of prior pregnancy among childless women by examining the cervix. He also

noted that even after several years of observing hospital admittances in
New Ireland, he saw few miscarriages.

Unrepresentativeness

Surveys frequently suffer from the problem of unrepresentativeness. Often they study only hospital or clinic patients or persons
living in low-fertility areas. Frequently the disease has taken a different
course in these persons than in members of the general population. For
example, autopsy studies of men who died of or with a recognized case
of TB suggested that in *all* cases of male genital TB the kidneys were
infected first. However, observation of ''well'' men with genital TB revealed that the epididymis was the first, and sometimes the only, urogenital structure to be involved. Furthermore, the incidence of disease
in a survey population is not the same as the incidence of disease in the
general population. Even for the particular subgroup that is being surveyed the data may be skewed. Henin (1969:189) noted VD in 40% of
women he examined for his study of nomads in the Sudan, but cautioned that these women do not represent the total nomadic population
because only infertile women presented for examination.

Absence of Normal Values

The problem of getting fertile members of a population to submit
to examination, in order to establish baseline values of certain criteria
such as sperm count, serum prolactin levels, etc. for that population, is
frequently encountered. It is natural that persons are reluctant to par-
ticipate in tests that are unpleasant or even painful when the results will
not benefit them. (And in some areas examining the genitals and obtaining specimens, even blood samples, is particularly difficult because
of cultural taboos and suspicions.) Scragg (1957:98) wanted to get semen
samples from fertile men in New Ireland to see whether the very low
semen volumes he observed in infertile men were a sign of pathology
or normal for that population. But the fertile men were unwilling to
cooperate. As he explained (1957:99), ''they declined as they knew they
were fertile and the matter must affront even the mind of the sterile
natives.'' Similarly, Ledward (1980:118) found that serum prolactin levels were elevated, at least by European standards, in his infertile patients in Saudi Arabia, many of whom were not ovulating. Because the
average prolactin level for fertile women in this population was unknown, however, it was not determined if the levels found in the infertile women were the cause of ovulatory failure.

Proxy Prevalence Data

The prevalence of a disease or of subfecundity in a population subgroup or territorial subdivision often cannot be estimated accurately from national data or from data from another subgroup or subdivision. This is particularly true in the developing world. The reason is that both disease and subfecundity vary substantially by subgroup and place. In Uganda, for instance, the frequency of subfecundity and its causes, including disease, vary widely from district to district (*Uganda Atlas of Disease Distribution* 1968). Similarly, in the Congo, where the crude birthrate is about 45, district birthrates range from 20 to 60, depending largely on the prevalence of subfecundity (Romaniuk 1968:337). And Scragg (1957:63) found great variability (4–45%) among New Ireland population groups in the percentage infecund. At least in the developing world, subfecundity must be studied on a relatively small scale. (For additional input on this point, see the section, "Variability of Response to a Disease by Population".)

Effect of the Social Setting on Disease and Subfecundity Prevalence

When studying the impact of a disease on the fertility of a particular population, many aspects of the social setting must be taken into consideration. For example, it cannot be assumed that the prevalence of disease or subfecundity is reduced simply because new programs or treatments are introduced into society. The researcher must consider the quality of the new treatment, the effectiveness of the program, and the target population's awareness and acceptance of these developments. A model of this approach already exists.

The VD hypothesis states that the rise in U.S. black fertility that began in 1936 was due to a fall in VD prevalence resulting from the discovery of superior treatment methods in the 1930s and their simultaneous application to many blacks through the creation of government VD programs. In evaluating the hypothesis McFalls (1973:9–12) showed how important it was to determine whether these VD programs and new treatment methods were actually available to blacks and how blacks responded to these developments in those places where they were available. The answers to these questions indicated that most blacks did not benefit from these programs and treatment methods until after the fertility rise was well under way, a finding that seriously undermined the plausibility of this part of the VD hypothesis.

Persistent Myths

A number of incorrect notions exist in fertility research. Some have shown remarkable staying power, persisting long after the medical and scientific communities have refuted them. Perhaps the most persistent of these myths is the notion that a woman with syphilis has only a slim chance of ever bearing a healthy infant when, in fact, a woman with untreated syphilis will experience an adverse pregnancy outcome only during the first 2 years following infection—that is, while she has spirochetes in her blood that can be transmitted transplacentally to the fetus. Spirochetemia is rare 2 years postinfection, and after this time an infected woman has every reason to expect the birth of an unaffected child.

Other myths have prompted researchers to initiate projects they otherwise might not have pursued. Weisbrod *et al.* (1973), for example, accepting the view that schistosomiasis causes mass chronic invalidism, sought to quantify its negative effect on natality (and other parameters) in Saint Lucia. Their study did not find any negative effect on natality (and little effect on the other parameters studied), and they had to conclude that schistosomiasis, even in an area of moderately severe endemicity, has only a modest effect on physical and mental health.

Such myths persist in the population literature often because population researchers consult either outdated medical sources or a recent population source that contains the myth. Even some current sources in the medical literature recount outdated notions about a disease. To avoid these problems, population students should consult several of the most recent studies available.

Relying on Indirect Evidence

Another pitfall to avoid is relying too heavily on indirect evidence. Bullough (1976:820–821) asked us to do this when he proposed that schistosomiasis causes reproductive failure because 41% of infertile women and only 21% of fertile women in his study were positive for schistosomal infection of the bladder or colon. But infection of these organs is no guarantee of genital tract involvement. He would have been on firmer ground, however, if he had shown that in the infected women the intensity of the bladder infection was high, because there is a much greater chance of genital tract involvement in such cases.

Variability of Response to a Disease by Population

The last pitfall encountered in fecundity research is not understanding the disease as it affects the study population. Many things about a population can alter its response to disease: the prevailing strain or species of organism and vector found in a locale and a population's immunity level, disease status, nutritional status, racial composition, and genetic makeup. The impact of a particular disease on fecundity therefore varies from population to population depending on the mix of these factors.

Species, Strain, and Vector

The particular strain or species of organism found in an area and/or its vector are very important in determining the impact of the disease on fecundity. With respect to malaria, *Plasmodium falciparum* is an important subfecundity factor whereas other *Plasmodia* species such as *P. ovale* and *P. vivax* are not. Similarly African sleeping sickness caused by the subspecies *T. b. rhodesiense* of *Trypanosoma brucei* is more important than that caused by *T. b. gambiense* in depressing fecundity during the early stages of disease, although both are important during the advanced stage. And *Schistosoma haematobium* is much more likely than *S. mansoni* to affect the genitals because of differences between the two parasites in the favored sites of egg laying. Different strains of organisms are also responsible for different reactions to infection. In Bancroftian filariasis, for example, differences among populations in the severity of diseases have been attributed to different strains of *Wuchereria bancrofti*. And differences in the anatomic sites affected by filariasis have been attributed to differences in the biting habits of its vectors. Therefore, in areas where the vector bites primarily below the waist a greater impact in fecundity would be expected.

Immunity Level

Immunity to a particular disease may be inherited or acquired. Inherited immunity is genetically determined and will be discussed in the section "Racial and Genetic Makeup." Acquired immunity is of two types: the transient immunity seen in newborns because of maternal antibodies acquired transplacentally and the immunity that individuals build on their own upon exposure to an infectious organism.

Population immunity to a particular disease is positively correlated to the endemicity of that disease in the population. In areas of hyperendemic malaria, for example, repeated exposure at short intervals to the parasite ensures the development of high antibody levels by adult life, whereas in mesoendemic areas less intense exposure results in lower antibody levels. Not only do persons living in areas of mesoendemic malaria have lower antibody levels, but so too do migratory populations, regardless of the endemicity levels they encounter. Even in areas of hyperendemic malaria nomads are never able to develop the protective levels of immunity of their settled counterparts because they are continuously exposed to different strains of *P. falciparum* and are never able to build high levels of antibody to any one strain.

In each population the impact of fecundity varies with the endemicity level and how this is mitigated by levels of acquired immunity (antibody) and inherited immunity (e.g., sickle hemoglogin). It is a complicated affair because not every one of the three concomitants of malaria infection that affect fecundity—fever, anemia, and placental parasitization—is more frequent or more severe in the less immune. Placental parasitization, for example, is common in highly immune women living in hyperendemic areas, but is rare in nonimmunes. And fevers of a height and duration capable of causing male infertility are present even in immune men living in hyperendemic areas. On the other hand, fevers capable of causing pregnancy loss are rare in hyperendemic areas but are common in mesoendemic areas. (See Chapter 4 for an in-depth discussion.)

The endemicity level of a disease also influences the age at which most persons are initially infected, which can substantially alter subfecundity effects. If a disease such as schistosomiasis, filariasis, or malaria is highly endemic, most persons are infected very early in life; in areas of lower endemicity a fair number of persons escape infection until early adult life. In diseases such as schistosomiasis, where chronicity of infection means a reduced host reaction to infecting organisms and less tissue pathology and where the genitals are not very vulnerable to infection until they become highly vascularized during puberty, initial infection in childhood may mean less effect on fecundity than does initial infection in young adulthood.

Not every disease offers protection to those who are repeatedly exposed, however. Gonorrhea offers no such protection. Neither does African sleeping sickness. And with some diseases such as filariasis it is the repeated exposure that results in fecundity-compromising sequelae such as hydrocele and genital elephantiasis. Each disease must therefore be considered separately to determine the exact relationship among immunity, chronicity, and subfecundity.

Disease Status

The disease status of a population is also very important in determining the impact of a particular subfecundity factor. It is a frequent observation that in persons with severe anemia infections are more frequent and more severe. Iron-deficiency anemia secondary to hookworm disease is common in developing countries, and it has been noted that affected persons are particularly susceptible to infection with malaria (Masawe *et al.* 1974). And certainly persons infected with a large number of different organisms are likely to suffer more serious sequelae from any one organism because of the tremendous drain on the body's ability to defend itself. The situation is somewhat similar to that following infection with African sleeping sickness, where the body is challenged by successive waves of parasites, each with a different antigenic profile, leading to exhaustion of the immune system. Local immunity may also be compromised by certain diseases. Workers have suggested that women with genital filariasis or genital schistosomiasis are more likely to develop PID because of a dimunition in the ability of affected tissue to defend itself against bacterial invasion.

In some cases this reduced ability to respond to an organism may mean that some negative aspects of a disease will also be reduced. In diseases such as schistosomiasis and filariasis where host hypersensitivity is the major factor responsible for the observed tissue pathology, concomitant infection with other organisms, especially those organisms which are known to exhaust the immune system, may mean less tissue pathology. Animal experiments have shown that the tissue reaction to schistosome eggs is less if the animal is already infected with malaria. Indeed, malaria does seem to be an immunosuppressive, dampening the body's ability to mount an immune response to other infectious organisms. It has been suggested that African Burkitt's lymphoma, a tumor of young children whose geographical distribution is the same as *falciparum* malaria, is caused by a virus that is relatively harmless in immunocompetent individuals but expresses an oncogenic potential in persons whose immune response is suppressed by concomitant malaria.

Nutritional Status

Nutritional status is also an important factor in the disease–subfecundity relationship. Deficiencies of a specific nutrient, folic acid, can cause a type of anemia (megaloblastic) that Masawe *et al.* (1974) have shown greatly increases the risk of bacterial infection. The risk of infection is also greatly increased by a lack of dietary protein. Hence, in persons suffering from such deficiencies there is an increased risk of gonorrhea and other subfecundity-producing diseases. Nutritional deficiencies are also responsible for a large proportion of pelvic abnormalities, which frequently lead to difficulties in childbirth (cephalo–pelvic disproportion) and high rates of morbidity and mortality in both the mother and child. Vitamin D deficiency is responsible for rickets in children and osteomalacia in adults, and a general malnutrition is responsible for the contracted pelvises seen so frequently in the developing world. Therefore, in areas where diets are poor, higher rates of disease-related subfecundity would be expected.

Racial and Genetic Makeup

The impact of a particular disease on subfecundity also varies by race. Blacks are more likely to develop extrapulmonary forms of TB, such as genital TB, than are whites. On the other hand, schistosomiasis is a more serious disease in whites, as is African sleeping sickness; very high fevers are noted in whites but not blacks with early-stage Gambian disease.

Some of these differences may be dose-related. That is, persons of a particular race may, because of their occupations or socioeconomic status, be more likely to come into contact with large doses of infectious organisms producing serious disease, whereas persons of another race are more likely to be exposed to small, subinfective doses allowing the gradual development of protective levels of immunity.

But some of these differences may, in fact, be inherited. Mourant *et al.* (1978) have written a fascinating book about blood groups and disease that shows the differential distribution of many diseases by blood group. And now, by determining the proteins on the surface of an individual's cells (so- called histocompatibility antigens) scientists can predict to some extent those diseases individuals are likely to get and those they are not likely to get.

In regard to blood group and diseases that affect fecundity, workers have found that persons of blood group A are more susceptible to schistosomiasis and persons of blood group B are more susceptible to gonorrhea. Because more blacks than whites are type B, this is one nonsociological reason for the higher rates of gonorrhea among blacks.

Certain inherited red cell abnormalities such as glucose-6-phosphate dehydrogenase (G6PD) deficiency and sickle (S) hemoglobin may also affect disease susceptibility and/or severity and therefore any subsequent effect on fecundity. G6PD deficiency may, in women heterozygous for the trait, confer some protection against the more serious sequelae of *falciparum* malaria. A much stronger protection is conferred by sickle hemoglobin, hemoglobin SA (HbSA) persons enjoying both a mortality and a fertility advantage over normal HbAA individuals. This is because the growth of *P. falciparum* is retarded in red cells containing hemoglobin S. Parasitemia levels are therefore lower in HbSA persons and so too are the fevers that adversely affect male and female fecundity.

VI

Appendixes

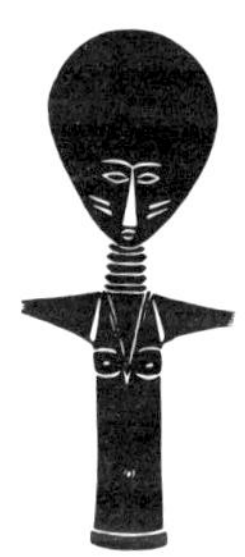

Diabetes

Diabetes is a common metabolic disease characterized by an absolute or relative deficiency in the supply of insulin secreted by the pancreas. The result is that sugar (glucose) in the diet is not broken down correctly, causing a high level of sugar in the blood and urine. The condition, which is largely inherited, can be controlled by diet, exercise, and/or regular injections of insulin, but cannot be cured.

Diabetes significantly depresses fecundity, but because it usually does not appear until after age 40 only a small proportion of the population will be affected during their reproductive years.

Impotence is a serious problem in diabetic men. About 50% of diabetic men are impotent (Carver and Oaks 1976:175). This amounts to 1 million men in the United States alone. There is no treatment available and the problem is not likely to correct itself. The occurrence of impotence is not correlated with control, duration, or severity of the disease. In fact, preliminary evidence from Masters and Johnson (1970:187) suggested that diabetes may be the etiological factor in impotent men who give an abnormal glucose tolerance test but have no other signs of disease.

Conceptive failure is an important feature of diabetes. Before insulin was discovered in 1921 few diabetic women conceived; 50% were amenorrheic (had no menstrual bleeding) and another 15% had menstrual problems (Gold 1968:221). In those who did conceive, maternal mortality rates approached 50%. Now, with the use of insulin, diabetic woman have no trouble conceiving (Marble *et al.* 1971:584) and maternal mortality rates are low. However, diabetic men, even those treated with insulin, may develop ejaculatory problems and thus be unable to bring about conception (Israel 1967:547).

Before the discovery of insulin in the early 1920s, babies born to diabetic women suffered extremely high perinatal mortality rates. Although the rates fell steadily thereafter, they remained quite high until the 1960s, at which time diabetic pregnancies, at least those in developed countries, began to receive full medical supervision. Nevertheless, even with the best medical care 4–7% of babies carried by diabetic mothers die just before or after birth;[1] under less favorable circumstances the rate is much higher (Peel 1972:391). Perinatal mortality rates are also higher than normal for those mothers over 25 who are ''gestational'' diabetics, diabetic only during pregnancy (O'Sullivan *et al.* 1973: 902). (Many of these women will eventually develop full-blown diabetes.) Such women, however, are only 2–4% of all women having babies.

Given the reproductive problems that diabetics experience, how could diabetes persist at relatively high rates, especially in the days before insulin? It has been hypothesized that when food supplies are chronically short, as in the past and still in some developing societies, those persons who would develop overt diabetes in an environment of plenty have an advantage (Medawar 1971:303). It has been noted, for example, that women with a hereditary tendency to diabetes begin to menstruate earlier and are more fertile (Mourant *et al.* 1978:32). But when persons with a tendency to diabetes begin to get more food, the disease develops and its negative aspects appear.

Overt diabetes is thus becoming common in many parts of the world where rapid social change is being accompanied by substantial dietary changes. Research among the San (Bushmen) of the Kalahari Desert in Africa, who live on a sparse but by no means starvation diet, has shown that their fasting blood sugar levels are normal but reach values that hint of diabetes when they are given a dose of glucose (Jenkins *et al.* 1974, cited in Mourant *et al.* 1978:32). Similarly, in South Africa diabetes rates among the tribal peoples still in their villages remain low, but are very high for those who have moved into the cities (Jackson 1972:394, 396). And in Nauru, a tiny island in the North Pacific where rapid development changed life-styles most abruptly—the annual per-capita in-

---

[1]Women suffering from severe diabetes and its complications were, until very recently, advised against pregnancy because of grave risks to both mother and child. However, some medical centers now offer these women an excellent chance of bearing a live, healthy infant. For these women full medical supervision must begin by the eighth week of pregnancy, and hospitalization for at least the last trimester is usually required. But with such measures doctors report that no matter how bad the mother's kidneys or her circulatory problems, the offspring are healthy.

come in the late 1970s was $30,000—31% of the 7300 inhabitants have diabetes (Willcox 1980a:175).

When the changeover to a richer diet occurs in developing societies, the genes for diabetes may be bred out if insulin is not available and the negative effects of the disease begin to outweigh its positive aspects. But in the United States insulin is plentiful and its widespread use has ensured that diabetes is likely to become even more common.

Sickle-Cell Hemoglobin

A surprising number of genetic factors related to the red blood cell pose serious threats to fecundity. Among these are the inherited anemias—sickle-cell anemia and the related diseases sickle-cell hemoglobin C disease and sickle-cell beta thalassemia. Under certain conditions red cells containing sickle hemoglobin bend into an inflexible sicklelike or new-moon shape, in contrast to the round shape of a normal red blood cell. This prevents the cells from moving easily through the circulatory system and thus they mass together and obstruct the flow of blood to the organs, causing pain and tissue destruction. So far there is no cure for the condition.

Sickle-cell-C disease and sickle-cell beta thalassemia are rare anemias found almost exclusively in the tropics. They can seriously depress fecundity. Pregnancy loss has been reported at anywhere from 16 to 62% among women with sickle-cell-C disease (Horger 1972:877; Pritchard *et al.* 1973:664), and up to 24% for those suffering from sickle-cell beta thalassemia (Morrison *et al.* 1973:39; Pritchard *et al.* 1973:665).

For the relatively more comon sickle-cell anemia, pregnancy loss can reach 57% (Horger 1972:875; Pritchard *et al.* 1973:663). Moreover, the anemia itself is often exacerbated by pregnancy and the risk of maternal death is significant. Males with the disease have been noted to have low sperm counts or hypogonadism (Friedman *et al.* 1974:1020). Another possible complication of sickle-cell anemia is priapism (Karayalcin *et al.* 1972:289), a persistent painful erection of the penis that makes coitus impossible. Unfortunately, surgery to correct priapism often leaves the patient permanently impotent (Seeler 1973:360).

Without exemplary medical care, 20–40% of the victims of sickle-cell anemia die before reaching reproductive age. Fertility rates for those who do survive are very low. Despite this weeding out the *S* gene still persists and, in fact, is carried by about 30% of persons in those parts of Africa where malaria is endemic. This is because persons with the sickle-cell trait (that is, those persons with only one gene for sickle hemoglobin, *AS*) stand a better chance of surviving malaria than the normal *AA* genotypes, 10–15% better in the case of the most dangerous of malaria parasites, *Plasmodium falciparum* (Cavalli-Sforza 1974:44).

Some experts believe that this survival advantage in malarious areas is not the only explanation for the high frequency of the *S* gene seen in some parts of Africa. Could it be that the *AS* genotype is also more fecund and thus more fertile? This may indeed be the case, because in areas where malaria is mesoendemic *AS* women have higher birthrates than *AA* women (Firschein 1961:250) (see Chapter 4 for a discussion of the relationships among endemicity of *falciparum* malaria, sickle-cell trait, and pregnancy loss).

Men with *AS* hemoglobin may also have a fecundity (and fertility) advantage in malarious areas (Eaton and Mucha 1971:456). Where malaria is rife, even adults who have built up high levels of immunity from repeated infections usually suffer the fevers of malaria twice a year. In normal *AA* men, these fevers are of sufficient height and duration to depress sperm counts for 1 to 2 months. In *AS* hemoglobin males, malarial fevers are shorter and less intense and sperm counts remain pretty much unaffected (see Chapter 4 for a detailed discussion of this point). Thus, whereas the *AA* male is relatively infertile 2–4 months of the year, the fertility of the *AS* male is unaltered.

Any such fecundity (and fertility) advantage for the *AS* genotype disappears in nonmalarious areas. In the United States, for example, pregnancy histories are essentially the same for the 10% of black American women who have the sickle-cell trait and the vast majority who do not (Blank and Freedman 1969:129), with the exception of a suggested increase in rates of prematurity and low-birth-weight infants among women with sickle-cell trait (Brown *et al.* 1972:1405; Rimer 1975:6).

Smallpox

Smallpox is an acute viral disease marked by a 2- to 4-day prodromal illness of fever, malaise, headache, and prostration. This is followed by a deep-seated rash that progresses from macules to pustules and finally to scabs that fall off at the end of the third or fourth week, frequently leaving scars.[1] Smallpox may have been present in Egypt or India or China about 1000 B.C. Indeed, the Egyptian pharoah Ramses V may have died of it. It was certainly present by the beginning of the Christian Era, and by the seventeenth century was very common. A pandemic was reported in 1614 and epidemics occurred throughout the seventeenth century.

The first step in the control of smallpox came in 1796 when Edward Jenner showed that the disease could be prevented by inoculation with serum prepared from cattle recovering from a similar disease called cowpox. Following this remarkable discovery smallpox began to recede in many parts of the world. Because of widespread vaccination programs, the United States and other developed countries have been troubled only by sporadic outbreaks since the 1950s. However, up until the late 1960s smallpox continued to take millions of lives in Africa, Asia, and other developing areas where economic and social conditions precluded widespread vaccination programs. Hence, in 1967 the World Health Organization undertook a global eradication program. At that time the dis-

---

[1]There are two types of smallpox, variola major or classical smallpox and variola minor or alastrim. The latter is associated with a less-severe systemic reaction and a mortality rate of only 1% or less (Benenson 1975:289).

ease was endemic in thirty countries, including most of the countries in sub–Saharan Africa, Afghanistan, India, Indonesia, Nepal, Pakistan, and Brazil. That year alone it struck approximately 2.5 million persons. The campaign was enormously successful. By the early 1970s only four countries—Pakistan, India, Bangladesh, and Ethiopia—still recorded smallpox, and on October 26, 1977, the last case of smallpox was recorded in the Horn of Africa. Smallpox had been eradicated.

Smallpox is a significant determinant of population growth. It is an important cause of mortality; 20–40% of all cases are fatal (Benenson 1975:289). It is also an important cause of subfecundity, causing both male conceptive failure and pregnancy loss, and several workers (e.g., Razzell 1977; Tabah 1977) have felt that it may have depressed fertility levels in some societies.

Smallpox is a significant cause of male conceptive failure. Phadke *et al.* (1973:803) noted that "the association of a history of smallpox infection with the occurrence of obstructive azoospermia is of proverbial frequency." Their study of infertile men attending a clinic in Bombay bore out this clinical impression. Of 8000 Indian men investigated for infertility, 895 (11%) had a history of smallpox. These men were matched against 895 infertile men with no history of the disease. Azoospermia occurred in 43% of the smallpox series, and 80% of this was due to obstruction. In the control series only 18% were azoospermic, and only 40% of this was due to obstruction. (The site of the obstruction was at the lower end of the epididymis; the testes seemed to have escaped the brunt of the disease as spermatogenic function was usually intact.) The authors concluded that in India smallpox is the most important cause of obstructive azoospermia (Phadke *et al.* 1973:802–804).

Smallpox is also a very important cause of pregnancy loss. Indeed, it is rare for pregnancy to continue in the wake of maternal smallpox, especially in severe cases. Maternal mortality is particularly high; 40% of pregnant women with smallpox die as compared to 12% of nonpregnant women (Harris 1974:1005). Fetal loss is also very common and due to the high fever and/or fever infection. Even in those children who are born alive, if there is a congenital infection the child is likely to die in the neonatal period, particularly if the child is premature (Bass 1959:627; Harris 1974:1005; Lawson 1967c:49–50). In Ibadan, Nigeria, during a 1957 epidemic there were 52 offspring recorded among 50 pregnant women with smallpox. Of these, 6 were spontaneously aborted, 12 were stillborn, 7 died neonatally, and 4 women died undelivered. Only 23 (44%) of the offspring survived (Lawson 1967c:50).

There are mixed opinions about whether or not vaccination constitutes a threat to the fetus. Although no increased risk was reported in a large series in New York City, in Scotland there was an increased incidence of spontaneous abortions and stillbirths in mothers vaccinated during early pregnancy (Barrett-Connor 1969:279). Lawson (1967c:51–52) also stated that vaccination is a threat during the first trimester. Concensus is that, if possible, vaccination should be avoided throughout pregnancy (Benenson 1975:293).

In sum, before eradication smallpox was a significant cause of subfecundity in both men and women. Its impact on fecundity (and fertility) varied with endemicity. In areas where smallpox was endemic, as it was in India before its eradication in the late 1970s, the ever-present nature of the disease meant that most infections occurred in children. Hence, male conceptive failure due to smallpox in childhood (which averts many births) would have been more frequent than pregnancy loss (which averts only one birth). Naturally, the greater the endemicity level, the greater the impact on fecundity (and fertility). In areas where smallpox was not a constant feature of life and epidemics occurred, persons of all ages were affected in approximately equal numbers. In such areas male conceptive failure (due to infection in either childhood or adulthood) and pregnancy loss would have been seen with approximately equal frequency. The impact of smallpox on population fecundity (and fertility) in such areas depended on the frequency and severity of epidemics.

References

Aal, H., A. El Atribi, A. Abdel Hafiz, and M. Aidaros. 1975. Azoospermia in bilharziasis and the presence of sperm antibodies. *Journal of Reproduction and Fertility*, **42**, 403.

Abdel-Wahab, M., K. Powers, S. Mahmoud, and W. Good. 1974. Suppression of schistosome granuloma formation by malaria in mice. *American Journal of Tropical Medicine and Hygiene*, **23**, 915.

Acosta, A., C. Mabray, and R. Kaufman. 1971. Intrauterine pregnancy and coexistent pelvic inflammatory disease. *Obstetrics and Gynecology*, **37**, 282.

Acton, H., and S. Rao. 1930. Factors which determine the differences in the types of lesions produced by *Filaria bancrofti* in India. *Indian Medical Gazette*, **65**, 620.

Adadevoh, B. (ed.). 1974. *Sub-fertility and infertility in Africa*. Ibadan, Nigeria: Caxton Press.

Adler, M. 1980. The terrible peril: An historical perspective on the venereal diseases. *British Medical Journal*, **2**, 206.

Agarwal, A. 1980. Waging war on the superpest. *Earthwatch*, **1**, 5.

Ajaegbu, H., and C. Mann. 1972. Human population and the disease factor in the development of Nigeria. In R. Moss and R. Rathbone (eds.), *The population factor in African studies*, pp. 123–138. New York: Africana.

Akerlund, M., P. Mardh, and L. Westrom. 1975. On the diagnosis and aetiology of infections of the lower genital tract in the female. In D. Danielsson *et al.* (eds.), *Genital infections and their complications*, pp. 169–175. Stockholm: Almqvist and Wiksell International.

Alausa, K., and A. Osoba. 1980. Epidemiology of gonococcal vulvovaginitis among children in the tropics. *British Journal of Venereal Diseases*, **56**, 239.

Alexander, E., J. Chandler, T. Pheifer, S. Wang, M. English, and K. Holmes. 1977. Prospective study of perinatal *Chlamydia trachomatis* infection. In D. Hobson and K. Holmes (eds.), *Nongonococcal urethritis and related infections*, pp. 148–152. Washington, DC: American Society for Microbiology.

Allison, A. 1954. Protection afforded by the sickle-cell trait against subtertian malarial infection. *British Medical Journal*, **1**, 290.

Allman, J. 1980. Natural fertility in North Africa and the Middle East. Paper presented at the Population Association of America Meetings, Denver, April.

Allman, J., and J. May. 1979. Fertility, mortality, migration and family planning in Haiti. *Population Studies*, **33**, 505.

Ambrose, K. 1964. *Recent advances in venerology.* London: Churchill.

Amelar, R. 1966. *Infertility in men: Diagnosis and treatment.* Philadelphia: Davis.

Amelar, R., and L. Dubin. 1977. Other factors affecting male fertility. In R. Amelar *et al.* (eds.), *Male infertility,* pp. 69–101. Philadelphia: Saunders.

Amelar, R., L. Dubin, and P. Walsh. 1977. *Male infertility.* Philadelphia: Saunders.

American Social Health Association. 1981. Some questions and answers about VD. Palo Alto, CA: American Social Health Association.

American Social Health Association. Undated. Body pollution. An environmental impact report on harmful by-products of the sexual revolution. Palo Alto, CA: American Social Health Association.

Ampofo, D. 1977. Socio-cultural and medical perspectives of infertility in Ghana. In *Family welfare and development in Africa,* pp. 101–111. London: International Planned Parenthood Federation.

Amstey, M. 1973. Current concepts of herpesvirus infection in the woman. *American Journal of Obstetrics and Gynecology,* **117**, 717.

Amstey, M. 1974. Herpes VD: A serious problem in pregnancy. *Medical Aspects of Human Sexuality,* **8**, 128.

Amstey, M. and G. Monif. 1974. Genital herpesvirus infection in pregnancy. *Obstetrics and Gynecology,* **44**, 394.

Apted, F. 1970. Clinical manifestations and diagnosis of sleeping sickness. In H. Mulligan and W. Potts (eds.), *The African trypanosomiases,* pp. 661–683. London: Allen and Unwin. (a)

Apted, F. 1970. The epidemiology of Rhodesian sleeping sickness. In H. Mulligan and W. Potts (eds.), *The African trypanosomiases,* pp. 645–660. London: Allen and Unwin. (b)

Apted, F. 1970. Treatment of human trypanosomiasis. In H. Mulligan and W. Potts (eds.), *The African trypanosomiases,* pp. 684–710. London: Allen and Unwin. (c)

Arean, V. 1956. Lesions caused by *Schistosoma mansoni* in the genitourinary tract of men. *American Journal of Clinical Pathology,* **26**, 1010. (a)

Arean, V. 1956. Manson's schistosomiasis of the female genital tract. *American Journal of Obstetrics and Gynecology,* **72**, 1038. (b)

Arean, V. 1976. American trypanosomiasis. In G. Hunter *et al.* (eds.), *Tropical medicine* (5th edition), pp. 440–450. Philadelphia: Saunders.

Armagnac, C., and A. Retel-Laurentin. 1981. Relations between fertility, birth intervals, foetal mortality and maternal health in Upper Volta. *Population Studies,* **35**, 217.

Aronson, J. 1931. Incidence of tuberculous infection in some communities of the south. *American Journal of Hygiene,* **14**, 374.

Arora, K., B. Cohen, and A. Beaudoin. 1979. Fetal and placental responses to artifically induced hyperthermia in rats. *Teratology,* **19**, 251.

Arowolo, O. 1978. A demographic note on relative infertility in Nigeria. Unpublished paper derived from Segment 1 of the Changing African Family Project in Nigeria.

Arriaga, E. 1982. Changing trends in mortality in developing countries. Paper presented at the Population Association of America Meetings, San Diego, March.

Arya, O., and J. Lawson. 1977. Sexually transmitted diseases in the tropics. Epidemiological, diagnostic, therapeutic, and control aspects. *Tropical Doctor,* **7**, 51.

Arya, O., H. Nsanzumuhire, and S. Taber. 1973. Clinical, cultural, and demographic aspects of gonorrhoea in a rural community in Uganda. *Bulletin of the World Health Organization,* **49**, 587.

Arya, O., and S. Taber. 1974. Some observations on venereal disease and infertility in the

Teso district of Uganda: A brief communication. In B. Adadevoh (ed.), *Sub-fertility and infertility in Africa*, pp. 78–80. Ibadan, Nigeria: Caxton Press.

Arya, O., and S. Taber. 1975. Correlates of venereal disease and fertility in rural Uganda. Paper presented at the Medical Society for the Study of Venereal Diseases, Malta, April. World Health Organization, WHO/VDT/RES/GON/75.96.

Assaad, M. 1980. Female circumcision in Egypt: Social implications, current research, and prospects for change. *Studies in Family Planning*, **11**, 3.

Auerbach, S. 1976. First step toward malaria cure. *Washington Post*, June 21, A9.

Ayres, M., F. Salzano, M. Helena, L. Franco, and R. de Souza Barros. 1976. The association of blood groups, ABH secretion, haptoglobins, and hemoglobins, with filariasis. *Human Heredity*, **26**, 105.

Aziz, F. 1980. Gynecologic and obstetric complications of female circumcision. *International Journal of Gynaecology and Obstetrics*, **17**, 560.

Azm, T., S. Saad, A. Arafa, and M. Al Ghorab. 1977. Can bilharziasis of the seminal vesicles be a cause of obstructive infertility? *Fertility and Sterility*, **28**, 775.

Babson, S. and R. Benson. 1971. *Management of high-risk pregnancy and intensive care of the neonate*. St. Louis, MO: Mosby.

Baer, A., L. Lie-Injo, Q. Welch, and A. Lewis. 1976. Genetic factors and malaria in the Temuan. *American Journal of Human Genetics*, **28**, 179.

Bai, K., K. Rao, and B. Vijayalakshmi. 1972. Congenital syphilis. *Indian Pediatrics*, **9**, 174.

Baird, D. 1979. Endocrinology of female infertility. *British Medical Bulletin*, **35**, 193.

Baker, J. 1970. Techniques for the detection of trypanosome infections. In H. Mulligan and W. Potts (eds.), *The African trypanosomiases*, pp. 67–88. London: Allen and Unwin.

Baker, J. 1974. Epidemiology of African sleeping sickness. In *Trypanosomiasis and leishmaniasis with special reference to Chagas' disease*, Ciba Foundation Symposium No. 20, pp. 29–43. Amsterdam: Associated Scientific Publishers.

Barlovatz, A. 1955. Sterility in central Africa. *Fertility and Sterility*, **6**, 363.

Barlow, D. 1979. *Sexually transmitted diseases. The facts*. Oxford: Oxford University Press.

Barrett-Connor, E. 1969. Infections and pregnancy: A review. *Southern Medical Journal*, **62**, 275.

Barrett-Connor, E. 1978. Latent and chronic infections imported from Southeast Asia. *Journal of the American Medical Association*, **239**, 1901.

Basch, P. 1978. *International Health*. New York: Oxford University Press.

Bass, M. 1959. Viral and parasitic diseases of the pregnant woman affecting the fetus. *Clinical Obstetrics and Gynecology*, **2**, 627.

Basson, W., M. Page, and D. Myburgh. 1977. Human trypanosomiasis in southern Africa. *South African Medical Journal*, **51**, 453.

Beaver, P. 1970. Filariasis without microfilaremia. *American Journal of Tropical Medicine and Hygiene*, **19**, 181.

Behrman, S., and R. Kistner. 1968. *Progress in infertility*. Boston: Little, Brown.

Bell, D. 1980. Introduction. *Social Science and Medicine*, **14C**, 63.

Belsey, M. 1976. The epidemiology of infertility: A review with particular reference to sub-Saharan Africa. *Bulletin of the World Health Organization*, **54**, 319.

Belsey, M. 1977. Biological factors other than nutrition and lactation which may influence natural fertility: Additional notes with particular reference to sub-Saharan Africa. Paper presented at the International Union for the Scientific Study of Population Seminar on Natural Fertility, Paris, March.

Belsey, M. 1978. Infertility: Etiology and natural history (Part 1). Paper presented at the Regional Multidisciplinary Consultative Meeting on Human Reproduction, Yaounde, Cameroon, December.

Belsey, M. 1979. Biological factors other than nutrition and lactation which may influence natural fertility: Additional notes with particular reference to sub-Saharan Africa. In H. Leridon and J. Menken (eds.), *Natural fertility,* pp. 253–272. Liège, Belgium: Ordina.

Benenson, A. (ed.). 1975. *Control of communicable diseases in man.* Washington, DC: American Public Health Association.

Benirschke, K. 1974. Syphilis—The placenta and the fetus. *American Journal of the Diseases of Children,* **128,** 142.

Bennett, F. 1962. The social determinants of gonorrhoea in an East African town. *East African Medical Journal,* **39,** 332.

Bennett, F. 1965. The social, cultural, and emotional aspects of sterility in women in Buganda. *Fertility and Sterility,* **16,** 243.

Berger, R., E. Alexander, G. Monda, J. Ansell, G. McCormick, and K. Holmes. 1978. *Chlamydia trachomatis* as a cause of "idiopathic" epididymitis. *New England Journal of Medicine,* **298,** 301.

Bhuyan, U. 1976. Immune responses in protein-calorie malnutrition. *Journal of the All India Institute of Medical Sciences,* **1,** 275.

Birdsall, N. 1980. *Population growth and poverty in the developing world.* Washington, DC: Population Reference Bureau.

Bittencourt, A. 1976. Congenital Chagas' disease. *American Journal of Diseases of Children,* **130,** 97. (a)

Bittencourt, A. 1976. Pathogenic aspects of congenital transmission of *T. cruzi.* In *New approaches in American trypanosomiasis research,* Pan American Health Organization, Scientific Publication No. 318, pp. 216–220. Proceedings of an International Symposium, Belo Horizonte, Minas Gerais, Brazil, March 1975. (b)

Blacker, J. 1962. Population growth and differential fertility in Zanzibar protectorate. *Population Studies,* **15,** 258.

Blackman, A. 1975. Baby boom not likely now. *Philadelphia Bulletin,* November 2, WA1.

Blackwood, L. 1981. Alaska Native fertility trends, 1950–1978. *Demography,* **18,** 173.

Blake, J. 1961. *Family structure in Jamaica.* New York: Free Press of Glencoe.

Bland, P. 1919. Influenza in its relation to pregnancy and labor. *American Journal of Obstetrical Diseases of Women and Children,* **79,** 184.

Bland, K., and M. Gelfand. 1970. The effect of schistosomiasis in the fallopian tubes in the African female. *Journal of Obstetrics and Gynaecology of the British Commonwealth,* **77,** 1024.

Blank, A., and W. Freedman. 1969. Sickle cell trait and pregnancy. *Clinical Obstetrics and Gynecology,* **12,** 123.

Blatt, J., J. Mulvihill, J. Ziegler, R. Young, and D. Poplack. 1980. Pregnancy outcome following cancer chemotherapy. *American Journal of Medicine,* **69,** 828.

Blattner, R. 1961. Syphilis is still a problem. *Journal of Pediatrics,* **59,** 625.

Bloomfield, R., J. Suarez, and A. Malangit. 1978. Transplacental transfer of Bancroftian filariasis. *Journal of the National Medical Association,* **70,** 597.

Bonafos, N. Laliam, and Cherfils. 1967. Sterility of the tubes due to tuberculosis. In B. Westin and N. Wiqvist (eds.), *Fertility and Sterility: Proceedings of the Fifth World Congress,* pp. 308–310. Amsterdam: Excerpta Medica.

Bongaarts, J. 1976. Intermediate fertility variables and marital fertility rates. *Population Studies,* **30,** 227.

Bongaarts, J. 1978. A framework for analyzing the proximate determinants of fertility. *Population and Development Review,* **4,** 105.

Bongaarts, J. 1980. Does malnutrition affect fecundity? A summary of evidence. *Science,* **208,** 564.

Bongaarts, J. 1982. Infertility after age 30: A false alarm. *Family Planning Perspectives,* **14,** 75.

Boreham, P., L. Gall, L. Goodwin, C. Hoare, B. Maegraith, H. Mulligan, W. Ormerod, and N. Wedderburn. 1970. Discussion following L. Goodwin's "The pathology of African trypanosomiasis." *Transactions of the Royal Society of Tropical Medicine and Hygiene,* **64,** 813.

Botella-Llusia, J. 1967. Tuberculosis of the endometrium. In B. Westin and N. Wiqvist (eds.), *Fertility and Sterility: Proceedings of the Fifth World Congress,* pp. 514–520. Amsterdam: Excerpta Medica.

Bottini, E., F. Gloria-Bottini, and G. Maggioni. 1978. On the relation between malaria and G-6-PD deficiency. *Journal of Medical Genetics,* **15,** 363.

Bougeois-Pichat, J. 1965. The general development of the population of France since the eighteenth century. In D. Glass and D. Eversley (eds.), *Population in history,* pp. 474–493. Chicago: Aldine.

Bowie, W. 1980. Urethritis and infections of the lower urogenital tract. *Urologic Clinics of North America,* **7,** 17.

Bowie, W., S. Wang, E. Alexander, and K. Holmes. 1977. Etiology of nongonococcal urethritis. In D. Hobson and K. Holmes (eds.), *Nongonococcal urethritis and related infections,* pp. 19–29. Washington, DC: American Society for Microbiology.

Boyce, W., and V. Politano. 1970. Infections and diseases of the scrotum and its contents. In M. Campbell and J. Harrison (eds.), *Urology, Vol. 1* (3rd edition), pp. 585–640. Philadelphia: Saunders.

Brass, W. 1968. The demography of French speaking territories covered by special sample inquiries: Upper Volta, Dahomey, Guinea, North Cameroon, and other areas. In W. Brass *et al.* (eds.), *The demography of tropical Africa.* Princeton: Princeton University Press.

Brisset, C. 1979. Excision condemned. *People* (UK), **6,** 2, 40.

British Medical Journal. 1972. Immunological control of schistosomiasis. **3,** 366. (a)

British Medical Journal. 1972. Infertility after the pill. **1,** 59. (b)

British Medical Journal. 1975. Promiscuity and infertility. **3,** 501.

British Medical Journal. 1976. African trypanosomiasis. **1,** 1298. (a)

British Medical Journal. 1976. New look at malaria. **1,** 1029. (b)

British Medical Journal. 1979. Non-specific genital infection. **2,** 161.

British Medical Journal. 1980. Genital herpes. **1,** 1335.

Brody, J. 1980. The continuing spread of herpes. *New York Times,* November 11, C1.

Brooks, G., W. Darrow, and J. Day. 1978. Repeated gonorrhea: An analysis of importance and risk factors. *Journal of Infectious Diseases,* **137,** 161.

Brothwell, D., and A. Sandison. 1967. *Diseases in antiquity.* Springfield, IL: Thomas.

Brown, H. (ed.). 1975. *Basic clinical parasitology* (4th edition). New York: Appleton-Century-Crofts.

Brown, S., A. Merkow, M. Wiener, and J. Khajezadeh. 1972. Low birth weights in babies born to mothers with sickle cell trait. *Journal of the American Medical Association,* **221,** 1404.

Brown, W., J. Donohue, N. Axnick, J. Blount, O. Jones, and N. Ewen. 1970. *Syphilis and other venereal diseases.* Cambridge, MA: Harvard University Press.

Browne, O. 1943. Tuberculosis of the female genital tract. *Journal of Obstetrics and Gynaecology of the British Empire,* **50,** 128.

Bruce, L. 1970. The incidence of genito-urinary tuberculosis in the western region of Scotland. *British Journal of Urology,* **42,** 637.

Bullough, C. 1976. Infertility and bilharziasis of the female genital tract. *British Journal of Obstetrics and Gynaecology,* **83,** 819.

Buyst, H. 1973. The diagnosis of sleeping sickness. *Tropical Doctor,* **3,** 110. (a)

Buyst, H. 1973. Pregnancy complications in Rhodesian sleeping sickness. *East African Medical Journal,* **50,** 19. (b)

Buyst, H. 1975. The treatment of *T. rhodesiense* sleeping sickness, with special reference to its physiopathological and epidemiological basis. *Annales de la Société Belge de Medecine Tropicale,* **55,** 95.

Buyst, H. 1976. Sleeping sickness research in Zambia. *East African Medical Journal,* **53,** 452.

Buyst, H. 1977. The epidemiology of sleeping sickness in the historical Luangwa Valley. *Annales de la Société Belge de Medecine Tropicale,* **57,** 349. (a)

Buyst, H. 1977. Sleeping sickness in children. *Annales de la Société Belge de Medecine Tropicale,* **57,** 201. (b)

Bwibo, N. 1971. Congenital syphilis. *East African Medical Journal,* **48,** 185.

Caldwell, J. 1974. The study of fertility and fertility change in tropical Africa. *World Fertility Survey Occasional Papers,* **No. 7.** Voorberg, the Netherlands: International Statistical Institute.

Caldwell, J. 1981. Fertility in Africa. In N. Eberstadt (ed.), *Fertility decline in the less developed countries,* pp. 101–122. New York: Praeger.

Camus, D., J. Bina, Y. Carlier, and F. Santoro. 1977. A, B, O blood groups and clinical forms of schistosomiasis mansoni. *Transactions of the Royal Society of Tropical Medicine and Hygiene,* **71,** 182.

Cannefax, G. 1965. Immunity in syphilis. *British Journal of Venereal Diseases,* **41,** 260.

Cannon, D. 1958. Malaria and prematurity in the western region of Nigeria. *British Medical Journal,* **2,** 877.

Cao, A., M. Melis, and R. Galanello. 1977. Fetal hemoglobin and malaria. *Lancet,* **1,** 202.

Carty, M., and W. Chatfield. 1972. The assessment of tubal patency by insufflation: A comparison with laparoscopic hydrotubation. *East African Medical Journal,* **49,** 1020.

Carty, M., J. Nzioki, and A. Verhagen. 1972. The role of gonococcus in acute pelvic inflammatory disease in Nairobi. *East African Medical Journal,* **49,** 376.

Carver, J. and W. Oaks. 1976. Sex and hypertension. In W. Oaks *et al.* (eds.), *Sex and the life cycle,* pp. 175–178. New York: Grune and Stratton.

Cassell, G., J. Younger, M. Brown, R. Blackwell, J. Davis, P. Marriott, and S. Stagno. 1983. Microbiologic study of infertile women at the time of diagnostic laparoscopy. *New England Journal of Medicine,* **308,** 502.

Cassen, R. 1978. Current trends in population change and their causes. *Population and Development Review,* **4,** 331.

Cates, W., H. Ory, R. Rochat, and C. Tyler. 1976. The intrauterine device and deaths from spontaneous abortion. *New England Journal of Medicine,* **295,** 1155.

Cates, W., K. Schulz, and D. Grimes. 1980. Dilatation and evacuation for induced abortion in developing countries; Advantages and disadvantages. *Studies in Family Planning,* **11,** 128.

Catterall, R. 1975. The situation of gonococcal and nongonococcal infections in the United Kingdom. In D. Danielsson *et al.* (eds.), *Genital infections and their complications,* pp. 5–13. Stockholm: Almqvist and Wiksell International.

Cavalli-Sforza, L. 1974. The genetics of human populations. In *The human population,* a Scientific American book, pp. 41–49. San Francisco: Freeman.

Cave, V., W. Harris, and E. Clark. 1971. Venereal diseases. *Encyclopaedia Britannica, 22,* 945.

Centers for Disease Control. 1982. Treatment guidelines for sexually transmitted diseases (STD), draft.

Cerisola, J. 1977. Chemotherapy of Chagas' infection in man. In *Chagas' disease,* Pan American Health Organization, Scientific Publication No. 347, pp. 35–47. Proceedings of an International Symposium held in conjunction with the Fifth International Congress on Protozoology, New York, June.

Charles, A., S. Cohen, M. Kass, and R. Richman. 1970. Asymptomatic gonorrhea in prenatal patients. *American Journal of Obstetrics and Gynecology, 108,* 595.

Charlewood, G. 1956. *Bantu gynaecology.* Johannesburg: Witwatersrand University Press.

Chatfield, W., P. Suter, A. Bremner, E. Edwards, and J. McAdam. 1970. The investigation and management of infertility in East Africa. *East African Medical Journal, 47,* 212.

Chedd, G. 1981. Who shall be born? *Science 81,* Jan.–Feb., 32.

Cheever, A., I. Kamel, A. Elwi, J. Mosimann, and R. Danner. 1977. *Schistosoma mansoni* and *S. haematobium* infections in Egypt. II. Quantitative parasitological findings at necropsy. *American Journal of Tropical Medicine and Hygiene, 26,* 702.

Cheever, A., I. Kamel, A. Elwi, J. Mosimann, R. Danner, and J. Sippel. 1978. *Schistosoma mansoni* and *S. haematobium* infections in Egypt. III. Extrahepatic pathology. *American Journal of Tropical Medicine and Hygiene, 27,* 55.

Christensen, W. 1974. Genitourinary tuberculosis. Review of 102 cases. *Medicine, 53,* 377.

Chukudebelu, W. 1978. The male factor in infertility—Nigerian experience. *International Journal of Fertility, 23,* 238.

Ciba Foundation Symposium No. 20. 1974. General discussion. In *Trypanosomiasis and leishmaniasis with special reference to Chagas' disease,* pp. 335–341. Amsterdam: Associated Scientific Publishers.

Clark, M. 1978. New hope for barren women. *Newsweek,* August 7, 70.

Clarren, S., D. Smith, M. Harvey, R. Ward, and M. Myrianthopoulos. 1979. Hyperthermia—A prospective evaluation of a possible teratogenic agent in man. *Journal of Pediatrics, 95,* 81.

Coale, A. 1974. The history of the human population. *Scientific American, 231,* 3, 40.

Coale, A. 1978. Reply to L. Stedman's "Third world development: A rebuttal." *Foreign Affairs,* Fall, 410.

Coale, A., and N. Rives. 1973. A statistical reconstruction of the black population of the United States, 1880–1970. *Population Index, 39,* 1.

Cohen, S. 1978. Development of a malaria vaccine. *Journal of the Royal Society of Medicine, 71,* 476.

Comhaire, F., G. Vershraegen, and L. Vermeulen. 1980. Diagnosis of accessory gland infection and its possible role in male infertility. *International Journal of Andrology, 3,* 32.

Comstock, G. 1975. Frost revisited: The modern epidemiology of tuberculosis. *American Journal of Epidemiology, 101,* 363.

Connor, D., R. Neafie, and J. Dooley. 1976. African trypanosomiasis. In C. Binford and D. Connor (eds.), *Pathology of tropical and extraordinary diseases,* pp. 252–257. Washington, DC: Armed Forces Institute of Pathology.

Cook, J., P. Jordan, and R. Bartholomew. 1977. Control of *Schistosoma mansoni* transmission by chemotherapy in St. Lucia. I. Results in man. *American Journal of Tropical Medicine and Hygiene, 26,* 887.

Copenhaver, W. (Revisor). 1964. *Bailey's Textbook of histology.* Baltimore: Williams and Wilkins.

Correa, P. 1969. Features of primary and secondary human sterility in the African region. Report of the scientific group on basic, clinical, and public health aspects of sub-fertility and sterility, Geneva, September, World Health Organization, HR/SS/69.5.

Corsaro, M., and C. Korzeniowsky. 1980. *STD: A commonsense guide.* New York: St. Martin's.

Council on Environmental Quality and the United States Department of State. 1981. *The global 2000 report to the President: Entering the twenty-first century.* Washington, DC: US Govt. Printing Office.

Cox, C., and M. Barber. 1974. Oxygen uptake by *Treponema pallidum. Infection and Immunity,* **10,** 123.

Crain, A., M. Sussman, and W. Weil. 1971. Effects of a diabetic child on marital integration and related measures of family functioning. In C. Crawford (ed.), *Health and family,* pp. 243–256. New York: Macmillan.

Crooks, R., and K. Baur. 1980. *Our sexuality.* Menlo Park, CA: Benjamin/Cummings.

Cross, R. 1973. Management of sexual dysfunction in family practice. Paper presented at the meeting of the Post-Graduate Medical Association of North America, Chicago, November.

Cruickshank, E. 1967. Nutrition in pregnancy and lactation. In J. Lawson and D. Stewart (eds.), *Obstetrics and gynaecology in the tropics and developing countries,* pp. 11–28. London: Edward Arnold.

Curran, J. 1979. Management of gonococcal pelvic inflammatory disease. *Sexually Transmitted Diseases,* **6,** 2, (Supplement), 174.

Curran, J. 1980. Economic consequences of pelvic inflammatory disease in the United States. *American Journal of Obstetrics and Gynecology,* **138,** 848.

Curran, J., R. Rendtorff, R. Chandler, W. Wiser, and H. Robinson. 1975. Female gonorrhea. Its relation to abnormal uterine bleeding, urinary tract symptoms, and cervicitis. *Obstetrics and Gynecology,* **45,** 195.

Curtis, A., and J. Huffman. 1950. *A textbook of gynecology.* Philadelphia: Saunders.

Cushman, P., and C. Sherman. 1974. Biologic false-positive reactions in serologic tests for syphilis in narcotic addiction. Reduced incidence during methadone maintenance treatment. *American Journal of Clinical Pathology,* **61,** 346.

Cusick, A. 1981. Population figures reveal USSR's continuing health crisis. *Intercom,* **9,** 4, 11.

Cutler, W., C. Garcia and A. Krieger. 1979. Infertility and age at first coitus: A possible relationship. *Journal of Biosocial Science,* **11,** 425. (a)

Cutler, W., C. Garcia, and A. Krieger. 1979. Luteal phase defects: A possible relationship between short hyperthermic phase and sporadic sexual behavior in women. *Hormones and Behavior,* **13,** 214. (b)

Cutler, W., C. Garcia, and A. Krieger. 1979. Sexual behavior frequency and menstrual cycle length in mature premenopausal women. *Psychoendocrinology,* **4,** 297. (c)

Cutright, P., and E. Shorter. 1979. The effects of health on the completed fertility of nonwhite and white U.S. women born between 1867 and 1935. *Journal of Social History,* **13,** 191.

Czernobilsky, B. 1968. Pathology of septic abortion. In R. Schwarz (ed.), *Septic abortion,* pp. 23–54. Philadelphia: Lippincott.

Daling, J., and I. Emanuel. 1975. Induced abortion and subsequent outcome of pregnancy. *Lancet,* **3,** 170.

Daling, J., L. Spadoni, and I. Emanuel. 1981. Role of induced abortion in secondary infertility. *Obstetrics and Gynecology,* **57,** 59.

Danielsson, D. 1975. Aspects on the indigenous flora and established and probable pathogens of the genital tract, with special regard to bacteria and their L-phases. In D. Danielsson *et al.* (eds.), *Genital infections and their complications,* pp. 29–37. Stockholm: Almqvist and Wiksell International.

Danielsson, D., V. Falk, and L. Forslin. 1975. Acute salpingitis and gonorrhoeae in a gynaecological ward. In D. Danielsson *et al.* (eds.), *Genital infections and their complications,* pp. 151–156. Stockholm: Almqvist and Wiksell International.

Dankoussou, I., S. Diarra, D. Laya, and D. Pool. 1975. Niger. In J. Caldwell (ed.), *Population growth and socioeconomic change in west Africa,* pp. 670–693. New York: Columbia University Press.

Davidson, S., R. Passmore, J. Brock, and A. Truswell. 1975. *Human nutrition and dietetics.* New York: Churchill Livingstone.

Davis, C., and M. Feshbach. 1980. Rising Soviet infant mortality. *Intercom,* **8,** 7, 12.

Davis, J. 1970. Treatment of epididymitis. *Modern Treatment,* **7,** 1036.

Davis, J., M. Clyman, A. Decker, W. Oker, and M. Roland. 1967. Varicocele as contributing factor in male infertility. In B. Westin and N. Wiquist (eds.), *Fertility and Sterility: Proceedings of the Fifth World Congress,* pp. 842–844. Amsterdam: Excerpta Medica.

Davis, K., and J. Blake. 1956. Social structure and fertility: An analytic framework. *Economic Development and Cultural Change,* **4,** 211.

de Carle, D. 1955. Pelvic tuberculosis: Its relationship to sterility, present and future. *Fertility and Sterility,* **6,** 534.

Decker, A., and S. Loebl. 1978. *Why can't we have a baby?* New York: Dial.

de Leon, R. 1973. Syphilis and gonorrhea. *Journal of the American Pharmaceutical Association,* **NS13,** 190.

De Lora, J., C. Warren, and C. Ellison. 1981. *Understanding sexual interaction.* Boston: Houghton Mifflin.

Denham, D., and G. Nelson. 1976. Pathology and pathophysiology of nematode infections of the lympathic system and blood vessels. In E. Soulsby (ed.), *Pathophysiology of parasitic infections,* pp. 115–132. New York: Academic Press.

DeRaadt, P. 1974. Immunity and antigenic variation: Clinical observations suggestive of immune phenomena in African trypanosomiasis. In *Trypanosomiasis and leishmaniasis with special reference to Chagas' disease,* Ciba Foundation Symposium No. 20, pp. 199–216. Amsterdam: Associated Scientific Publishers.

DeRaadt, P. 1976. African sleeping sickness today. *Transactions of the Royal Society of Tropical Medicine and Hygiene,* **70,** 114.

Desai, S., M. Cohen, M. Khatamee, and E. Leiter. 1980. *Ureaplasma urealyticum* (T-mycoplasma) infection: Does it have a role in male infertility? *Journal of Urology,* **124,** 469.

Devereux, G. 1976. *A study of abortion in primitive societies.* New York: International Universities Press.

Di Musto, J., D. Bohjalian, and M. Millar. 1973. *Mycoplasma hominis* Type 1 infection and pregnancy. *Obstetrics and Gynecology,* **41,** 33.

Dippel, A. 1944. The relationship of congenital syphilis to abortion and miscarriage, and the mechanism of intrauterine protection. *American Journal of Obstetrics and Gynecology,* **47,** 369.

Dogliotti, M. 1971. The incidence of syphilis in the Bantu: Survey of 587 cases from Baragwanath Hospital. *South African Medical Journal,* **45,** 8.

Dogliotti, M. 1975. Survey of skin disorders in the urban black population of South Africa. *British Journal of Dermatology,* **92,** 259.

Dorland's Medical Dictionary. Various years. Philadelphia: Saunders.

Downes, J. 1939. The effect of tuberculosis on the size of family. *Milbank Memorial Fund Quarterly,* **17,** 274.

544 References

Dreifus, C. 1980. "Ideal" contraceptive dangerous? *Philadelphia Bulletin*, June 15, D1.

DuBois, W. 1967. *The Philadelphia negro.* New York: Schocken. (Originally published 1899)

Duggan, A. 1973. The treatment of African trypanosomiasis. *Tropical Doctor*, **4**, 162.

Duke, B. 1980. Problems of chemotherapy with diethylcarbamazine citrate in lymphathic filariasis. World Health Organization, WHO/FIL/80.158, 1.

Dunn, H. 1944. The magnitude of the abortion problem. In *The abortion problem*, pp. 1–14. Baltimore: Williams and Wilkins.

Durgamba, K., S. Swany, and C. Rao. 1972. Genital tuberculosis. *Indian Journal of Chest Diseases*, **14**, 32.

Dvorak, J. 1977. Host-parasite relationships at the cellular level in *Trypanosoma cruzi* infections. In *Chagas' disease*, Pan American Health Organization Scientific Publication No. 347, pp. 1–10. Proceedings of an International Symposium held in conjunction with the Fifth International Congress on Protozoology, New York, June.

Dyson, T. 1980. Review of *Demography of the Dobe !Kung*, by N. Howell. *Population Studies*, **34**, 411.

Easterlin, R., R. Pollack, and M. Wachter. 1976. Toward a more general economic model of fertility determination: Endogenous preferences and natural fertility. *U-NBER Conference on Economic and Demographic Change in Less Developed Countries*, Philadelphia, September.

Eaton, J., J. Eckman, E. Berger, and H. Jacob. 1976. Suppression of malaria infection by oxidant-sensitive host erythrocytes. *Nature*, **264**, 758.

Eaton, J., and A. Mayer. 1954. *Man's capacity to reproduce. The demography of a unique population.* Glencoe, IL: Free Press.

Eaton, J., and J. Mucha. 1971. Increased fertility in males with sickle cell trait. *Nature*, **231**, 456.

Eaton, J., and R. Weil. 1955. *Culture and mental disorders.* Glencoe, IL: Free Press.

Edeson, J. 1972. Filariasis. *British Medical Bulletin*, **28**, 60.

Edgcomb, J., and C. Johnson. 1976. American trypanosomiasis. In C. Binford and D. Connor (eds.), *Pathology of tropical and extraordinary diseases*, pp. 244–251. Washington, DC: Armed Forces Institute of Pathology.

Edington, G., I. Nwabuabo, and T. Junaid. 1975. The pathology of schistosomiasis in Ibadan, Nigeria with special reference to the appendix, brain, pancreas, and genital organs. *Transactions of the Royal Society of Tropical Medicine and Hygiene*, **69**, 153.

Edstrom, K. 1975. Early complications and late sequelae of induced abortion: A review of the literature. *Bulletin of the World Health Organization*, **52**, 123.

Edstrom, K. 1978. Infertility: Diagnostic and service aspects. Regional Multidisciplinary Consultative Meeting on Human Reproduction, December, Part II. World Health Organization, HRP/RMC/78.7, 31.

Edwards, M., and R. Kinsie. 1940. Illegal and unethical practices in the diagnosis and treatment of syphilis and gonorrhea. *Journal of Venereal Disease Information*, **21**, 1.

Eisenberg, L. 1973. Syphilis in the Bantu of Soweto. A serologic study. *South African Medical Journal*, **47**, 2181.

Eliasson, R. 1975. Pathophysiology of the male accessory glands. In D. Danielsson *et al.* (eds.), *Genital infections and their complications*, pp. 113–119. Stockholm: Almqvist and Wiksell International.

El-Mahgoub, S. 1972. Antispermal antibodies in infertile women with cervicovaginal schistosomiasis. *American Journal of Obstetrics and Gynecology*, **112**, 781.

El-Mofty, A. 1962. Clinical aspects of bilharziasis. In G. Wolstenholme and M. O'Connor (eds.), *Bilharziasis*, Ciba Foundation Symposium, pp. 174–197. Boston: Little, Brown.

Elsdon-Dew, R. 1962. The pathognomy of bilharziasis. In G. Wolstenholme and M.

O'Connor (eds.), *Bilharziasis*, Ciba Foundation Symposium, pp. 207–214. Boston: Little, Brown.

Elsdon-Dew, R. 1975. Parasitic infections and the genitourinary tract. *Practitioner,* **214**, 75.

Ely, J. 1979. Herpes treatment a success. *Forum,* **9**, 42.

Epelboin, S., and A. Epelboin. 1979. Dangers of infection, pain and death. *People* (UK), **6**, 1, 26.

Ericksen, J., E. Ericksen, J. Hostetler, and G. Huntington. 1979. Fertility patterns and trends among the Old Order Amish. *Population Studies,* **33**, 255.

Eschenbach, D. 1980. Epidemiology and diagnosis of acute pelvic inflammatory disease. *Obstetrics and Gynecology,* **55, Supplement 5,** 142S.

Eschenbach, D., T. Buchanan, H. Pollock, P. Forsyth, E. Alexander, J. Lin, S. Wang, B. Wentworth, W. McCormack, and K. Holmes. 1975. Polymicrobial etiology of acute pelvic inflammatory disease. *New England Journal of Medicine,* **293**, 166.

Eschenbach, D., J. Harnisch, and K. Holmes. 1977. Pathogenesis of acute pelvic inflammatory disease: Role of contraception and other risk factors. *American Journal of Obstetrics and Gynecology,* **128**, 838.

Eschenbach, D., and K. Holmes. 1975. Acute pelvic inflammatory disease: Current concepts of pathogenesis, etiology, and management. *Clinical Obstetrics and Gynecology,* **18**, 35.

Eugenical News. 1936. Brief communication. **6**, 147.

Evans, B. 1979. Non-specific genital infection [letter]. *British Medical Journal,* **2**, 441.

Eversley, D. 1963. Population in England in the eighteenth century: An appraisal of current research. *Proceedings of the International Population Conference, New York, 1961, Vol. 1,* pp. 573–581. London: International Union for the Scientific Study of Population.

Fair, W. 1977. Epididymitis and prostatitis. In D. Hobson and K. Holmes (eds.), *Nongonococcal urethritis and related infections,* pp. 55–63. Washington, DC: American Society for Microbiology.

Falk, V. 1965. Treatment of acute non-tuberculous salpingitis with antibiotics alone and in combination with glucocorticoids. *Acta Obstetricia et Gynecological Scandinavica* (Suppl. b), **44**, 1.

Falk, V., K. Ludviksson, and G. Agren. 1980. Genital tuberculosis in women. *American Journal of Obstetrics and Gynecology,* **138**, 974.

Family Planning Perspectives. 1979. Repeated abortions increase risk of miscarriage, premature births and low-birth-weight babies. **11**, 39.

Family Planning Perspectives. 1980. Bacterial infection from actinomyces, though rare, is found to be a problem among some IUD users. **12**, 306. (a)

Family Planning Perspectives. 1980. IUD users may have higher risk of contracting PID, studies find; pill may have protective effect. **12**, 206. (b)

Family Planning Perspectives. 1980. Pill, IUD users run no increased risk of ectopics, malformation, miscarriage in planned pregnancies. **12**, 156. (c)

Family Planning Perspectives. 1981. IUD users have fewer ectopic pregnancies than non-contraceptors. **13**, 150. (a)

Family Planning Perspectives. 1981. No increased risk of spontaneous abortion found among women with a previous induced abortion. **13**, 238. (b)

Family Planning Perspectives. 1981. PID risk increased sharply among IUD users, British cohort, U.S. case-control studies affirm. **13**, 182. (c)

Family Planning Perspectives. 1982. Pill users protected against PID if they have used OCs for longer than one year. **14**, 32.

Farley, R. 1970. *Growth of the black population.* Chicago: Markham.

Faust, E., and P. Russell. 1964. Craig and Faust's *Clinical parasitology* (7th edition). Philadelphia: Lea and Febiger.

Feldman, J. 1977. Effects of tuberculosis on sexual functioning. *Medical Aspects of Human Sexuality*, **11**, 29.

Felman, Y., and J. Nikitas. 1981. Nongonococcal urethritis. A clinical review. *Journal of the American Medical Association*, **245**, 381.

Firschein, I. 1961. Population dynamics of the sickle-cell trait in the black Caribs of British Honduras, Central America. *American Review of Human Genetics*, **13**, 233.

Fisher, R. 1967. Criminal abortion. In H. Rosen (ed.), *Abortion in America*, pp. 3–11. Boston: Beacon Press.

Fiumara, N. 1974. Acquired syphilis in three patients with congenital syphilis. *New England Journal of Medicine*, **290**, 1119.

Fleming, A. 1973. Maternal anemia and fetal outcome in pregnancies complicated by thalassemia minor and "stomatocytosis." *American Journal of Obstetrics and Gynecology*, **116**, 309.

Florman, A., A. Gershon, P. Blackett, and A. Nahmias. 1973. Intrauterine infection with herpes simplex virus. *Journal of the American Medical Association*, **225**, 129.

Fogel, R., and S. Engerman. 1974. *Time on the cross*. Boston: Little, Brown.

Forrest, J., C. Tietze, and E. Sullivan. 1978. Abortion in the United States, 1976–1977. *Family Planning Perspectives*, **10**, 271.

Foster, M., and A. Labrum. 1976. Relation of infection with *Neisseria gonorrhoeae* to ABO blood groups. *Journal of Infectious Diseases*, **133**, 329.

Francis, W. 1964. Female genital tuberculosis. *Journal of Obstetrics and Gynaecology of the British Commonwealth*, **71**, 418.

Frank, E., C. Anderson, and D. Rubinstein. 1978. Frequency of sexual dysfunction in normal couples. *New England Journal of Medicine*, **299**, 111.

Frank, O. 1983. Infertility in sub-Saharan Africa: Estimates and implications. *Population and Development Review*, **9**, 137.

Frazier, C., and L. Hung-Chuing. 1948. *Racial variations in immunity to syphilis*. Chicago: University of Chicago Press.

Freedman, R. 1963. *The sociology of human fertility*. Oxford: Basil Blackwell.

Freedman, R., P. Whelpton, and A. Campbell. 1959. *Family planning, sterility, and population growth*. Princeton: Princeton University Press.

Friberg, J., and H. Gnarpe. 1974. Mycoplasma infections and infertility. In R. Mancini and L. Martini (eds.), *Male fertility and sterility*, pp. 327–335. New York: Academic Press.

Friedman, G., R. Freeman, R. Bookchin, R. Boyar, G. Murthy, and L. Hellman. 1974. Testicular function in sickle cell disease. *Fertility and Sterility*, **25**, 1018.

Frisch, R. 1975. Demographic implications of the biological determinants of female fecundity. *Social Biology*, **22**, 17.

Fritjofsson, A., and S. Kollberg. 1973. The incidence of urogenital tuberculosis in Sweden. *International Urology and Nephrology*, **5**, 291.

Frost, O. 1975. Bilharzia of the fallopian tube. *South African Medical Journal*, **49**, 1201.

Fuller, J. 1974. *Fever! The hunt for a new killer virus*. New York: Ballantine.

Fullerton, W. 1971. Methods of abortion. *Journal of Biosocial Science*, **3**, 128.

Gall, S., A. Kohan, D. Ayres, C. Hughes, W. Addison, and G. Hill. 1981. Intravenous metroniridazole or clindamycin with tobramycin for therapy of pelvic infections. *Obstetrics and Gynecology*, **57**, 51.

Gallagher, R. 1969. *Diseases that plague modern man*. Dobbs Ferry, NY: Oceana.

Galton, L. 1980. VD: Outbreak of a new variety. *Parade*, February 24, 16.

Gantt, H. 1926. Medical review of Soviet Russia, Vol. IV. Changes in type and incidence of disease. *British Medical Journal*, **2**, 303.

Gardner, H. 1979. Herpes genitalis: Our most important venereal disease. *American Journal of Obstetrics and Gynecology*, **135**, 553.

Gear, J. 1974. The occurrence and diagnosis of malaria. *South African Medical Journal*, **48**, 1078.

Gebhard, P. 1965. Situational factors affecting human sexual behavior. In F. Beach (ed.), *Sex and behavior*, pp. 483–495. New York: Wiley.

Gelfand, M. 1976. The pattern of disease in Africa and the western way of life. *Tropical Doctor*, **6**, 173.

Gelfand, M., C. Ross, D. Blair, W. Castle, and M. Weber. 1970. Schistosomiasis of the male pelvic organs. Severity of infection as determined by digestion of tissue and histologic methods in 300 cadavers. *American Journal of Tropical Medicine and Hygiene*, **19**, 779.

Gelfand, M., M. Ross, D. Blair, and M. Weber. 1971. Distribution and extent of schistosomiasis in female pelvic organs, with special reference to the genital tract, as determined at autopsy. *American Journal of Tropical Medicine and Hygiene*, **20**, 846.

Gelfand, M., E. Taube, and A. Wolhuter. 1973. A survey of the forms of tuberculosis encountered at Haare Hospital, Rhodesia, 1967–1969. *Central African Journal of Medicine*, **19**, 65.

Gibbons, R. 1977. Adherence of bacteria to host tissue. In D. Schlessinger (ed.), *Microbiology-1977*, pp. 395–406. Washington, DC: American Society for Microbiology.

Giglioli, G. 1972. Changes in the pattern of mortality following eradiction of hyperendemic malaria from a highly susceptible community. *Bulletin of the World Health Organization*, **46**, 181.

Gilbert, B. 1943. Schistosomiasis (bilharziasis) of the female genital tract and neighbouring tissues. *Journal of Obstetrics and Gynaecology of the British Empire*, **50**, 317.

Gill, C. 1940. The influence of malaria on natality with special reference to Ceylon. *Journal of the Malaria Institute of India*, **3**, 201.

Glass, D. 1965. Population and population movements in England and Wales, 1700 to 1850. In D. Glass and D. Eversley (eds.), *Population in history*, pp. 221–246. Chicago: Aldine.

Glover, T. 1974. Recent progress in the study of male physiology: Testis stimulation; sperm formation; transport and maturation (epididymal physiology); semen analysis, storage and artificial insemination. In R. Greep (ed.), *Reproductive physiology*, pp. 221–277. Baltimore: University Park Press.

Gnarpe, H., and J. Friberg. 1972. Mycoplasma and human reproductive failure. I. The occurrence of different mycoplasmas in couples with reproductive failure. *American Journal of Obstetrics and Gynecology*, **114**, 727.

Goble, F. 1970. South American trypanosomes. In G. Jackson *et al.* (eds.), *Immunity to parasitic animals*, Vol. 2, pp. 597–689. New York: Appleton-Century-Crofts.

Gold, J. (ed.). 1968. *Gynecologic endocrinology.* New York: Harper and Row.

Goldsmith, R., I. Kagan, R. Zarate, M. Reyes-Gonzalez, and J. Cedeno-Ferreira. 1978. Epidemiologic studies of Chagas' disease in Oaxaca, Mexico. *Bulletin of the Pan American Health Organization*, **12**, 236.

Goodwin, L. 1970. The pathology of African trypanosomiasis. *Transactions of the Royal Society of Tropical Medicine and Hygiene*, **64**, 797.

Goodwin, L. 1974. The African scene: Mechanisms of pathogenesis of trypanosomiasis. In *Trypanosomiasis and leishmaniasis with special reference to Chagas' disease*, Ciba Foundation Symposium No. 20, pp. 107–119. Amsterdam: Associated Scientific Publishers.

Gordon, L. 1977. *Woman's body, woman's right*. New York: Penguin Books.

Gorman, J. 1982. New hope for the childless. *Discover Magazine*, March, 62.

Gotwald, W., and G. Golden. 1981. *Sexuality: The human experience*. New York: Macmillan.

Gow, J. 1970. Results of treatment in a large series of genitourinary tuberculosis and the changing pattern of the disease. *British Journal of Urology*, **42**, 647.

Gow, J. 1971. Genito-urinary tuberculosis. *Practitioner*, **207**, 609.

Grabill, W., C. Kiser, and P. Whelpton. 1958. *The fertility of American women*. New York: Wiley.

Grady, W. 1981. National Survey of Family Growth, cycle II: Sample design, estimation procedures, and variance estimation. *Vital and Health Statistics*, National Center for Health Statistics, DHHS (NCHS), Series 2, No. 87.

Gratama, S. 1966. *Onchocerciasis in the south-eastern territories of Liberia*. Zwolle, Netherlands: Willink.

Gratama, S. 1969. The aetiology of hydrocele in the south-eastern territories of Liberia. *Tropical and Geographical Medicine*, **21**, 269. (a)

Gratama, S. 1969. The pathogenesis of hydrocele in filarial infections. *Tropical and Geographical Medicine*, **21**, 254. (b)

Gray, A. 1976. Immunological research and the problem of immunization against African trypanosomiasis. *Transactions of the Royal Society of Tropical Medicine and Hygiene*, **70**, 119.

Gray, R. 1974. The decline of mortality in Ceylon and the demographic effects of malaria control. *Population Studies*, **28**, 205.

Gray, R. 1977. Biological factors other than nutrition and lactation which may influence natural fertility: A review. Paper presented at the International Union for the Scientific Study of Population Seminar on Natural Fertility, Paris, March.

Gray, R. 1979. Biological factors other than nutrition and lactation which may influence natural fertility: A review. In H. Leridon and J. Menken (eds.), *Natural fertility*, pp. 217–251. Liège, Belgium: Ordina.

Grech, E., J. Everett, and F. Mukasa. 1973. Epidemiological aspects of acute pelvic inflammatory disease in Uganda. *Tropical Doctor*, **3**, 123.

Greenberg, S. 1979. Male reproductive tract sequelae of gonococcal and nongonococcal urethritis. *Archives of Andrology*, **3**, 317.

Greenwood, B., D. Stratton, W. Williamson, and I. Mohammed. 1978. A study of the role of immunological factors in the pathogenesis of the anaemia of acute malaria. *Transactions of the Royal Society of Tropical Medicine and Hygiene*, **72**, 378.

Gremillion, D., R. Geckler, R. Kuntz, and R. Marraro. 1978. Schistosomiasis in Saudi Arabian recruits. A morbidity study based on quantitative egg excretion. *American Journal of Tropical Medicine and Hygiene*, **27**, 924.

Greve, F. 1982. Experts want to test gonorrhea vaccine on 10,000 soldiers. *Philadelphia Inquirer*, March 11, 4A.

Griffith, H. 1963. Gonorrhea and fertility in Uganda. *Eugenics Review*, July, 201.

Grimble, A. 1972. Gonorrhea. *Practitioner*, **209**, 614.

Grossman, B., and editors. 1971. Rickets. *Encyclopaedia Britannica*, **19**, 318.

Grove, D., F. Valeza, and B. Cabrera. 1978. Bancroftian filariasis in a Phillippine village: Clinical, parasitological, immunological, and social aspects. *Bulletin of the World Health Organization*, **56**, 975.

Gubler, D. and N. Bhattacharya. 1974. A quantitative approach to the study of bancroftian filariasis. *American Journal of Tropical Medicine and Hygiene*, **23**, 1027.

Guest, I. 1978. Infertility in Africa. *People* (UK), **5**, 23.

Gupta, S. 1957. Pelvic tuberculosis in women. *Journal of Obstetrics and Gynaecology of India,* **7,** 181.

Gutteridge, W. 1976. Chemotherapy of Chagas' disease. *Transactions of the Royal Society of Tropical Medicine and Hygiene,* **70,** 123.

Guttmacher, A. 1967. The shrinking non-psychiatric indications for therapeutic abortion. In H. Rosen (ed.), *Abortion in America,* pp. 12–21. Boston: Beacon Press.

Guttmacher, M. 1967. The legal status of therapeutic abortions. In H. Rosen (ed.), *Abortion in America,* pp. 175–186. Boston: Beacon Press.

Gwatkin, D. 1977. Health and population: What's known and what's needed. Mimeographed. November.

Gwatkin, D. 1980. Indications of change in developing country mortality trends: The end of an era? *Population and Development Review,* **6,** 615.

Gwatkin, D. 1981. Mortality change and slowed population growth in developing countries. *Intercom,* **9,** 6, 8.

Habakkuk, H. 1965. English population in the eighteenth century. In D. Glass and D. Eversley (eds.), *Population in history,* pp. 269–284. Chicago: Aldine.

Hacker, K. 1976. Why infertility is increasing. *Philadelphia Bulletin,* February 19, D14.

Hacker, K. 1981. Failed pregnancy. *Philadelphia Bulletin,* November 8, D1.

Hackett, C. 1967. The human treponematoses. In D. Brothwell and A. Sandison (eds.), *Diseases in antiquity,* pp. 152–169. Springfield, IL: Thomas.

Hager, W., and P. Wiesner. 1977. Selected epidemiologic aspects of acute salpingitis: A review. *Journal of Reproductive Medicine,* **19,** 47.

Haggan, M. 1944. Sexual desire in tuberculous women. *American Review of Respiratory Diseases,* **49,** 53.

Haines, M. 1958. Tuberculous salpingitis as seen by the pathologist and the surgeon. *American Journal of Obstetrics and Gynecology,* **75,** 472.

Hajj, S. 1978. Does sterilization prevent pelvic infection? *Journal of Reproductive Medicine,* **20,** 289.

Halbrecht, I. 1956. Latent genital tuberculosis as the main cause of tubal occlusion in primary sterility. *International Journal of Fertility,* **1,** 367.

Haldane, J. 1949. Disease and evolution. *La Ricerca Sci.* (Suppl.), **19,** 2.

Hall, P. 1976. The treatment of malaria. *British Medical Journal,* **1,** 323.

Hallo, H. 1971. Female genital tuberculosis. In R. Kleinman and V. Pickles (eds.), *Fertility and Sterility: Abstracts of papers presented at the Seventh World Congress,* p. 138. Amsterdam: Excerpta Medica.

Hamilton, P., D. Gebbie, N. Wilks, and F. Lothe. 1972. The role of malaria, folic acid deficiency and haemoglobin AS in pregnancy in Mulago [Uganda] Hospital. *Transactions of the Royal Society of Tropical Medicine and Hygiene,* **66,** 594.

Handsfield, H., W. Hodson, and K. Holmes. 1973. Neonatal gonococcal infection. I. Orogastric contamination with *Neisseria gonorrhoeae. Journal of the American Medical Association,* **225,** 697.

Handsfield, H., T. Lipman, J. Harnisch, E. Tronca, and K. Holmes. 1974. Asymptomatic gonorrhea in men. *New England Journal of Medicine,* **290,**117.

Haney, D. 1982. Herpes treatment called ineffective in recurrences. *Philadelphia Inquirer,* June 5, 1B.

Hang, L., D. Boros, and K. Warren. 1974. Induction of immunological hyporesponsiveness to granulomatous hypersensitivity in *Schistosoma mansoni* infection. *Journal of Infectious Diseases,* **130,** 515.

Hansluwka, H. 1975. Health, population, and socio-economic development. In L. Tabah (ed.), *Population growth and economic development in the third world*. Liège, Belgium: Ordina.

Hanson, W. 1977. Immune response and mechanisms of resistance in *Trypanosoma cruzi*. In *Chagas' disease*, Pan American Health Organization Scientific Publication No. 347, pp. 22–34. Proceedings of an International Symposium held in conjunction with the Fifth International Congress on Protozoology, New York, June.

Hansson, H. and I. Juhlin. 1975. Clinical patterns of uncomplicated gonococcal infections. In D. Danielsson *et al.* (eds.), *Genital infections and their complications*, pp. 73–76. Stockholm: Almqvist and Wiksell International.

Harahap, M. 1980. Sexually transmitted diseases in Indonesia. *British Journal of Venereal Diseases*, **56**, 282.

Harris, R. 1974. Viral teratogenesis: A review with experimental and clinical perspective. *American Journal of Obstetrics and Gynecology*, **119**, 996.

Harrison, K. 1974. Malaria transmission and fetal growth. *British Medical Journal*, **4**, 229.

Harrison, K., and P. Ibeziako. 1973. Maternal anemia and fetal birth weight. *Journal of Obstetrics and Gynaecology of the British Commonwealth*, **80**, 798.

Harrison, M. 1977. *Infertility: A couple's guide to causes and treatments*. Boston: Houghton Mifflin.

Harrison, R., J. de Louvois, M. Blades, and R. Hurley. 1975. Doxycycline treatment and human infertility. *Lancet*, **1**, 605.

Harter, C. 1970. The fertility of sterile and subfecund women in New Orleans. *Social Biology*, **17**, 195.

Harter, C., and K. Benirschke. 1976. Fetal syphilis in the first trimester. *American Journal of Obstetrics and Gynecology*, **124**, 705.

Haupt, A. 1980. Africa faces new population challenges. *Intercom*, **8**, 5, 1.

Hawking, F. 1975. The distribution of human filariasis throughout the world. Part IV. America. World Health Organization, WHO/FIL/75.136, 1.

Hawthorn, G. 1970. *The sociology of fertility*. London: Collier-Macmillan.

Hedberg, E. 1965. Gonorrheal salpingitis, views on treatment and prognosis. *Fertility and Sterility*, **16**, 125.

Hedberg, E., and S. Spetz. 1958. Acute salpingitis: Views on prognosis and treatment. *Acta Obstetricia et Gynecologica Scandinavica*, **37**, 131.

Hellman, L., J. Pritchard, and R. Wynn (eds.). 1971. *Williams' obstetrics* (14th edition). New York: Appleton-Century-Crofts.

Hendershot, G., W. Mosher, and W. Pratt. 1982. Infertility and age: An unresolved issue. *Family Planning Perspectives*, **14**, 287.

Henig, R. 1981. The child savers. *New York Times Magazine*, March 22, 34.

Henin, R. 1969. The patterns and causes of fertility differentials in the Sudan. *Population Studies*, **23**, 171.

Henry-Suchet, J., and V. Loffredo. 1980. Chlamydiae and mycoplasma genital infection in salpingitis and tubal sterility. *Lancet*, **1**, 539.

Hesser, J., B. Blumberg, and J. Drew. 1976. Hepatitis B surface antigen, fertility and sex ratio: Implications for health planning. In B. Kaplan (ed.), *Anthropological studies of human fertility*, pp. 73–81. Detroit: Wayne State University Press.

Hiatt, R., and M. Gebre-Medhin. 1977. Morbidity of *Schistosoma mansoni* infections: An epidemiologic study based on quantitative analysis of egg excretion in Ethiopian children. *American Journal of Tropical Medicine and Hygiene*, **26**, 473.

Hoare, C. 1970. Systematic description of the mammalian trypanosomes of Africa. In H. Mulligan and W. Potts (eds.), *The African trypanosomiases*, pp. 24–59. London: Allen and Unwin.

Hoff, R., K. Mott, M. Milanesi, A. Bittencourt, and H. Barbosa. 1978. Congenital Chagas' disease in an urban population: Investigation of infected twins. *Transactions of the Royal Society of Tropical Medicine and Hygiene,* **72,** 247.

Hofsten, E., and H. Lundstrom. 1976. *Swedish population in history: Main trends from 1750 to 1970.* Stockholm: National Central Bureau of Statistics.

Holder, W., and J. Knox. 1972. Syphilis in pregnancy. *Medical Clinics of North America,* **56,** 1151.

Holmes, K. 1975. Average risk of gonorrheal infection after exposure. *Medical Aspects of Human Sexuality,* **9,** February, 83.

Holmes, K., and D. Hobson. 1977. Introduction. In D. Hobson and K. Holmes (eds.), *Nongonococcal urethritis and related infections,* pp. 1–5. Washington, DC: American Society for Microbiology.

Holmes, K., and M. Puziss. 1980. News from the National Institute of Allergy and Infectious Diseases. Recommendations of the Study Group for Research and Training in Sexually Transmitted Diseases. *Journal of Infectious Diseases,* **142,** 639.

Holtz, F. 1930. Klinische studien uber die nicht tuberkulose salpingoophoritis. *Acta Obstetricia et Gynecologica Scandinavica* (Suppl.), **10,** 5.

Hopcraft, M., A. Verhagen, S. Nigigi, and E. Haga. 1973. Genital infections in developing countries: Experience in a family planning clinic. *Bulletin of the World Health Organization,* **48,** 581.

Horger, E. 1972. Sickle cell and sickle cell-hemoglobin C disease during pregnancy. *Obstetrics and Gynecology,* **39,** 873.

Horton, P., and G. Leslie. 1974. *The sociology of social problems.* Englewood Cliffs, NJ: Prentice Hall.

Hotelling, H., and F. Hotelling. 1931. Causes of birth rate fluctuations. *Journal of the American Statistical Association,* **26,** 135.

Houba, V. 1981. Immune complexes in malaria and their immunopathological significance. World Health Organization, WHO/MAL/81.963, 1.

Hovelius, B., I. Thelin, and P. Mardh. 1979. *Staphylococcus saprophyticus* in the aetiology of nongonococcal urethritis. *British Journal of Venereal Diseases,* **55,** 369.

Howard, J. 1976. Clinical aspects of congenital Chagas' disease. In *New approaches in American trypanosomiasis research,* Pan American Health Organization Scientific Publication No. 318, pp. 212–215. Proceedings of an International Symposium, Belo Horizonte, Minas Gerais, Brazil, March 1975.

Howe, G. (ed.). 1977. *A world geography of human diseases.* London: Academic Press.

Howe, M. 1974. For Brazil's tribes, a new will to live. *New York Times,* August 2, 29.

Howell, N. 1979. *Demography of the Dobe !Kung.* London: Academic Press.

Hull, T., and Tukiran. 1976. Regional variations in the prevalence of childlessness in Indonesia. *The Indonesian Journal of Geography,* **6,** 32, 1.

Hunter, G., J. Swartzwelder, and D. Clyde (eds.). 1976. *Tropical medicine* (5th edition). Philadelphia: Saunders.

Hyde, J. 1979. *Understanding human sexuality.* New York: McGraw-Hill.

Ibeziako, P. 1974. Age and infertility with particular reference to VVF [vesicovaginal fistula]. In B. Adadevoh (ed.), *Sub-fertility and infertility in Africa,* pp. 92–93. Ibadan, Nigeria: Caxton Press.

Ikede, B. 1974. Subfertility and infertility in Africa: The role of trypanosomiasis. In B. Adadevoh (ed.), *Sub-fertility and infertility in Africa,* pp. 87–89. Ibadan, Nigeria: Caxton Press.

Intercom. 1976. World liberalizing abortion views. **4,** 4, 9.

Intercom. 1977. Malaria still a killer—vaccine near? **5,** 1, 11. (a)

Intercom. 1977. Sleeping sickness vaccine near. **5,** 4, 13. (b)

Intercom. 1978. Across the border for abortion—to China. **6,** 12, 5. (a)

Intercom. 1978. Population hearings look at impact of U.S. immigration. **6,** 5, 13. (b)

Intercom. 1978. Select committee focuses on population, development aid. **6,** 6 12. (c)

Intercom. 1978. U.S. hearings take official look at status of Depo-Provera. **6,** 9, 9. (d)

Intercom. 1979. Fertility in Kenya: Alarmingly high and continuing to rise. **7,** 10, 3.

Intercom. 1980. Making an end run around blocked fallopian tubes. **8,** 11, 2.

Intercom. 1982. Depo-Provera still waiting for U.S. government approval. **10,** 1, 14.

International Family Planning Perspectives and Digest. 1978. No apparent harmful effect from legal abortion on later pregnancies; D and C possible exception. **4,** 23.

Isaac, V. 1971. Genital tuberculosis and infertility in South Indian patients. In R. Kleiman and V. Pickles (eds.), *Fertility and Sterility: Abstracts of papers presented at the Seventh World Congress,* p. 97. Amsterdam: Excepta Medica.

Isley, R. 1980. Medical, socio-cultural, economic and psychological correlates of childlessness in Africa. RTI Concept Paper No. 24-CP-80-01, Research Triangle Institute, Research Triangle Park.

Israel, S. 1967. *Diagnosis and treatment of menstrual disorders and sterility.* New York: Harper and Row.

Iturregui-Pagan, J., R. Fortuno, and M. Noy. 1976. Genital manifestations of filariasis. *Urology,* **8,** 207.

Jackson, W. 1972. Diabetes and related variables among the five main racial groups in South Africa: Comparisons from population studies. *Postgraduate Medical Journal,* **48,** 391.

Jacobs, D. 1978. Syphilis in Australian aborigines in the northern territory. *Medical Journal of Australia,* **1,** 10.

Jacobson, L. and L. Westrom. 1969. Objectivized diagnosis of acute pelvic inflammatory disease. *American Journal of Obstetrics and Gynecology,* **105,** 1088.

Jacobsson, L., B. von Schoultz, and F. Solheim. 1976. Repeat aborters—first aborters, a social-psychiatric comparison. *Social Psychiatry,* **11,** 75.

Jain, A., and B. Moots. 1977. Fecundability following the discontinuation of IUD use among Taiwanese women. *Journal of Biosocial Science,* **9,** 137.

Jansen, L. 1952. Measuring family solidarity. *American Sociological Review,* **17,** 727.

Jeansson, S. and L. Molin. 1975. Genital herpes simplex infection. In D. Danielsson *et al.* (eds.), *Genital infections and their complications,* pp. 189–191. Stockholm: Almqvist and Wiksell International.

Jedberg, H. 1950. A study on genital tuberculosis in women. *Acta Obstetricia et Gynecologica Scandinavica,* **31,** Supplement 1, 130.

Jelliffe, D. 1967. Prematurity. In J. Lawson and D. Stewart (eds.), *Obstetrics and gynaecology in the tropics and developing countries,* pp. 253–276. London: Edward Arnold.

Jelliffe, E. 1967. Placental malaria and foetal growth failure. In G. Wolstenholme and M. O'Connor (eds.), *Nutrition and infection,* Ciba Foundation Study Group No. 31, pp. 18–40. Boston: Little, Brown.

Jelliffe, E. 1975. Malarial chemoprophylaxis for pregnant women. *Journal of Pediatrics,* **86,** 820.

Johnson, F. 1977. Chemoprophylaxis of malaria. *British Medical Journal,* **1,** 1535.

Johnston, F. 1974. Control of age at menarche. *Human Biology,* **46,** 159.

Jonas, G. 1978. Africa: Taming the tsetse. *R. F.* [Rockefeller Foundation] *Illustrated,* **4,** 1, 1.

Jones, A. 1967. *Introduction to parasitology.* Reading, MA: Addison-Wesley.

Jordan, A. 1976. Tsetse control—present and future. *Transactions of the Royal Society of Tropical Medicine and Hygiene*, **70**, 128.

Jordan, P. 1960. Bancroftian filariasis in Tanganyika: Observations on elephantiasis, microfilarial density, genital filariasis and microfilaraemia rates. *Annals of Tropical Medicine and Parasitology*, **54**, 132.

Jordan, P. 1972. Epidemiology and control of schistosomiasis. *British Medical Bulletin*, **28**, 55.

Jordan, P., and G. Webbe. 1969. *Human schistosomiasis*. London: William Heinemann.

Josey, W., A. Nahmias, and Z. Naib. 1969. Viral and virus-like infections of the female genital tract. *Clinical Obstetrics and Gynecology*, **12**, 161.

Journal of the American Medical Association. 1981. The silent clap. **245**, 609.

Journal of Tropical Medicine and Hygiene. 1977. Editorial: WHO Weekly Epidemiological Review 1977 No. 41, **80**, 229.

Juhlin, L., and J. Wallin. 1972. Factors which increase the spread of gonorrhea. *Postgraduate Medical Journal*, January Supplement, 12.

Kamel, I., A. Elwi, A. Cheever, J. Moismann, and R. Danner. 1978. *Schistosoma mansoni* and *S. haematobium* infections in Egypt. IV. Hepatic lesions. *American Journal of Tropical Medicine and Hygiene*, **27**, 931.

Kampmeier, R. 1974. Final report on the "Tuskegee Syphilis Study." *Southern Medical Journal*, **67**, 1349.

Karayalcin, G., M. Imran, and F. Rosner. 1972. Priapism in sickle cell disease: Report of five cases. *American Journal of Medical Science*, **264**, 289.

Katchadourian, H., and D. Lunde. 1980. *Biological aspects of human sexuality*. New York: Holt, Rinehart, and Winston.

Kerslake, D., and D. Casey. 1967. Abortion induced by means of uterine aspiration. *Obstetrics and Gynecology, N.Y.*, **30**, 35.

Keyfitz, N. 1981. Evaluation of the International Union for Scientific Study of Population Seminar on Population and Biology. *IUSSP Newsletter*, **14**, September, 14.

King, B. 1944. Early filariasis diagnosis and clinical findings: A report of 268 cases in American troops. *American Journal of Tropical Medicine*, **24**, 285.

King, T., and R. Burkman. 1977. Pelvic inflammatory disease. In R. de Alvarez (ed.), *Textbook of gynecology*, pp. 413–429. Philadelphia: Lea and Febiger.

Kiple, K., and V. King. 1981. *Another dimension to the black diaspora. Diet, disease, and racism*. New York: Cambridge University Press.

Kiraly, K. 1973. The venereal disease problem around the world. *Journal of Reproductive Medicine*, **11**, 119.

Kirk, D. 1971. A new demographic transition? In *Rapid population growth: Consequences and policy implications. Vol. 2*, pp. 123–147. National Academy of Sciences. Baltimore: Johns Hopkins University Press.

Kiser, C. 1939. Voluntary and involuntary aspects of childlessness. *Milbank Memorial Fund Quarterly*, **17**, 50.

Kissane, J. 1975. *Pathology of infancy and childhood* [2ⁿᵈ edition]. St. Louis, MO: Mosby.

Kissane, J., and M. Smith. 1967. *Pathology of infancy and childhood*. St. Louis, MO: Mosby.

Kleegman, S. 1967. Planned parenthood: Its influence on public health and family welfare. In H. Rosen (ed.), *Abortion in America*, pp. 254–265. Boston: Beacon Press.

Klein, T., J. Richmond, and D. Mishell. 1976. Pelvic tuberculosis. *Obstetrics and Gynecology*, **48**, 99.

Klimas, A. 1982. A comparison of the mortality of reservation and non-reservation Indians. Paper presented to the Population Association of America meetings, San Diego, March.

Knodel, J. 1974. *The decline of fertility in Germany, 1871–1939.* Princeton: Princeton University Press.

Knodel, J., and C. Wilson. 1981. The secular increase in fecundity in German village populations: An analysis of reproductive histories of couples married 1750–1899. *Population Studies,* **35,** 53.

Knopf, S. 1915. Birth control and tuberculosis. *Survey,* **34,** 345.

Knopf, S. 1932. Birth control in disease. *The Nation,* **134,** 109.

Koberle, F. 1974. Pathogenesis of Chagas' disease. In *Trypanosomiasis and leishmaniasis with special reference to Chagas' disease,* Ciba Foundation Symposium No. 20, pp. 137–152. Amsterdam: Associated Scientific Publishers.

Kondo, A. 1971. Treatment of male genital tuberculosis. In R. Kleinman and V. Pickles (eds.), *Fertility and Sterility: Abstracts of papers presented at the Seventh World Congress,* p. 139. Amsterdam: Excerpta Medica.

Kotulak, R. 1981. Syphilis test draws bad blood. *Philadelphia Inquirer,* December 6, 14H.

Krahn, H., A. Tessler, and R. Hotchkiss. 1963. Studies of the effect of hydrocele upon scrotal temperature, pressure, and testicular morphology. *Fertility and Sterility,* **14,** 226.

Kraus, S. 1972. Complications of gonococcal infection. *Medical Clinics of North America,* **56,** 1115.

Krause, J. 1963. English population movements between 1700 and 1850. *Proceedings of the International Population Conference, New York, 1961.* Vol. 1, pp. 585–590. London: International Union for the Scientific Study of Population.

Krishna, U., A. Sathe, H. Mehta, S. Wagle, and V. Purandare. 1979. Tubal factors in sterility. *Journal of Obstetrics and Gynaecology of India,* **29,** 663. (a)

Krishna, U., S. Sheth, and N. Motashaw. 1979. Place of laparoscopy in pelvic inflammatory disease. *Journal of Obstetrics and Gynaecology of India,* **29,** 505. (b)

Kuhr, M. 1973. Fetal risks in rubella vaccination. *Journal of the American Medical Association,* **226,** 1357.

Lachman, E. 1973. The anatomy of male gonorrhea. *Medical Times,* **101,** 47.

Ladipo, O. 1980. Seminal analysis in fertile and infertile Nigerian men. *Journal of the National Medical Association,* **72,** 785.

Lambert, S. 1934. *The depopulation of Pacific races.* Honolulu: Bishop Museum, Special Publication 23.

Lancet. 1978. Malaria and immunology. 2, 974. (a)

Lancet. 1978. New leads for trypanosomiasis chemotherapy. 2, 1190. (b)

Lancet. 1979. Malaria—The Phoenix with drug resistance. 1, 1328.

Langford, C. 1981. Fertility change in Sri Lanka since the war: An analysis of the experience of different districts. *Population Studies,* **35,** 285.

Lantum, D. 1971. The malaria problem in Cameroon in 1969. (A demographic perspective). *West African Medical Journal,* **20,** 285.

Lantum, D. 1979. *Population dynamics of rural Cameroon and its public health repercussions.* Yaounde, Cameroon Public Health Unit, University Centre for Health Sciences, University of Yaounde.

Laser, H., and R. Klein. 1979. Haemoglobin S. and *P. falciparum* malaria. *Nature,* **280,** 613.

Lawson, J. 1967. Anaemia in pregnancy. In J. Lawson and D. Stewart (eds.), *Obstetrics and gynaecology in the tropics and developing countries,* pp. 73–99. London: Edward Arnold. (a)

Lawson, J. 1967. Chronic lymphoedema and elephantiasis of the vulva. In J. Lawson and D. Stewart (eds.), *Obstetrics and gynaecology in the tropics and developing countries,* pp. 466–480. London: Edward Arnold. (b)

Lawson, J. 1967. Infections complicating pregnancy. In J. Lawson and D. Stewart (eds.), *Obstetrics and gynaecology in the tropics and developing countries,* pp. 43–58. London: Edward Arnold. (c)

Lawson, J. 1967. Malaria and pregnancy. In J. Lawson and D. Stewart (eds.), *Obstetrics and gynaecology in the tropics and developing countries,* pp. 59–72. London: Edward Arnold. (d)

Lawson, J. 1967. Obstructed labor. In J. Lawson and D. Stewart (eds.), *Obstetrics and gynaecology in the tropics and developing countries,* pp. 172–202. London: Edward Arnold. (e)

Lawson, J. 1967. Sequelae of obstructed labour. In J. Lawson and D. Stewart (eds.), *Obstetrics and gynaecology in the tropics and developing countries,* pp. 203–218. London: Edward Arnold. (f)

Lawson, J., and D. Stewart (eds.). 1967. *Obstetrics and gynaecology in the tropics and developing countries.* London: Edward Arnold.

Learmonth, A. 1972. Atlases in medical geography 1950–70: A review. In N. McGlashan (ed.), *Medical geography,* pp. 133–152. London: Metheun.

Leary, W. 1982. Good effect of legal abortion on U.S. health is spelled out. *Philadelphia Inquirer,* July 11, 4A.

Ledward, R. 1980. Infertility in Saudi Arabia: Initial experience in a new gynaecological unit. *Tropical Doctor,* **10,** 117.

Lee, P. 1977. Review of Thomas McKeown's "The modern rise of population." *Studies in Family Planning,* **9,** 295.

Lee, R. 1977. Methods and models for analyzing historical series of births, deaths, and marriages. In R. Lee (ed.), *Population patterns in the past,* pp. 337–370. New York: Academic Press.

Leke, R. and B. Nash. 1981. Biological and socio-cultural aspects of infertility and subfertility in Africa. In United Nations Economic Commission for Africa (UNECA), *Population dynamics: Fertility and mortality in Africa,* pp. 488–498. ST/ECA/SER.A/1; UNFPA Project No. RAF/78/P17. Addis Ababa, Ethiopia, UNECA, May.

Lepes, T. 1981. Malaria—A global health problem. World Health Organization, WHO/MAL/81.949.

Leridon, H. 1973. *Aspects biométriques de la fécondité humaine.* Paris: Presses Universitaires de France. (a)

Leridon, H. 1973. *Natalité, saisons et conjoncture économique.* Paris: Presses Universitaires de France. (b)

Leridon, H. 1977. *Human fertility: The basic components.* Chicago: University of Chicago Press.

Leridon, H. 1982. Stérilité, hypofertilité et infécondité en France. *Population,* **37,** 807.

Leridon, H., and J. Menken (eds.). 1979. *Natural fertility.* Liège, Belgium: Ordina.

Lessa, W. 1955. Depopulation of Ulithi. *Human Biology,* **27,** 161.

Lessa, W., and G. Myers. 1962. Population dynamics of an atoll community. *Population Studies,* **15,** 752.

Lesthaeghe, R. 1977. *The decline of Belgian fertility, 1880–1970.* Princeton: Princeton University Press.

Levy, N. 1978. Sexual factors and rehabilitation. *Dialysis and Transplantation,* **7,** 591.

Lewis, R., N. Lauersen, and S. Birnbaum. 1973. Malaria associated with pregnancy. *Obstetrics and Gynecology,* **42,** 696.

Lich, R., and L. Howerton. 1970. Anatomy and surgical approach to the urogenital tract in the male. In M. Campbell and J. Harrison (eds.), *Urology, Vol. 1* (3rd edition), pp. 1–38. Philadelphia: Saunders.

Livi-Bacci, M. 1971. *A century of Portuguese fertility.* Princeton: Princeton University Press.

Livi-Bacci, M. 1977. *A history of Italian fertility.* Princeton: Princeton University Press.

Livingstone, F. 1957. Sickling and malaria. *British Medical Journal,* **1**, 762.

Livingstone, F. 1971. Malaria and human polymorphisms. *Annual Review of Genetics,* **5**, 33.

Llewellyn-Jones, D. 1974. *Human reproduction and society.* New York: Pitman.

Logie, D., I. McGregor, D. Rowe, and W. Billewicz. 1973. Plasma immunoglobin concentrations in mothers and newborn children with special reference to placental malaria. *Bulletin of the World Health Organization,* **49**, 547.

Logrillo, V., P. Luickenton, G. Therriault, and M. Ellrott. 1980. Effect of induced abortion on subsequent reproductive function. Final report on research carried out by the New York State Department of Health, Office of Biostatistics under Contract No. NO1-HD-6-2802, National Institute of Child Health and Human Development. Albany, New York: New York State Health Department.

Long, E. 1971. Tuberculosis. *Encyclopaedia Britannica,* **20**, 298.

Lowell, A., L. Edwards, and C. Palmer. 1969. *Tuberculosis.* Cambridge, MA: Harvard University Press.

Lucas, J. 1972. The national venereal disease problem. *Medical Clinics of North America,* **56**, 1073.

Lumsden, W. 1976. Chagas' disease—A survey of the present position. *Transactions of the Royal Society of Tropical Medicine and Hygiene,* **70**, 121.

Luzzatto, L. 1974. Genetic factors in malaria. *Bulletin of the World Health Organization,* **50**, 195.

Luzzatto, L. and U. Bienzle. 1979. The malaria/G-6-PD hypothesis. *Lancet,* **1**, 1183.

Lwanga, C. 1977. Infertility and subfertility in Africa. In *Family welfare and development in Africa,* pp. 61–73. London: International Planned Parenthood Federation.

Macgregor, J., and J. Avery. 1974. Malaria transmission and fetal growth. *British Medical Journal,* **3**, 433.

Mackie, T., G. Hunter, and C. Worth (eds.). 1954. *A manual of tropical medicine* (2nd edition). Philadelphia: Saunders.

Maekelt, G. 1970. Seroepidemiology of Chagas' disease. *Journal of Parasitology,* **5**, 557.

Maekelt, G. 1974. Discussion following Koberle. In *Trypanosomiasis and leishmaniasis with special reference to Chagas' disease,* Ciba Foundation Symposium No. 20, pp. 152–158. Amsterdam: Associated Scientific Publishers.

Magdi, I. 1967. Bilharziasis (schistosomiasis) of the female genital tract. In J. Lawson and D. Stewart (eds.), *Obstetrics and gynaecology in the tropics and developing countries,* pp. 416–431. London: Edward Arnold.

Magnuson, H., E. Thomas, S. Olansky, B. Kaplan, L. de Mello, and J. Cutler. 1956. Inoculation syphilis in human volunteers. *Medicine,* **35**, 33.

Mahler, H. 1979. An interview with Halfdan Mahler entitled, ''Rescue mission for tomorrow's health.'' *People* (UK), **6**, 2, 25.

Mahmoud, A. 1977. Schistosomiasis. *New England Journal of Medicine,* **297**, 1329.

Mahoney, L., and J. Kessel. 1971. Treatment failure in filariasis in mass treatment programmes. *Bulletin of the World Health Organization,* **45**, 35.

Maize, K. 1978. 20 million children who need vaccination. *Parade,* March 26, 22.

Malaviya, A. 1976. Discussion following the paper, Secondary immuno-deficiency in tuberculosis. *Journal of the All India Institute of Medical Sciences,* **1**, 198.

Mansfield, J. 1978. Immunobiology of African trypanosomiasis. *Cellular Immunology,* **39**, 204.

Manson-Bahr, P. 1966. *Manson's tropical medicine* (16th edition). Baltimore: Williams and Wilkins.

Marano, H. 1971. She may look clean. *Emergency Medicine*, **3**, 99.

Marble, A., P. White, R. Bradley, and L. Krall (eds.). 1971. *Joslin's diabetes mellitus* (11th edition). Philadelphia: Lea and Febiger.

Marcy, P. 1981. Factors affecting the fecundity and fertility of historical populations: A review. *Journal of Family History*, **6**, 309.

Mardh, P. 1980. An overview of infectious agents of salpingitis, their biology, and recent advances in methods of detection. *American Journal of Obstetrics and Gynecology*, **138**, 933.

Mardh, P., I. Lind, L. Svensson, L. Westrom, and B. Moller. 1981. Antibodies to *Chlamydia trachomatis*, *Mycoplasma hominis*, and *Neisseria gonorrhoeae* in sera from patients with acute salpingitis. *British Journal of Venereal Diseases*, **57**, 125.

Mardh, P., T. Ripa, L. Svensson, and L. Westrom. 1977. *Chlamydia trachomatis* infection in patients with acute salpingitis. *New England Journal of Medicine*, **296**, 1377.

Mardh, P., L. Westrom, and S. Colleen. 1975. Infections of the genital and urinary tracts with mycoplasmas and ureaplasmas. In D. Danielsson *et al.* (eds.), *Genital infections and their complications*, pp. 53–62. Stockholm: Almqvist and Wiksell International.

Marsden, P. 1971. South American trypanosomiasis. *International Review of Tropical Medicine*, **4**, 97.

Marsden, P. 1974. South American trypanosomiasis. *Tropical Doctor*, **1**, 12.

Martin, D., L. Koutsky, D. Eschenbach, J. Daling, E. Alexander, J. Benedetti, and K. Holmes. 1982. Prematurity and perinatal mortality in pregnancies complicated by maternal *Chlamydia trachomatis* infections. *Journal of the American Medical Association*, **247**, 1585.

Martin, S., L. Miller, D. Alling, V. Okoye, G. Esan, B. Osunkoya, and M. Deane. 1979. Severe malaria and glucose-6-phosphate dehydrogenase deficiency: A reappraisal of the malaria/G-6-PD hypothesis. *Lancet*, **1**, 524. (a)

Martin, S., L. Miller, C. Hicks, A. David-West, C. Ugbode, and M. Deane. 1979. Frequency of blood group antigens in Nigerian children with falciparum malaria. *Transactions of the Royal Society of Tropical Medicine and Hygiene*, **73**, 216. (b)

Masawe, A., J. Muindi, and G. Swai. 1974. Infections in iron deficiency and other types of anaemia in the tropics. *Lancet*, **2**, 314.

Masnick, G., and J. McFalls. 1976. A new perspective on the twentieth-century American fertility swing. *Journal of Family History*, **1**, 217.

Masnick, G., and J. McFalls. 1978. Those perplexing U.S. fertility swings. *PRB* [Population Reference Bureau] *Report*, November 1.

Masters, W., and V. Johnson. 1966. *Human sexual response*. Boston: Little, Brown.

Masters, W., and V. Johnson. 1970. *Human sexual inadequacy*. Boston: Little, Brown.

Masters, W., V. Johnson, and R. Kolodny. 1982. *Human sexuality*. Boston: Little, Brown.

Mati, J., A. Hatimy, and D. Gibbie. 1971. The importance of anaemia of pregnancy in Nairobi, and the role of malaria in the aetiology of megaloblastic anaemia. *Journal of Tropical Medicine, and Hygiene*, **74**, 1.

Matthews, C., R. Elmslie, K. Clapp, and J. Svigos. 1975. The frequency of genital mycoplasma infection in human fertility. *Fertility and Sterility*, **26**, 988.

Mazor, M. 1979. Barren couples. *Psychology Today*, May, 101.

McCullough, F. 1980. Organization of schistosomiasis control in the African region. World Health Organization, WHO/SCHISTO/80.48.

McFalls, J. 1973. Impact of VD on the fertility of the U.S. black population, 1880–1950. *Social Biology*, **20**, 2.

McFalls, J. 1979. Frustrated fertility: A population paradox. *Population Bulletin*, **34**, 2 (a)

McFalls, J. 1979. *Psychopathology and subfecundity*. New York: Academic Press. (b)

McFalls, J., and G. Masnick. 1981. Birth control and the fertility of the U.S. black population, 1880 to 1980. *Journal of Family History*, **6**, 89.

McFalls, J., and S. Tolnay. Forthcoming. *Black fertility in the United States: A social demographic history*. Durham, NC: Duke University Press.

McFee, J. 1973. Anemia: A high-risk complication of pregnancy. *Clinical Obstetrics and Gynecology*, **16**, 153.

McGregor, I. 1974. Mechanisms of acquired immunity and epidemiological patterns of antibody response in malaria in man. *Bulletin of the World Health Organization*, **50**, 259.

McKay, J. 1981. Diabetics find pregnancy worth the risk. *Philadelphia Bulletin*, May 24, B4.

McKelvy, J., and T. Turner. 1934. Syphilis and pregnancy. *Journal of the American Medical Association*, **102**, 503.

McKeown, T. 1976. *The modern rise of population*. New York: Academic Press.

McKeown, T. 1978. Fertility, mortality, and causes of death: An examination of issues related to *The modern rise of population*. *Population Studies*, **32**, 535.

McKusick, V. 1964. *Human genetics*. Englewood Cliffs, NJ: Prentice-Hall.

McNeill, W. 1976. *Plagues and people*. Garden City, NY: Doubleday.

Medawar, P. 1971. Do advances in medicine lead to genetic deterioration? In C. Bajema (ed.), *Natural selection in human populations*, pp. 300–308. New York: Wiley.

Medlar, E. 1955. *The behavior of pulmonary tuberculosis lesions*. New York: Metropolitan Life Insurance Company.

Medlar, E., D. Spain, and R. Holliday. 1949. Post-mortem compared with clinical diagnosis of genito-urinary tuberculosis in adult males. *Journal of Urology*, **61**, 1078.

Meheus, A., R. Ballard, M. Dlamini, E. Van Dyck, and P. Piot. 1980. Epidemiology and aetiology of urethritis in Swaziland. *International Journal of Epidemiology*, **9**, 239.

Melo, J. 1979. Nongonococcal urethritis. *Journal of the Kentucky Medical Association*, **77**, 520.

Menken, J. 1972. The health and social consequences of teenage childbearing. *Family Planning Perspectives*, **4**, 3, 45.

Menken, J. 1979. Introduction. In H. Leridon and J. Menken (eds.), *Natural fertility*, pp. 1–12. Liège, Belgium: Ordina.

Menken, J., J. Trussel, and S. Watkins. 1981. The nutrition-fertility link: An evaluation of the evidence. *Journal of Interdisciplinary History*, **11**, 425.

Meuwissen, J. 1966. Natality and marital infertility in Ghana. *Tropical and Geographical Medicine*, **18**, 153.

Meuwissen, J. 1967. Human infertility in Ghana. *Fertility and Sterility*, **18**, 223. (a)

Meuwissen, J. 1967. Human infertility in Ghana. In B. Westin and N. Wiquist (eds.), *Fertility and Sterility: Proceedings of the Fifth World Congress*, pp. 1203–1205. Amsterdam: Excerpta Medica. (b)

Middlemiss, J. 1972. Radiology of the urinary tract in the tropics. *British Medical Bulletin*, **28**, 255.

Miles, M. 1976. Human behavior and the propagation of Chagas' disease. *Transactions of the Royal Society of Tropical Medicine and Hygiene*, **70**, 521.

Millar, J. 1973. The national venereal disease problem. *Journal of Reproductive Medicine*, **11**, 111.

Miller, L., S. Mason, D. Clyde, and M. McGinniss. 1976. The resistance factor to *Plasmodium vivax* in blacks. *New England Journal of Medicine*, **295**, 302.

Mohr, J. 1978. *Abortion in America. The origins and evolution of national policy, 1800–1900*. New York: Oxford University Press.

Moller, B., E. Freundt, F. Black, and P. Frederiksen. 1978. Experimental infection of the genital tract of female grivet monkeys by *Mycoplasma hominis*. *Infection and Immunity*, **20**, 248.

Moller, B., and P. Mardh. 1980. Experimental salpingitis in grivet monkeys by *Chlamydia trachomatis*. *Acta Pathologica et Microbiologica Scandinavica Sect. B*, **88**, 107.

Money, J. 1967. Sexual problems of the chronically ill. In C. Wahl (ed.), *Sexual problems*, pp. 266–288. New York: Free Press.

Monif, G. 1974. *Infectious diseases in obstetrics and gynecology*. Hagerstown: Harper and Row.

Monif, G. 1980. Significance of polymicrobial bacterial superinfection in the therapy of gonococcal endometritis–salpingitis–peritonitis. *Obstetrics and Gynecology*, **55** (Supplement 5), 154S.

Montefiore, D., A. Sogbetun, and C. Anong. 1980. *Herpesvirus hominis* type 2 infection in Ibadan. *British Journal of Venereal Diseases*, **56**, 49.

Mooney, E. 1979. The white plague. *American Heritage*, **30**, 54.

Morishima, H., B. Glaser, W. Niemann, and L. James. 1975. Increased uterine activity and fetal deterioration during maternal hyperthermia. *American Journal of Obstetrics and Gynecology*, **121**, 531.

Morley, D., M. Woodland, and W. Cuthbertson. 1964. Controlled trial of pyrimethamine in pregnant women in an African village. *British Medical Journal*, **1**, 667.

Morris, C., F. Boxall, and H. Cayton. 1970. Genital tract tuberculosis in subfertile women. *Journal of Medical Microbiology*, **3**, 85.

Morrison, J., P. Roe, R. Stahl, W. Whybrew, E. Bocovaz, W. Wiser, A. Kraus, and S. Fish. 1973. Heterozygous thalassemia and pregnancy: A twenty-five year experience. *Journal of Reproductive Medicine*, **11**, 35.

Morse, D. 1967. Tuberculosis. In D. Brothwell and A. Sandison (eds.), *Diseases in antiquity*, pp. 249–271. Springfield, IL: Thomas.

Mosher, W. 1982. Fertility and family planning in the 1970s: The National Survey of Family Growth. *Family Planning Perspectives*, **14**, 314. (a)

Mosher, W. 1982. Infertility trends among U.S. couples: 1965–1976. *Family Planning Perspectives*, **14**, 22. (b)

Mosher, W., and S. Aral, 1983. Factors related to infertility in the U.S., 1965–1976. Unpublished manuscript.

Mosher, W., and W. Pratt. 1982. Reproductive impairments among married couples: United States. *Vital and Health Statistics*, National Center for Health Statistics, Public Health Service. Washington, DC: US Govt. Printing Office.

Mosk, C. 1981. The evolution of the pre-modern demographic regime in Japan. *Population Studies*, **35**, 28.

Mosley, W. (ed.). 1978. *Nutrition and human reproduction*. New York: Plenum.

Mosley, W. 1983. Review of R. Waife and M. Burkhart's *The nonphysician and family health in sub-Saharan Africa*. *Family Planning Perspectives*, **15**, 49.

Mosley, W., L. Werner, and S. Becker. 1982. *The dynamics of birth spacing and marital fertility in Kenya*. World Fertility Survey Scientific Report No. 30. Voorsburg, Netherlands, International Statistical Institute, August.

Mott, F., and S. Mott. 1980. Kenya record population growth: A dilemma of development. *Population Bulletin*, **35**, 3.

Mourant, A., A. Kopic, and K. Domaniewska-Sobczak. 1978. *Blood groups and disease*. New York: Oxford University Press.

Muir, D., and M. Belsey. 1980. Pelvic inflammatory disease and its consequences in the developing world. *American Journal of Obstetrics and Gynecology*, **138**, 913.

Mukherjee, C. 1967. Osteomalacia. In J. Lawson and D. Stewart (eds.), *Obstetrics and gynaecology in the tropics and developing countries*, pp. 29–42. London: Edward Arnold.

Muller, R., 1975. *Worms and disease. A manual of medical helminthology*. London: Heinemann.

Mulligan, H., and W. Potts (eds.). 1970. *The African trypanosomiases*. London: Allen Unwin.

Munisi, S. 1979. Problems exaggerated [Letters]. *People* (UK), **6**, 2, 2.

Murray, J. 1979. Problems exaggerated [Letters]. *People* (UK), **6**, 2, 2.

Myers, J., and J. Steele. 1969. *Bovine tuberculosis control in man and animals.* St. Louis, MO: Green.

Myrdal, G. 1972. *An American dilemma.* New York: Pantheon. (Originally published 1944)

Nag, M. 1962. *Factors affecting human fertility in nonindustrial societies: A cross-cultural study.* New Haven: Yale University Publications in Anthropology.

Nag, M. 1968. *Factors affecting human fertility in nonindustrial societies: A cross-cultural study.* New Haven: Yale University Publications in Anthropology.

Nag, M. 1980. How modernization can also increase fertility. *Current Anthropology,* **21,** 571.

Nahmias, A., W. Josey, and Z. Naib. 1975. Clinical and laboratory aspects of genital herpes simplex virus infections. In D. Danielsson *et al.* (eds.), *Genital infections and their complications,* pp. 183–188. Stockholm: Almqvist and Wiksell International. (a)

Nahmias, A., W. Josey, and Z. Naib. 1975. Viral infections of the urogenital tract. In D. Danielsson *et al.* (eds.), *Genital infections and their complications,* pp. 63–68. Stockholm: Almqvist and Wiksell International. (b)

Nahmias, A., W. Josey, Z. Naib, M. Freeman, R. Fernandez, and J. Wheeler. 1971. Perinatal risk associated with maternal genital herpes simplex virus infection. *American Journal of Obstetrics and Gynecology,* **110,** 825.

Narkavonnakit, T. and T. Bennett. 1981. Health consequences of induced abortion in rural northeast Thailand. *Studies in Family Planning,* **12,** 58.

Nasah, B., M. Azefor, and B. Ondoa. 1974. Clinical and pathological conditions affecting fertility in Cameroon. In B. Adadevoh (ed.), *Sub-fertility and infertility in Africa,* pp. 75–78. Ibadan, Nigeria: Caxton Press.

Nasah, B., and J. Cox. 1978. Vascular lesions in testes associated with male infertility in Cameroon. *Virchows Archiv: Pathological Anatomy and Histology,* **377,** 225.

Nass, G., R. Libby, and M. Fisher. 1981. *Sexual choices.* Belmont, CA: Wadsworth.

Nathanson, B. 1979. *Aborting America.* New York: Doubleday.

National Tuberculosis and Respiratory Disease Association. 1969. *Diagnostic standards and classification of tuberculosis.* New York: National Tuberculosis and Respiratory Disease Association.

Nelson, G. 1979. Current concepts in parasitology. Filariasis. *New England Journal of Medicine,* **300,** 1136.

Nelson, H. 1978. Malaria vaccine set for human testing. *Philadelphia Inquirer,* October 28, D1.

Neves, H., and L. Scaff. 1952. Microfilaremia, congenita. Paper presented at the X Congresso Brazileiro de Hygiene.

Newman, P. 1970. Malaria control and population growth. *Journal of Development Studies,* **6,** 133.

Newsweek. 1947. Pregnancy and TB. July 26, 53.

Newsweek. 1972. VD—The epidemic. January 24, 46.

Newsweek. 1976. Fertility rites. October 11, 61.

Newton, B. 1974. The chemotherapy of trypanosomiasis and leishmaniasis: Towards a more rational approach. In *Trypanosomiasis and leishmaniasis with special reference to Chagas' disease,* Ciba Foundation Symposium No. 20, pp. 285–301. Amsterdam: Associated Scientific Publishers.

New York Times. 1978. Low birth rate in Central Africa causes concern. January 22, 8.

Nickerson, C. 1973. Gonorrhea amnionitis. *Obstetrics and Gynecology,* **42,** 815.

Nicol, C. 1971. Venereal disease in women—I. *British Medical Journal,* **2,** 328. (a)

Nicol, C. 1971. Venereal disease in women—II. *British Medical Journal*, **2**, 383. (b)

Novak, E., and J. Woodruff. 1967. *Novak's gynecologic and obstetric pathology*. Philadelphia: Saunders.

Ogunmodede, E. 1979. End this mutilation. *People* (UK), **6**, 1, 30.

Ojo, O., A. Onifade, E. Akande, and R. Bannerman. 1971. The pattern of female genital tuberculosis in Ibadan. *Israel Journal of Medical Science*, **7**, 280.

Okojie, S. 1976. Induced illegal abortion in Benin City, Nigeria. *International Journal of Gynaecology and Obstetrics*, **14**, 517.

Olusanya, P. 1974. Reduced fertility and associated factors in the Western State of Nigeria. In B. Adadevoh (ed.), *Sub-fertility and infertility in Africa*, pp. 43–53. Ibadan, Nigeria: Caxton Press.

Omran, A. 1971. The epidemiological transition: A theory of the epidemiology of population change. *Milbank Memorial Fund Quarterly*, **49**, 509.

O'Rear, H. 1947. Hazards of bovine tuberculosis as a matter of public health significance and potential lung infections with bovine tubercle bacilli. *Diseases of the Chest*, **13**, 381.

Oriel, J. 1977. *Chlamydia trachomatis* and postgonococcal genital infection. In D. Hobson and K. Holmes (eds.), *Nongonococcal urethritis and related infections*, pp. 230–232. Washington, DC: American Society for Microbiology. (a)

Oriel, J. 1977. Treatment of nongonococcal urethritis. In D. Hobson and K. Holmes (eds.), *Nongonococcal urethritis and related infections*, pp. 38–42. Washington, DC: American Society for Microbiology. (b)

Ormerod, W. 1970. Pathogenesis and pathology of trypanosomiasis in man. In H. Mulligan and W. Potts (eds.), *The African trypanosomiases*, pp. 587–601. London: Allen and Unwin.

O'Sullivan, J., D. Charles, C. Mahan, and R. Dandrow. 1973. Gestational diabetes and perinatal mortality rate. *American Journal of Obstetrics and Gynecology*, **116**, 901.

Ottesen, E. 1980. The clinical spectrum of lymphatic filariasis and its immunological determinants. World Health Organization, WHO/FIL/80.160.

Paavonen, J., P. Saikku, E. Vesterinen, and P. Lehtovirta. 1979. Infertility and cervical *Chlamydia trachomatis* infections. *Acta Obstetricia et Gynecologica Scandinavica*, **58**, 301.

Padubidri, V., L. Baijal, P. Prakash, and K. Chandra. 1980. The detection of endometrial tuberculosis in cases of infertility by uterine aspiration cytology. *Acta Cytologica*, **24**, 320.

Pan American Health Organization. 1976. Discussion. In *New approaches in American trypanosomiasis research*, Scientific Publication No. 318, pp. 221–222. Proceedings of an International Symposium, Belo Horizonte, Minas Gerais, Brazil, March 1975.

Pantelakis, S., G. Papadimitriou, and S. Doxiadis. 1973. Influence of induced abortion and spontaneous abortion on the outcome of subsequent pregnancies. *American Journal of Obstetrics and Gynecology*, **116**, 799.

Pape, J., B. Liautaud, F. Thomas, J. Mathurin, M. St. Amand, M. Boncy, V. Pean, M. Pamphile, A. Laroche, and W. Johnson. 1983. Characteristics of the Acquired Immune Deficiency Syndrome (AIDS) in Haiti. *New England Journal of Medicine*, **309**, 943.

Pariser, H. 1972. Asymptomatic gonorrhea. *Medical Clinics of North America*, **56**, 1127.

Parkes, A. 1976. *Patterns of sexuality and reproduction*. London: Oxford University Press.

Parran, T. 1937. *Shadow on the land—Syphilis*. New York: Reynald and Hitchcock.

Pasvol, G., D. Weatherall, and R. Wilson. 1978. Cellular mechanism for the protective effect of haemoglobin S against *P. falciparum* malaria. *Nature*, **274**, 701.

Pasvol, G., D. Weatherall, R. Wilson, D. Smith, and H. Gilles. 1976. Fetal haemoglobin and malaria. *Lancet*, **1**, 1269.

Paulsen, C. 1977. Regulation of male fertility. In R. Greep and M. Koblinsky (eds.), *Frontiers in reproduction and fertility control*, pp. 458–465. Cambridge, MA: MIT Press.

Payne, H. 1949. The problem of tuberculosis control among American negroes. *American Review of Tuberculosis*, **60**, 332.

Pearl, R. 1939. *The natural history of population*. New York: Oxford University Press.

Peel, J. 1972. An historical review of diabetes and pregnancy. *Journal of Obstetrics and Gynaecology of the British Commonwealth*, **79**, 385.

Pelouze, P. 1939. *Gonorrhea in the male and female*. Philadelphia: Saunders.

Penrose, L. 1971. Congenital malformations in man and natural selection. In C. Bajema (ed.), *Natural selection in human populations*, pp. 110–118. New York: Wiley.

People (UK). 1979. Female circumcision. **6**, 1, 24.

Petana, W. 1978. American typanosomiasis (Chagas' disease) in the Caribbean. *Bulletin of the World Health Organization*, **12**, 45.

Peter, K. 1981. The decline of population growth among the Hutterites. *Intercom*, **9**, 5, 8.

Peters, W. 1974. Drug resistance in trypanosomiasis and leishmaniasis. In *Trypanosomiasis and leishmaniasis with special reference to Chagas' disease*, Ciba Foundation Symposium No. 20, pp. 309–326. Amsterdam: Associated Scientific Publishers.

Peters, W. 1977. Current concepts in parasitology. Malaria. *New England Journal of Medicine*, **297**, 1261.

Petersen, W. 1975. *Population*. New York: Macmillan.

Pettigrew, T. 1964. *A profile of the negro American*. Princeton: Van Nostrand.

Phadke, A., N. Samant, and S. Dewal. 1973. Smallpox as an etiologic factor in male infertility. *Fertility and Sterility*, **24**, 802.

Philadelphia Bulletin. 1980. Soviet infant mortality on rise. February 6, A3. (a)

Philadelphia Bulletin, 1980. TB in immigrants. A new worry for U.S. March 31, A1. (b)

Philadelphia Bulletin. 1980. VD report: Males list other men. March 3, A2. (c)

Philadelphia Bulletin. 1981. Flu, pneumonia cause decline in newborn's life expectancy. October 8, A4. (a)

Philadelphia Bulletin. 1981. Root of sickle-cell anemia and malaria is—a yam. November 10, A15. (b)

Philadelphia Bulletin. 1982. Struggle to survive takes its toll on baby rescued by Reagan. January 6, A3.

Philadelphia Inquirer. 1981. Hodgkin's disease and pregnancy. October 31, 3D.

Philadelphia Inquirer. 1982. VD linked to fetal and baby deaths. March 19, 13D.

Pieters, G., and A. Lowenfels. 1977. Infibulation in the Horn of Africa. *New York State Journal of Medicine*, **77**, 729.

Pieterse, H. 1973. Some aspects of urological disease among the indigenous peoples of South West Africa. *South African Medical Journal*, **47**, 2415.

Platt, H. 1971. Effect of maternal sickle-cell trait on perinatal mortality. *British Medical Journal*, **4**, 334.

Pleet, H., J. Graham, and D. Smith. 1981. Central nervous system and facial defects associated with maternal hyperthermia four to 14 weeks' gestation. *Pediatrics*, **67**, 785.

Pollard, J. 1979. Factors affecting mortality and length of life. IUSSP Conference on Population Science in the Service of Mankind, Vienna, 53. Liege, Belgium: International Union for the Scientific Study of Population.

Poltera, A., R. Owor, and J. Cox. 1977. Pathological aspects of human African trypanosomiasis (HAT) in Uganda. A post-mortem survey of fourteen cases. *Virchows Archiv: Pathological Anatomy and Histology*, **373**, 249.

Pomerol, J., and S. Marina. 1974. Urological aspects on the treatment of infertile men. In

R. Mancini and L. Martini (eds.). *Male fertility and sterility*, pp. 497–515. New York: Academic Press.

Popline. 1981. IUD safety is acclaimed. **3,** 9, 2.

Population Reference Bureau. 1982. World population data sheet. Washington, DC: Population Reference Bureau.

Population Reports. 1973. Copper IUDs—Performance to date. Series B, No. 1, December.

Population Reports. 1974. Menstrual regulation update. Series F, No. 4, May.

Population Reports. 1977. Cervical dilatation—A review. Series F, No. 6, September.

Population Reports. 1979. Age at marriage and fertility. Series M, No. 4, November. (a)

Population Reports. 1979. IUDs—Update on safety, effectiveness, and research. Series B, No. 3, May. (b)

Population Reports. 1980. Complications of abortion in developing countries. Series F, No. 7, July. (a)

Population Reports. 1980. Traditional midwives and family planning. Series J, No. 22, May. (b)

Population Reports. 1983. Infertility and sexually transmitted disease: A public challenge. Series L, No. 4, July.

Portnoy, J., J. Mendelson, B. Clecner, and L. Heisler. 1974. Asymptomatic gonorrhea in the male. *Canadian Medical Association Journal,* **110,** 169.

Poston, D., and K. Kramer. 1980. Patterns of voluntary and involuntary childlessness in the United States, 1955–1973. Texas Population Research Center Papers, Series 3.

Potts, D. 1970. Termination of pregnancy. *British Medical Bulletin,* **26,** 65.

Potts, M., P. Diggory, and J. Peel. 1977. *Abortion.* New York: Cambridge University Press.

Potts, M., and P. Selman. 1979. *Society and fertility.* Plymouth, England: Macdonald and Evans.

Presser, H. 1971. The timing of the first birth, female roles and black fertility. *Milbank Memorial Fund Quarterly,* **49,** 329.

Preston, S. (ed.). 1978. *The effects of infant and child mortality on fertility.* New York: Academic Press.

Pritchard, J., D. Scott, P. Whalley, F. Cunningham, and R. Mason. 1973. The effects of maternal sickle cell hemoglobinopathies and sickle cell trait on reproductive performance. *American Journal of Obstetrics and Gynecology,* **117,** 662.

Procci, W., K. Hoffman, and S. Chatterjee. 1978. Sexual functioning of renal transplant recipients. *Journal of Nervous and Mental Disease,* **166,** 402.

Prothero, R. 1972. Problems of public health among pastoralists: A case study from Africa. In N. McGlashan (ed.), *Medical geography,* pp. 105–118. London: Methuen.

Raeburn, P. 1981. 20 million Americans may have hidden herpes. *Philadelphia Bulletin,* November 29, E14.

Rajan, N., P. Parekh, and I. Shah. 1974. Tuberculous endometritis. *Journal of Postgraduate Medicine,* **20,** 10.

Rankin, J. 1970. Pelvic inflammatory disease. In D. Charles (ed.), *Modern treatment,* pp. 756–778. New York: Harper and Row.

Razzell, P. 1962. An interpretation of the modern rise of population in Europe—A critique. *Population Studies,* **28,** 5.

Razzell, P. 1977. *The conquest of smallpox: The impact of inoculation on smallpox mortality in eighteenth century Britain.* Firle, Sussex, England: Caliban.

Reddy, C., P. Rao, and K. Rajakumari. 1974. Filarial worms in organs. *Indian Journal of Medical Science,* **28,** 494.

Rée, G. 1977. Schistosomiasis. In G. Howe (ed.), *A world geography of human diseases,* pp. 17–31. London: Academic Press.

Rees, E., and E. Annels. 1969. Gonococcal salpingitis. *British Journal of Venereal Diseases,* **45,** 205.

Rees, E., I. Tait, D. Hobson, and F. Johnson. 1977. Perinatal chlamydial infection. In D. Hobson and K. Holmes (eds.), *Nongonococcal urethritis and related infections,* pp. 140–147. Washington, DC: American Society for Microbiology.

Reese, R., W. Trager, J. Jensen, D. Miller, and R. Tantravahi. 1978. Immunization against malaria with antigen from *Plasmodium falciparum* cultivated *in vitro. Proceedings of the National Academy of Science U.S.A.,* **75,** 5665.

Reinhardt, M., P. Ambroise-Thomas, R. Cavallo-Serra, C. Meylan, and R. Gautier. 1978. Malaria at delivery in Abidjan. *Helvetica Paediatrica Acta,* **33, Supplement, 41,** 65.

Rendle-Short, C., and D. Stewart. 1967. Pelvic inflammatory disease. In J. Lawson and D. Stewart (eds.), *Obstetrics and gynaecology in the tropics and developing countries,* pp. 398–415. London: Edward Arnold.

Rendtorff, R. 1975. Some economic aspects of venereal diseases. *Clinical Obstetrics and Gynecology,* **18,** 233.

Retel-Laurentin, A. 1972. *Infécondité et Maladies, les Nzakara.* Paris: Institute National de la Statistique et des Etudes Economiques.

Retel-Laurentin, A. 1974. Subfertility in Black Africa—The case of the Nzakara in Central African Republic. In B. Adadevoh (ed.), *Sub-fertility and infertility in Africa,* pp. 69–75. Ibadan, Nigeria: Caxton Press.

Retel-Laurentin, A. 1978. Appraising the role of certain diseases in sterility. *Population,* **33,** 101.

Revillard, J. 1971. Potential and actual clinical applications of *in vitro* tests for cell-mediated immunity. In J. Revillard (ed.), *Cell-mediated immunity: In vitro correlates,* pp. 154–201. Baltimore: University Park Press.

Rich, A. 1951. *The pathogenesis of tuberculosis.* Springfield, IL: Thomas.

Richmond, S., and S. Clarke. 1977. Problems in assigning a causative role to chlamydiae isolated in nongonococcal urethritis. In D. Hobson and K. Holmes (eds.), *Nongonococcal urethritis and related infections,* pp. 43–46. Washington, DC: American Society for Microbiology.

Ridley, J. 1981. Fecundity status. The extent of sterility and subfecundity in the low fertility cohort. Unpublished.

Ridley, J., M. Sheps, J. Lingner, and J. Menken. 1967. The effects of changing mortality on natality. *Milbank Memorial Fund Quarterly,* **45,** 77.

Rimer, B. 1975. Sickle-cell trait and pregnancy: A review of a community hospital experience. *American Journal of Obstetrics and Gynecology,* **123,** 6.

Ringelhann, B., M. Hathorn, P. Jilly, F. Grant, and G. Parniczky. 1976. A new look at the protection of hemoglobin AS and AC genotypes against *Plasmodium falciparum* infection: A census tract approach. *American Journal of Human Genetics,* **28,** 270.

Roberts, D., and R. Tanner. 1959. A demographic study in an area of low fertility in northeast Tanganyika. *Population Studies,* **13,** 61.

Roberts, G. 1957. *The population of Jamaica.* London: Cambridge University Press.

Roberts, G. 1965. Fertility. Paper No. 483 presented at the World Population Conference, Belgrade, August.

Robitscher, J. 1973. *Eugenic sterilization.* Springfield, IL: Thomas.

Romaniuk, A. 1967. *La fécondité des populations Congolaises.* Paris: Mouton.

Romaniuk, A. 1968. The demography of the Democratic Republic of the Congo. In W. Brass *et al.* (eds.), *The demography of tropical Africa,* pp. 241–341. Princeton: Princeton University Press.

Romaniuk, A. 1974. Modernization and fertility: The case of the James Bay Indians. *Canadian Review of Sociology and Anthropology*, **11**, 344.

Romaniuk, A. 1980. Comment on M. Nag's "How modernization can also increase fertility." *Current Anthropology*, **21**, 584. (a)

Romaniuk, A. 1980. Increase in natural fertility during the early stages of modernization: Evidence from an African case study. *Population Studies*, **34**, 293. (b)

Romaniuk, A. 1981. Increase in natural fertility during the early stages of modernization: Canadian Indians case study. *Demography*, **18**, 157.

Ronda, C., G. Vazquez, R. Bermudez, and P. Harrington. 1980. Sexually transmitted diseases. Part I. Gonococcal infections. *Boletin Asociacion Medica de Puerto Rico*, **72**, 251.

Rosen, Y., and B. Kim. 1974. Tubal gestation associated with *Schistosoma mansoni* salpingitis. *Obstetrics and Gynecology*, **43**, 413.

Rosenback, L., and C. Gangemi. 1956. Tuberculosis and pregnancy. *Journal of the American Medical Association*, **161**, 1035.

Ross, J., J. Gow, and C. St. Hill. 1961. Tuberculous epididymitis. *British Journal of Surgery*, **48**, 663.

Roth, E., M. Friedman, Y. Ueda, I. Tellez, W. Trager, and R. Nagel. 1978. Sickling rates of human AS red cells infected *in vitro* with *Plasmodium falciparum* malaria. *Science*, **202**, 650.

Roundy, R. 1976. Altitudinal mobility and disease hazards for Ethiopian populations. *Economic Geography*, **52**, 103.

Rozat, M. 1980. Review of *Un pays à la dérive. Une société en régression démographique. Loes Nzakara de l'est Centraafricain*. *Population Studies*, **34**, 418.

Rozin, S. 1968. Genital tuberculosis. In S. Behrman and R. Kistner (eds.), *Progress in infertility*, pp. 209–239. Boston: Little, Brown.

Ruffer, M. 1967. Note on the presence of "Bilharzia Haematobia" in Egyptian mummies of the twentieth dynasty. In D. Brothwell and A. Sandison (eds.), *Diseases in antiquity*, p. 177. Springfield, IL: Thomas.

Ryder, N. 1959. Fertility. In P. Hauser and O. Duncan (eds.), *The study of population*. Chicago: Chicago University Press.

Ryder, N., and C. Westoff. 1971. *Reproduction in the United States, 1965*. Princeton: Princeton University Press.

Sadun, E., A. Johnson, R. Nagle, and R. Duxbury. 1973. Experimental infections with African trypanosomes. V. Preliminary parasitological, clinical, hematological, serological, and pathological observations in rhesus monkeys infected with *Trypanosoma rhodesiense*. *American Journal of Tropical Medicine and Hygiene*, **22**, 323.

Sala-Diakanda, M. 1981. Problems of infertility and sub-fertility in west and central Africa. In *International Population Conference, Vol. 3* (Papers of the 19th General Conference of the IUSSP), pp. 643–666. Liège, Belgium: Ordina.

Salo, O., K. Aho, E. Nieminen, and P. Hormila. 1969. False-positive serological tests for syphilis in pregnancy. *Acta Dermatovenereologica*, **49**, 332.

Sandison, A. 1967. Parasitic diseases. In D. Brothwell and A. Sandison (eds.), *Diseases in antiquity*, pp. 178–183. Springfield, IL: Thomas.

Sandison, A., and C. Wells. 1967. Diseases of the reproductive system. In D. Brothwell and A. Sandison (eds.), *Diseases in antiquity*, pp. 498–520. Springfield, IL: Thomas.

Sanjurjo, L. 1970. Parasitic diseases of the genitourinary system. In M. Campbell and J. Harrison (eds.), *Urology, Vol. 1* (3rd edition), pp. 480–511. Philadelphia: Saunders.

Santamarina, B., and T. Klein. 1970. Treatment of septic abortion and septic shock. *Modern Treatment*, **7**, 779.

Sarrel, P., and K. Pruett. 1968. Symptomatic gonorrhea during pregnancy. *Obstetrics and Gynecology*, **32**, 670.

Sartwell, P. 1965. Tuberculosis. In P. Sartwell (ed.), *Preventive medicine and public health*, pp. 210–224. New York: Appleton-Century-Crofts.

Satti, M., and O. Abdul Nur. 1974. Bancroftian filariasis in the Sudan. *Bulletin of the World Health Organization*, **51**, 314.

Savane, M. 1979. Mothers before all else. *People* (UK), **6**, 1, 7.

Savitt, T. 1978. *Medicine and slavery. The diseases and health care of blacks in antebellum Virginia*. Urbana: University of Illinois Press.

Schacher, J., and P. Sahyoun. 1967. A chronological study of the histopathology of filarial disease in cats and dogs caused by *Brugia pahangi* (Buckley and Edeson, 1956). *Transactions of the Royal Society of Tropical Medicine and Hygiene*, **61**, 234.

Schaefer, G. 1964. Full term pregnancy following genital tuberculosis. *Obstetric and Gynecologic Survey*, **19**, 81.

Schaefer, G., and S. Birnbaum. 1956. Diagnosis of female genital tuberculosis. *Obstetrics and Gynecology*, **7**, 180.

Schifrin, B., S. Erez, and J. Moore. 1973. Teen-age endometriosis. *American Journal of Obstetrics and Gynecology*, **116**, 973.

Schmeck, H. 1978. Tropical diseases may be gaining on humanity. *New York Times*, July 9, 18E.

Schofield, C., and R. Shanks. 1971. Gonococcal opthalmia neonatorum despite treatment with antibacterial eye-drops. *British Medical Journal*, **1**, 257.

Schultz, M. 1977. Current concepts in parasitology. Parasitic diseases. *New England Journal of Medicine*, **297**, 1259.

Schut, N. 1971. Tuberculous salpingitis and tubal pregnancy. In R. Kleinman and V. Pickles (eds.), *Fertility and Sterility: Abstracts of papers presented at the Seventh World Congress*, p. 139. Amsterdam: Excerpta Medica.

Schwartz, D., and M. Mayaux. 1982. Female fecundity as a function of age. *New England Journal of Medicine*, **307**, 404.

Scott, D. 1970. The epidemiology of Gambian sleeping sickness. In H. Mulligan and W. Potts (eds.), *The African trypanosomiases*, pp. 614–644. London: Allen and Unwin.

Scott, R., and M. Winston. 1976. The health and welfare of the black family in the United States. *American Journal of Diseases of Children*, **130**, 704.

Scragg, R. 1957. *Depopulation in New Ireland*. Port Moresby, Papua: Administration of Papua and New Guinea.

Seeler, R. 1973. Intensive transfusion therapy for priapism in boys with sickle cell anemia. *Journal of Urology*, **110**, 360.

Sha'ked, A. 1978. *Human sexuality in physical and mental disabilities*. Bloomington: Indiana University Press.

Shapiro, S., E. Schlesinger, and R. Nesbitt. 1968. *Infant, perinatal, maternal, and childhood mortality in the United States*. Cambridge, MA: Harvard University Press.

Shearer, L. 1980. Quintuplets. [Intelligence report] *Parade*, August 31, 31. (a)

Shearer, L. 1980. Tricky pill. [Intelligence report] *Parade*, May 11, 14. (b)

Shepard, M. 1970. Nongonococcal urethritis associated with human strains of "T" mycoplasmas. *Journal of the American Medical Association*, **211**, 1335.

Siegler, S. 1944. *Fertility in women; Causes, diagnosis, and treatment of impaired fertility*. Philadelphia: Lippincott.

Silverstein, A. 1962. Congenital syphilis and the timing of immunogenesis in the human fetus. *Nature*, **194**, 196.

Siongok, T., A. Mahmoud, J. Ouma, K. Warren, A. Muller, A. Handa, and H. Houser.

1976. Morbidity in schistosomiasis mansoni in relation to intensity of infection: Study of a community in Machakos, Kenya. *American Journal of Tropical Medicine and Hygiene,* **25,** 273.

Smith, A. 1972. Malaria in pregnancy. *British Medical Journal,* **4,** 793.

Smith, C. 1972. Changing patterns of disease in the tropics. *British Medical Journal,* **28,** 3.

Smith, J., J. Dyck, and D. Connor. 1976. Autopsy analysis of disease frequency in Kinshasa, Republic of Zaire. *American Journal of Tropical Medicine and Hygiene,* **25,** 637.

Smith, J., H. Torky, N. Mansour, and A. Cheever. 1974. Studies on egg excretion and tissue egg burden in urinary schistosomiasis. *American Journal of Tropical Medicine and Hygiene,* **23,** 163.

Smith, M., and R. Soderstrom. 1976. Salpingitis: A frequent response to intrauterine contraception. *Journal of Reproductive Medicine,* **16,** 159.

Smith, T. 1960. The Cocos-Keeling Islands: A demographic laboratory. *Population Studies,* **14,** 94.

Snaith, L., and T. Barns. 1962. Fertility in pelvic tuberculosis. *Lancet,* **1,** 712.

Songhaprasert, P., B. Rungpitarangsi, and S. Phansomboon. 1972. The incidence of syphilis in Thailand. *Journal of Clinical Pathology,* **25,** 555.

Spangler, D., G. Jones, and H. Jones. 1971. Infertility due to endometriosis. *American Journal of Obstetrics and Gynecology,* **109,** 850.

Sparling, F. 1971. Diagnosis and treatment of syphilis. *New England Journal of Medicine,* **284,** 642.

Sparling, F. 1972. Antibiotic resistance in *Neisseria gonorrhoeae. Medical Clinics of North America,* **56,** 1133.

Spence, M. 1973. Gonorrhea in a military prenatal population. *Obstetrics and Gynecology,* **42,** 233.

Spencer, J. 1974. Surgical aspects of filariasis. *Tropical Doctor,* **1,** 26.

Spingarn, C., and M. Edelman. 1965. Parasitic diseases in relation to pregnancy. In J. Rovinsky and A. Guttmacher (eds.), *Medical, surgical, and gynecologic complications of pregnancy,* pp. 692–719. Baltimore: Williams and Wilkins.

Spitz, A. 1959. Malaria infection of the placenta and its influence on the incidence of prematurity in Eastern Nigeria. *Bulletin of the World Health Organization,* **21,** 242.

Stallworthy, J. 1963. Fertility and genital tuberculosis. *Fertility and Sterility,* **14,** 284.

Stewart, D. 1967. Complications of the puerperium. In J. Lawson and D. Stewart (eds.), *Obstetrics and gynaecology in the tropics and developing countries,* pp. 242–252. London: Edward Arnold. (a)

Stewart, D. 1967. Extra-uterine pregnancy. In J. Lawson and D. Stewart (eds.), *Obstetrics and gynaecology in the tropics and developing countries,* pp. 371–384. London: Edward Arnold. (b)

Stewart, D. 1967. Tuberculosis of the female genital tract. In J. Lawson and D. Stewart (eds.), *Obstetrics and gynaecology in the tropics and developing countries,* pp. 451–460. London: Edward Arnold. (c)

Stix, R. 1941. Syphilis and uncontrolled fertility. *American Journal of Obstetrics and Gynecology,* **42,** 296.

Stokes, J. 1919. *Today's world problem in disease prevention.* Washington, DC: United States Public Health Service.

Stokes, J. 1935. *Dermatology and syphilology for nurses.* Philadelphia: Saunders.

Stone, A. 1954. Biological factors influencing human fertility. In *Proceedings of the 1954 World Population Conference,* Rome, Meeting No. 6, **1,** 737.

Stray-Pedersen, B., A. Bruu, and K. Molne. 1982. Infertility and uterine colonization with *Ureaplasma urealyticum. Acta Obstetricia et Gynecologica Scandinavica,* **61,** 21.

Subak-Sharpe, G. 1978. The venereal disease of the new morality. In *Readings in health 78/79*, pp. 155–156. Guilford, CT: Dushkin.

Summary of Progress. 1978. A prospective study of the effects of induced abortion on subsequent reproductive function. Preliminary report on research carried out by the New York State Department of Health, Office of Biostatistics under Contract No. NO1-HD-6-2802, National Institute of Child Health and Human Development. Albany, New York: New York State Health Department.

Sutherland, A. 1960. Genital tuberculosis in women. *American Journal of Obstetrics and Gynecology*, **79**, 486.

Sutherland, I. 1977. Tuberculosis and leprosy. In G. Howe (ed.), *A world geography of human diseases*, pp. 175–196. London: Academic Press.

Swartz, S. 1977. Diagnosis of nongonococcal urethritis. In D. Hobson and K. Holmes (eds.), *Nongonococcal urethritis and related infections*, pp. 15–18. Washington, DC: American Society for Microbiology.

Sweeney, W. 1968. Inflammations in infertility. In S. Behrman and R. Kistner (eds.), *Progress in infertility*, pp. 239–254. Boston: Little, Brown.

Tabah, L. 1977. World population growth at the turning point. *Intercom*, **5**, 6, 7.

Tabah, L. 1980. World population trends, a stocktaking. *Population and Development Review*, **6**, 355.

Tabbarah, R. 1971. Toward a theory of economic development. *Economic Development and Cultural Change*, **19**, 257.

Tabutin, D. 1982. Évolution régionale de la fécondité dans l'ouest du Zaïre. *Population*, **37**, 29.

Tachon, P., and R. Borojevic. 1978. Mother-child relation in human schistosomiasis man soni: Skin test and cord blood reactivity to schistosomal antigen. *Transactions of the Royal Society of Tropical Medicine and Hygiene*, **72**, 605.

Tafari, N., S. Ross, R. Naeye, D. Judge, and C. Marboe. 1976. Mycoplasma T strains and perinatal death. *Lancet*, **1**, 108.

Taha, O., M. Ali, E. Omer, M. Ahmed, and S. Abbaro. 1979. Studies of STDs in patients attending venereal disease clinics in Khartoum, Sudan. *British Journal of Venereal Diseases*, **55**, 313.

Tanner, J. 1973. Growing up. In *Life and death and medicine*, a Scientific American book, pp. 17–28. San Francisco: Freeman.

Tatum, H. 1977. Intrauterine contraception. In R. Greep and M. Koblinsky (eds.), *Frontiers in reproduction and fertility control*, pp. 188–202. Cambridge, MA: MIT Press.

Tatum, H., and F. Schmidt. 1977. Contraceptive and sterilization practices and extrauterine pregnancy: A realistic perspective. *Fertility and Sterility*, **28**, 407.

Taussig, F. 1944. Effects of abortion on the general health and reproductive function of the individual. In *The abortion problem*, pp. 39–48. Baltimore: Williams and Wilkins.

Taylor, C., J. Newman, and N. Kelly. 1976. Interactions between health and population. *Studies in Family Planning*, **7**, 94.

Taylor, C., J. Wyon, and J. Gordon. 1958. Economic determinants of population growth. *Milbank Memorial Fund Quarterly*, **36**, 107.

Taylor-Robinson, D., and W. McCormack. 1980. The genital mycoplasmas (First of two parts). *New England Journal of Medicine*, **302**, 1003. (a)

Taylor-Robinson, D., and W. McCormack. 1980. The genital mycoplasmas (Second of two parts). *New England Journal of Medicine*, **302**, 1063. (b)

Teixeira, A. 1977. Immunoprophylaxis against Chagas' disease. In L. Miller *et al.* (eds.), *Advances in experimental medicine and biology*, Vol. 93, pp. 243–280. New York: Plenum Press.

Tekse, K. 1968. *A study of fertility in Jamaica.* Kingston, Jamaica: Department of Statistics, Demography and Vital Statistics Section.

Termini, B., and S. Music. 1972. The natural history of syphilis: A review. *Southern Medical Journal,* **65,** 241.

Thompson, S., and W. Hager. 1977. Acute pelvic inflammatory disease. *Sexually Transmitted Diseases,* **4,** 105.

Thompson, W., and P. Whelpton. 1933. *Population trends in the United States.* New York: McGraw-Hill.

Tietze, C., and S. Lewit. 1977. Legal abortion. *Scientific American,* **236,** 21.

Time. 1973. The case against herpes. April, 23, 55.

Time. 1978. The Cinderella disease. July 17, 73. (a)

Time. 1978. Risky abortions. November 27, 52. (b)

Time. 1980. Herpes: The new sexual leprosy. July 28, 76. (a)

Time. 1980. I.U.D. debate. May 26, 60. (b)

Time. 1981. The battle over abortion. April 6, 20. (a)

Time. 1981. Doubts about vasectomies. February 9, 63. (b)

Time. 1981. A son's rite. August 31, 57. (c)

Time. 1982. Malaria hope. July 19, 67.

Time. 1983. Made-to-order vaccines. October 31, 82.

Tolnay, S. 1980. Black fertility in decline: Urban differentials in 1900. *Social Biology,* **27,** 249.

Torchia, M. 1977. Tuberculosis among American negroes: Medical research on a racial disease, 1830–1950. *Journal of the History of Medicine and Allied Sciences,* **32,** 252.

Toth, A., M. Lesser, C. Brooks, and D. Labriola. 1983. Subsequent pregnancy among 161 couples treated for T-mycoplasma genital-tract infection. *New England Journal of Medicine,* **308,** 505.

Traub, N., P. Hira, C. Chintu, and C. Mhango. 1978. Congenital trypanosomiasis: Report of a case due to *Trypanosoma brucei rhodesiense. East African Medical Journal,* **55,** 477.

Treharne, J., K. Ripa, P. Mardh, L. Svensson, L. Westrom, and S. Darougar. 1979. Antibodies to *Chlamydia trachomatis* in acute salpingitis. *British Journal of Venereal Diseases,* **55,** 26.

Trichopoulos, D., N. Handanos, J. Danezis, A. Kalandidi, and V. Kalapothaki. 1976. Induced abortion and secondary infertility. *British Journal of Obstetrics and Gynaecology,* **83,** 645.

Trussell, R., E. Grech, and J. Galea. 1968. Maternal mortality. In *Uganda Atlas of Disease Distribution,* pp. 144–152. Kampala, Uganda: Makerere University College.

Tyson, J., and P. Felig. 1971. Medical aspects of diabetes in pregnancy and the diabetogenic effects of oral contraceptives. *Medical Clinics of North America,* **55,** 947.

Uganda Atlas of Disease Distribution. 1968. Kampala, Uganda: Makerere University College Press.

United Nations Monthly Bulletin of Statistics. 1979. **Vol. XXXIII,** No. 7. New York: United Nations.

United States Bureau of the Census. 1940. *Sixteenth census of the United States: 1940, population, differential fertility: 1940, fertility for states and large cities.* Washington, DC: US Govt. Printing Office.

United States Bureau of the Census. 1944. *Vital Statistics, Special Reports,* 15, 21. Washington, DC: US Govt. Printing Office. (a)

United States Bureau of the Census. 1944. *Vital Statistics, Special Reports,* 16, 7. Washington, DC: US Govt. Printing Office. (b)

United States Public Health Service. 1968. *Syphilis: A synopsis.* Public Health Service Publication No. 1660. Washington, DC: US Govt. Printing Office.

Urquhart, J. 1979. Effect of the venereal disease epidemic on the incidence of ectopic pregnancy—Implications for the evaluation of contraceptives. *Contraception,* **19,** 455.

U.S. News and World Report. 1976. The war against disease: Many gains—But setbacks, too. In *Readings in health 78/79,* pp. 130–133. Guilford, CT: Dushkin.

Valaoras, V., A. Polychronopoulou, and D. Trichopoulou. 1969. Greece: Postwar abortion experience. *Studies in Family Planning,* **46,** 10.

Van den Bossche, H. 1978. Chemotherapy of parasitic infections. *Nature,* **273,** 626.

van de Walle, E. 1974. *The female populatin of France in the nineteenth century: A reconstruction of 82 departments.* Princeton: Princeton University Press.

van de Walle, E. 1980. Comment on M. Nag's "How modernization can also increase fertility." *Current Anthropology,* **21,** 584.

van de Walle, E., and J. Knodel. 1980. Europe's fertility transition. *Population Bulletin,* **34,** 6, 1.

Verhagen, A. 1974. Gonorrhea. In L. Vogel *et al.* (eds.), *Health and disease in Kenya,* pp. 375–380. Nairobi, Kenya: East African Literature Bureau.

Verzin, J. 1975. Sequelae of female circumcision. *Tropical Doctor,* **5,** 163.

Vessey, M., M. Meisler, R. Flavel, and D. Yeates. 1979. Outcome of pregnancy in women using different methods of contraception. *British Journal of Obstetrics and Gynaecology,* **86,** 548.

Vessey, M., N. Wright, K. McPherson, and P. Wiggins. 1978. Fertility after stopping different methods of contraception. *British Medical Journal,* **1,** 265.

Victor, J. 1981. *Human sexuality.* Englewood Cliffs, NJ: Prentice-Hall.

Voller, A. 1974. Immunopathology of malaria. *Bulletin of the World Health Organization,* **50,** 177.

Vonderlehr, R., and L. Usilton. 1942. Syphilis among men of draft age in the United States. *Journal of the American Medical Association,* **120,** 1369.

Wang, S., C. Kuo, and J. Grayston. 1975. Biological properties and immunotypes of trachoma-LGV organisms with some comments on laboratory diagnosis. In D. Danielsson *et al.* (eds.), *Genital infections and their complications,* pp. 39–52. Stockholm: Almqvist and Wiksell International.

Warren, K. 1978. The pathology, pathobiology and pathogenesis of schistosomiasis. *Nature,* **273,** 609.

Warren, K., A. Mahmoud, P. Cummings, D. Murphy, and H. Houser. 1974. Schistosomiasis mansoni in Yemeni in California: Duration of infection, presence of disease, and therapeutic management. *American Journal of Tropical Medicine and Hygiene,* **23,** 902.

Warren, K., R. Pelley, and A. Mahmoud. 1977. Immunity and immunopathology following reinfection of mice cured of chronic schistosomiasis mansoni. *American Journal of Tropical Medicine and Hygiene,* **26,** 957.

Wartman, W. 1947. Filariasis in American armed forces in World War II. *Medicine,* **26,** 333.

Watson, R. 1979. Gonorrhea and acute epididymitis. *Military Medicine,* **144,** 785.

Webster, B. 1982. Methods disputed in fertility study. *New York Times,* March 21, 33.

Weekly Epidemiological Record. 1983. World malaria situation 1981. A synopsis of Nos. 25–30. Geneva: World Health Organization.

Weeks, A., and C. Hutchins. 1976. Ectopic pregnancy: A five year review. *British Journal of Clinical Practice,* **30,** 104.

Weisbrod, B., R. Andreano, R. Baldwin, E. Epstein, and A. Kelley. 1973. *Disease and eco-*

nomic development. The impact of parasitic diseases in St. Lucia. Madison: University of Wisconsin Press.

Weller, T. 1976. Manson's schistosomiasis; Frontiers *in vivo, in vitro,* and in the body politic. *American Journal of Tropical Medicine and Hygiene,* **25**, 208.

Westrom, L. 1975. Effect of acute pelvic inflammatory disease on fertility. *American Journal of Obstetrics and Gynecology,* **121**, 707.

Westrom, L., and P. Mardh. 1975. Acute salpingitis. Aspects on aetiology, diagnosis, and prognosis. In D. Danielsson *et al.* (eds.), *Genital infections and their complications,* pp. 157–167. Stockholm: Almqvist and Wiksell International.

Westrom, L., and P. Mardh. 1977. Epidemiology, etiology, and prognosis of acute salpingitis: A study of 1,457 laparoscopically verified cases. In D. Hobson and K. Holmes (eds.), *Nongonococcal urethritis and related infections,* pp. 84–90. Washington, DC: American Society for Microbiology.

Westrom, L., and P. Mardh. 1978. Pelvic inflammatory disease. I. Epidemiology, diagnosis, clinical manifestations and sequelae. World Health Organization Group on Nongonococcal Urethritis and Other Selected Sexually Transmitted Diseases of Public Health Importance. INT/VDT/78.347. November, 1.

Whelpton, P. 1944. Frequency of abortion. In *The abortion problem,* pp. 15–27. Baltimore: Williams and Wilkins.

Whelpton, P., A. Campbell, and J. Patterson. 1966. *Fertility and family planning in the United States.* Princeton: Princeton University Press.

Whelpton, P., and C. Kiser. 1946–1958. *Social and psychological factors affecting fertility.* New York: Milbank Memorial Fund. (1946, 1950, 1952, 1954, 1958)

White, A., P. Handler, and E. Smith (eds.). 1964. *Principles of biochemistry.* New York: McGraw-Hill.

Wiesner, P., and K. Holmes. 1975. Current view of the epidemiology of sexually transmitted diseases in the United States. In D. Danielsson *et al.* (eds.), *Genital infections and their complications,* pp. 15–24. Stockholm: Almqvist and Wiksell International.

Wigfield, A. 1972. How infectious is gonorrhea? *British Medical Journal,* **4**, 672.

Wijers, D., and J. McMahon. 1976. Early signs and symptoms of bancroftian filariasis in males at the East African coast. *East African Medical Journal,* **53**, 57.

Willcox, R. 1977. Venereal diseases. In G. Howe (ed.), *A world geography of human diseases,* pp. 201–254. New York: Academic Press.

Willcox, R. 1980. Venereal diseases in the islands of the North Pacific. *British Journal of Venereal Diseases,* **56**, 173. (a)

Willcox, R. 1980. Venereal diseases in the Pacific islands. Papua New Guinea. *British Journal of Venereal Diseases,* **56**, 277. (b)

Williams, A. 1967. Pathology of schistosomiasis of the uterine cervix due to *S. haematobium. American Journal of Obstetrics and Gynecology,* **98**, 784.

Williams, J., and K. Sun. 1926. A statistical study of the incidence and treatment of labor complicated by contracted pelvis in the obstetric service of the Johns Hopkins Hospital from 1896 to 1924. *American Journal of Obstetrics and Gynecology,* **11**, 737.

Williamson, J. 1976. Chemotherapy of African trypanosomiasis. *Transactions of the Royal Society of Tropical Medicine and Hygiene,* **70**, 117.

Williamson, W., and B. Greenwood. 1978. Impairment of the immune response to vaccination after acute malaria. *Lancet,* **1**, 1328.

Wilson, D. 1967. The abortion problem in the general hospital. In H. Rosen (ed.), *Abortion in America,* pp. 189–197. Boston: Beacon Press.

Wilson, J., G. Pasvol, and D. Weatherall. 1977. Invasion and growth of *Plasmodium fal-*

ciparum in different types of human erythrocytes. *Bulletin of the World Health Organization*, **55**, 179.

Witters, W., and P. Jones-Witters. 1980. *Human sexuality: A biological perspective.* New York: Van Nostrand.

Wolfe, M., and M. Aslamkhan. 1972. Bancroftian filariasis in two villages in Dinajpur District, East Pakistan. I. Infections in man. *American Journal of Tropical Medicine and Hygiene*, **21**, 22.

Woodall, M. 1982. A contraceptive device again gives birth to controversy. *Philadelphia Inquirer*, March 28, 1K.

Woodruff, A., V. Ansdell, and L. Pettitt. 1979. Cause of anaemia in malaria. *Lancet*, **1**, 1055.

Woodruff, A., J. Ziegler, A. Hathaway, and T. Gwata. 1973. Anaemia in African trypanosomiasis and 'big spleen disease' in Uganda. *Transactions of the Royal Society of Tropical Medicine and Hygiene*, **67**, 329.

World Health Organization. 1966. Immunological aspects of human reproduction. *World Health Organization Technical Report Series*, **334**, 1.

World Health Organization. 1967. WHO expert committee on filariasis *Wuchereria* and *Brugia* infections. *World Health Organization Technical Report Series*, **359**, 1.

World Health Organization. 1969. Comparative studies of American and African Trypanosomiasis. *World Health Organization Technical Report Series*, **411**, 1.

World Health Organization. 1973. Schistosomiasis control. *World Health Organization Technical Report Series*, **515**, 1.

World Health Organization. 1974. The malaria situation in 1973. *WHO Chronicle*, **28**, 479. (a)

World Health Organization. 1974. WHO expert committee on filariasis. *World Health Organization Technical Report Series*, **542**, 1. (b)

World Health Organization. 1975. The epidemiology of infertility. *World Health Organization Technical Report Series*, **582**, 1.

World Health Organization. 1976. The epidemiology of infertility. *WHO Chronicle*, **30**, 229.

World Health Organization. 1978. Epidemiology and control of schistosomiasis: Present situation and priorities for further research. *Bulletin of the World Health Organization*, **56**, 361. (a).

World Health Organization. 1978. Induced abortion. *World Health Organization Technical Report Series*, **623**, 1. (b)

World Health Organization. 1978. Malaria control—A reoriented strategy. *WHO Chronicle*, **32**, 226. (c)

World Health Organization. 1978. The malaria situation in 1976. *WHO Chronicle*, **32**, 9. (d)

World Health Organization. 1979. The African trypanosomiases. *World Health Organization Technical Report Series*, **635**, 1.

World Health Organization. 1980. *Sixth report on the world health situation.* Part I and Part II. Geneva: World Health Organization.

World Health Organization. 1981. Abstracts of papers related to filariasis either in press or submitted for publication. WHO/FIL/81.163. (a)

World Health Organization. 1981. Report of the sixth meeting of the Scientific Working Group on Filariasis: Lymphatic filariasis—Diagnosis of infection and evaluation of control. TDR/FIL/SWG(6)/81.3. Colombo, October. (b)

World Health Organization. 1982. Control of sleeping sickness due to *Trypanosoma brucei gambiense. Bulletin of the World Health Organization*, **60**, 821.

World Health Organization Task Force on Psychosexual Research in Family Planning. 1982.

Hormonal contraception for men: Acceptibility and effects on sexuality. *Studies in Family Planning,* **13,** 328.

World Health Organization, World Bank, and United Nations. 1982. *Newsletter: Special Programme for Research and Training in Tropical Diseases,* **18,** May.

Wright, C. 1972. Immunological control of schistosomiasis. *British Medical Journal,* **3,** 697.

Wright, N., and P. Laemmle. 1968. Acute pelvic inflammatory disease in an indigent population. *American Journal of Obstetrics and Gynecology,* **10,** 979.

Yorke, J., H. Hethcote, and A. Nold. 1978. Dynamics and control of transmission of gonorrhea. *Sexually Transmitted Diseases,* **5,** 51.

Young, A. 1972. Herpes genitalis. *Medical Clinics of North America,* **56,** 1175.

Young, M., and W. Taliaferro. 1971. Malaria. *Encyclopaedia Britannica,* **14,** 669.

Zeledon, R. 1974. Epidemiology, modes of transmission and reservoir hosts of Chagas' disease. In *Trypanosomiasis and leishmaniasis with special reference to Chagas' disease,* Ciba Foundation Symposium No. 20, pp. 51–77. Amsterdam: Associated Scientific Publishers.

Zellweger, H. 1974. Anticonvulsants during pregnancy: A danger of the developing fetus? *Clinical Pediatrics,* **13,** 338.

Zinsou, R., C. Quennum, and E. Alihonou. 1967. Role of bilharziasis in female sterility. In B. Westin and N. Wiqvist (eds.), *Fertility and Sterility: Proceedings of the Fifth World Congress,* pp. 281–283. Amsterdam: Excerpta Medica.

Index

Numbers in italics indicate that the entry indexed is a figure.

O

P

STUDIES IN POPULATION

Under the Editorship of: H. H. WINSBOROUGH

Department of Sociology
University of Wisconsin
Madison, Wisconsin

Doreen S. Goyer. International Population Census Bibliography: *Revision and Update, 1945-1977.*

David L. Brown and John M. Wardwell (Eds.). New Directions in Urban–Rural Migration: *The Population Turnaround in Rural America.*

A. J. Jaffe, Ruth M. Cullen, and Thomas D. Boswell. The Changing Demography of Spanish Americans.

Robert Alan Johnson. Religious Assortative Marriage in the United States.

Hilary J. Page and Ron Lesthaeghe. Child-Spacing in Tropical Africa.

Dennis P. Hogan. Transitions and Social Change: *The Early Lives of American Men.*

F. Thomas Juster and Kenneth C. Land (Eds.). Social Accounting Systems: *Essays on the State of the Art.*

M. Sivamurthy. Growth and Structure of Human Population in the Presence of Migration.

Robert M. Hauser, David Mechanic, Archibald O. Haller, and Taissa O. Hauser (Eds.). Social Structure and Behavior: *Essays in Honor of William Hamilton Sewell.*

Valerie Kincade Oppenheimer. Work and the Family: *A Study in Social Demography.*

Kenneth C. Land and Andrei Rogers (Eds.). Multidimensional Mathematical Demography.

John Bongaarts and Robert G. Potter. Fertility, Biology, and Behavior: *An Analysis of the Proximate Determinants.*

Randy Hodson. Workers' Earnings and Corporate Economic Structure.

Ansley J. Coale and Paul Demeny. Regional Model Life Tables and Stable Populations, Second Edition.

Mary B. Breckenridge. Age, Time, and Fertility: *Applications of Exploratory Data Analysis.*

Neil G. Bennett (Ed.). Sex Selection of Children.

Rodolfo A. Bulatao and Ronald D. Lee (Eds.). Determinants of Fertility in Developing Countries. Volume 1: *Supply and Demand for Children;* Volume 2: *Fertility Regulation and Institutional Influences.*

Joseph A. McFalls, Jr., and Marguerite Harvey McFalls. Disease and Fertility.

In preparation

Kenneth G. Manton and Eric Stallard. Recent Trends in Mortality Analysis.